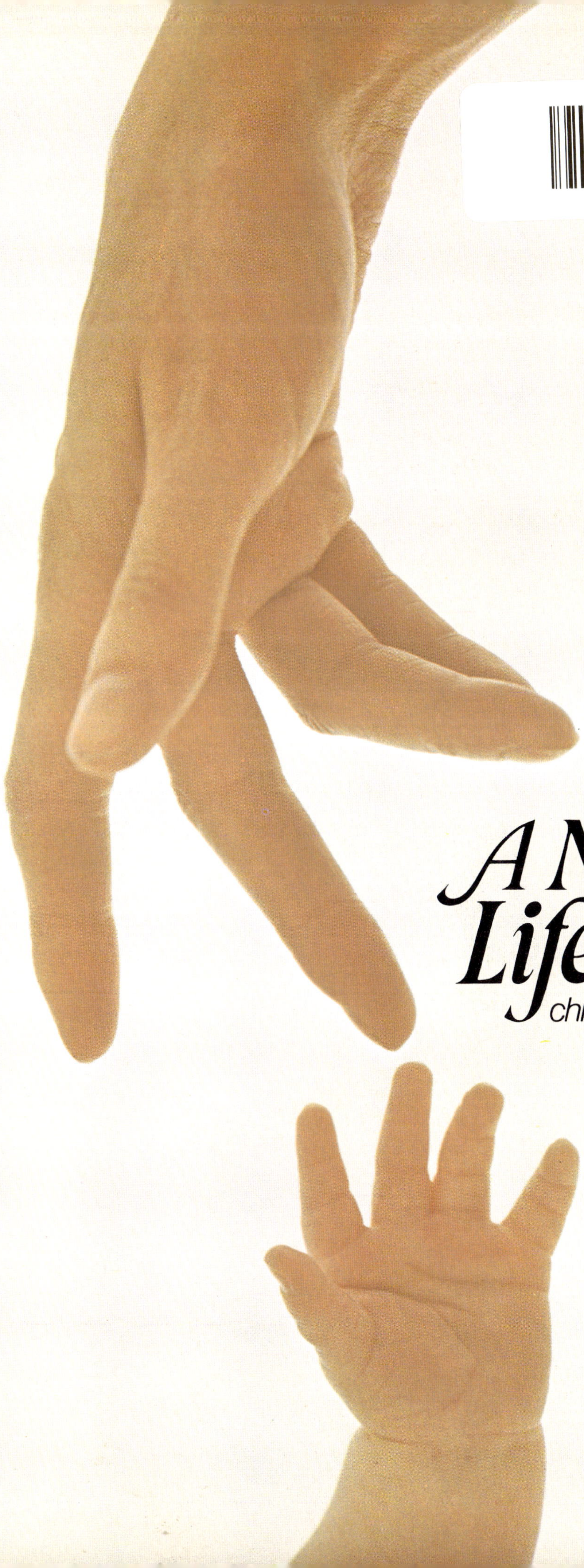

A New Life

Pregnancy, birth, and your child's first year

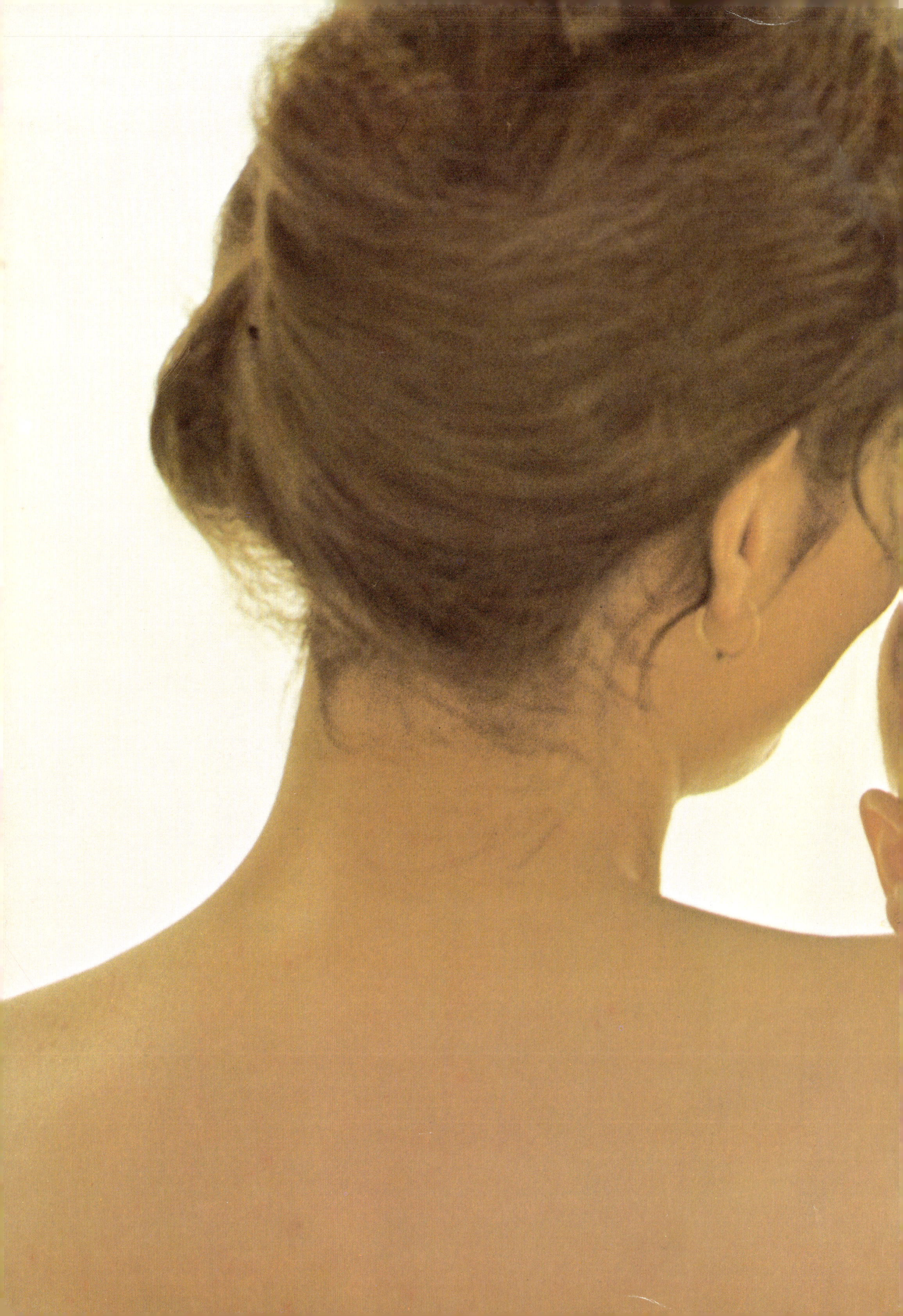

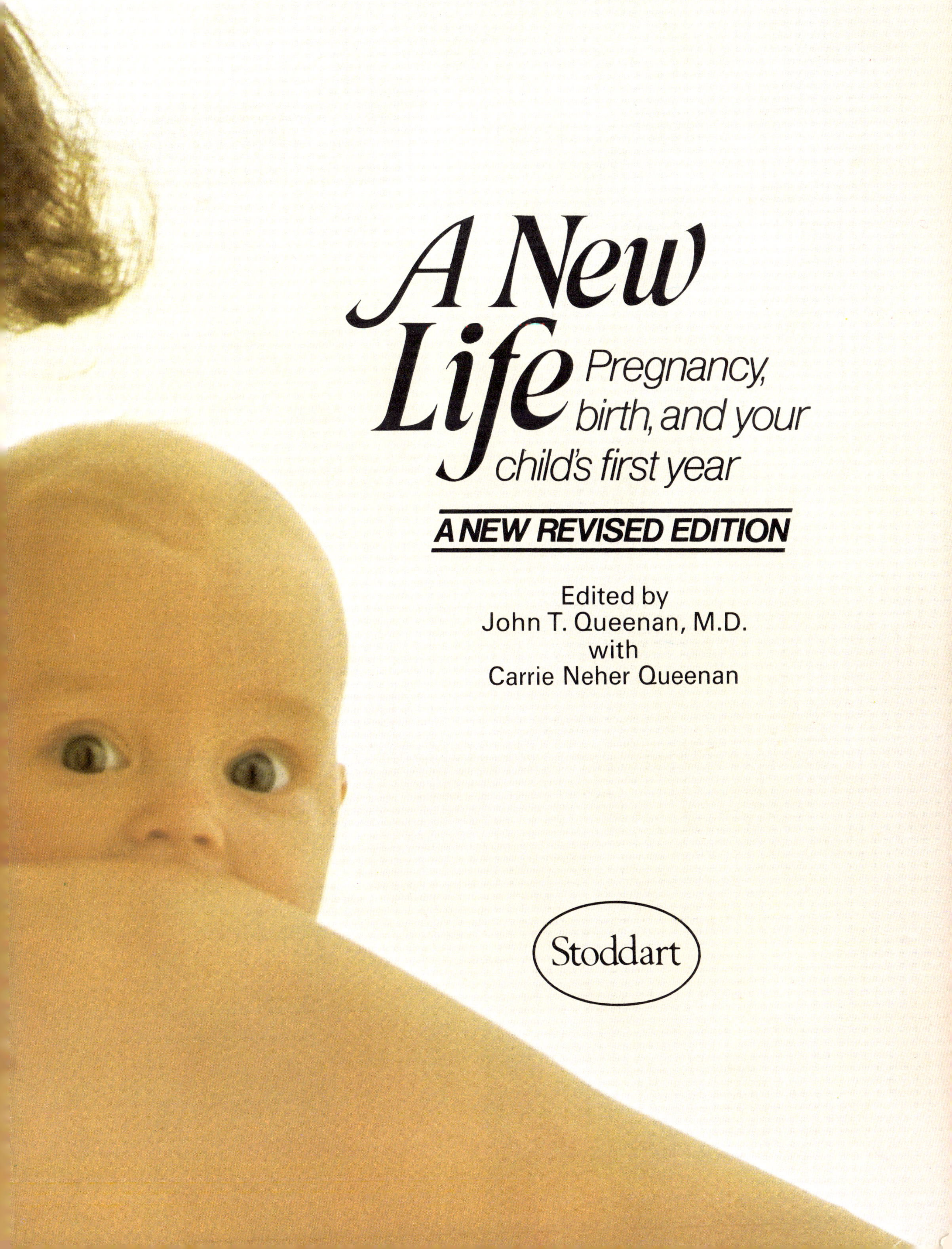

A New Life

Pregnancy, birth, and your child's first year

A NEW REVISED EDITION

Edited by
John T. Queenan, M.D.
with
Carrie Neher Queenan

Stoddart

First published in 1986 by
Stoddart Publishing Co. Limited
34 Lesmill Road
Toronto, Canada
M3B 2T6

Reprinted 1989

First published in the United Kingdom by
Marshall Cavendish Books Limited
58 Old Compton Street
London W1V 5PA
England

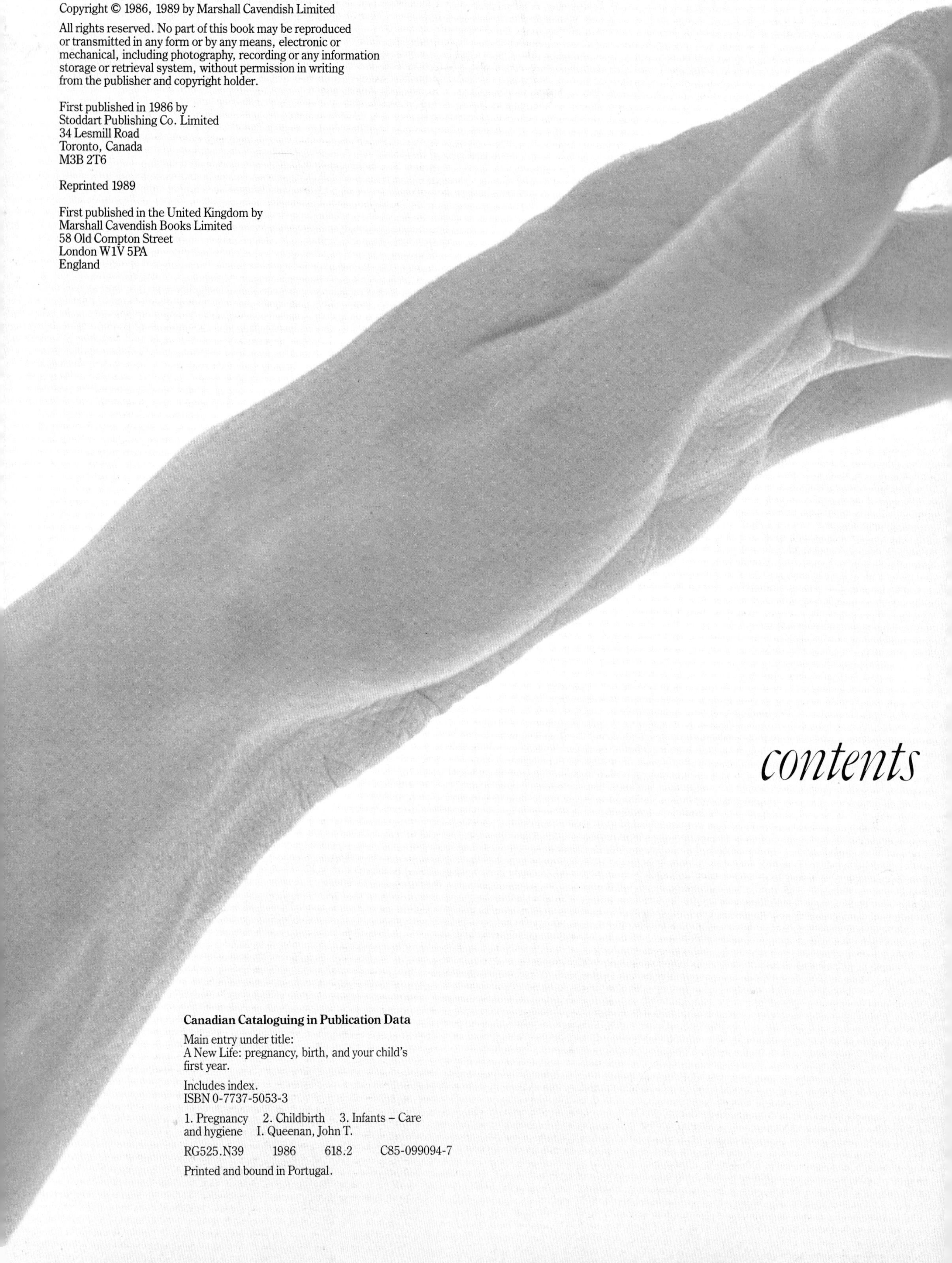

contents

Canadian Cataloguing in Publication Data

Main entry under title:
A New Life: pregnancy, birth, and your child's first year.

Includes index.
ISBN 0-7737-5053-3

1. Pregnancy 2. Childbirth 3. Infants – Care and hygiene I. Queenan, John T.

RG525.N39 1986 618.2 C85-099094-7

Printed and bound in Portugal.

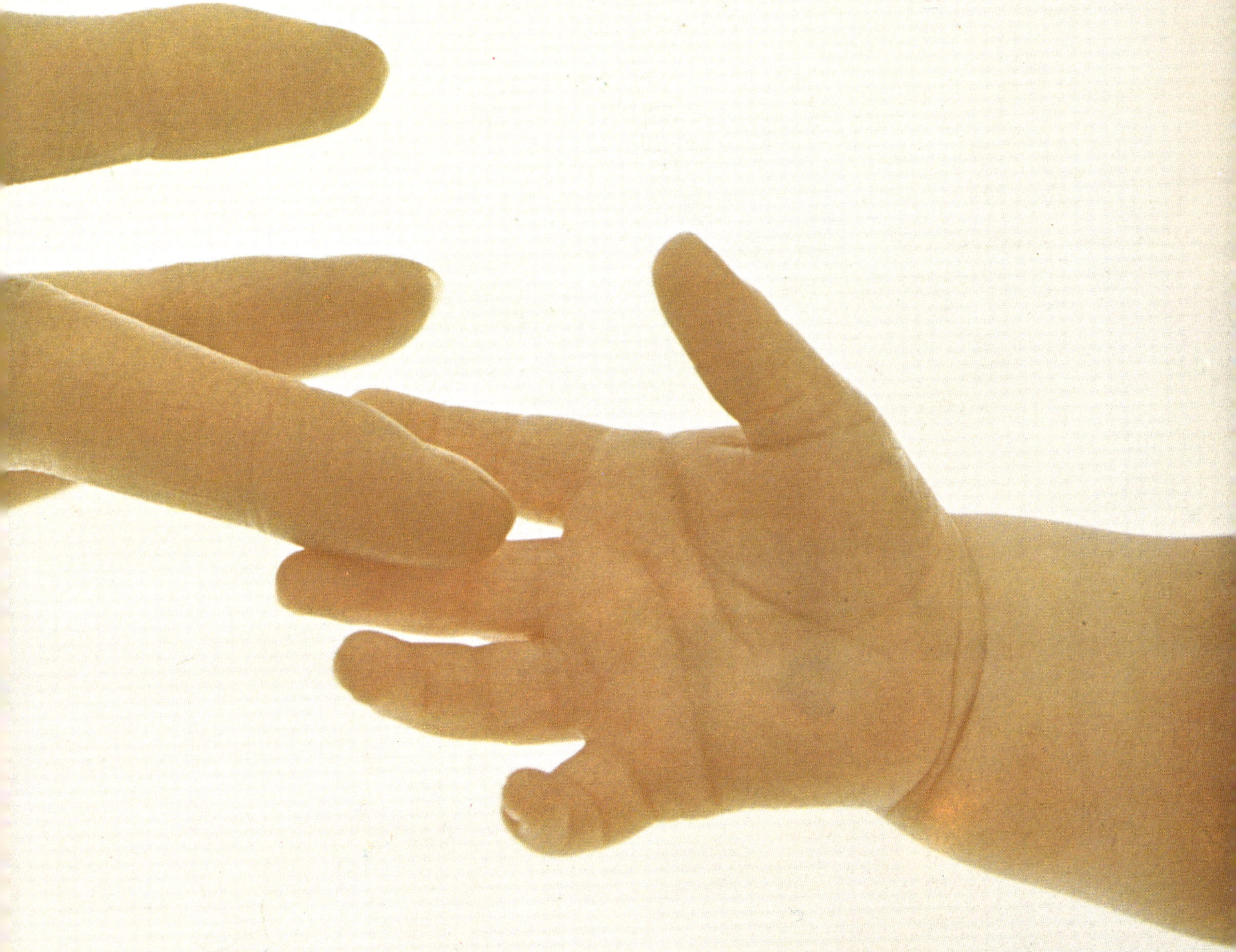

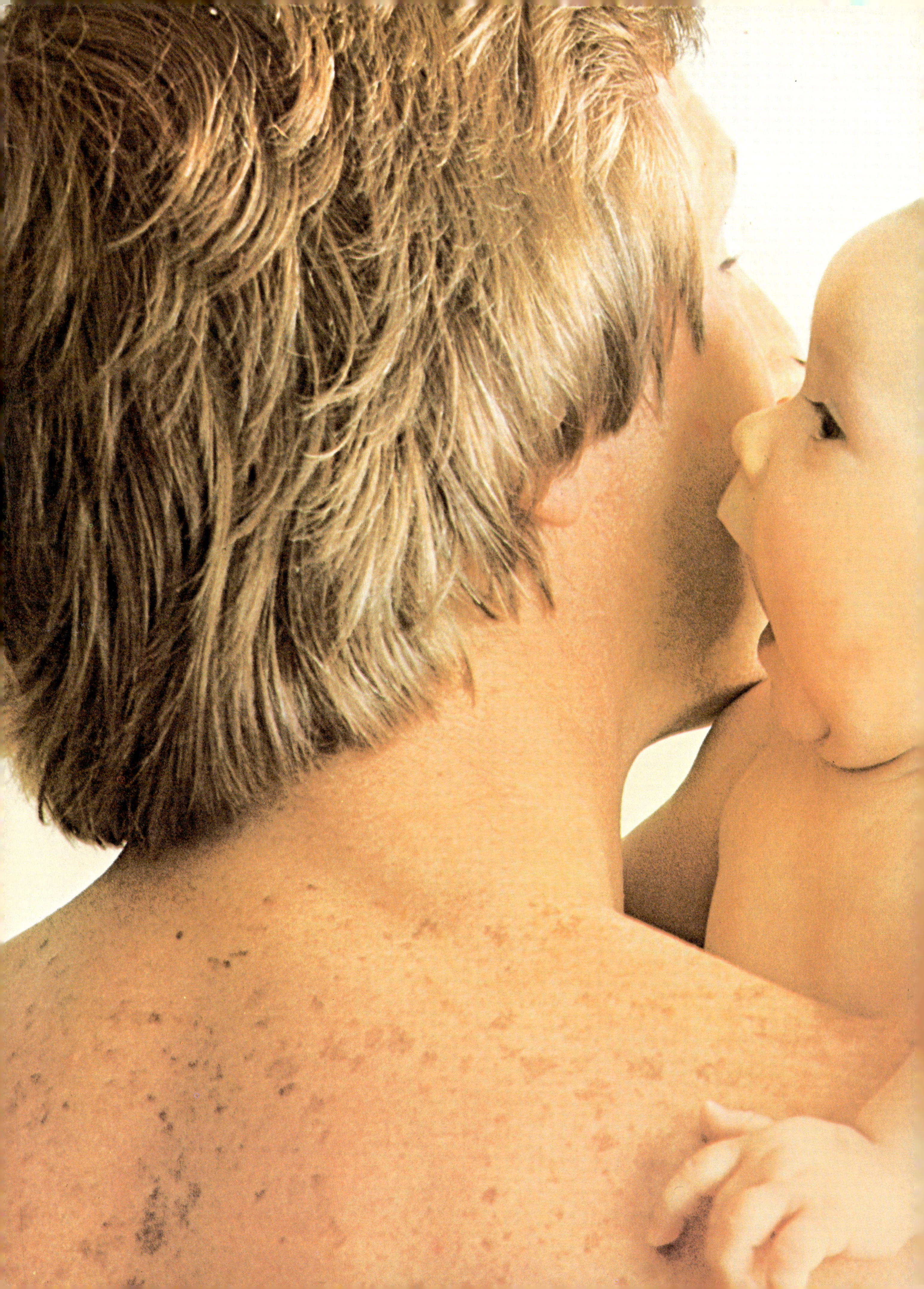

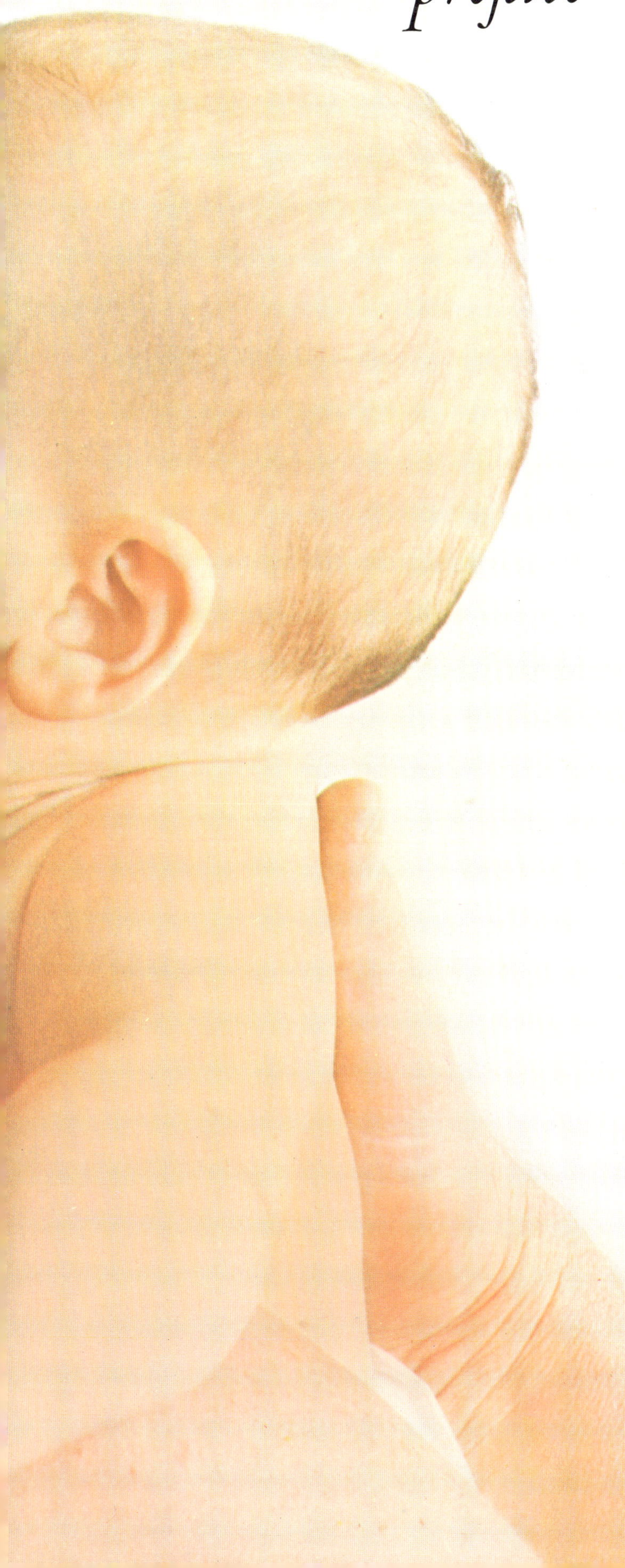

preface

The intention of this book is to provide an overview of pregnancy, delivery and the early growth and development of your child. The original British text was compiled and edited by Dr. David Harvey, a Professor of Pediatrics at Queen Charlotte's Maternity Hospital, London. This is our second edition of the United States version, and we have expanded and updated the text specifically for the American reader. This includes such things as adding a comprehensive section on Cesarean delivery, to reflect the changing birthing patterns in the United States.

One might think that having a baby in England would be similar to having a baby in the United States. After all, the anatomy and physiology are identical. But the similarity stops there. In preparing this book for the United States we made many changes. There are considerable differences in personal attitudes, delivery of care, and in the practice of obstetrics and pediatrics. The language alone presented many interesting variations. The expected differences in spelling such as oedema, foetus and labour for edema, fetus and labor added flavor, but were distracting. There were the more substantive differences in syntax, for example teat for nipple, wind for gas and back passage for rectum. Next, there were differences that were delightfully confounding like dummy for pacifier, nappy for diaper and "top and tail" for washing the baby's face and bottom. And finally, some frankly humorous differences like "wind your baby" for "burp your baby" and "knock up your health visitor" for "phone the visiting nurse."

The presentations are frank and straightforward. We have made the assumption that if you bought this book you are intelligent and wish to be highly informed. The text is carefully constructed, in order not to talk down to the reader. For instance, fetus and uterus are used whereas other texts might refer to the unborn baby and the womb.

The book is not written from an advocacy standpoint. The only causes espoused are good health care and healthy babies. Though breast-feeding may be excellent for some, it might not be best for others. The Lamaze technique may be ideal for some couples but others may prefer conduction anesthesia. It is our hope that this book is sufficiently comprehensive to cover most options.

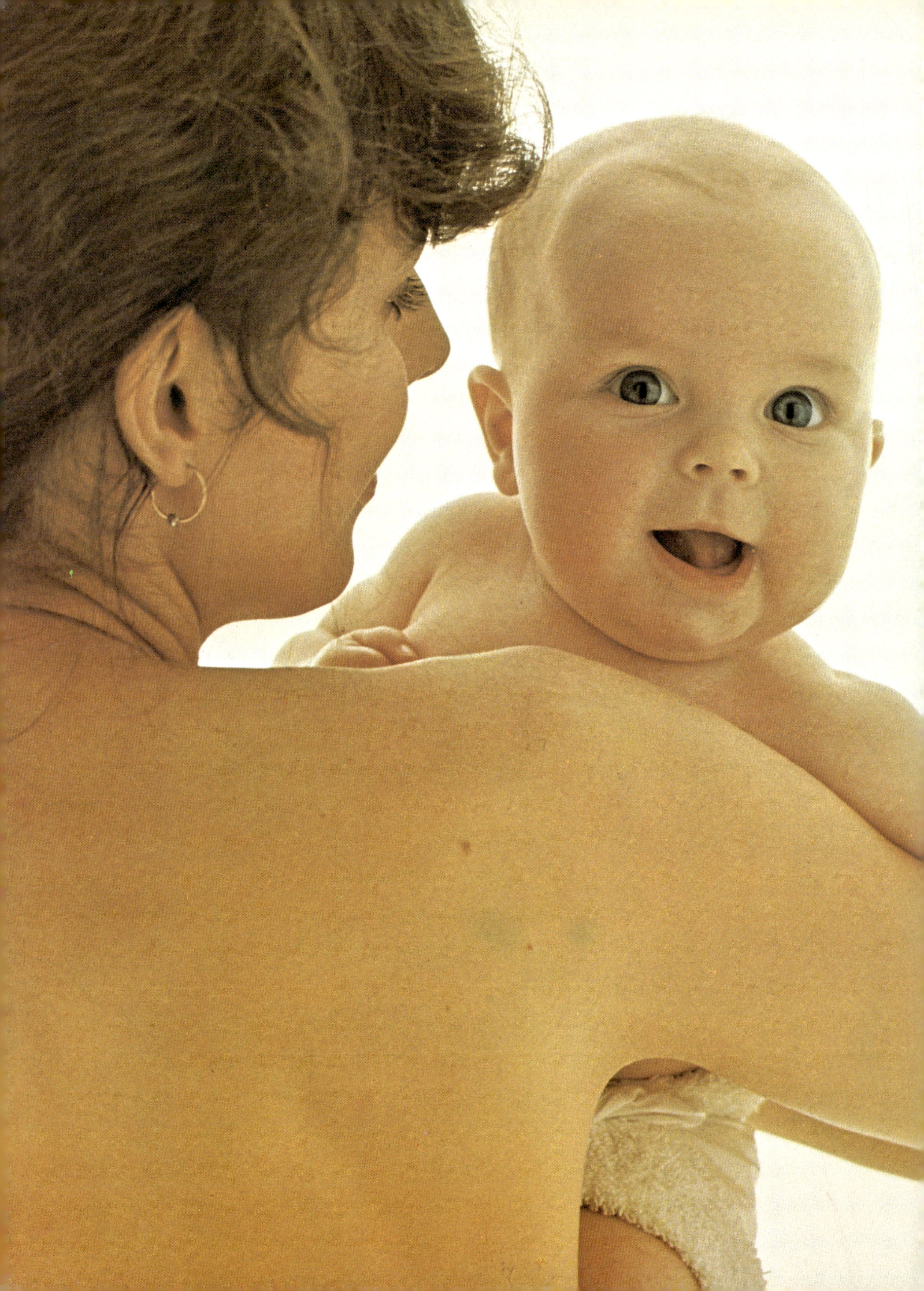

introduction

Today, a couple having a baby has so many things in their favor. The many choices in contraception make it possible to avoid pregnancy until they want a baby. A couple can plan a pregnancy when psychological and physical conditions are optimal. Then, there are a myriad of choices in the types of obstetrical and pediatric care.

Just two decades ago, unplanned and unwanted pregnancies were common. The options for preventing a pregnancy were not as many because safe and effective contraception was not as available as today.

Now the couple has an excellent opportunity of participating in health care delivery. Preparation for childbirth education, the father present during labor and delivery, birthing rooms, rooming-in units, sibling visitation and a healthier attitude toward couples participating in the reproductive process make having a baby a humanistic experience. In the past, the father was commonly excluded from the labor and delivery rooms. During postpartum visits he was treated as if his very presence would communicate some dread disease to the newborn. Ironically, a few days later when the mother and baby were discharged the baby would be thrust upon him. He was likely to be totally unprepared to handle the baby.

Today, an enlightened approach to having a baby blends understanding and caring with scientific advances. We have a vast and diverse country, and our health care system is complex and variable. Different options and opportunities are available in various parts of the United States. Obstetrical care has never been more sophisticated and efficient. Whether your pregnancy is normal and uncomplicated or a high-risk one, you have facilities available to provide optimal care. If your pregnancy is normal community hospitals are adequate for care. If you have a complex medical situation then a medical center for high-risk pregnancies would be preferable.

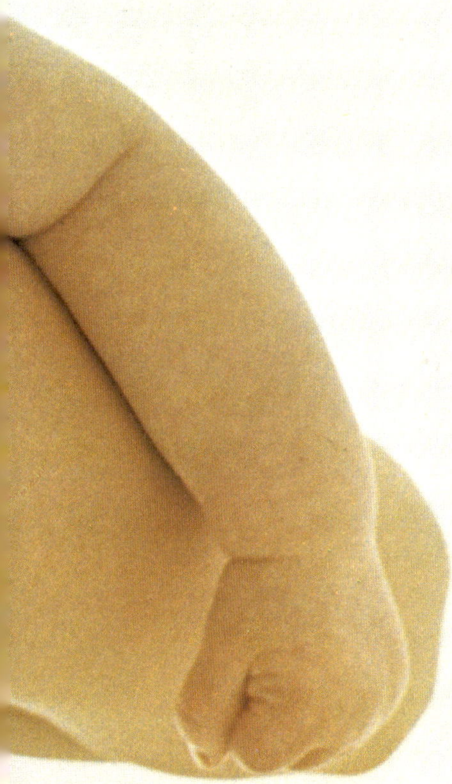

With the marked increase in scientific technology it is very important to emphasize the need to treat the whole patient and not just the problems or the complications. Fortunately, due to the efforts of determined consumers a new attitude has developed. There is increased sensitivity of the medical personnel for the stresses of the parents. Procedures done merely as routine have been markedly curtailed. There is a strong feeling that this is a team effort with the couple and the medical personnel working together for a humanistic and satisfying experience.

Creating a new life can be a couple's most fulfilling experience. It combines the selflessness of enduring inconvenience and physical difficulty, with the selfishness of creating something precious for yourselves. It requires a special kind of sharing – a sharing at the highest level of human activity. It seems miraculous to be able to create a new life directly from your own bodies. First, the child often has remarkable similarity due to inheritance. Then, the child grows even more in the image and likeness of the parents because of imitation fostered by love and attention.

Indeed, the growth and development of a young child seems awesome. Can you truly be qualified for such a daunting responsibility? There are no people better qualified! As parents, you can best give such things as love, attention and consistency. These have an enormously positive impact on the development of a child.

In the past, concepts and practices for raising a new baby were very rigid. Babies had to be fed on a schedule, the milk had to be warmed, and toilet training was started at a specific age. Such regimentation caused great anxieties and feelings of inadequacy on the part of the parents. After all, no two babies are alike. Today the art of raising a new baby is much more flexible and determined by the needs of the individual child. The basis for it is common sense. For instance, why still sterilize a formula at a stage when your baby is crawling and sampling things off the floor? Today's approach – the commonsense approach – is more creative and satisfying for the parents. Undoubtedly, the baby benefits also.

The vast majority of pregnancies are normal and proceed without a problem. Therefore, pregnancy should be looked upon as a normal state – not as an illness. A small percentage of expectant mothers will have a problem or a complication. The more knowledge the couple has the better they can cope with the problem. The sections in this book devoted to problems and complications are not meant to cause apprehension for the reader. They are intended to facilitate early recognition of problems so patients can seek appropriate solutions. Additionally, a full understanding of a problem will permit the best opportunity to develop a positive and creative attitude toward this problem.

This book presents a comprehensive overview of a new life: the conception, pregnancy, delivery, newborn baby and the early growth and development of the child. It does not just present the anatomy and physiology of having a baby. It presents educational, psychological, social and interpersonal aspects as well. We believe the more informed you are, the richer will be your experience.

Since having a baby is a delightful experience and since the chances of having no serious problems are overwhelmingly in your favor, we take this opportunity to say: having a baby is a uniquely favorable situation. We hope this book helps you enjoy life's most fulfilling experience.

Finally, a word about the preparation of *A New Life*. A book never gets to the market as the work of a single individual, and a book as complex as this demands all the creative efforts of a large team of dedicated people. Unfortunately, proper credit can never adequately be given to all, but we should like to give special thanks to just a few. To Elizabeth Longley whose help in preparing the text and planning the first and second editions was invaluable; she has our gratitude and admiration. To Dennis Hovell and Brenda Morrison, for maintaining the integrity and quality of both text and illustration. And to Richard Hayes, for his vision all those years ago.

If in reading this book you have suggestions or comments, we should welcome hearing from you.

And in closing – this is for you, John and Lynne – may this project increase your knowledge, understanding and excitement about life!

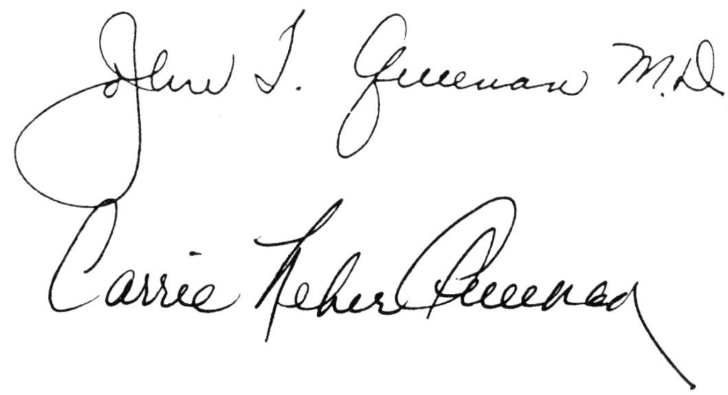

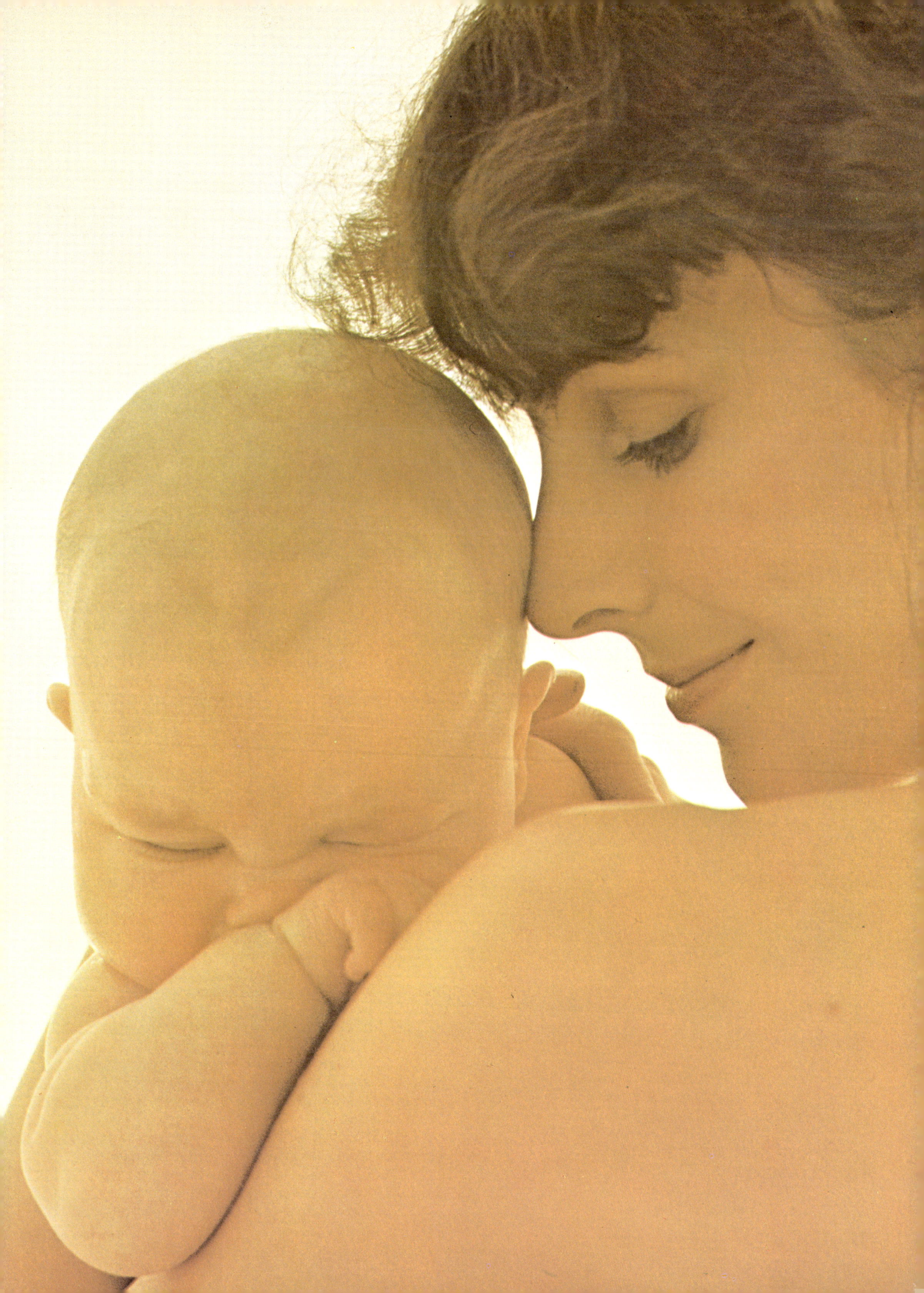

Fertility and conception

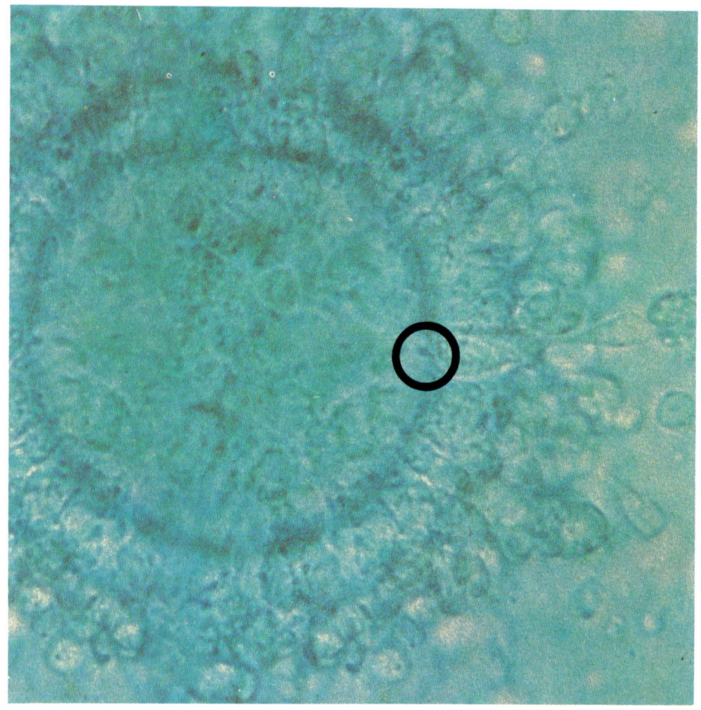

CHAPTER 1

Scientific knowledge about human reproduction is expanding rapidly, and in the last several decades it has become more and more feasible to control the process, making it more than ever possible for parents to understand what is involved. This chapter describes the male and female reproductive organs and their functions, and explains how fertilization takes place and the way in which the fertilized egg is implanted in the uterus. It also looks at the woman's menstrual cycle and the ways in which modern contraception works, as well as the problems of infertility and the process of inheritance.

Although the basic anatomy of the male and female reproductive organs has been known for hundreds of years, the most dramatic advances in the science of physiology (the study of the functions of living things) have been made during this century. During the first fifty years, the hormones, or chemical messengers, which play such a central part in reproduction, were discovered. Hormones act on enzymes – the molecules in every human cell that govern the chemical reactions of the body – and these in turn are determined by the genes that an individual inherits from his parents.

The underlying principles of inheritance have been understood for only a hundred years. In recent years scientists have discovered the mechanisms which transfer inherited characteristics from generation to generation via the man's sperm and the woman's ova. The list of characteristics that can be identified as genetically determined continues to grow as research into the subject continues.

In 1956 it was clearly established that every normal human cell contains 46 chromosomes. It is these chromosomes, half of which come from the

Cross references

See also	Chapter
Contraception	8
Fetal abnormalities	3
Fetal development	3
The placenta	3
Pregnancy	2, 4
Rh babies	2

The moment of conception.
A sperm (ringed) penetrates the wall of an ovum. The actual diameter of a human ovum ready for fertilization is approximately $\frac{1}{200}$ in (0.12mm)

father and half of which come from the mother, that carry the genes. The important and rapidly developing new science of cytogenetics is concerned with these matters and is highly relevant to childbearing. Some of the ways in which chromosomes act are now understood. For example, it is known that many abnormalities are determined by defects in the chromosomes or, more commonly, by defects in single enzymes within the cells. This new knowledge enables couples to be given a more realistic picture of the risks of conceiving children with various particular genetic defects.

At the same time as developments in genetics have enabled couples to make more rational decisions about whether to have children, contraception has made it possible to choose when to have them. Contraception of one sort or another has, of course, been practiced throughout history. Coitus interruptus has always been used; the ancient Egyptians apparently used a vaginal paste made of crocodile dung and honey; and barrier methods of contraception have been employed for over 400 years. But these methods were inefficient and were frequently socially unacceptable. For example, as recently as 1877, English authors who described contraceptive techniques were sent to prison.

The first half of this century saw contraception gaining social acceptance and in the 1950s efficient oral contraceptives were produced for the first time. Shortly thereafter, intrauterine devices were reintroduced in a modern form. These two methods have become very popular, and the complications sometimes associated with them are now being fully appreciated. As a result, contraceptives have been modified and they have come to be treated with more caution than was at first the case. Male and female sterilization have also become more widespread in recent years, largely because of the problems which arise if the modern methods of contraception are used over a long period of time. But sterilization must be approached as an irreversible procedure, and there is still a long way to go before the ideal contraceptive method is perfected.

One result of widely practiced contraception and abortion is an acute shortage of babies for couples to adopt. This in turn accentuates the plight of couples who are infertile. Fortunately great progress has also been made in the treatment of infertility in the last ten years. Methods of inducing ovulation when it fails to occur naturally are improving all the time and the ability to measure hormone levels has made it possible to diagnose the problem more accurately. There are still, however, many women with damaged fallopian tubes which are difficult to treat. Today, there is great progress in overcoming this problem. Work is being done on replacing and repairing the damaged tubes and on by-passing the problem by in vitro fertilization and embryo transfer. Male infertility is also receiving more serious consideration and clinics for this problem are increasing in number.

All this modern scientific knowledge, and the increased ability to plan, should not obscure the fact that reproduction remains a natural process and sexuality is instinctive. Knowledge of what is involved should never interfere with the spontaneity of lovemaking. Indeed, anxiety can be an important factor: with some infertile couples, a pregnancy is eventually only achieved when they relax and stop consciously trying to have a child.

The female reproductive organs

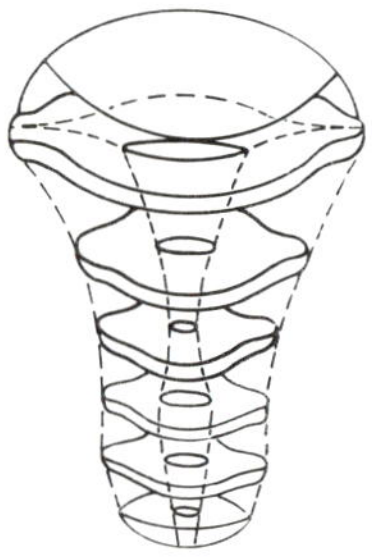

A reconstruction of the uterus (above) reveals its narrow central cavity and thick muscular walls.

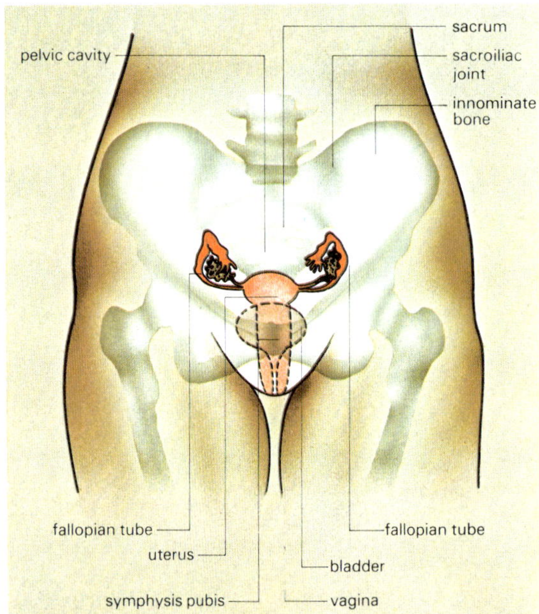

The bones of the pelvic girdle link the backbone to the legs and at the same time create a cavity which is wide enough to hold the pelvic organs and to allow a baby to pass through (above right).

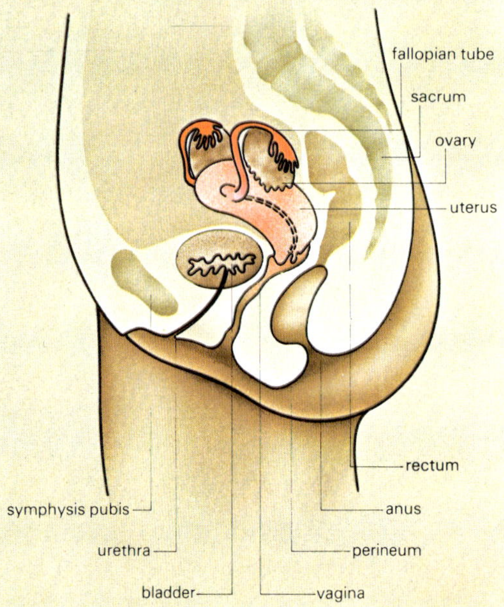

The pelvic organs (the bladder, uterus and rectum) lie within the pelvic girdle between the sacrum at the back and the symphysis pubis at the front. In passing down the birth canal the baby turns first toward and then away from the spine, passing through an angle of 90°.

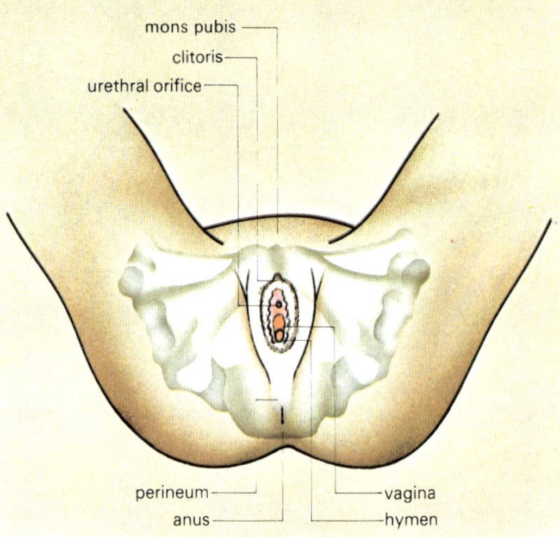

The position of the external reproductive organs is shown on this diagram. Their shape and size varies from woman to woman. The bones of the pelvic girdle are also shown. The cavity between them, through which the baby's head must pass during delivery, is clearly visible from this angle.

A woman's body is designed to enable her to sustain the complex process of childbearing as well as all the other necessary human functions. In particular her reproductive organs and the pelvic girdle within which they lie possess an extraordinary capacity to expand in pregnancy and childbirth.

The pelvic girdle and pelvic floor

The pelvic girdle consists of three bones. The lowest part of the spine, the sacrum, is joined on either side by the sacroiliac joints to the two innominate bones, which curve outward to form the hip bones, and down to form the ridge of the pubic bone in front. Here they are connected by a small piece of cartilage called the symphysis pubis. Since the pelvis links the spine to the legs the joints between the bones have to carry the whole weight of the body, and for this reason they are usually rigidly fixed. During the last stages of pregnancy, however, the supporting ligaments of the joints soften, allowing the birth canal to widen a little.

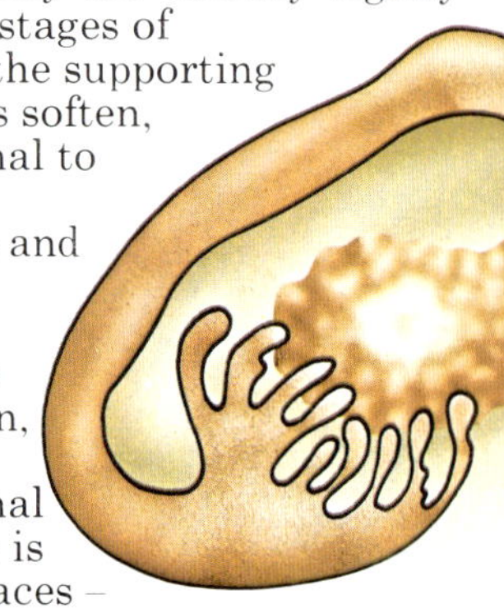

The layer of muscle and fibrous tissue, known as the pelvic floor, which runs across the bottom of the abdomen, is able to support the weight of the abdominal organs even though it is perforated in three places – by the urethra, vagina and anal canal. It is also, however, flexible enough to allow the vagina to stretch during birth. The levator ani muscles are the most important elements of the pelvic floor, making this dual function possible. When extra pressure is exerted on the pelvis, during coughing for example, they contract to give extra support. During birth they relax, folding back against the walls of the birth canal as the baby's head passes through. Their strength and tone can be restored by post-natal exercises (*see* p. 116).

The external organs and the vagina

The external reproductive organs, known collectively as the vulva, extend from the mons pubis, a soft mound of flesh covered with pubic hair, to the perineum, the area between the vagina and the anus. Between them on either side run two folds of skin, the labia minora and the labia majora. At the front, where the labia minora meet, is the clitoris, the center of sexual excitement, and behind it the urethra, which carries the urine down from the bladder. The vaginal entrance, edged by the hymen, a fold of skin which usually narrows the entrance in a virgin, lies just behind the urethra.

The vagina is the passage leading from the vulva to the uterus. The skin which lines it produces an acid environment during the fertile years which acts as a barrier to infection. During childbirth the vagina expands to allow the passage of the baby's head.

The womb, or uterus, in which the fetus grows is a hollow, pear-shaped organ, with two parts: the body above, and the narrower cervix which protrudes into the vagina below. The uterine end of the cervical canal is called the internal os and the vaginal end of the canal is called the external os.

Glands opening into the canal secrete a mucous plug which seals the canal against infection but becomes thinner at ovulation to allow sperm to pass through. In most women the uterus is anteverted, or tilted forward, though in about one in five it is retroverted, or tilted backwards. Like all the pelvic organs it moves freely. For example, when the bladder fills, the uterus changes its position quite noticeably.

The narrow cavity within the uterus contains a lining which is known as the endometrium, which varies in thickness and composition with the menstrual cycle. The thick walls of the uterus are made largely of muscle which makes it possible to push out the fetus at birth. The whole organ is normally only about the size of a clenched fist, but it expands to many times this size by the end of pregnancy (*see* p. 31).

The fallopian tubes run from the top corners of the uterus to the ovaries and are lined with tiny projections, the plicae, covered with little hairs known as cilia, which move the ova down the tube. Along these tubes the sperm swim to meet the ovum, and the lining of the tubes secretes material to nourish the sperm and fertilized ovum during their respective journeys. The outer end of each tube opens out into a funnel fringed with fingerlike projections, known as fimbriae, which help to catch the ovum after its release from the nearby ovary.

The ovaries, a pair of white oval bodies which lie on either side of the uterus, have two functions. They produce and release ova and send out chemical messengers (hormones) which play an important part in the menstrual cycle. They are as tender as testicles if they are knocked. The surface of the ovaries is white and smooth but gradually becomes ridged with tiny scars caused by the release of ova.

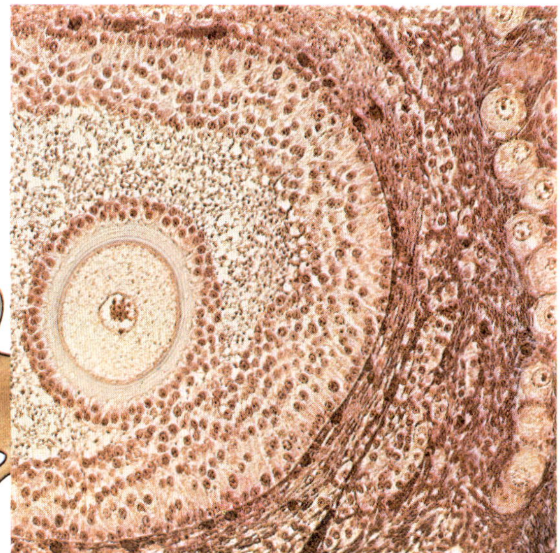

A cross-section of the follicle within an ovary shows a spherical egg attached to the inside of a pale, fluid-filled cavity by a ring of cells (right). The cells at the edge of the picture will later secrete the female hormones which sustain pregnancy.

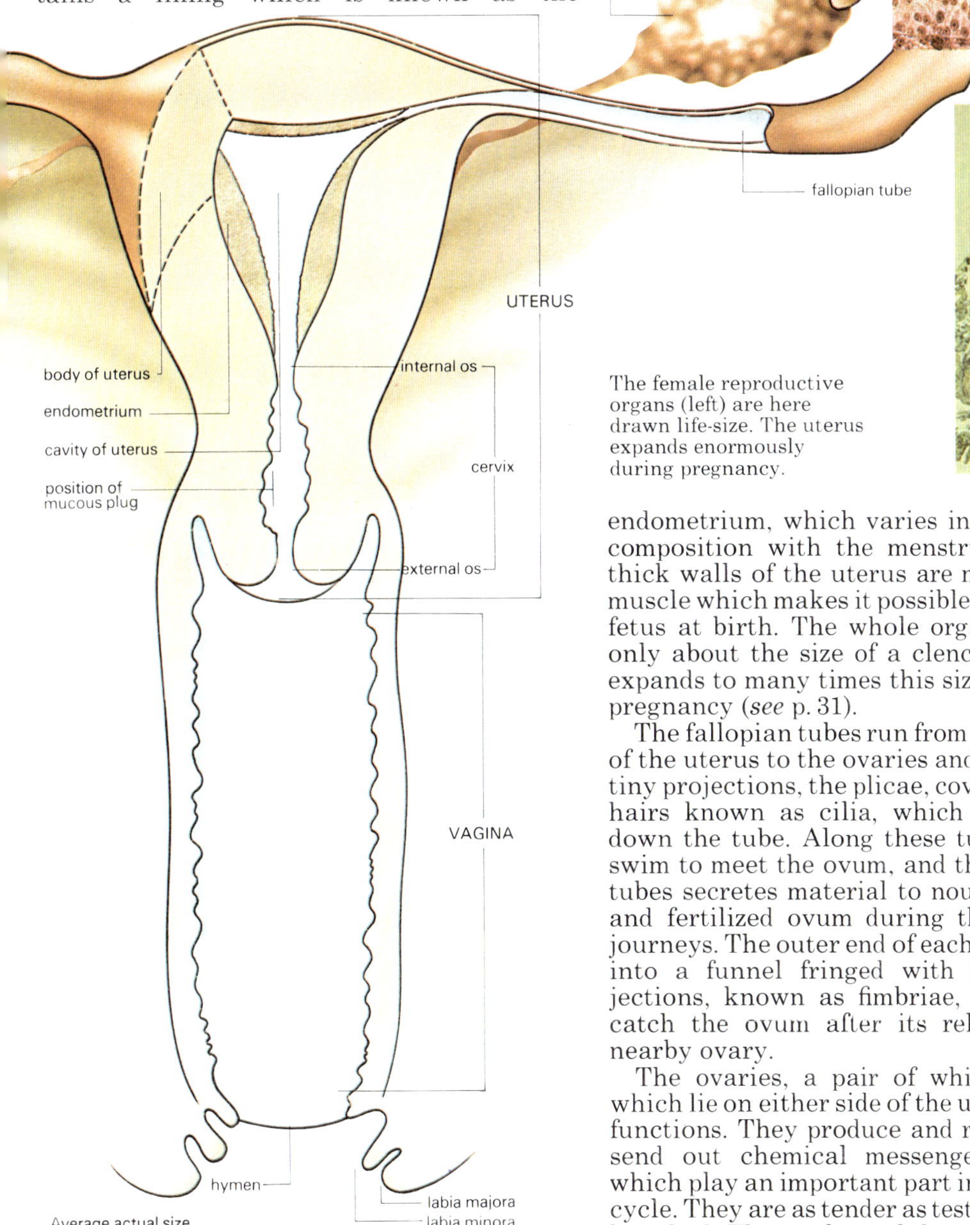

The female reproductive organs (left) are here drawn life-size. The uterus expands enormously during pregnancy.

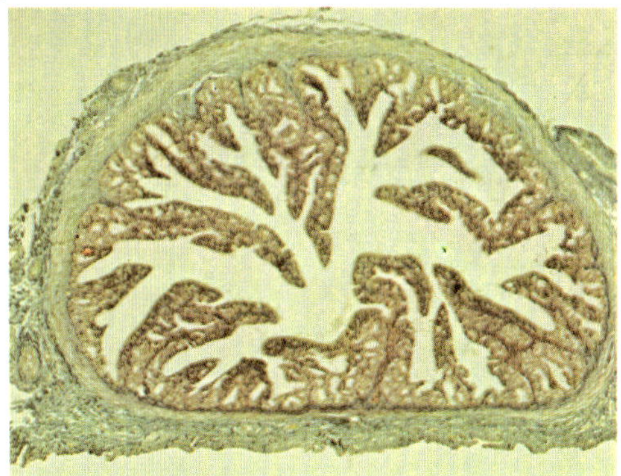

A fallopian tube (seen above in cross-section and stained to display its features) is made up of three layers; an outer wall, a middle layer of muscle and an inner ring of delicate projections, the plicae, which extend into the center of the tube.

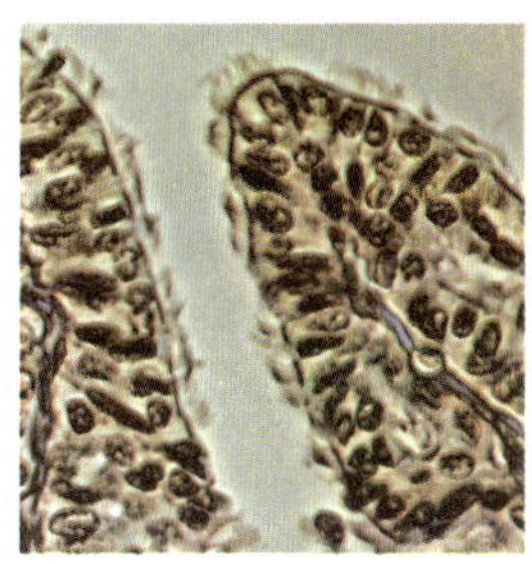

The cilia which cover the plicae in the fallopian tubes (above, part of a plicae enlarged) regulate the movement of the fertilized ovum along the tube. They pulsate, setting up a current in the direction of the uterus, and prevent the ovum moving too fast, ensuring that it is ready for implantation when it reaches the uterus.

The menstrual cycle

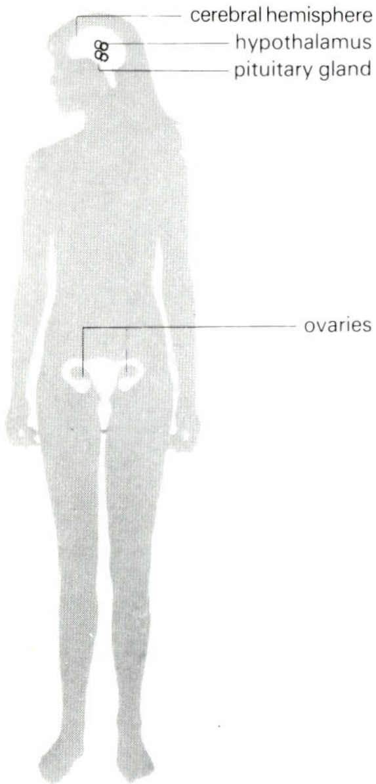

The hypothalamus, a part of the brain regulates the hormones secreted by the pituitary gland during the menstrual cycle.

The menstrual cycle is a process whereby an egg ripens in the ovaries and is released for fertilization while changes occur in the endometrium, the lining of the uterus, to prepare it for the implantation of a fertilized egg. If fertilization does not take place the endometrium breaks down, producing the menstrual flow (or period) and the cycle begins again. The different stages of the process are triggered by four hormones, or chemical messengers, two of which are secreted by the pituitary gland and two by the ovaries. The initial signal for the start of the cycle is given by the hypothalamus, a part of the brain which possesses its own clock mechanism. The menstrual cycle usually lasts for one month but in some women it takes up to six weeks or is irregular. The cycle can also be affected by mental and physical stress and weight loss. Something as simple as long-distance travel or a new job can suppress the cycle.

At birth the ovaries contain thousands of immature follicles each of which encloses an immature egg, or ovum. At the start of each menstrual cycle, several follicles are stimulated into growth by the follicle-stimulating hormone (F.S.H.), produced by the pituitary gland in response to a signal from the hypothalamus. Though several ova may start to develop, normally only one ripens each month and the rest degenerate. Where two ova ripen and both are fertilized fraternal, or non-identical, twins will be conceived.

As the follicle is growing, the ovaries send out a second hormone, estrogen. This causes the endometrium to thicken and acts on the pituitary gland via the hypothalamus, triggering a surge of luteinizing hormone (L.H.). This causes ovulation, the release of the ovum into the abdominal cavity.

The empty follicle from which the ovum has split may bleed a little and this sometimes causes a sharp pain. The follicle then heals, developing into the corpus luteum which produces more estrogen and the fourth hormone, progesterone. Under their influence the nature of the endometrium changes so that it is capable of receiving and nourishing a fertilized ovum. After two weeks, if the woman has not conceived, the corpus luteum degenerates. The level of estrogen and progesterone falls, causing the outer layer of the endometrium to be shed as the period or menstrual flow, and a new cycle begins.

OVULATION

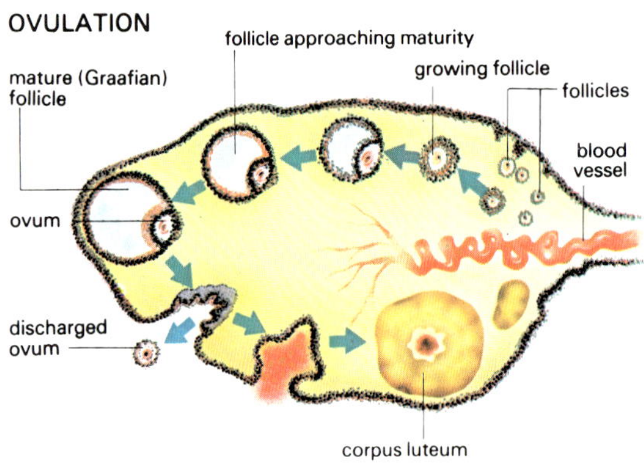

At the start of the menstrual cycle several follicles in the ovary begin to grow. Usually only one matures, producing a ripe ovum. At ovulation the ovum is released into the abdominal cavity. The empty follicle bleeds a little and develops into the corpus luteum. Unless fertilization occurs, the corpus luteum withers away after two weeks.

Hormones and the life cycle

The major changes which occur in women at puberty and the menopause are the result of the influence of the hormones F.S.H. and estrogen. During childhood a gradual rise in the hormone F.S.H., controlled by the hy-

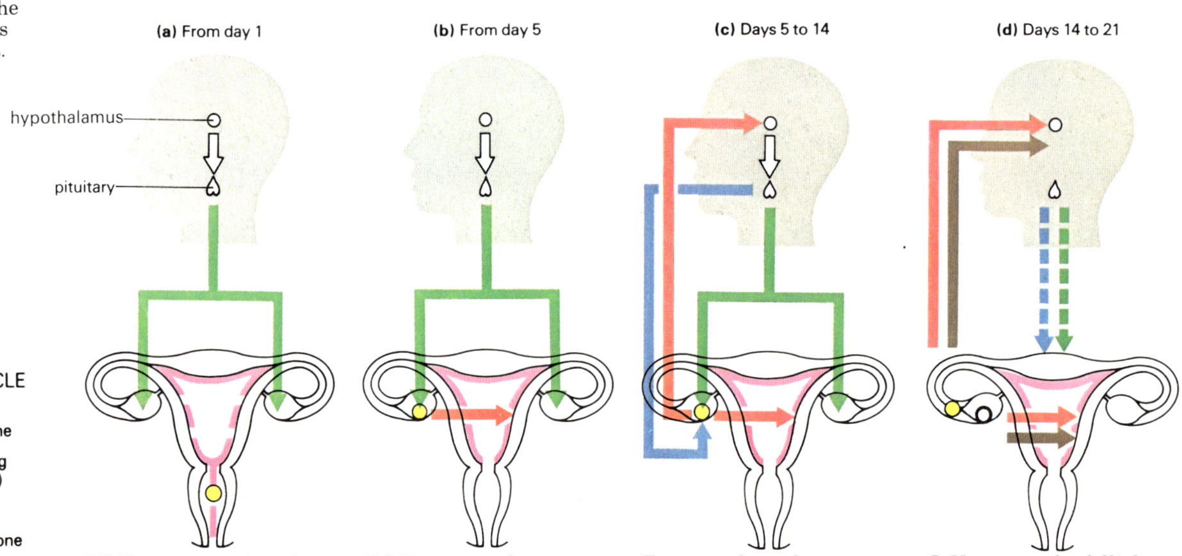

(a) While menstruation, the last stage of the cycle, is still going on, the first stage of a new cycle is initiated by the hypothalamus, which signals to the pituitary gland to release F.S.H. into the bloodstream.

(b) F.S.H. acts on the immature follicles in the ovaries causing several of them to begin to develop. Usually only one ripens in each cycle; the rest degenerate. Estrogen from the ovaries stimulates the lining of the uterus.

(c) Estrogen from the ovary acts on the hypothalamus, controlling the secretion of F.S.H. and triggering the release of L.H. by the pituitary gland. It also causes thickening of the endometrium.

(d) L.H. causes the follicle to rupture and release the ovum. The empty follicle forms the corpus luteum. This secretes estrogen and progesterone, which prepare the endometrium for implantation and stop the flow of F.S.H. and L.H.

THE MENSTRUAL CYCLE

- Releasing hormone
- Follicle stimulating hormone (F.S.H.)
- Estrogen
- Luteinizing hormone (L.H.)
- Progesterone
- Human chorionic gonadotrophin (H.C.G.)
- Endometrium
- Ovum
- Corpus luteum

pothalamus, produces a rise in the level of estrogen. By puberty, usually between 11 and 13 years, the estrogen level reaches a point where it causes enlargement of the breasts, uterus, vagina and external genital organs and triggers the first menstrual period. Small amounts of male hormones, called androgens, are also produced in women, mainly by the adrenal gland, and these hormones are responsible for the appearance of abnormal pubic, facial and axillary hair.

A woman's reproductive years usually last until her mid-forties or early fifties when her supply of eggs runs out. At this point, which is known as the menopause, or "change of life" hormones produced by the pituitary gland fail to elicit any response from the ovaries. There is therefore a drop in the level of estrogen circulating in the bloodstream and all the organs sensitive to this hormone are affected. There is also a marked increase in F.S.H. which is no longer being suppressed by estrogens. The symptoms associated with the menopause, including hot flashes and dry skin, are the result of this changing balance of hormones within the body. Many women, however, pass through the menopause without these symptoms, all of which can be relieved by taking estrogen and a progestin.

In the years leading up to the menopause, follicles may develop but fail to ovulate, causing irregular and sometimes heavy bleeding. Medical advice should always be sought in such cases. Even when menstruation has stopped, however, sporadic ovulations still sometimes occur and it is therefore advisable to use contraception until two years after menstrual periods have ceased.

How "the pill" works

Most contraceptive pills contain some form of estrogen and progestin and are known as "combined" pills. They maintain a blood level of these hormones which prevents the development of follicles and ovulation by suppressing the production of F.S.H. and L.H. In addition, the progestin acts to thicken the cervical mucus, making it impenetrable to sperm. The combined pill can also be an effective cure for menstrual pains since these often occur only in ovulating women.

When a woman stops taking the pill the level of estrogen and progesterone falls and the endometrium is shed as in normal menstruation. It may, however, take some weeks or even months for spontaneous ovulation and menstruation to begin again. Indeed, it is very common for it to take longer than the length of the usual menstrual cycle for the first period to occur. This may make it difficult to calculate expected date of delivery if conception occurs at the first ovulation (*see* p. 63).

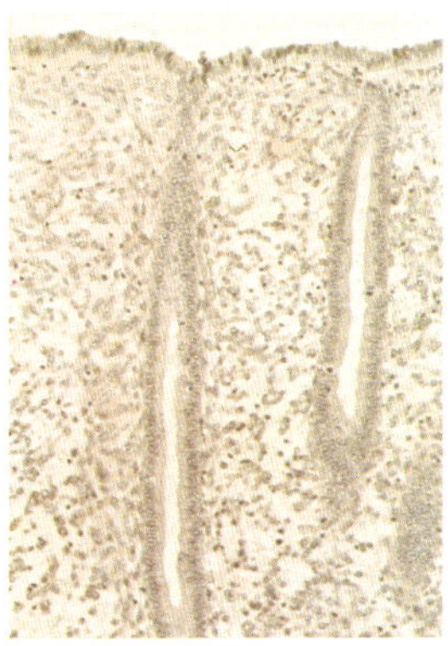

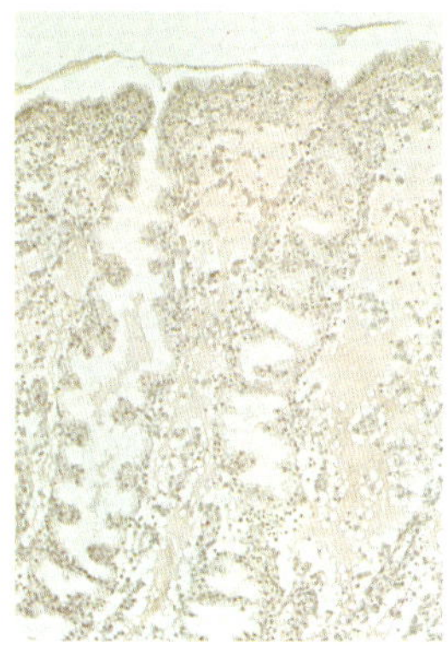

During the first two weeks of the menstrual cycle, the endometrium is thickening rapidly. Its appearance under the microscope is shown, far left, during this proliferative phase, stage (c) in the diagrams below.

After ovulation, the secretory phase, in which the endometrium secretes hormones, begins. The endometrium is seen, left, at the end of this phase, stage (e) in the diagrams below.

(e) Days 21 to 28

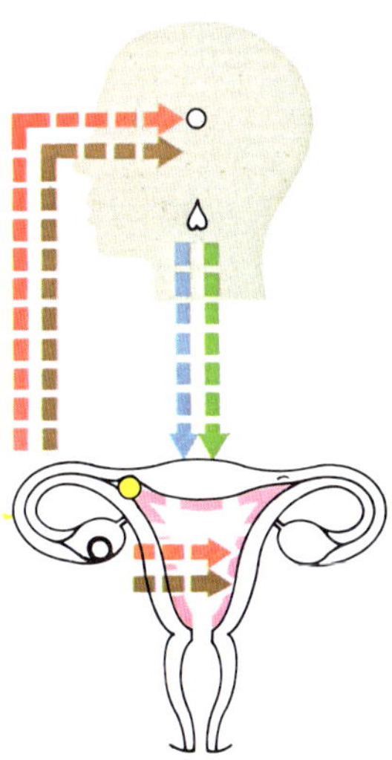

If the ovum is not fertilized, the corpus luteum degenerates and the level of estrogen and progesterone therefore falls rapidly, causing the outer layer of the endometrium to break down and be shed as the period, or menstrual flow.

(f) From day 26

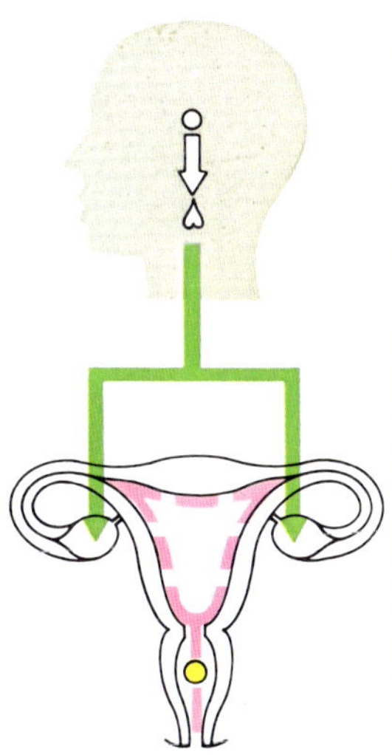

The hypothalamus once more signals the release of F.S.H. from the pituitary, causing the next menstrual cycle to begin.

PREGNANCY

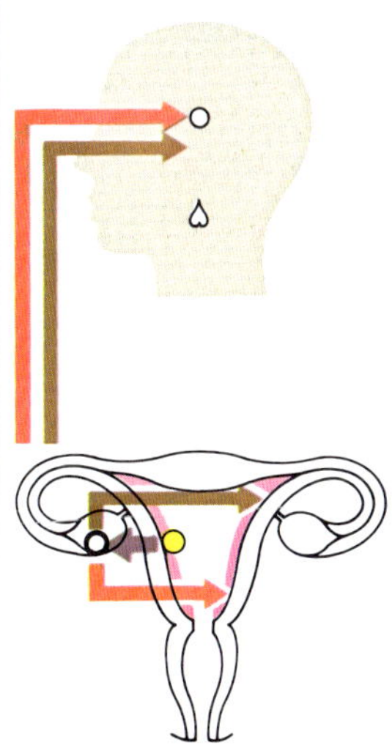

If the ovum is fertilized, a fifth hormone (H.C.G.) is produced by the blastocyst and this maintains the corpus luteum. Thus the production of estrogen and progesterone continues, sustaining the endometrium and preventing a new cycle.

THE CONTRACEPTIVE PILL

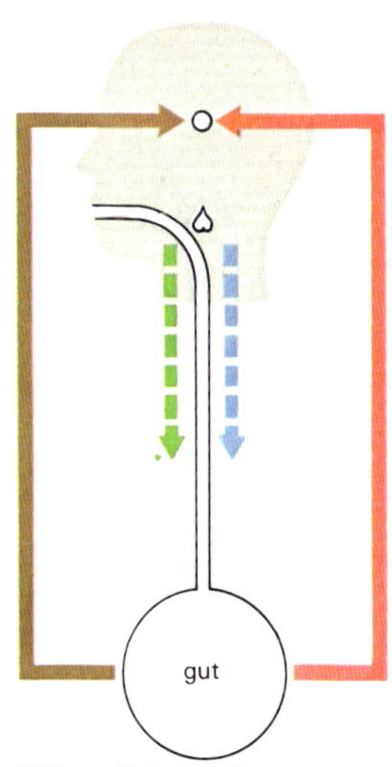

"The pill" usually contains estrogen and a form of progestin which act on the hypothalamus to prevent it triggering the release of F.S.H. and L.H. by the pituitary gland.

The male reproductive organs / Fertilization

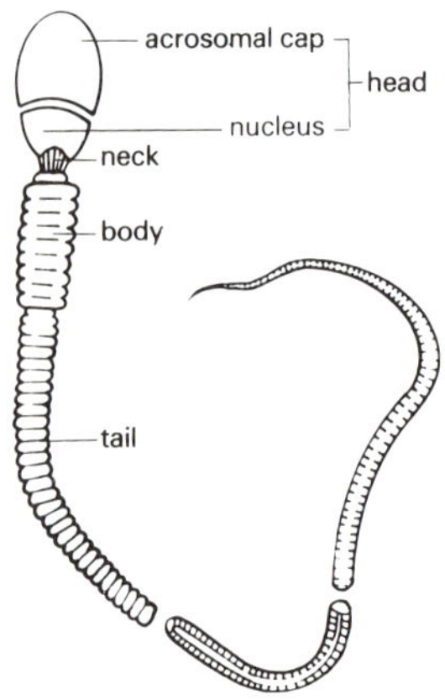

The sperm head, covered by the acrosomal cap, contains the nucleus which carries the genetic material. The body, joined to the head by the neck, supplies energy to the tail, which drives the sperm along.

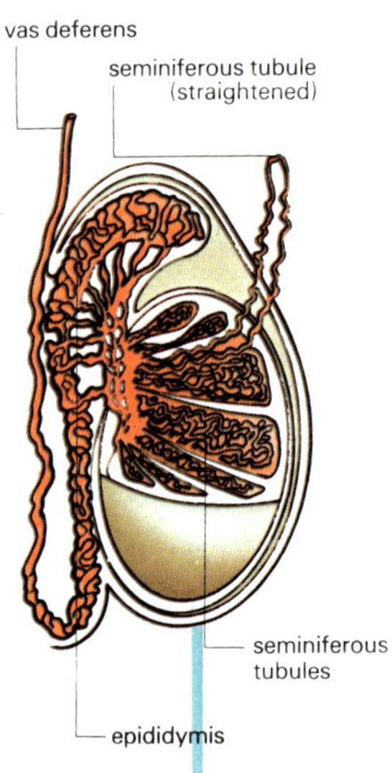

A cross-section of a testis shows the seminiferous tubules where sperm are manufactured (one is straightened to indicate its length), and the epididymis where they mature.

The central feature of the male reproductive organs is the testicles, or testes, the site of sperm production and the male counterpart of the ovaries. The testes are a pair of oval-shaped glands that hang outside the body below the penis in a loose pouch of skin called the scrotum. This serves to keep the testes at the optimum temperature for sperm production, a few degrees below the normal internal body temperature. When the testes hang loosely, evaporation from the closely packed sweat glands in the scrotum lowers their temperature. In cold conditions, a lining of muscle within the scrotum draws them close against the body. From puberty to old age the testes manufacture sperm.

The adult testis is around 2 in long by $1\frac{1}{4}$ in wide (5 cm by 3 cm). It is surrounded by a tough white fibrous coat called the tunica albuginea. It is divided into some 300 compartments, each containing one to three seminiferous tubules. The total length of these is estimated to be about 1300 feet, or 400 meters.

The production of sperm

Sperm are tadpole-shaped. The genetic material of the cell nucleus is carried in the head, and the tail provides the needed propulsion. Sperm are manufactured by a process of cell division called meiosis from the spermatogonia, minute round cells found in the lining of the seminiferous tubules coiled within each testis (*see* p. 20).

Groups of cells lying between the seminiferous tubules in the testes secrete the male hormone, testosterone. Produced in response to interstitial cell stimulating hormone (I.C.S.H.), which is identical to luteinizing hormone (L.H.) in women, testosterone stimulates the development of the external male genital organs in utero as well as changes which occur during puberty: growth of body and facial hair, deepening of the voice and broadening of the shoulders.

Once sperm are formed they move along the seminiferous tubules and collect in the two epididymes, larger tubes coiled behind each testis. Here the sperm finally reach maturity, approximately 45 days after the original spermatogonia divided.

From each epididymis they pass along the vas deferens, a tube which loops up over the pubic bone, and down past the bladder where each is joined by a gland, the seminal vesicle, in which some sperm are stored. The duct thus formed passes through the prostate gland and joins the urethra.

The seminal fluid, or semen, in which sperm are ejaculated is secreted mainly by the prostate gland and the seminal vesicles, and usually contains between 200 and 400 million sperm, only 10 per cent of which are likely to reach the cervical canal.

The secretions which are produced from the glands are alkaline and serve to help neutralize the acid environment in the vagina when the sperm enter. They also contain fructose, which is a source of energy for the sperm.

The process of fertilization

Normally the penis hangs limply down in a position suitable for urination, but when a man is sexually excited it becomes erect, swelling to about double its normal size and rising away from the body. The erection is caused by blood pumping into the spongy erectile tissues within the penis.

Sexual excitement reaches a peak at orgasm when muscle contractions drive sperm out of the storage areas in each epididymis, mixing them with the various secretions to form the semen (i.e. ejaculate).

As the semen flows into the urethra the route to the bladder clamps shut and a series of contractions in the muscles around the spongy tissue of the penis drives the semen along the urethra and out.

After ejaculation the semen tends to form a small pool deep within the vagina, giving the sperm the maximum chance to penetrate the jellylike plug of mucus that blocks and protects the canal through the cervix. At the time

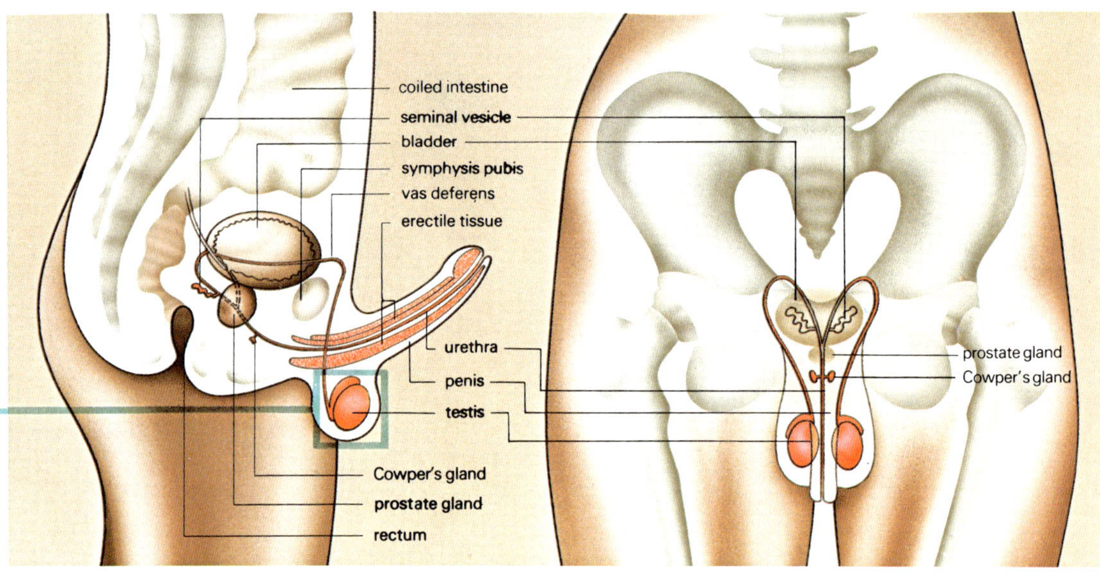

The male organs include the testes, where sperm and hormones are created, and a series of tubes which carry the sperm to the penis. The sperm mixes with secretions from the seminal vesicles, the prostate gland and Cowper's glands to form the semen. During sexual excitement blood pumps into the tissues of the penis, causing it to become erect (left).

of ovulation the mucous plug is thin and easy to penetrate.

Once the sperm have entered the uterus they swim up the fallopian tubes against the current which is set up by the beating of the hair-like cilia which line the tubes. The sperm arrive at the outer ends of the fallopian tubes within 30 minutes of ejaculation but they continue to break free from the cervical mucus and retain their fertilizing power for up to 18 hours.

If a newly-released egg, or ovum, enters the fallopian tube while sperm are still active, or is already within the tube, the sperm are attracted to it and cluster thickly around it. Altogether between 1000 and 3000 sperm may reach the ovum. The chemicals in the tip of each sperm help strip away the layers of ovarian cells that may still surround the egg until one sperm can reach and penetrate its smooth shell.

When a sperm has pierced the ovum a change in the lattice-like outer surface layer ensures no more can enter. Once through the shell, the head of the sperm splits off and fuses with the nucleus of the ovum.

For about three days after fertilization the new cell progresses along the fallopian tube, dividing and redividing to form a small clump of cells called the morula. For a further three or four days it floats in the uterus, still dividing until it becomes a hollow clump of about a hundred cells called the blastocyst. The dividing cells are nourished at this stage by secretions from the uterine glands known as the uterine milk.

Implantation

About seven or eight days after fertilization, the blastocyst settles on the wall of the uterus. At this point in the menstrual cycle the endometrium is particularly thick and rich in blood vessels and is ready for implantation. Some of the cells which cover the blastocyst, known as the trophoblast, begin to eat into the lining of the uterus and grow into cords that anchor the blastocyst to the wall of the uterus. Eventually the trophoblast develops into the placenta (*see* p. 46).

A fertilized egg which fails to implant will be swept out of the uterus during menstruation. In a few cases the fertilized egg implants in the fallopian tube, and begins to develop there. This is known as an ectopic pregnancy and has to be removed surgically.

The intrauterine contraceptive device (I.U.D.) prevents implantation but not fertilization. Its action may be due in part to increased movement within the fallopian tubes which forces the morula to arrive at the uterus before it is ready to implant. The I.U.D. also interferes with the process of implantation itself. The presence of an I.U.D. does not, however, preclude the possibility of an ectopic pregnancy particularly where there is tubal infection (*see* p. 22).

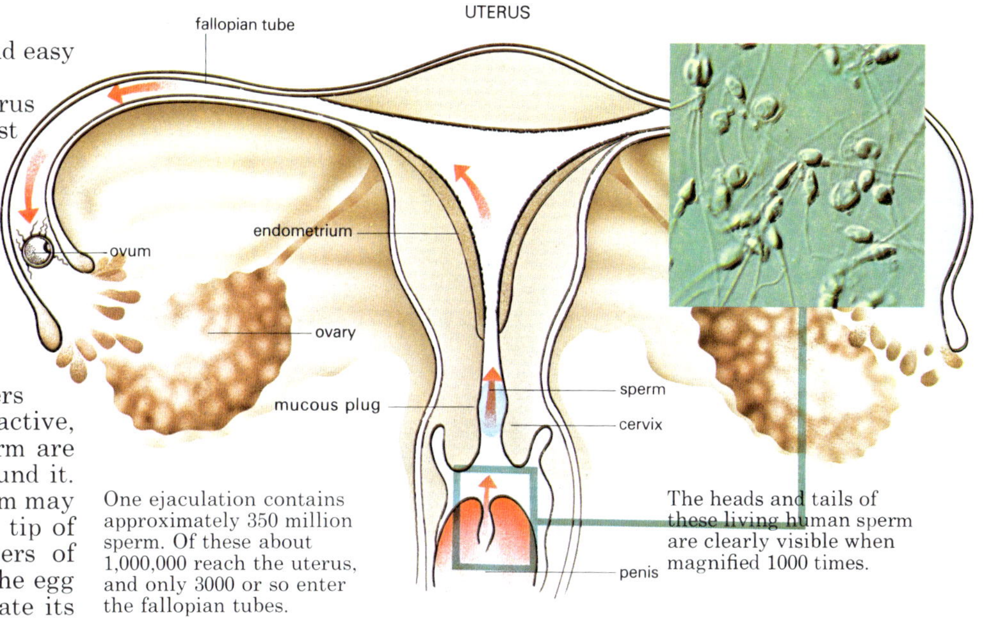

One ejaculation contains approximately 350 million sperm. Of these about 1,000,000 reach the uterus, and only 3000 or so enter the fallopian tubes.

The heads and tails of these living human sperm are clearly visible when magnified 1000 times.

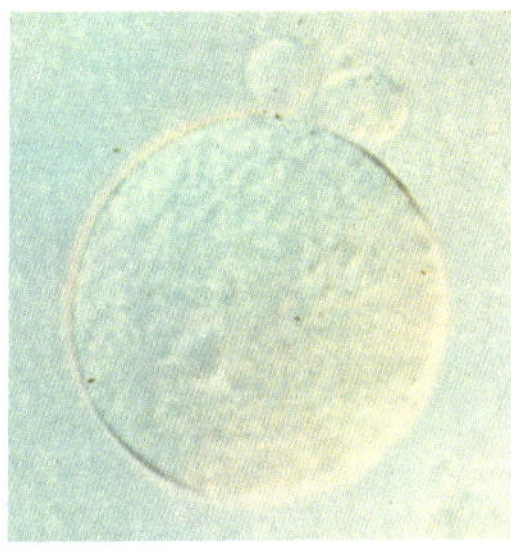

Seen here about 12 hours after ovulation, this ovum has been fertilized by one of the sperm which reached it as it traveled down the fallopian tube toward the uterus. The nuclei of the sperm and ovum have fused to form a single cell. The two polar bodies can still be seen in the top right-hand corner.

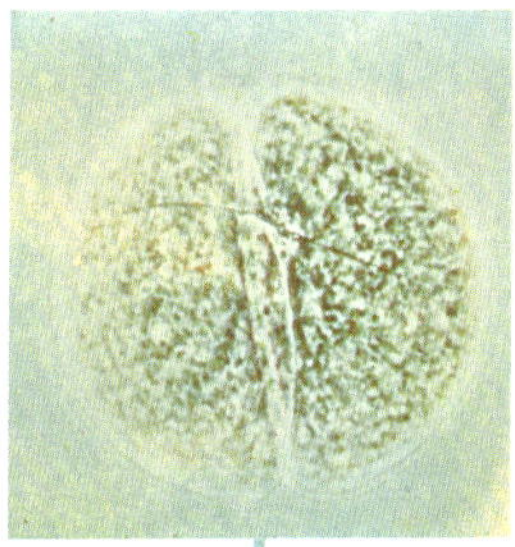

The first division occurs a few hours after the ovum has been fertilized.

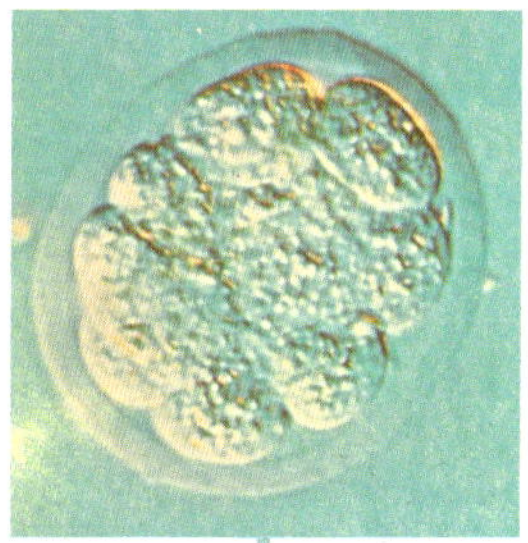

After three or four days further division produces a clump of cells known as the morula.

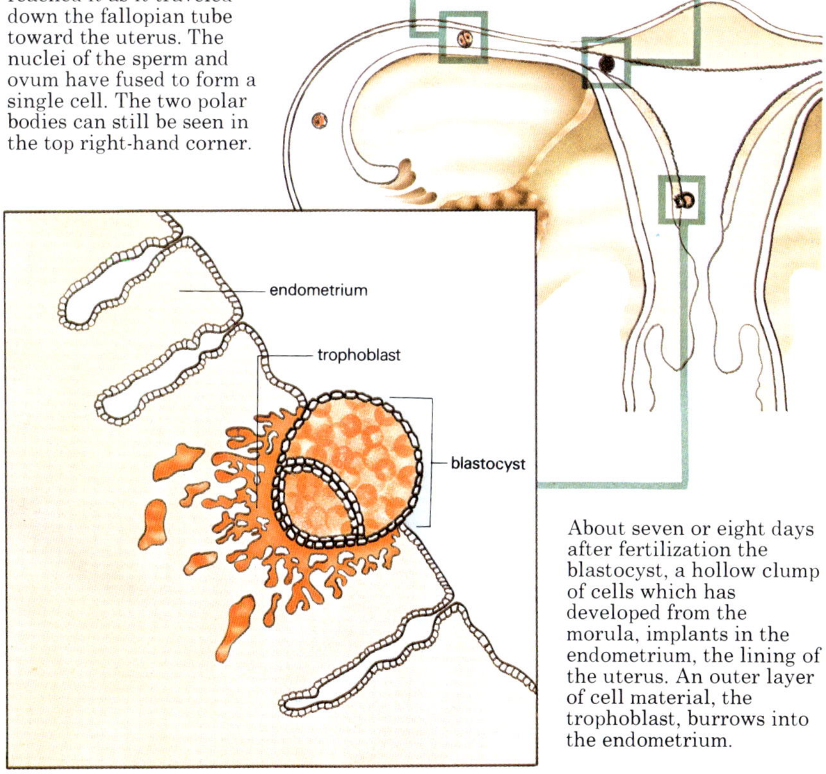

About seven or eight days after fertilization the blastocyst, a hollow clump of cells which has developed from the morula, implants in the endometrium, the lining of the uterus. An outer layer of cell material, the trophoblast, burrows into the endometrium.

Genetics and inheritance

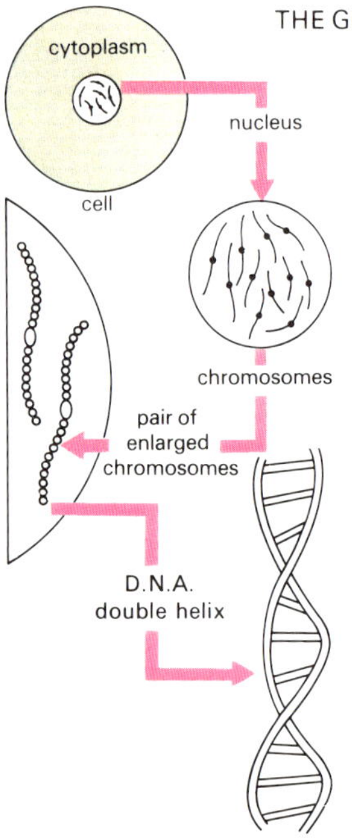

Inheritance is governed by the D.N.A. molecule found in the nucleus of each cell.

THE GROWTH OF NEW CELLS (MITOSIS)

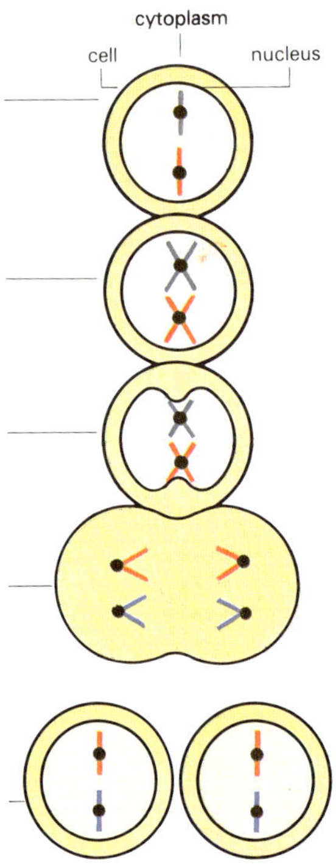

(1) 46 chromosomes are contained in the nucleus of every human cell. (Only two are represented here.)

(2) When a cell is going to divide, each chromosome doubles, reproducing exactly the same genetic code.

(3) The doubled chromosomes then line up along the center of the cell.

(4) Each chromosome splits in half and the two complete sets of chromosomes group at either end of the cell.

(5) The whole cell then divides, creating two daughter cells each with the same genetic code as the parent cell.

Environment and heredity combine to mold our mental and physical characteristics but the first cell, the fertilized egg, already contains all the inherited information needed to construct a new and unique human being.

The basic unit of the body is the cell, made of cytoplasm – a jellylike material – and a nucleus. The nucleus contains 46 chromosomes, which themselves carry thousands of genes, the vehicles for the transmission of inherited characteristics. The fundamental constituent of the genes (and therefore of the chromosomes) is a molecule of a chemical called deoxyribonucleic acid (D.N.A.), shaped like a long, intertwined double helix. The genetic code for the entire body is contained in the D.N.A. helixes and depends on the order of molecules in them.

The growth of a new cell

Each cell in the body contains 46 chromosomes which can be arranged in 23 pairs. One chromosome from each pair is inherited from each parent. Two of the chromosomes, the twenty-third pair, determine sex. In a woman the sex chromosomes appear as two Xs; in a man as an X and a Y. Human growth involves increasing the number of cells by a process of division known as mitosis. In this process each

PRODUCTION OF SPERM AND OVA (MIOSIS)

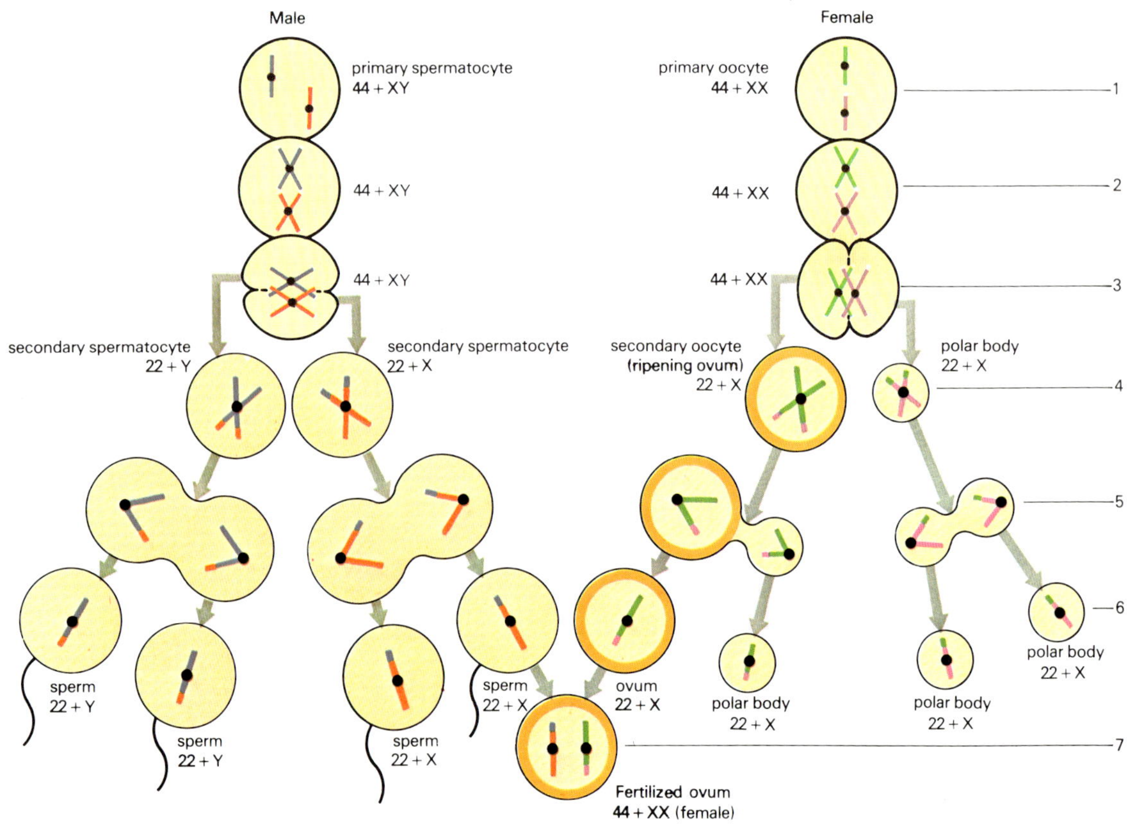

The germ cells of a man (the primary spermatocytes) each contain 46 chromosomes including two sex chromosomes, one X and one Y. The germ cells of a woman (the primary oocytes) contain 46 chromosomes including two X sex chromosomes. The chromosomes are paired, one of each pair being derived from the person's mother and one from the father. Here only two chromosomes (one pair) are shown. The colors stand for the genetic code. Numbers (1) to (7) refer to both sides of the diagram.
The chromosomes within the germ cells pair off (1). The paired chromosomes duplicate themselves (2). They then intertwine and exchange genetic material (called "crossing over") (3). When they separate each contains material from both parents.
The cells divide to form two new cells (the two secondary spermatocytes in the male and one secondary oocyte and a polar body in the female). One chromosome from each pair goes to each new cell, which therefore contains only 23 chromosomes. Both female cells contain X sex chromosomes. One of the male cells contains an X chromosome; the other a Y chromosome (4).

At the next stage, the two daughter cells split again, this time by the same process as that involved in ordinary cell division, mitosis (5 and 6).

Only one ovum ripens, the other cells (the polar bodies) disappear. Half of the sperm created contain an X sex chromosome; the other half a Y.

The fertilized ovum contains 23 chromosomes from each parent (7). However, because of the crossing over (3), the arrangement of genes is new and unique. If the ovum is fertilized by a sperm containing a Y chromosome, a boy is conceived; if by one with an X (as here), a girl.

chromosome in the nucleus, followed by the whole cell, divides into two. As a result, two daughter cells are produced each carrying 46 chromosomes and each having exactly the same genetic code as the parent cell.

Sperm and ova

The creation of sperm and eggs, or ova, differs in two ways from the standard process of cell division. First, each chromosome intertwines with its pair and the two exchange genetic material, a process known as "crossing over". This gives each chromosome a new and unique genetic code, albeit one made up of the same elements as the original chromosomes. Then, when the cells divide for the first time, each daughter cell receives only 23 chromosomes: 22 ordinary chromosomes, and one sex chromosome, always an X in the ovum and either an X or a Y in the sperm.

When conception occurs, the 23 chromosomes of the sperm combine with the 23 chromosomes of the egg to form a new cell with a full complement of 46 chromosomes. The new cell from which the child will grow therefore contains genes from both parents, but because of the mixing of genes that has taken place each child is unique. Where an ovum splits by chance after fertilization and two embryos develop from one egg the result is two children who are exactly alike. For this reason they are called identical twins.

Dominant and recessive genes

Most ordinary characteristics like height and coloring are governed by combinations of several different genes. Moreover, traits may show in one generation but not in the next and still appear in grandchildren. Inheritance over generations is therefore very complex. The interaction of several genes on each other is rarely understood but it is possible, for example, in the case of red hair to give some idea of how a girl can inherit her maternal grandmother's hair color when her own mother did not.

Inherited traits can be dominant or recessive, and for any one trait genes from one parent act in relation to those inherited from the other parent. Thus for a trait carried by a dominant gene a child will show the trait even if it has been inherited from only one parent. By contrast a recessive gene must be passed on by both parents for the trait to show in the child.

Red hair is controlled by a recessive gene. Thus parents who both have brown hair but also carry a red hair gene, while far more likely to produce a brown-haired child, still may produce one with red hair. On the other hand, if one parent has red hair, and the other has brown but carries no red hair gene, none of their children will have red hair.

DOMINANT AND RECESSIVE GENES

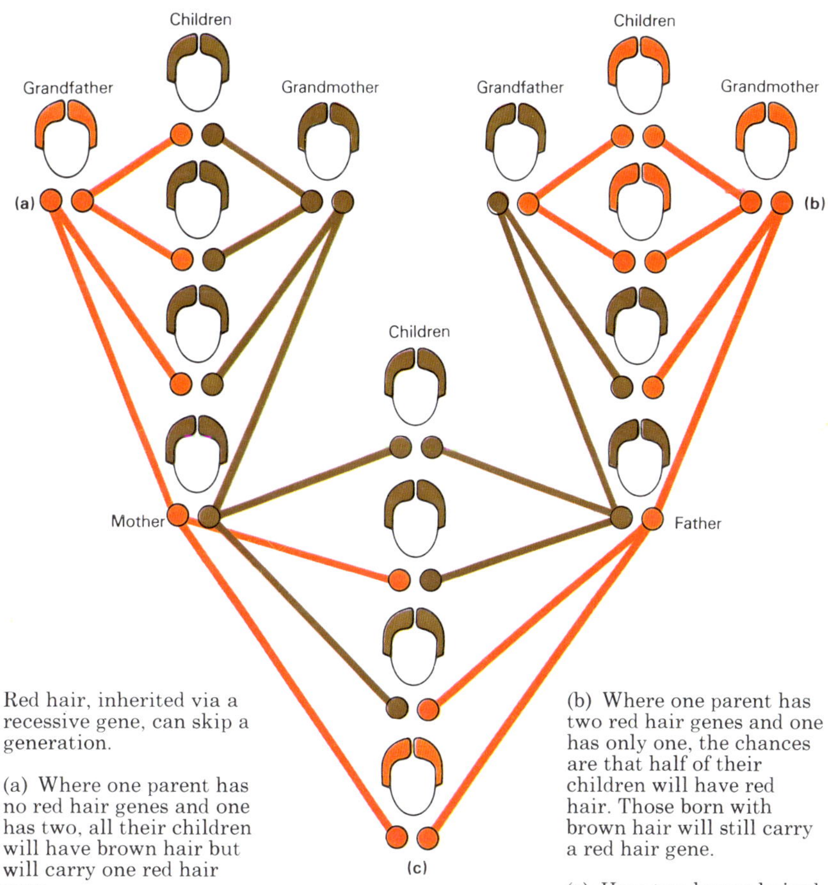

Red hair, inherited via a recessive gene, can skip a generation.

(a) Where one parent has no red hair genes and one has two, all their children will have brown hair but will carry one red hair gene.

(b) Where one parent has two red hair genes and one has only one, the chances are that half of their children will have red hair. Those born with brown hair will still carry a red hair gene.

(c) Here two brown-haired parents of the next generation both carry one red hair gene. They have a one in four chance of giving birth to a red-haired child.

Blood groups, like other characteristics, are inherited. The main blood groups are A, B, AB, and O. A and B behave like dominant genes. Blood group O means the absence of A or B genes. Matching of blood groups is essential to successful blood transfusion. For the couple wishing to conceive, however, the most critical blood characteristic is the Rh factor.

All blood is either Rh positive or Rh negative, the former transmitted by a dominant gene, the latter by a recessive gene. The factor only assumes significance when an Rh-negative woman conceives an Rh-positive child. In this case there is the danger that if the fetal and maternal blood mix during pregnancy the mother may develop antibodies which will attack and damage the blood of the fetus in the current and future pregnancies. Fortunately, it is now possible to prevent this by treating the mother during and immediately after an unaffected pregnancy (*see* p. 33).

Some recessive characteristics are linked to sex. For example, hemophilia, a condition which prevents the blood from clotting, is carried on the X sex chromosome but affects

When analyzing the chromosomes of a human cell geneticists arrange them in pairs in order of decreasing size numbering the pairs from 1 to 23. The 23rd pair determines sex. In this case the pair is XY and the cell is therefore male.

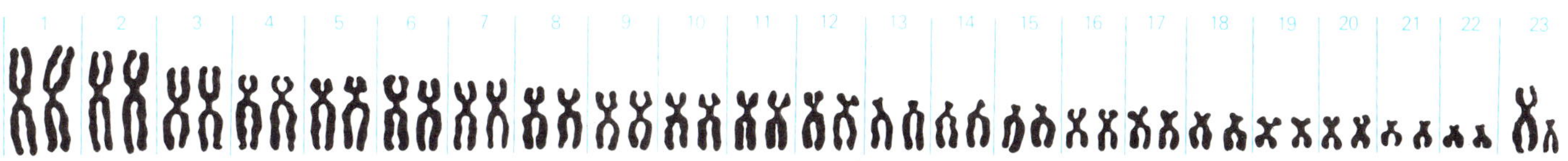

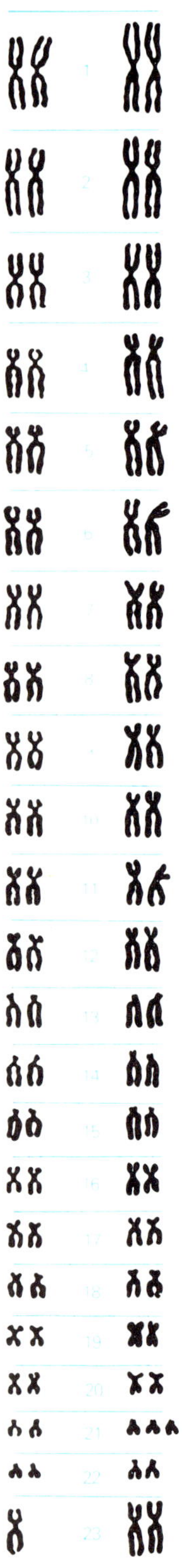

Certain chromosomal abnormalities are clearly seen when chromosomes are lined up in their pairs. Turner's syndrome is the result of a missing sex chromosome (number 23, left) in a woman. Down's syndrome is produced by three chromosomes at number 21 (right) instead of the usual pair.

only boys. Although women may carry the gene they do not suffer from hemophilia because the abnormal gene is balanced by a normal dominant gene carried on the second X chromosome. In men, however, the smaller Y sex chromosome lacks any balancing gene.

Genetic abnormalities

The normal human has 23 pairs of chromosomes but chromosomal abnormalities which produce particular conditions do sometimes occur. The most common is Down's syndrome, or "mongolism", a condition of mental deficiency in which there are three of a certain type of chromosome (number 21) instead of the usual pair in each cell. The incidence rises with maternal age. The incidence at age 30 is 1: 885, whereas at age 40 it is 1:109.

Turner's syndrome is an example of an even rarer chromosomal abnormality. Caused by the absence of a second X or of the Y sex chromosome, it results in a female child who is short and infertile. Some abnormalities are caused by the presence of an extra sex chromosome. The Klinefelter's syndrome is the most common sex chromosome abnormality, ocurring in 1 in 700 live-born males. These individuals have three sex chromosomes, two Xs and one Y. They are generally tall with a tendency to long limbs. The testicles are soft and atrophic. Spermatogenesis may be reduced or absent. They have IQs that are significantly below those of their siblings.

Individual genes carried on the chromosomes also produce abnormalities and occasionally genes undergo spontaneous change. Such changes, known as mutations, are often lethal but in certain rare instances their effect will be good.

An increasing number of genetic abnormalities and diseases are now known and genetic counseling is available for prospective parents. This means that couples with a family history of congenital abnormalities who are thinking of having a baby can often find out how likely they are to conceive an abnormal child. Women already pregnant can be tested by amniocentesis to discover whether the fetus has any chromosomal abnormality.

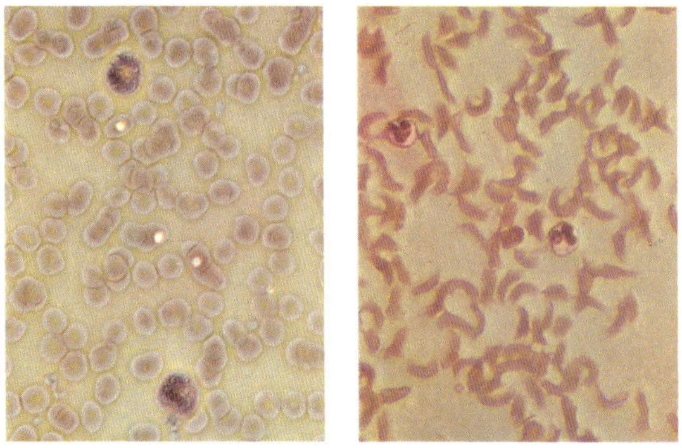

Normal blood cells have a rounded shape (left). In sickle-cell anemia, an hereditary condition found in 1 out of 600 blacks, the blood cells are sickle-shaped (right) and carry less oxygen.

Infertility

Most young couples conceive within the first six months of trying but, even without any abnormality, conception can take up to two years. It is reasonable to start infertility investigations after a year, although a shorter time is appropriate in older women or if there is reason to suppose that there may be some abnormality. There are a large number of possible causes of infertility, some simple to remedy, others more difficult. It is almost as common for the problem to be due to a male as a female factor.

The causes of infertility

Since the sperm has to meet the ovum at a particular moment in the menstrual cycle for conception to occur infertility may simply be due to infrequent intercourse. The couple may not be aware of the fertile time in the menstrual cycle and if they seldom have intercourse they may keep missing the best time.

Infertility in men can result from an inability to get or maintain an erection or from a failure to ejaculate during intercourse. Anxiety about sexual performance or other psychological problems may be the cause and some form of therapy may help.

It may, however, be the case that the testicles are not working properly. If they are undescended – that is, if they do not hang down in the scrotum – they can fulfill their hormonal function but do not produce sperm. The same is true if corrective surgery for undescended testicles or for a hernia has interfered with the blood supply, or there is a knot of varicose veins in the scrotum. Mumps sometimes causes inflammation of the testes, and if both are affected this may cause a low sperm count. Lastly the XXY chromosomal abnormality usually produces small and inadequate testicles and sterility.

Failure to ovulate is a relatively common cause of infertility in a woman. In most cases the absence of ovulation or infrequent ovulation is not due to any specific abnormality. But it may be caused by loss of weight, thyroid disease, premature menopause, overproduction of the milk-producing hormone (prolactin) by the pituitary gland or by a pituitary tumor. It can also be the result of taking "the pill". A woman who has infrequent periods probably should not take the pill if she wishes to conceive soon after discontinuing it.

Damage to the fallopian tubes, another source of infertility, can arise from an infection within the tubes (salpingitis) or from some external effect on them. Of the latter, a pelvic abscess caused by appendicitis is the most common. This leads to adhesions which kink the tubes and interfere with the passage of the ovum into the open end of the tube. Salpingitis may be caused by venereal disease or, rarely, tuberculosis. It may also be caused by an infection which ascends to the fallopian tubes, often after a delivery, miscarriage or termination of pregnancy.

Fertilization may take place but fail. A poorly functioning corpus luteum will mean that the levels of estrogen and progesterone fall too soon so that menstruation occurs and the fertilized ovum is washed away. Another possible cause of infertility in women is cervical hostility, in which the cervical mucus is impenetrable to sperm.

Investigation and treatment of infertility
When investigating infertility it is usually best to rule out the possibility of problems in the man before subjecting the woman to extensive tests. A semen analysis is the first step. Normal semen should have more than 30 million sperm per ml, 50 per cent of which should be moving and 60 per cent of normal appearance. If the sperm are few or defective, hormone therapy or wearing looser underwear may be beneficial. If there are no sperm at all, tests can establish whether this is due to testicle failure or to a blockage in the tubules that carry the sperm. The former cannot be treated; the latter can sometimes be corrected by surgery. When the sperm count is low or when the couple fails to have intercourse or in cases of cervical hostility, the husband's sperm may be used for artificial insemination (A.I.H.). However, if the man's semen specimen is incapable of fertilization, artificial insemination by a donor (A.I.D.) may be acceptable to the couple.

Investigation of the woman starts with simple tests. A daily chart of the early morning body temperature should show a rise on the day following ovulation. Whether or not a woman is ovulating can therefore be established. In addition, since fertilization has to occur soon after ovulation, intercourse timed for the day before the temperature rise should increase the chances of conception. If the woman's menstrual cycle is irregular, however, it may prove difficult to get the timing right. Once the day of ovulation can be predicted, a postcoital test conducted by a doctor can then be made. A little cervical mucus is collected on the predicted day of ovulation, between 6 and 12 hours after intercourse. A positive test will reveal the normal mucus as thin and clear, teeming with live sperm. A negative test may be the result of abnormalities of the sperm or of the cervical mucus or indicate a failure to ovulate.

The failure to ovulate can often be treated with drugs. The drug clomiphene is used to stimulate the pituitary gland to produce the hormones F.S.H. and L.H. which cause the ovary to ovulate. If this fails the pituitary gland itself may be defective and the next stage is to inject the hormones themselves. Clomiphene is associated with a slightly higher than usual chance of having twins. Hormone injections, such as Pergonal, increase the risk of multiple ovulations leading to quadruplets or even more babies, and therefore have to be administered very carefully.

Two tests are commonly used to discover whether the fallopian tubes are blocked or damaged. The simplest involves taking an X ray while a radio-opaque fluid is injected through the cervical canal. This type of test is known as a hysterosalpingogram. If the tubes are open, the dye is seen to pass along them and out into the abdominal cavity. If there is a blockage its location can be pinpointed.

Further information can be obtained by diagnostic laparoscopy, which is performed under anesthetic. A slender telescope-like instrument is passed through a small incision made in the abdominal wall. The pelvic organs can then be seen and, if the fallopian tubes are open, a blue dye injected through the cervix is observed spilling out of the ends of the tubes.

Tubal blockage is the most common cause of female infertility. Unfortunately, it is difficult to treat successfully, and the more the tubes are damaged, the smaller the chances of success. If the fallopian tubes are normal, any pelvic adhesions caused, for example, by appendicitis can often be divided successfully, thus freeing the tubes. Internal tubal infection is, on the other hand, frequently much more serious: the infection is likely to have destroyed the delicate cellular lining of the tubes as well as causing blockage. There is, however, a higher success rate if the infection is confined to the uterine end of the tube.

Tubal surgery involves a major operation and, except in cases of minimal damage, the very low success rate – less than five per cent – makes it probably not worthwhile. Even if the tube is opened there will be a much higher than normal risk of an ectopic, or tubal, pregnancy because the ovum may lodge in the tube on its way to the uterus, stopping the pregnancy at an early stage or leading to rupture of the fallopian tube and severe internal bleeding.

If the fallopian tubes are blocked or absent, pregnancy can still be achieved by in-vitro fertilization or embryo transfer. In the former, clomiphene is used to stimulate follicle development in the ovaries. The ova are retrieved by laparoscopy or ultrasound-guided needle aspiration. The ova are fertilized by the husband's sperm and are instilled into the uterus on day 4–5.

With embryo transfer a "donor" woman is artificially inseminated with the husband's sperm. The fertilized egg is flushed out of the donor's uterus and instilled into the mother's uterine cavity.

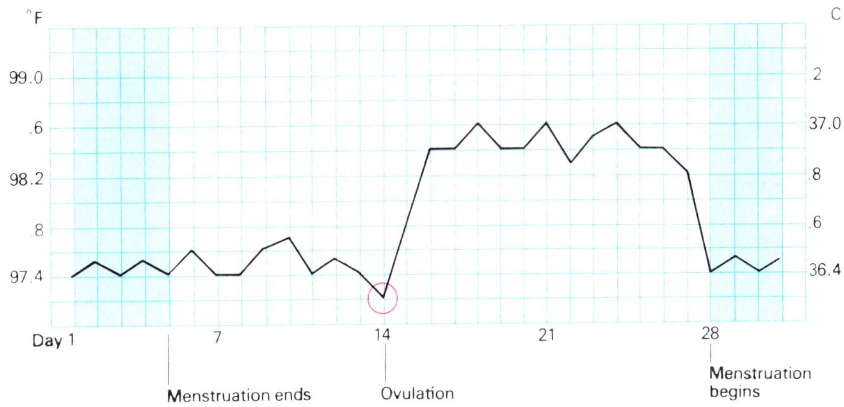

A chart of a woman's temperature taken each morning during the menstrual cycle shows that her temperature rises sharply just after ovulation.

INFERTILITY CHECKLIST

There are several causes of infertility. Either or both partners may be responsible. Below is a list of the most common causes.

BOTH PARTNERS
1. Infrequent intercourse

MEN
1. Impotence
2. Low sperm count
3. Poor sperm
4. No sperm because:
   a. failure of production
   b. blockage of transport

WOMEN
1. Cervical hostility
2. Failure to ovulate
3. Damaged fallopian tubes
4. Poor corpus luteum
5. Sexual disfunction

The mother in pregnancy

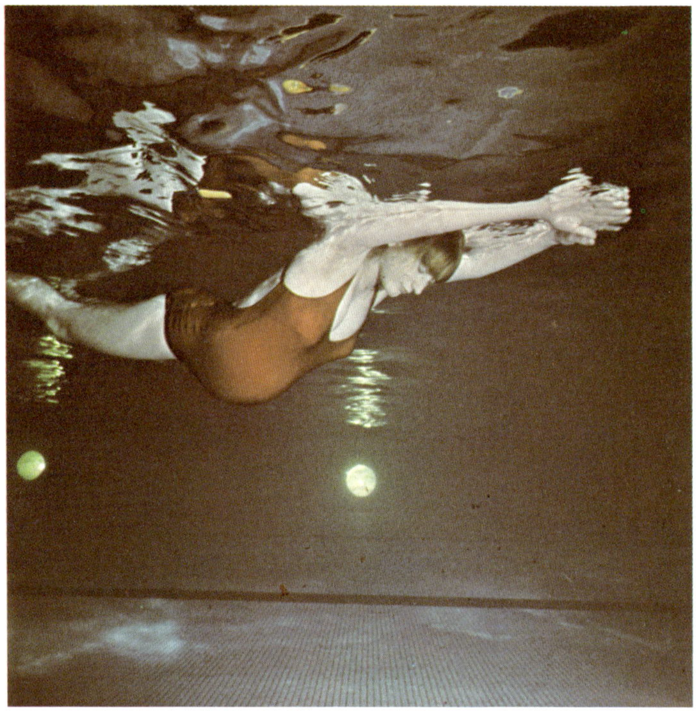

CHAPTER 2

Cross references

See also	Chapter
Problems in pregnancy	4
Hormones	1
Preparing for labor	5
Health of the fetus	3
Drugs and the fetus	3
Losing weight	8

Most of our understanding of what happens to the mother during pregnancy is very recent. At the time of the birth of our nation, in 1776, only one hospital existed in the United States. Over the next few decades there was a proliferation of hospitals but obstetrical problems were not considered important enough to be managed in a hospital. It was not uncommon for women to die in childbirth. They rarely had the luxury of medical care. Indeed often couples lost two or three children during childbirth or the first year of life.

In 1910, the first antenatal clinic was established in Adelaide, Australia. Others soon followed. Over the next few decades the outcome of pregnancies continued to improve such that the loss of the mother was a relatively uncommon event. But, puerperal sepsis, obstetrical hemorrhage and death due to anesthesia were still major problems. By the Second World War, the advent of antibiotics was responsible for the first inroads in conquering puerperal sepsis. Then transfusion technology offered an answer to maternal hemorrhage. Additionally, improved obstetrical anesthesia markedly reduced maternal deaths. The maternal mortality rate which was 799/100,000 live births in 1920, decreased to 83 by 1950, and to 21 in 1970. Today a mother stands only a 1/7000 chance of dying due to pregnancy. But most of these deaths occur in patients who have major predisposing factors. The prospects for the normal healthy patient are overwhelmingly favorable.

In the last three decades, the prognosis of the fetus and the newborn has been markedly improved. Approximately three decades ago, major breakthroughs occurred in the management of prematurity. The infants born between 25 and 36 weeks of gestation,

For pregnant women swimming produces a marvelous sense of lightness, as the extra weight is supported by the water. It is also very good exercise.

generally have a very difficult time in overcoming the handicaps of immature organ systems. The development of neonatal intensive care units has made the survival of a 2lb (1 kg) baby possible today. Furthermore, with good care and provided no extraordinary complications occur, the long-term problems with these babies have now proven to be minimal.

Improved antepartum care for the mother has decreased the frequency of prematurity. Improved delivery techniques have decreased the incidence of trauma to the newborn. Prophylactic measures like Rh immune prophylaxis and rubella vaccines have almost eliminated the chance of babies suffering from Rh disease and congenital malformations.

One of the major advances in the last 15 years has been the development of the high risk pregnancy concept. This approach places a high priority on antenatal care. The patient who has maternal or fetal factors that can adversely influence the outcome of pregnancy is referred to a high risk pregnancy center where many diagnostic tests are available to evaluate the condition of the fetus.

Couples are increasingly aware that preparation for pregnancy is important. It is quite common for a patient to visit her physician and ask what measures she may take to prepare herself for a healthy pregnancy. A growing emphasis has been placed on proper nutrition during pregnancy.

Many reports have shown the link between smoking and decreased growth of the fetus. Expectant mothers are now seriously encouraged not to smoke. Additionally, ingestion of alcohol has been shown to cause fetal alcohol syndrome in some instances. Many doctors warn their patients to be abstemious or not drink at all during pregnancy.

Major improvements in the outcome of pregnancy must also be credited to enlightened family planning. Today the mother becomes pregnant because of a desire to have a child. She generally has the number of children she wants. Mothers who have severe complications and who lose babies have effective means of birth control available so that they do not have to risk another pregnancy.

We now know that an individual woman's pregnancy is affected by the number of previous pregnancies, her age and living conditions. Physique, diet and general health also affect the pregnancy.

Investigators have also shown that some fetal abnormalities are caused by viruses, like rubella (German measles) and by certain drugs, especially if taken in early pregnancy. There are many medications that have been in use many years and have been shown to be safe but it is still important for a woman who is pregnant to take only drugs approved by her doctor. New accurate methods of diagnosing pregnancy have made it easier to protect the fetus.

Ultrasound scans have replaced X rays as a way of looking at the development of the pregnancy in the uterus. Ultrasound is a safe technique which provides detailed information of the earliest changes in uterine growth and the development of the fetus.

First attempts at antenatal care tended to restrict the mother's activity and encourage a feeling that pregnancy was an artificial state requiring a protective approach. Mothers are now encouraged to lead normal active lives, often working until their baby is born, secure in the knowledge that the body accommodates to pregnancy in its own remarkable ways and that should something start to go wrong it will almost certainly be detected quickly.

Symptoms and diagnosis

THE TRIMESTERS

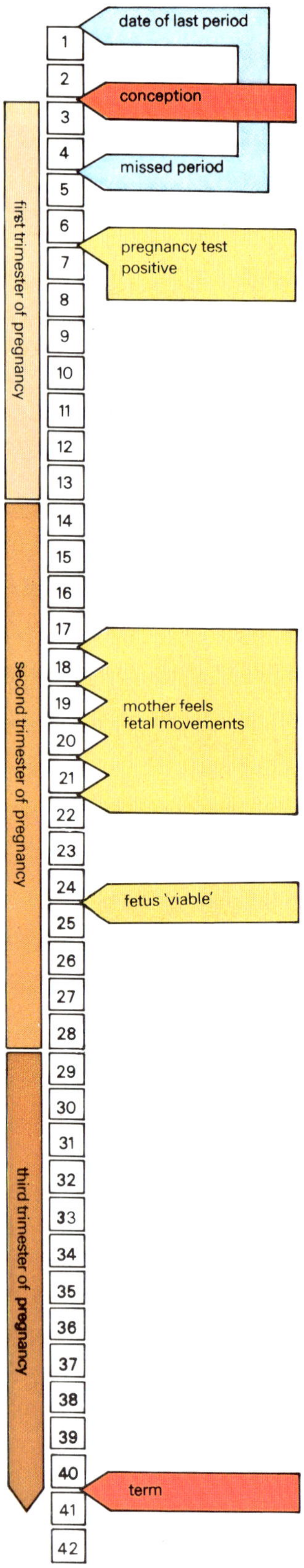

Above: the chronology of pregnancy, in weeks.

Pregnancy lasts for approximately nine months and can be divided into three roughly equal parts, called trimesters. The first trimester is the period in which all the various different parts of the baby are formed. During the second and third trimesters the organs needed for the baby to survive in the outside world develop and mature and the fetus continues to grow in size and weight.

The first signs

The first clear sign of pregnancy is a missed period although some women may already be convinced that they are pregnant and others may want to wait a little to see if their period is only delayed, particularly if their periods are irregular. The menstrual cycle is interrupted by fertilization and implantation of the embryo cell in the uterus (*see* pp. 16, 19), and at this time, about one week before the normal period, there may be a little bleeding. Even when a pregnancy is progressing, some women may still have a congested feeling as if a period is about to start.

Other signs of early pregnancy are nausea, passing urine more frequently and a sense of fullness or tenderness in the breasts, especially around the nipples.

Nausea usually occurs early in the day and then stops (hence the phrase "morning sickness") but it may last all day. Some women suffer from actual vomiting and should speak to their doctor about this. Women who are troubled by nausea during the day are advised to eat a little, or drink a glass of milk or some liquid at two-hour intervals. It is usual for both nausea and vomiting to cease after the first three months of pregnancy (*see* chapter 4).

Frequent passing of urine is caused by pressure of the enlarging uterus on the bladder, which lies just in front of it. Tenderness in the breasts may be quite marked and is due to the changing hormone levels in the body which serve to prepare the breasts for lactation. As pregnancy progresses the breasts grow larger and the areola, the pink area around the nipple, becomes wider and often darker. Changes in the breasts are dealt with in more detail on page 34.

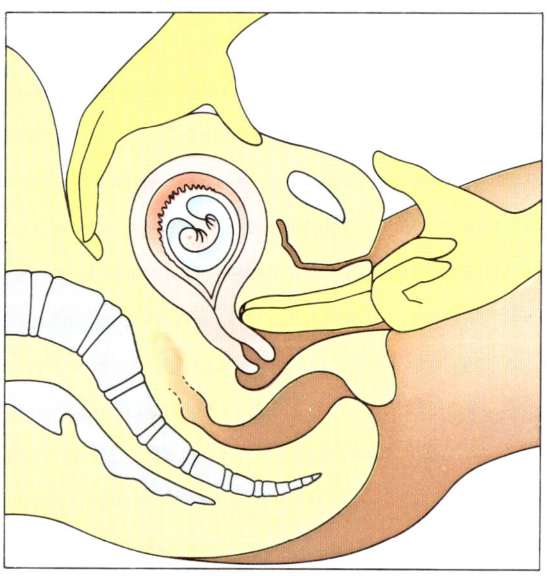

Hegar's sign: early in pregnancy the lower part of the uterus above the cervix becomes so soft that the doctor's fingers can nearly meet in the position shown. This test for pregnancy is being superseded by the urine test, which is painless and risk-free.

The pregnancy test

Once you suspect you are pregnant you should check to see if this is so by going to see your doctor who will examine you and may do a pregnancy test. Home test kits are also available from the pharmacy. The results of the test can be accurate as early as three days after a missed period. This is because of the heightened sensitivity of recently developed kits.

The pregnancy test makes use of the presence in the urine of the hormone H.C.G. which is produced as the pregnancy develops (*see* pp. 16, 17). Although several types of home test are marketed, all rely on the same mechanism, differing only in how the result is observed. A specimen of early morning urine is collected and mixed in the test tube provided with chemicals which react to the presence of H.C.G. In the most widely-used test, e.p.t., a woman is not pregnant if the chemical preparation mixed with the urine produces a ring. A positive result is indicated by a brown/yellowish overall color (*see* diagram). Clear instructions are given with every kit.

In each case you should read the instructions carefully before doing the test. False positive results are unlikely but false negative results can be found, particularly if less than six weeks has passed since the last period. It is difficult to confirm a pregnancy in this case since the level of H.C.G. will not normally be high enough to give a clear result. If you obtain a clear positive result you should then make an appointment to see your doctor.

Doctor's examination

Instead of having a home pregnancy test most women choose to go to their obstetrician/gynecologist. If you do you should take an early morning urine sample with you. You usually receive the results of the test during that office visit. The doctor will probably also want to examine you.

There are various signs that a doctor looks for. In a pregnant woman the breast tissue is firm and may be more tender than usual, and in a woman's first pregnancy the color of the nipples often changes from pink to brown. The doctor will also ask you to lie down on an examining table for an internal examination. This may include looking at the cervix with a smooth instrument called a speculum and in addition placing one or two fingers inside the vagina and the other hand on the abdomen. If you are pregnant the doctor will detect a change in the shape and size of the uterus and changes in the vaginal lining and cervix. In a pregnant woman the lining of the vagina

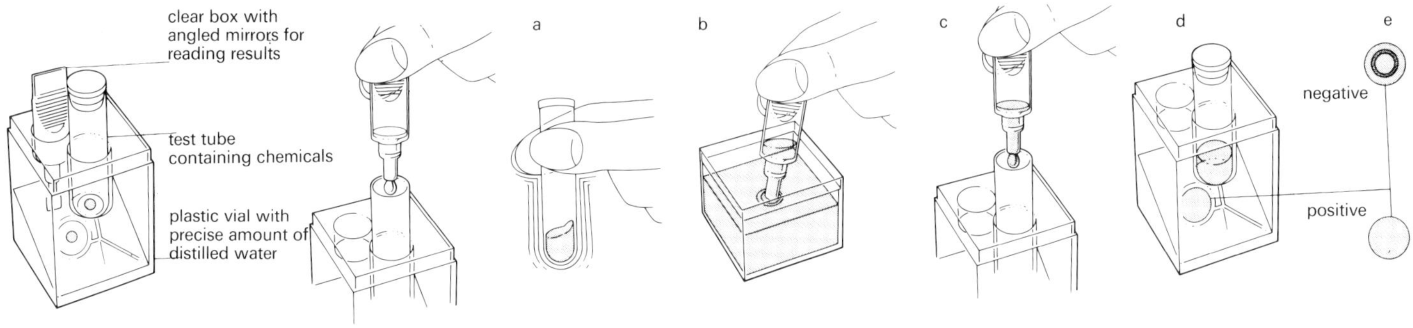

Home pregnancy test (e.p.t.)
a Remove rubber stopper from test tube and replace tube in holder. Twist top off plastic vial and squeeze contents into test tube.

b Replace stopper and shake test tube for at least 10 seconds until contents are well mixed.

c Fill empty vial with first morning urine.

d Carefully put one drop of urine into test tube.

e Replace stopper and shake test tube well. Put back into holder and stand box on flat surface with mirror facing you, away from sunlight and vibrations. Let stand for exactly two hours. Do not touch holder.

A brown yellow overall color means the urine contains H.C.G. and the woman is pregnant. A dark brown ring indicates a negative result.

becomes blue because of the increase in blood flowing to it, and the cervix softens so that it is possible to feel the rest of the uterus clearly through it. The uterus softens as well and becomes larger and rounder than usual. These signs of pregnancy are often very difficult to detect less than eight weeks from the last normal menstrual period.

During the first trimester the growth of the uterus is rapid and it is possible to estimate how many weeks pregnant a woman is; this is done more accurately by feeling the uterus at this stage than later in pregnancy. This is one of the main reasons for encouraging women to see their doctor early. There is of course some variation in the size of the uterus between women and in second and subsequent pregnancies the uterus is always slightly larger than in the first pregnancy.

If the doctor is uncertain whether you are pregnant, he can order a pregnancy test. This can be done quickly with a simple urine test in his office or with a sensitive blood test.

When will the baby be born?

On average a pregnancy lasts for 267 days, but as the date of conception itself is not normally known it is usual to calculate the date of delivery from the start of the last menstrual period. In a regular 28-day cycle, ovulation occurs on the fourteenth day. The estimated date of confinement (E.D.C.) can therefore be calculated by adding 281 days to the first day of the last period, or roughly 40 weeks. Where the average menstrual cycle is longer, it is necessary to add a few more days to the E.D.C.

It is not possible to predict exactly when the baby will arrive but you can easily make a good guess by adding seven days and subtracting three months from the first day of the last menstrual period. Thus if the last menstrual period began on July 23rd you should first add 7 days (July 30th) and then subtract three months, arriving at April 30th.

Because of the varying lengths of the months this date differs by one or two days from the date arrived at by counting 281 days, which is the method used in the chart below. The various methods used may explain why some women are given different dates.

Greater problems arise, however, when a mother fails to note the date of her last period or where she has been taking the pill and conceives before her periods have become clearly established once more. In these cases doctors may ask for an ultrasound examination (*see* p. 54) which gives remarkably accurate information on the age of the fetus. To avoid disappointment you should always be prepared for a slightly earlier or later delivery.

ESTIMATED DELIVERY DATE CHART

Jan.	1	2	3	4	5	6	7	8	9	10	11	12	13	14	15	16	17	18	19	20	21	22	23	24	25	26	27	28	29	30	31	Jan.
Oct.	**8**	**9**	**10**	**11**	**12**	**13**	**14**	**15**	**16**	**17**	**18**	**19**	**20**	**21**	**22**	**23**	**24**	**25**	**26**	**27**	**28**	**29**	**30**	**31**	**1**	**2**	**3**	**4**	**5**	**6**	**7**	**Nov.**
Feb.	1	2	3	4	5	6	7	8	9	10	11	12	13	14	15	16	17	18	19	20	21	22	23	24	25	26	27	28	—	—	—	Feb.
Nov.	**8**	**9**	**10**	**11**	**12**	**13**	**14**	**15**	**16**	**17**	**18**	**19**	**20**	**21**	**22**	**23**	**24**	**25**	**26**	**27**	**28**	**29**	**30**	**1**	**2**	**3**	**4**	**5**	—	—	—	**Dec.**
Mar.	1	2	3	4	5	6	7	8	9	10	11	12	13	14	15	16	17	18	19	20	21	22	23	24	25	26	27	28	29	30	31	Mar.
Dec.	**6**	**7**	**8**	**9**	**10**	**11**	**12**	**13**	**14**	**15**	**16**	**17**	**18**	**19**	**20**	**21**	**22**	**23**	**24**	**25**	**26**	**27**	**28**	**29**	**30**	**31**	**1**	**2**	**3**	**4**	**5**	**Jan.**
Apr.	1	2	3	4	5	6	7	8	9	10	11	12	13	14	15	16	17	18	19	20	21	22	23	24	25	26	27	28	29	30	—	Apr.
Jan.	**6**	**7**	**8**	**9**	**10**	**11**	**12**	**13**	**14**	**15**	**16**	**17**	**18**	**19**	**20**	**21**	**22**	**23**	**24**	**25**	**26**	**27**	**28**	**29**	**30**	**31**	**1**	**2**	**3**	**4**	—	**Feb.**
May.	1	2	3	4	5	6	7	8	9	10	11	12	13	14	15	16	17	18	19	20	21	22	23	24	25	26	27	28	29	30	31	May
Feb.	**5**	**6**	**7**	**8**	**9**	**10**	**11**	**12**	**13**	**14**	**15**	**16**	**17**	**18**	**19**	**20**	**21**	**22**	**23**	**24**	**25**	**26**	**27**	**28**	**1**	**2**	**3**	**4**	**5**	**6**	**7**	**Mar.**
June.	1	2	3	4	5	6	7	8	9	10	11	12	13	14	15	16	17	18	19	20	21	22	23	24	25	26	27	28	29	30	—	June
Mar.	**8**	**9**	**10**	**11**	**12**	**13**	**14**	**15**	**16**	**17**	**18**	**19**	**20**	**21**	**22**	**23**	**24**	**25**	**26**	**27**	**28**	**29**	**30**	**31**	**1**	**2**	**3**	**4**	**5**	**6**	—	**Apr.**
July	1	2	3	4	5	6	7	8	9	10	11	12	13	14	15	16	17	18	19	20	21	22	23	24	25	26	27	28	29	30	31	July
Apr.	**7**	**8**	**9**	**10**	**11**	**12**	**13**	**14**	**15**	**16**	**17**	**18**	**19**	**20**	**21**	**22**	**23**	**24**	**25**	**26**	**27**	**28**	**29**	**30**	**1**	**2**	**3**	**4**	**5**	**6**	**7**	**May**
Aug.	1	2	3	4	5	6	7	8	9	10	11	12	13	14	15	16	17	18	19	20	21	22	23	24	25	26	27	28	29	30	31	Aug.
May	**8**	**9**	**10**	**11**	**12**	**13**	**14**	**15**	**16**	**17**	**18**	**19**	**20**	**21**	**22**	**23**	**24**	**25**	**26**	**27**	**28**	**29**	**30**	**31**	**1**	**2**	**3**	**4**	**5**	**6**	**7**	**June**
Sept.	1	2	3	4	5	6	7	8	9	10	11	12	13	14	15	16	17	18	19	20	21	22	23	24	25	26	27	28	29	30	—	Sept.
June	**8**	**9**	**10**	**11**	**12**	**13**	**14**	**15**	**16**	**17**	**18**	**19**	**20**	**21**	**22**	**23**	**24**	**25**	**26**	**27**	**28**	**29**	**30**	**1**	**2**	**3**	**4**	**5**	**6**	**7**	—	**July**
Oct.	1	2	3	4	5	6	7	8	9	10	11	12	13	14	15	16	17	18	19	20	21	22	23	24	25	26	27	28	29	30	31	Oct.
July	**8**	**9**	**10**	**11**	**12**	**13**	**14**	**15**	**16**	**17**	**18**	**19**	**20**	**21**	**22**	**23**	**24**	**25**	**26**	**27**	**28**	**29**	**30**	**31**	**1**	**2**	**3**	**4**	**5**	**6**	**7**	**Aug.**
Nov.	1	2	3	4	5	6	7	8	9	10	11	12	13	14	15	16	17	18	19	20	21	22	23	24	25	26	27	28	29	30	—	Nov.
Aug.	**8**	**9**	**10**	**11**	**12**	**13**	**14**	**15**	**16**	**17**	**18**	**19**	**20**	**21**	**22**	**23**	**24**	**25**	**26**	**27**	**28**	**29**	**30**	**31**	**1**	**2**	**3**	**4**	**5**	**6**	—	**Sept.**
Dec.	1	2	3	4	5	6	7	8	9	10	11	12	13	14	15	16	17	18	19	20	21	22	23	24	25	26	27	28	29	30	31	Dec.
Sept.	**7**	**8**	**9**	**10**	**11**	**12**	**13**	**14**	**15**	**16**	**17**	**18**	**19**	**20**	**21**	**22**	**23**	**24**	**25**	**26**	**27**	**28**	**29**	**30**	**1**	**2**	**3**	**4**	**5**	**6**	**7**	**Oct.**

Using the E.D.C. chart (left), it is possible for the pregnant mother to estimate the date when her baby will be born, if she knows the date of her last period. The first day of the last period is shown in light type, and the estimated date of delivery will be found in heavy type immediately below it.

Antenatal care

Nature does a very good job with pregnancy and childbirth in most instances, but problems do sometimes arise. For this reason, it is essential to arrange for regular antenatal check-ups with your doctor. Physicians have been receiving specialized training in obstetrics and gynecology for over 60 years in the United States. Today, there are over 26,000 physicians who provide obstetrical care. Of this number, there are approximately 14,000 who have been certified by the American Board of Obstetrics and Gynecology. To receive this certification a physician must have completed four years of residency training in obstetrics and gynecology and pass a written examination. Following this the physician must practice two years and then pass an oral examination. This includes an evaluation of the management of all the patients that he has hospitalized during a one-year period.

In most instances patients will be followed by physicians in their offices. Generally, obstetricians practice in groups. That is to say, two or more obstetricians practice together in order to provide comprehensive coverage 24 hours a day, 365 days a year. In these groups a patient may be rotated among the doctors or she may be followed by one doctor throughout her pregnancy, seeing the other physicians one time to know who they are. Some doctors choose solo practice. Whenever they are sick or are on vacation, generally, they have the same physician cover the practice so that their patients will know who the substitute is.

If you have reason to contact your doctor outside of office hours your call will probably be answered by an answering service which will then locate your doctor and he will call you back. This may take 5-20 minutes. If you have an emergency situation, be sure to tell the person at the answering service, giving as many pertinent details as clearly as possible.

Some patients do not go to private doctors but to clinics. For the most part, these are in hospitals and provide excellent care. Commonly, in clinics the patient does not see the same doctor each antenatal visit.

At each antenatal visit the routine procedure includes a weight gain assessment, a blood pressure check (below) and measurement of the pregnant woman's abdomen to determine the growth of the fetus.

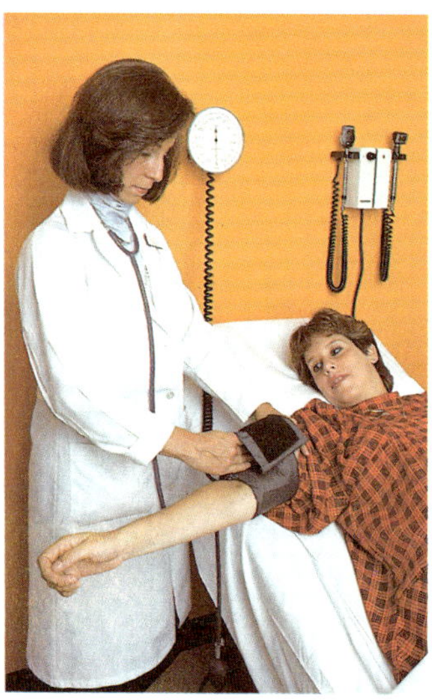

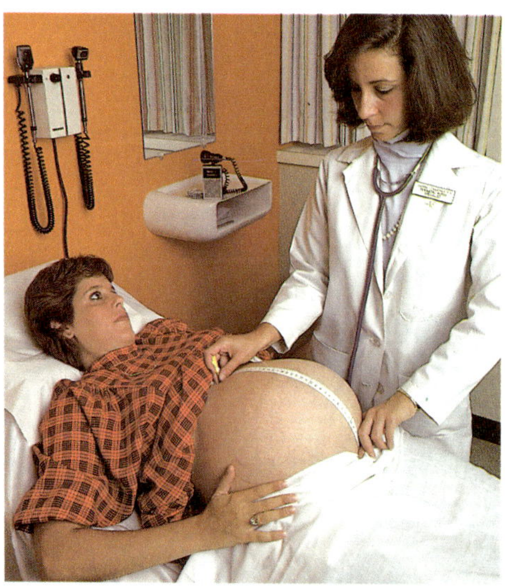

You should visit a doctor once you think you are pregnant, say six weeks from the end of your last period. At this visit the doctor will confirm the pregnancy, take a careful medical history, do a physical examination, give you instructions for the antenatal period, and tell you when your expected date of delivery is.

Visits to the doctor are then arranged on a monthly basis until about the twenty-eighth week, then every two weeks to the thirty-sixth week, and weekly in the last month. More frequent examinations may become necessary at any stage, and certain complications including vaginal bleeding, suddenly raised blood pressure and severe kidney infection may make admission to the hospital necessary (*see* chapter 4).

Since your baby will be born in the hospital, it is the practice in many communities for the patient and her husband to visit the hospital before delivery. During this visit a representative of the hospital often shows the couple the delivery and the postpartum floors so that they will feel at home when the patient is admitted in labor.

When the patient believes she is in labor, she calls her doctor's office. Outside of office hours the phone is usually answered by an answering service which will locate the doctor. If he decides that she should be admitted to the hospital, generally, she proceeds to the hospital entering through the emergency room. In the hospital, the patient and her husband may see nurses, aides and residents, who are members of the obstetrical team.

The pattern of care

At your initial visit to your doctor, obstetric and social histories are taken. Even if they are already well known they should be checked for accuracy. A physical examination is done, height and weight are recorded, blood pressure is checked and urine tested for glucose and protein. These last four are repeated at every visit because they can give a clue to problems which may show no symptoms.

Usually, at the first visit a test is made for infection in the urine, because it is important to give treatment for it. Some doctors also take vaginal swabs as a matter of routine to ensure that there is no vaginal infection.

A sample of blood is always taken at the first visit to test for anemia and any related problems, to determine blood group (A, B, O, AB) and Rh type (positive or negative) (*see* p. 33) and to detect syphilis, and determine if she is immune to rubella. This blood sample is also tested for antibodies in the maternal blood which could affect the baby.

A further blood test for alpha fetoproteins (A.F.P.) is now often made at about the sixteenth week of pregnancy to detect spina bifida and related rare fetal abnormalities, though these tests are still in the experimental stage. Blood tests for anemia and antibodies will also be repeated later in pregnancy, particularly in the case of mothers whose blood is Rh negative (*see* pp. 32–4).

At every visit the doctor will ask the mother if she has any worries or symptoms she wishes to raise. If he forgets to ask, remember to mention any unusual symptoms you have. It is a good idea to keep a diary in which to note symptoms, questions and worries as they occur. You can then make a short list to take to the doctor for discussion. There is no point in being diffident and hesitant about bothering the doctor: he is there to help. No doctor should be too busy to listen and dispel anxieties. The information which you can give might well be of help in your medical care. Most doctors welcome questions because they believe it helps the patient have a better experience in pregnancy. Occasionally, patients find that doctors are not receptive to discussion. In this case, you should consider changing your doctor.

Antenatal classes

Antenatal, or prenatal, education is very valuable; women want to know how their bodies change during pregnancy, what happens in labor and birth, and how they can best help themselves and the obstetric team. But it is equally clear that antenatal education is valuable for both parents. The father is a good labor companion and if he shares the training he is more likely to feel part of the whole experience and can be of great support.

Antenatal education should offer advice about labor and birth and preparation for parenthood. Women should be told about all the various methods of pain relief available and offered instruction in relaxation, neuromuscular control and a method of breathing. The latter are worth learning even if you decide to have medications during labor (*see* p. 82). Information should be given on the physiological and psychological effects of pregnancy and labor on the mother, and the development of the fetus. Advice on diet, medications, rest and exercise are also important. You should make sure you visit the labor and delivery suite, to see the equipment.

Courses should also include preparation for breast-feeding, information on bottle feeding and advice on handling and caring for a newborn baby. Lastly, "Question and Answer" sessions are usually included. Parents often find that these are most useful, because no course can cover everything you might want to know.

Generally, you meet other expectant parents in these classes. This provides an excellent opportunity for an exchange of ideas and a chance to discuss things you may not wish to talk about in class. Often couples who have recently had a baby will come to the class to relate their experience. You should take the opportunity to discuss with these couples any of your concerns or problems.

Throughout the United States education for the expectant parents is provided in many forms. It is widely available and is either offered free or for a nominal charge. Some courses are oriented toward taking no medications during labor, while others are more general and deal with the full spectrum of preparation for childbirth which would even embrace the mother who is having a first-time or repeat cesarean section.

Many hospitals offer education classes for expectant parents. Many physicians, particularly those in group practice, offer antenatal education classes. The organizations such as The American Association for Psychoprophylaxis in Obstetrics (ASPO) and International Childbirth Education Association (ICEA) offer courses for patients who wish to learn such techniques as Lamaze psychoprophylaxis for going through labor with little or no medication. Commonly, Planned Parenthood, YWCAs, or other humanitarian organizations hold childbirth education courses. The La Leche League holds regular courses in the practice of breast-feeding. Most hospitals provide educational courses postpartum to help teach the mother how to care for her baby. During the hospital stay the nurses help the mother at her bedside with instructions in breast-feeding, bottle feeding and general baby care.

The pattern of antenatal education varies. This class (below left and right) is part of a course run for couples at which fathers are trained to take an active part in all stages of labor.

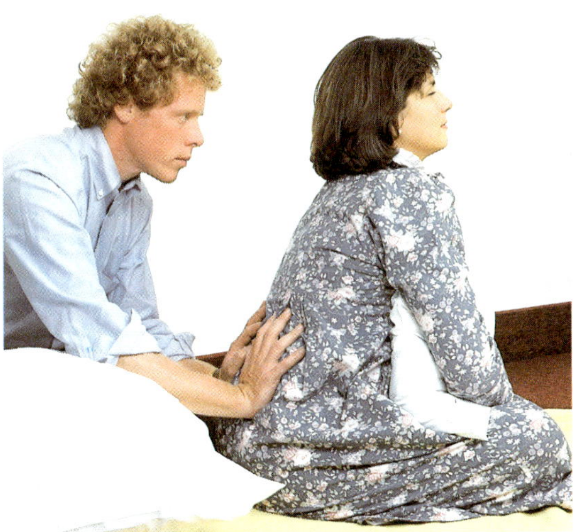

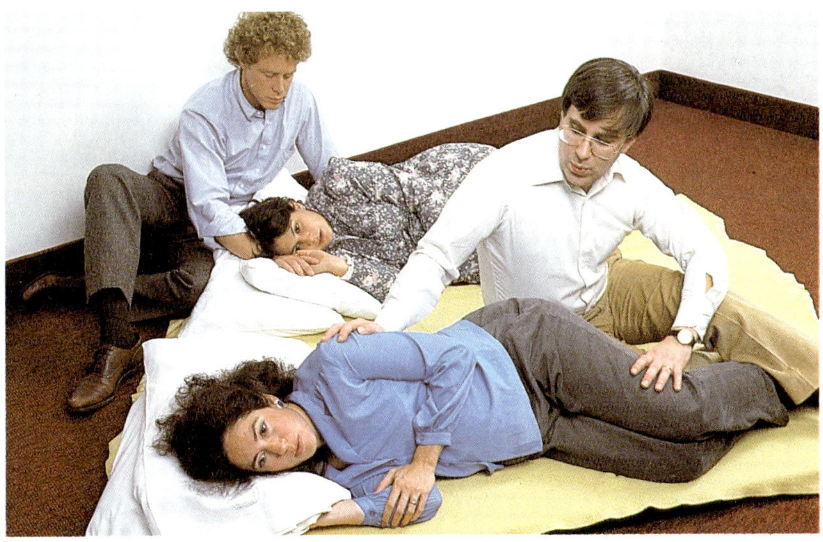

Major physical changes

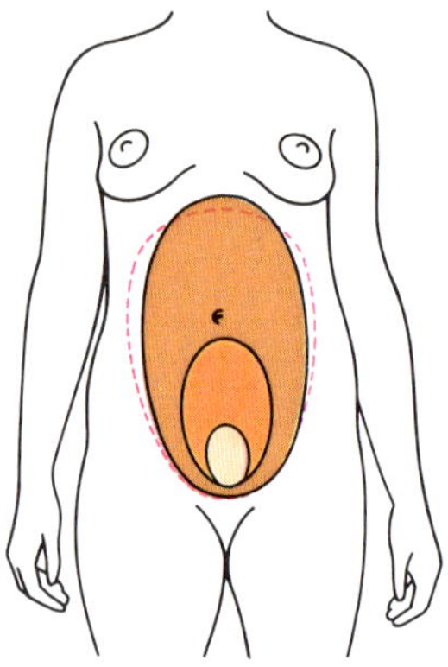

The position of the fundus – the upper surface of the uterus – at 12, 20 and 36 weeks. The dotted line shows its position after the baby's head has descended into the pelvis near the end of pregnancy.

The many changes that occur in a woman's body during pregnancy and the constant monitoring of her progress by doctors might persuade her that being pregnant is the same as being ill. Pregnancy is a remarkably normal state – one in which the body skillfully adapts to a great variety of new demands. The key to this process is a range of hormones, or chemical messengers (mentioned in chapter 1), which are secreted by glands and circulate in the blood.

Progesterone is the hormone most particularly associated with pregnancy. Secreted by one of the ovaries in the first weeks (*see* p. 16), it is produced thereafter by the placenta. Progesterone has a relaxing effect on a whole series of muscle fibers known as smooth (or involuntary) muscles which are found in the uterus, the gastrointestinal tract and the walls of veins.

The uterus is composed entirely of smooth muscle, and under the relaxing influence of progesterone it is able to grow and stretch to accommodate the growing fetus with a minimum risk of expelling the fetus prematurely. Progesterone also helps to improve the blood supply to all parts of the woman's body because it serves to relax the walls of the blood vessels, thus allowing them to carry a larger volume of blood. Blood volume increases by almost 40 per cent during pregnancy (*see* p. 32).

Unfortunately, because progesterone affects all smooth muscle fibers it also has some unwanted side effects. Relaxation of the ureters – the ducts leading from the kidneys to the bladder – increases the possibility of kidney infections, while the effect of progesterone on blood vessels may cause varicose veins. It loosens the sphincter muscle at the opening from the esophagus into the stomach and thus can allow the stomach contents to be regurgitated and cause heartburn. It slows down the movement of food which may result in constipation. This is particularly likely later in pregnancy. All these minor discomforts of pregnancy with their remedies are discussed in chapter 4.

Estrogen is the other major hormone of pregnancy and many of the effects obtained by it and progesterone depend on the relationship between the two. Estrogen plays a major role in the growth of the fetus and the placenta and in the development of the breasts.

In the non-pregnant woman, estrogen is secreted by the ovaries and to a lesser extent by the adrenal glands (*see* p. 16). In pregnancy it is produced in another form (estriol) through the complex interaction of the mother, fetus and placenta. Traces of estriol found in the urine of a pregnant woman can be used to test whether the fetus and placenta are developing well. This test, however, requires the collection of all urine passed over 24 hours and is thus a rather cumbersome procedure.

The hormone H.P.L. is produced by the placenta. The function of this hormone is still unclear but it too can be used to check that the placenta is working well simply by testing a sample of the mother's blood.

The hormone prolactin is also essential to pregnancy but its exact function is not yet

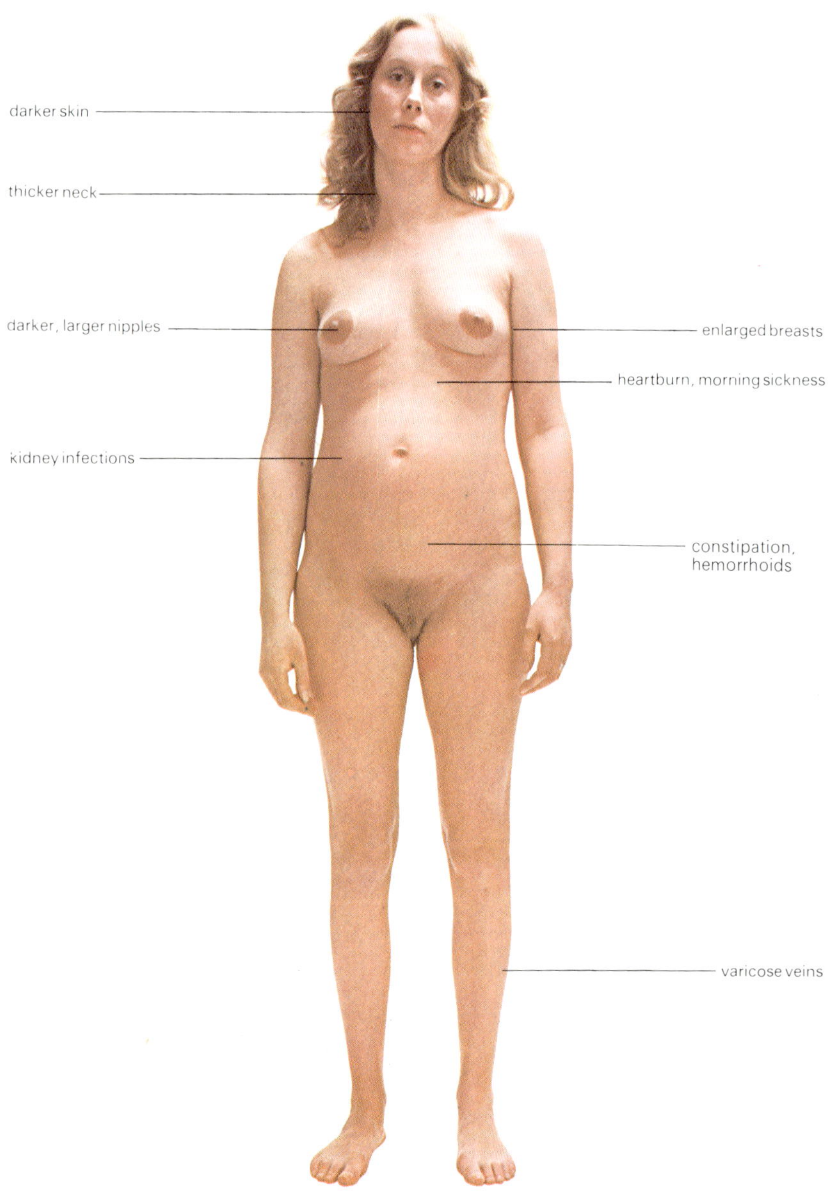

THE EFFECT OF HORMONES

A woman's body must undergo many changes during pregnancy – changes prompted by a range of hormones, or "chemical messengers". Progesterone and estrogen, the hormones which promote the development of the uterus, placenta and fetus, and prepare the breasts for milk production, also affect the body in other ways. For example, the relaxing effect of progesterone on smooth muscle fiber is not confined to the uterus, but affects the bowel and sphincter muscle too. This can lead, in the first case, to constipation and, in the second, to heartburn. Some of the changes and side effects a woman may expect are shown left, and are discussed in more detail in chapter 4.

clear, although it plays a part in the birth itself and in the production of milk. It is produced by the pituitary gland and possibly by the fetus and placenta as well. Raised levels of prolactin are found in early pregnancy and a high level is present at birth which then slowly falls, rising again each time the baby sucks milk from the breast.

Oxytocin, like prolactin, comes from the pituitary gland and is important in stimulating the contractions of labor. It can be synthesized and is available as a medication which is often given to mothers to stimulate labor which has stopped, or once the baby is born to aid the delivery of the placenta (*see* pp. 75, 103). This hormone also helps to trigger the flow of milk from the breasts.

The growing uterus

During pregnancy the uterus enlarges and changes its shape. It also grows heavier, though this is only one factor in the mother's weight gain. At the early antenatal visits the doctor can check the growth of the uterus quite quickly and accurately. During the first trimester the uterus is still confined within the pelvis but in the second trimester it begins to displace the intestines, pushing them upward (*see* below, diagrams 1 and 2). By 14 weeks the uterus can be felt by placing the hand on the abdomen, and the upper edge, or fundus, reaches the navel at about 20 weeks. The overall size and relative position of the uterus varies, however, from one woman to another depending on the number of previous pregnancies, the position of the navel and how fat the mother is. A larger (or smaller) than average amount of amniotic fluid, a twin or multiple pregnancy and the relative firmness of the abdominal muscles will all affect the size of the uterus and, therefore, make it difficult for the doctor to estimate the length of the pregnancy by checking fundal height alone.

Only the top part of the uterus expands. The lower part, the cervix, is composed of a band of muscle and remains tightly closed to keep the fetus inside the uterus.

Once the twenty-eighth week is reached, it is usually possible to begin to identify the different parts of the fetus and to feel how it is lying. Whether it is upright or head-down at this stage is unimportant: the fetus will usually settle into a head-down position between 32 and 34 weeks.

By the end of the thirty-sixth week the pregnant uterus takes up most of the abdominal cavity and pushes the front wall forward to make more space. At this time the intestines are pushed to the sides and the back, high up in the abdomen and just beneath the diaphragm (*see below*). The pressure beneath the diaphragm means that the lungs cannot expand completely and for this reason women may find themselves short of breath. At the same time, because of its position high in the center of the abdomen immediately beneath the diaphragm, the stomach gets compressed and the stomach contents may be forced back through the sphincter muscle into the esophagus, causing heartburn. This is more likely to happen because the sphincter muscle is relaxed.

In most cases when the mother is having her first baby, the baby's head descends into the pelvis in the last few weeks of pregnancy (*see* p. 53). This is called the engagement of the head and may cause the fundus to drop a little taking the pressure off the diaphragm and stomach. Generally, the mother can feel when the fetus has dropped. She may feel pressure in her pelvis and tend to walk with a broader base. Occasionally, engagement is accompanied by a scant amount of bloody show.

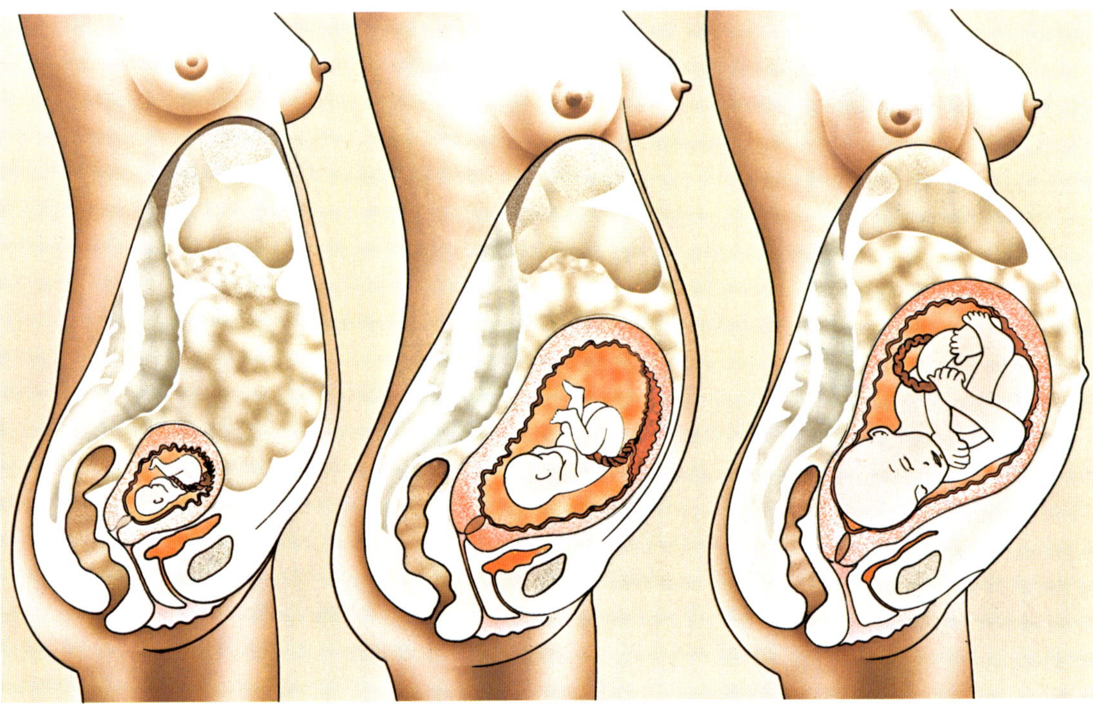

At 12 weeks the uterus takes up the whole pelvic space. By 20 weeks it has begun to displace the intestines. At 36 weeks most of the abdominal cavity is taken up; the intestines are pushed upward and sideways so that they press on the diaphragm and stomach.

The blood

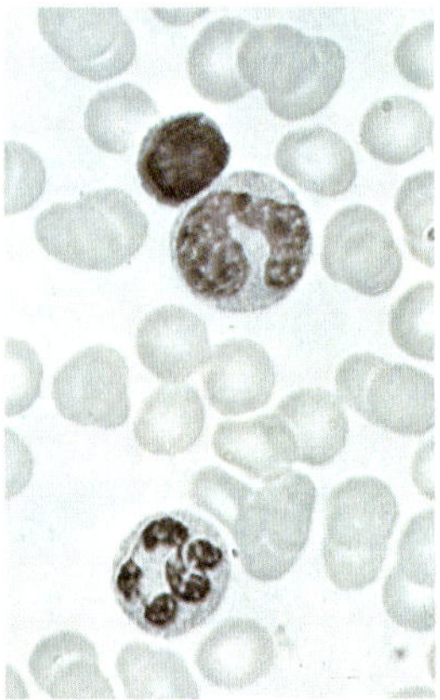

Blood seen under the microscope, showing white blood cells (with dark nuclei) and red blood cells.

Blood is the means by which all parts of the body receive the oxygen and food needed for growth and health. As the blood circulates it picks up oxygen from the lungs and fluid and dissolved nutrients from the intestines, and carries these substances to the cells throughout the body. At the same time carbon dioxide and waste products from the cells pass into the blood. The blood then returns to the lungs, where the carbon dioxide is removed. Waste products from the cells are carried to the kidneys and excreted in the urine.

During pregnancy the volume of the blood increases by nearly 40 per cent above the non-pregnant level. This happens as early as the eighth week and remains at that level until after delivery. During the early weeks of pregnancy the extra blood is largely directed toward the kidneys which receive up to 1 pint (500 ml) per minute more than before pregnancy. As the fetus begins to grow, the blood requirements of the uterus increase tenfold; although 50 ml per minute is an adequate blood flow before pregnancy, it reaches 500 ml per minute by the last month of pregnancy.

Other parts of the body have a share in the additional blood supply, in particular the lungs, breasts and peripheral skin vessels. An enormous increase in the volume of blood passing through the skin blood vessels raises the mother's surface temperature. Many pregnant women notice that they have warmer feet and hands than usual.

This increase in the blood supply during pregnancy makes it possible for the growing fetus to be supplied with all its needs and for the woman's body to adapt to the changes of pregnancy. However, despite the increase in output by the heart there is no natural increase in blood pressure as a result of this.

The placenta

The most significant change in the mother's blood system during pregnancy is that her blood now also serves to supply the fetus via the placenta. The placenta, which develops from the outer cells of the fertilized egg (*see* p. 19) has developed into a separate organ by the twelfth week of pregnancy. Within it the blood vessels of the fetus lie inside the mother's blood system, and though the two circulations never mix, vital substances from the mother and waste products from the fetus are exchanged.

The vital substances transferred to the fetus include oxygen and all the necessary nutrients. Waste products from the fetus include carbon dioxide, which is eventually breathed

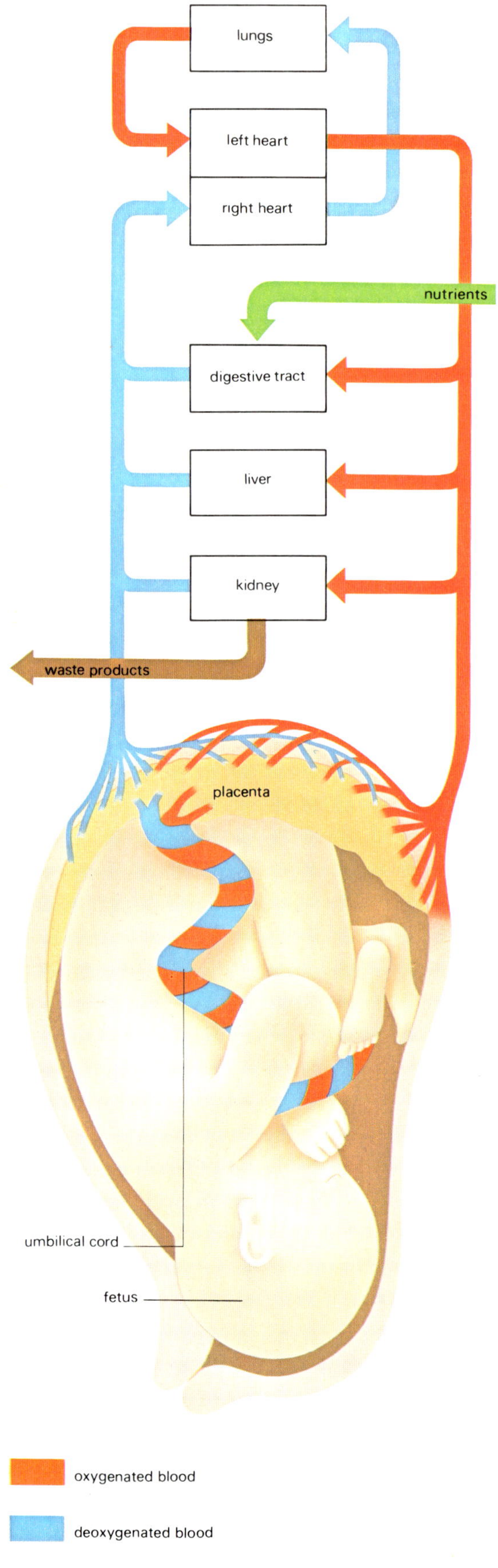

A simplified diagram of the mother's circulation. Oxygenated blood is pumped by the left heart around the body, and to the placenta, where oxygen and nutrients cross over into the circulation of the fetus; carbon dioxide and waste products from the fetus cross into the mother's circulation. This exchange enables the mother's lungs, kidneys, liver and digestive system to act for the fetus. Eventually the deoxygenated blood flows back to the right heart and is pumped into the lungs, where carbon dioxide is breathed out and oxygen is taken in.

out through the mother's lungs, and nitrogenous compounds, which are excreted through her kidneys in the urine. It also acts as a barrier to protect the fetus from potentially harmful substances (*see* p. 39) and produces hormones which help to maintain the pregnancy (*see* p. 48).

Blood components

Human blood consists of red cells, white cells and platelets, all of which are in a straw-colored fluid known as plasma.

The red cells are small discs containing hemoglobin, a substance which carries oxygen from the lungs to the body tissues. If the content of hemoglobin in the blood cells falls or the number of red cells is reduced, then anemia results. It is very important that this does not happen in pregnancy, firstly because it will hinder the transport of oxygen to the fetus, and secondly because any excessive loss of blood at delivery would leave the mother even more anemic.

Iron, which is vital for the formation of hemoglobin, is normally obtained from the diet. However, during pregnancy the fetus makes great demands on the mother's blood supply to produce all its blood cells while in the uterus, and builds up a store of iron for the period after the birth when he or she may be breast-fed. Because the mother does not menstruate during pregnancy she saves a little iron, but by the time of the birth, she usually has a slight iron deficiency. Particularly when one pregnancy rapidly follows another, a woman may find herself getting more and more anemic. For this reason iron pills are prescribed during pregnancy.

Folic acid is also important in the formation of the hemoglobin, and most iron pills prescribed during pregnancy contain some of this vitamin. In addition, some vitamin C is also required to build the blood cells of the fetus. For details of natural sources of iron, folic acid and vitamin C *see* p. 37.

Blood grouping: ABO and Rh

Each person's blood belongs to one of several blood groups and all mothers have their blood group determined early in pregnancy. There are two main systems of blood grouping, known as ABO and Rh. The ABO system has four major groups known as A, B, AB and O. The letters refer to the type of antigen on the red blood cells. There are two Rh types: Rh positive and Rh negative, both of which refer to a type of red blood cell. Safe blood transfusion requires matching the patient's ABO and Rh groups with the type of blood given. If the wrong type is given it will immunize the mother or cause a transfusion reaction.

Human blood groups are determined by observing the reaction between the antigens on the surface of the red cells and the antibodies that are found in the blood plasma. Antibodies are one of the many mechanisms which protect the body from invasion by foreign substances. An antigen is a substance

PREVENTION OF RH-DISEASE

If a woman with Rh-negative blood carries a fetus with Rh-positive blood (A), the possibility arises that the fetus in a subsequent pregnancy will have Rh-disease. During labor at the end of a pregnancy, some blood from the fetus may cross into the maternal circulation (B and C). If this blood is of an ABO group which is not compatible with that of the mother, the mother's blood will soon destroy the foreign cells. But if the fetal blood is of the same ABO group as the maternal blood, then the mother's blood becomes sensitized, i.e. develops the capacity to produce Rh-antibodies (D). In a later pregnancy, if the fetus is again Rh-positive, the maternal blood produces antibodies which attack and destroy the fetal blood, causing Rh-disease (E).

The chain of events can now be avoided. If the Rh-positive blood cells which enter the maternal circulation during pregnancy and at delivery can be destroyed immediately, the maternal blood will not become sensitized. Injections of anti-Rh gamma globulin at 28 weeks of pregnancy and within 72 hours of the birth ensure such destruction (F, G). As a result, no antibodies are produced by the mother's blood in a subsequent pregnancy and the fetal blood cells are safe from attack (H).

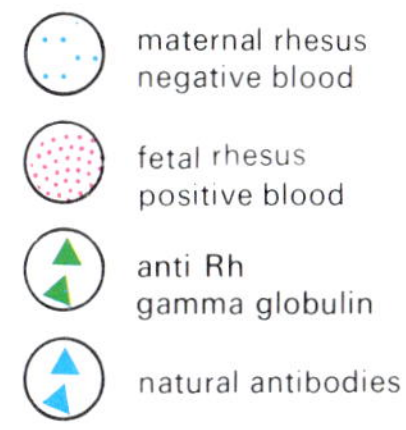

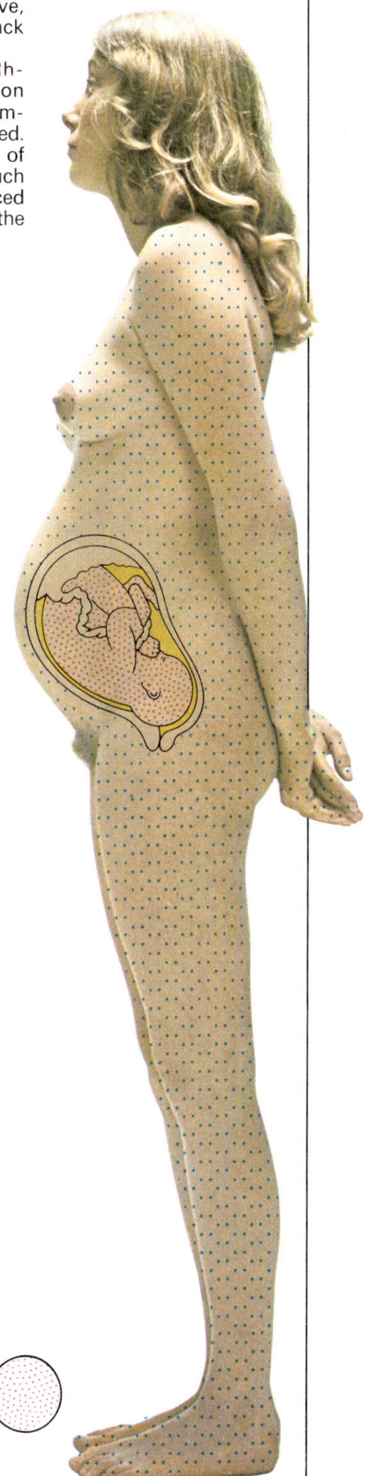

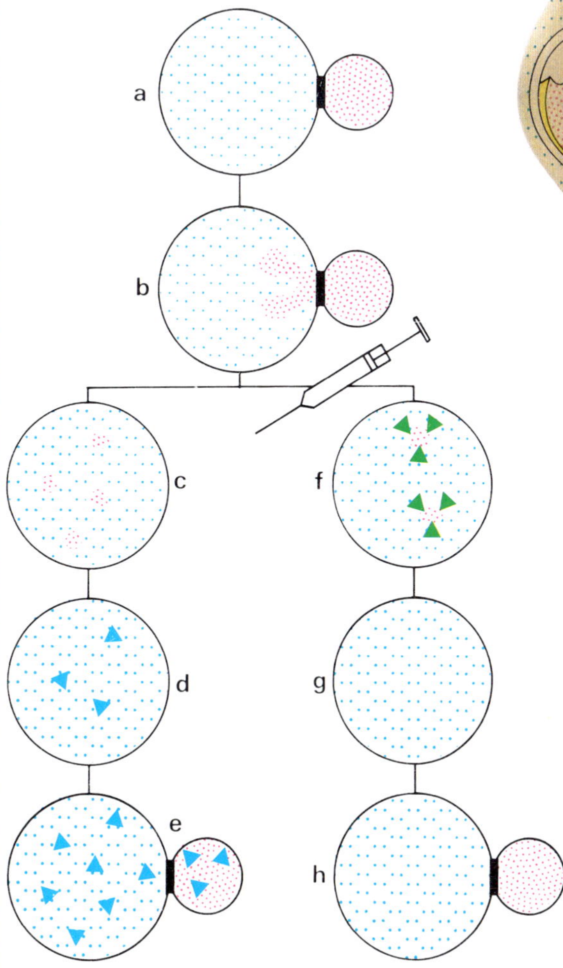

which is capable of stimulating the formation of antibodies. If a person lacks a red cell antigen, she may develop specific antibodies if exposed to that antigen.

The Rh system is particularly important in pregnancy because it explains the origin of a blood disease which can affect the fetus. Everybody's blood is either Rh positive or Rh negative; the former is transmitted by a dominant gene, the latter by a recessive gene (*see* chapter 1). About 15 per cent of white and 5 per cent of black women in the United States are Rh negative. The risk to the fetus occurs when one of them conceives a child with an Rh positive man. If the fetus is Rh positive, there is danger that the blood of the fetus will enter the Rh-negative mother's circulation. She may develop antibodies which will attack the blood of that fetus or subsequent Rh-positive fetuses.

It is now possible to avoid this danger by injecting the Rh-negative mother at 28 weeks' gestation and immediately after her delivery with Rh-immune globulin or Rhogam, that prevents the development of these antibodies.

Antibodies

When antigens enter the body, for example, through infection or through eating contaminated food, the white blood cells produce antibodies composed of large molecules of immunoglobulins (IgM), which act as a first line of defense but have a relatively short lifespan. The task of all antibodies is to penetrate the antigen and make it easier to destroy.

The body then produces much smaller molecules (IgG), which would not only have a much longer lifespan but provide the body with a "memory" of the structure of different antibodies. This allows the body to manufacture more antibodies rapidly at any time when it is exposed to an infection or an antigen for the second time.

During pregnancy some of the IgG molecules that a mother has previously encountered are transferred across the placenta and protect the baby during the first few weeks of life from infection. Breast milk also contains antibodies, produced in response to infections.

Rh-disease

When an Rh-negative woman has given birth to an Rh-positive child, if the preventive measures outlined above are not followed, antibodies in the mother's blood may attack the blood of a subsequent Rh-positive fetus. The effects vary from slight to very serious. The baby may be born slightly jaundiced; he may be severely jaundiced and anemic; or he may die *in utero* or soon after birth. The mother's history, and tests at the antenatal clinic, will warn doctors of Rh imcompatibility, and amniocentesis will provide information about whether, and how severely, the fetus is affected. The birth may be induced prematurely or a cesarean birth may be performed. The baby may need an exchange blood transfusion soon after birth to remove hostile antibodies and counteract anemia.

Breast care

During pregnancy the major change that a woman will notice in her breasts is that they grow larger to prepare for breast-feeding. Mothers who have their first baby before thirty usually have the greatest increase. Breast size, however, still varies from woman to woman; remember that small breasts are just as good at producing milk as large ones.

One of the earliest signs of pregnancy which a woman may notice is a sense of fullness and tenderness in the breasts due to hormone changes. During the early weeks extra fatty tissue grows around the milk-secreting tissues. At the same time, especially in a first pregnancy, the areola – the ring of darker skin around the nipple – gets larger and deeper in color, becoming a light or dark brown. At the same time, around the nipple a second ring of pigmentation appears called the secondary areola, which helps to improve the strength of the skin in preparation for breast-feeding.

The breasts have a rich supply of blood which increases during pregnancy and the veins which lie just below the skin tend to become more prominent as pregnancy advances. Sebaceous glands in the areolar

STRUCTURE OF THE BREAST

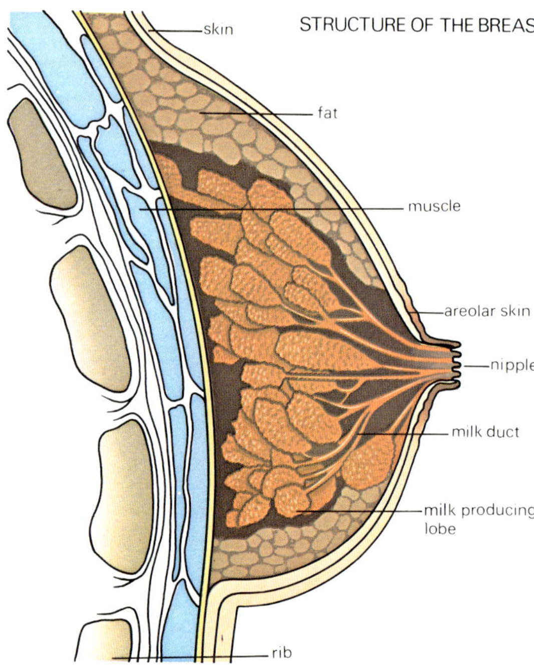

tissue, known as Montgomery's tubercles, produce an oily substance which protects the skin from moisture and for this reason it is unwise to try and wash the nipple too fastidiously because both the lubricant and its protective effect may be lost.

The structure of the breast

Each breast has an axillary "tail" which extends right up into the armpit. This extension may become apparent in the first few days of breast-feeding. The breast tissue lies in the fatty layer just beneath the skin and overlying the muscles of the chest wall.

Milk is produced in lobes of milk-secreting

tissue, called the alveoli, deep within the breast and is carried to the nipple in the milk ducts. The nipple is composed of erectile tissues surrounded by a ring of muscle and usually stands out from the breast when stimulated. If it does not, the nipple can be encouraged to stand out by repeated gentle traction during the antenatal period.

On the surface of the nipple are fifteen to twenty small openings, each of which is connected to one of the lobes of breast tissue, the centers of milk production. The lobes are arranged in a circle around the nipple and each lobe is made up of small lobules cushioned by fatty tissue. Milk is produced in the lobules and is carried from them by milk ducts to collect in the ducts immediately behind the areola. These ducts increase in capacity during pregnancy and in breast-feeding the pressure of the baby's gums on the areola stimulates the milk flow.

Each lobe is encased in a separate compartment which helps to support the breast tissue and serves the important function of preventing any infection from spreading from one lobe to another. Lobes can become infected if bacteria enter through the openings of the nipple or through a crack nearby (*see* p. 121).

Milk secretion is under the control of a hormone called prolactin which is secreted by the pituitary gland. The initial stimulus to produce the hormone is provided by a sharp fall in the estrogen level which accompanies the delivery of the baby.

The smooth muscle surrounding the ducts is contracted by oxytocin, another hormone secreted by the pituitary gland. Sucking or touching the nipples causes the lobules to let down milk into the ducts under the areola, and from there it is drawn out by the action of the baby's jaw and tongue. The nipple is in contact with the roof of the baby's mouth and its gums press on the areola, part of which will be drawn into the baby's mouth.

From about twelve weeks of pregnancy the breasts produce a protein-rich substance called colostrum. This fluid, which may be pale and colorless or thick and yellow, supplies all the nutritional needs of the newborn baby until the hormone levels settle and the milk appears on about the third day after the birth of the baby.

Preparation for breast-feeding

During pregnancy it is worth considering whether you want to breast-feed. This is a subject which can arouse strong feelings, so that mothers themselves may be reluctant to breast-feed, or they may feel that it is inconvenient because of the possible reaction of people in public places. Nevertheless, breast-feeding is most enjoyable, healthy for the baby and less bother than sterilizing bottles and mixing formulas.

One of the most important factors in successful breast-feeding is the shape of the nipple. The nipple must be long enough to reach the baby's palate to stimulate sucking. Most nipples protrude, or will come to do so as pregnancy progresses. Occasionally they are flat or retracted, sticking to the breast tissue. In such cases the nipple can be made more erect by placing the thumb and forefinger around the areola and gently drawing out the nipple. A good time to do this is when taking either a bath or a shower.

Sometimes quite a lot of colostrum is formed during the last weeks of pregnancy. Massage of the breast from the outer edge toward the nipple, followed by light squeezing of the areola between finger and thumb, is sometimes recommended to keep the colostrum moving and avoid duct blockage, but there is no evidence that it makes any difference to the success of breast-feeding. In view of its stimulating effect, handling such as this should not be done if breast-feeding is not contemplated.

Preparation is not vital to successful breast-feeding: it is possible to decide to feed this way as late as a day after delivery. An elaborate routine during the antenatal period is unnecessary and can even be harmful if the mother finds it "unnatural" or distasteful.

There is also no need to fear that breast-feeding will cause the breasts to lose their firmness and sag. After pregnancy the breasts are a little softer and less firm and pointed than before, but if a well-fitting bra is worn in the last weeks and for the first few weeks after the baby is born, a mother should have no problems in regaining her figure.

Actually, breast-feeding is a natural function. It does not require special training. However, most expectant mothers will benefit by readings and discussions on the subject.

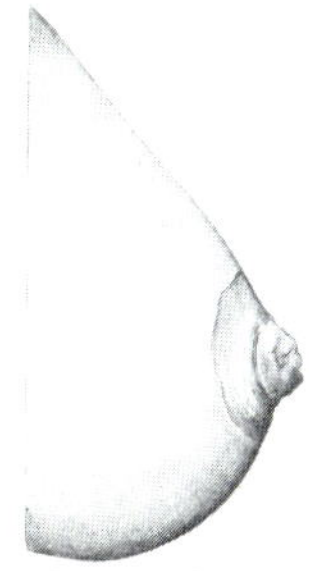

The nipple before stimulation.

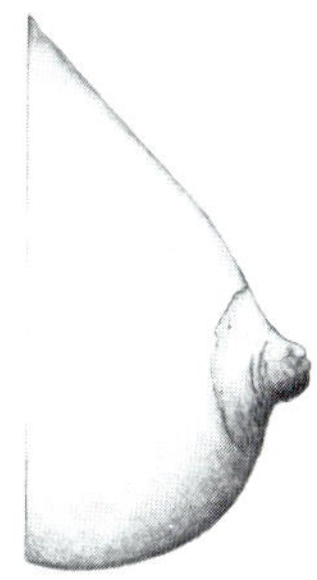

When stimulated, a normal nipple projects further.

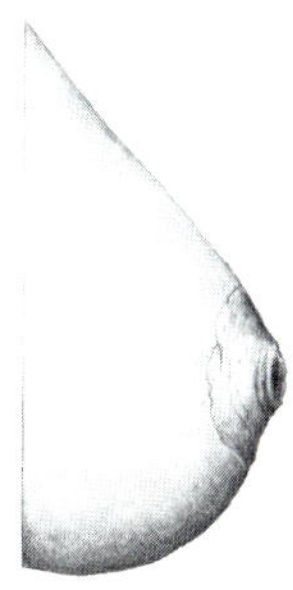

The nipple may retract when stimulated, or be permanently flat or retracted.

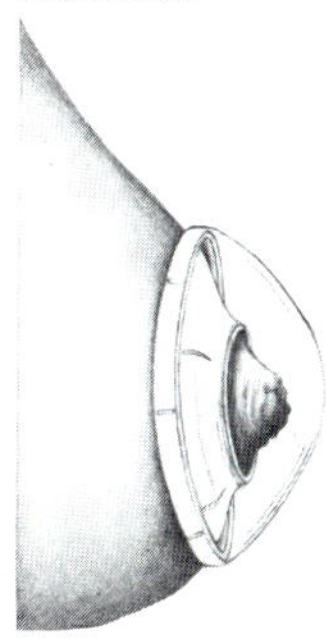

A breast shield encourages a retracted nipple to project.

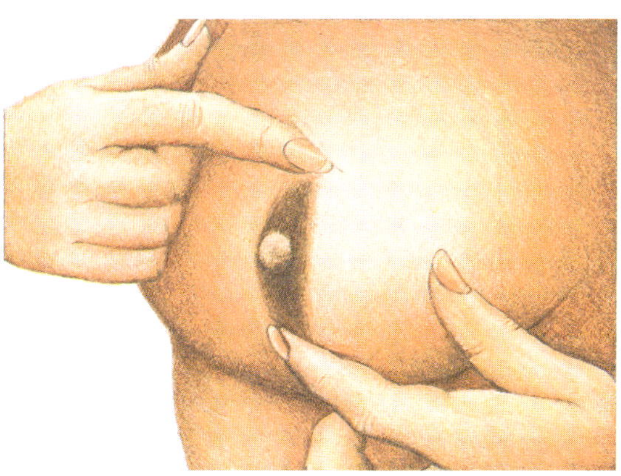

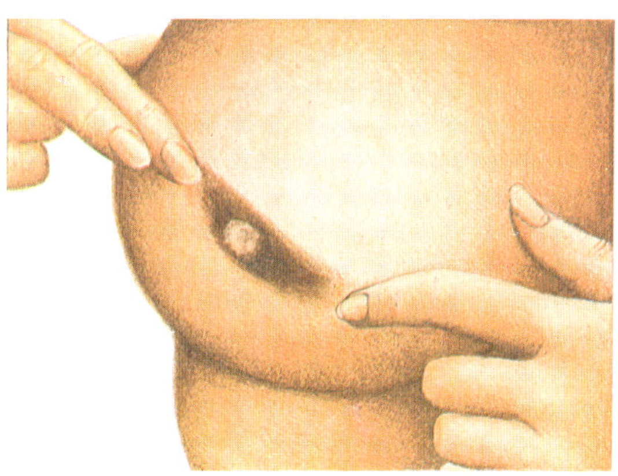

Hoffman's exercises (left) help to break down adhesions at the base of a retracted nipple. Most mothers with retracted nipples can breast-feed with the help of these simple and painless correctives.

Weight and diet

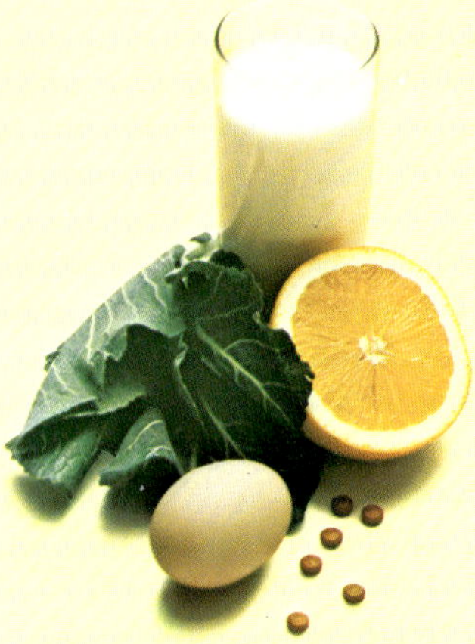

Calcium, found in milk, helps build strong bones. Iron, needed for the blood, is found in several foods but supplementary pills are often prescribed. Oranges contain vitamin C and eggs are one of the simplest sources of protein. Green vegetables are an important source of fiber.

As pregnancy progresses the mother's weight increases. This is partly due to the enlargement of the uterus and the breasts, partly to the weight of the fetus, and partly to the general changes that take place in the mother's body during pregnancy. It is not, however, true that the mother should "eat for two". You will probably require about 2500 calories per day.

The total weight gained in pregnancy should not be more than 25 – 28 lbs, and not more than 9 lb should be put on in the first 20 weeks. Excessive weight gain is not good for the mother or the baby and makes it more difficult to return to a normal figure after the birth. If you find you are putting on too much weight you should discuss this with your doctor. It is important in attempting to cut down on food that you do not affect the balance of your diet. A balanced diet contains the right proportions of the basic nutritional components: protein, carbohydrates, fats, vitamins, and minerals and fiber.

Protein is essential for the tissue construction of the breasts and the red blood cells of the mother as well as for the growth of the fetus, uterus and placenta. The greatest demand for protein occurs during the second half of pregnancy. Proteins are found both in animal foods and plants, though most animal foods are a better source of protein. Meat, fish, eggs, milk and cheese are all sources rich in protein but wheat, rice and other cereals, as well as beans, peas and nuts, contain some protein.

To save money you can easily combine animal proteins and the cheaper plant proteins in meals such as macaroni and cheese or breakfast cereal and milk. You can also obtain all your protein requirements by eating a mixture of plant proteins; meals combining plant proteins include baked beans and many varieties of vegetables.

Carbohydrates are necessary to provide energy, and when too few are eaten the body turns to its reserves of food, which are stored in the form of fat. This is what happens when a person eats less to lose weight, but it is not good for this to happen in pregnancy. Cereal products and starchy vegetables, like potatoes, are rich in carbohydrates as well as containing other nutrients.

Fat is a reserve fuel for the body: it is the most concentrated energy source which the diet can provide. All fats supply energy and in addition some – butter, for example – naturally contain vitamins A and D.

A SENSIBLE DAILY DIET FOR A VEGETARIAN

2 pints milk, including yogurt (or $1\frac{1}{2}$ pints and 2 eggs, or $1\frac{1}{2}$ pints, 1 egg and 1 helping cheese);
flour, bread, rice, or other cereal (3 helpings);
green vegetables or salad (2 helpings);
fresh fruit (2 portions, preferably citrus);
butter, margarine.
Additional vitamin D will be required.

A SENSIBLE DAILY DIET FOR A MEAT EATER

meat, fish, eggs, cheese (3 helpings);
milk (1 pint);
green, root and salad vegetables (2 helpings);
fresh fruit (2 portions, to include 1 citrus or its juice);
butter or margarine in moderation;
bread, 4/5 slices (or cereal, pasta or rice

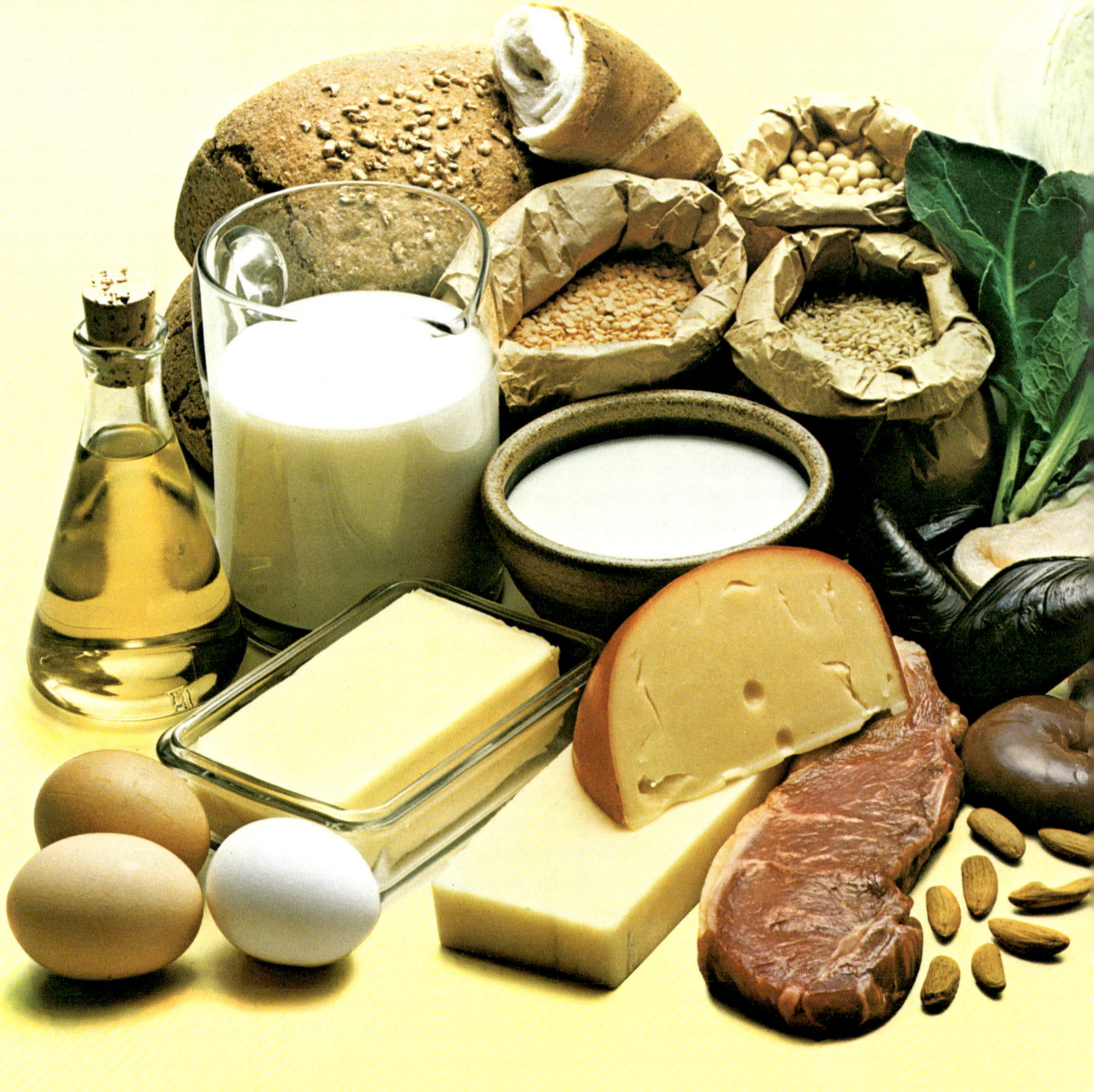

The vitamins play an important role in general health and often have quite specific functions. Vitamin A is essential for the development of the eyes, bones and many of the internal organs.

Vitamin D (together with calcium) is necessary for skeletal development, and lack of it can lead to rickets in children and soft bones in adults. A high proportion of our Vitamin D requirements come from the action of sunlight on the skin, but in countries with little sunshine a greater amount should come from the diet. During pregnancy more is needed than usual but supplements are not usually necessary except for strict vegetarians.

The B group of vitamins, which is important for tissue growth, is found in most meats, wholewheat bread, eggs, milk, green leafy vegetables and soybeans. Folic acid, one of the B group vitamins, is needed especially for the growth of red blood cells. It is mainly found in the same foods as iron (*see* below), but it is easily destroyed by overcooking. Because of the quantities required during pregnancy doctors often prescribe iron tablets with folic acid in them.

Vitamin B 12 is found only in animal foods, including milk, so it is very important for vegetarians to drink a quart of milk each day.

Vitamin C is found in citrus and many other fresh fruits, most vegetables, particularly green ones, and in tomatoes and potatoes. It too is very easily destroyed by overcooking.

Vitamin K, found in green leafy vegetables and cereals, is important in the development of the blood clotting mechanism. It is also produced in the body itself by the bacteria which inhabit the intestine.

Minerals are necessary for the proper functioning of the body, in particular, iron and calcium. Iron is essential to blood formation: it is the main component in hemoglobin. Iron is found naturally in liver, kidneys, red meat, egg yolks, dried fruit and green leafy vegetables. Many doctors prescribe iron pills

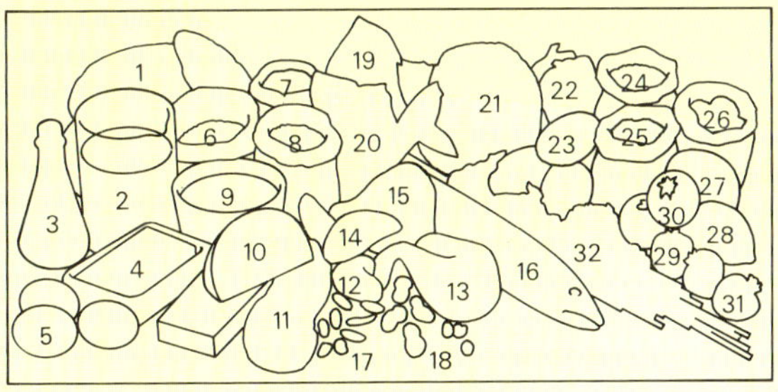

Eating a balanced diet depends on knowing the nutritional value of various foods. The key below sets out the major forms of nourishment found in the food shown left.

1 Bread (CB, FB – only) wholegrain
2 Milk (P, F, CAL)
3 Cooking oil (F)
4 Butter (F)
5 Eggs (P,I)
6 Lentils (P, I, FB)
7 Soybeans (P, I, FB)
8 Rice (CB)
9 Yogurt (P, CAL)
10 Cheese (P, F, CAL)
11 Red meat (P, F, I)
12 Kidney (P, I)
13 Chicken (P)
14 Mussels (P, I)
15 Cod (P)
16 Mackerel (P, F)
17 Almonds (P, F, FB)
18 Peanuts (P, F, FB)
19 Cabbage (CAL, I, C, FB)
20 Greens (CAL, I, FB)
21 Cauliflower (C)
22 Peppers (C)
23 Potatoes (CB, C)
24 Raisins (I, FB)
25 Currants (I, FB)
26 Dried apricots (I, FB)
27 Orange (C, FB)
28 Lemon (C, FB)
29 Lime (C, FB)
30 Tomatoes (C, FB)
31 Strawberries (C, FB)
32 Pasta (CB)

P = protein
CB = carbohydrates
F = fats
CAL = calcium
I = iron
C = vitamin C
FB = fiber

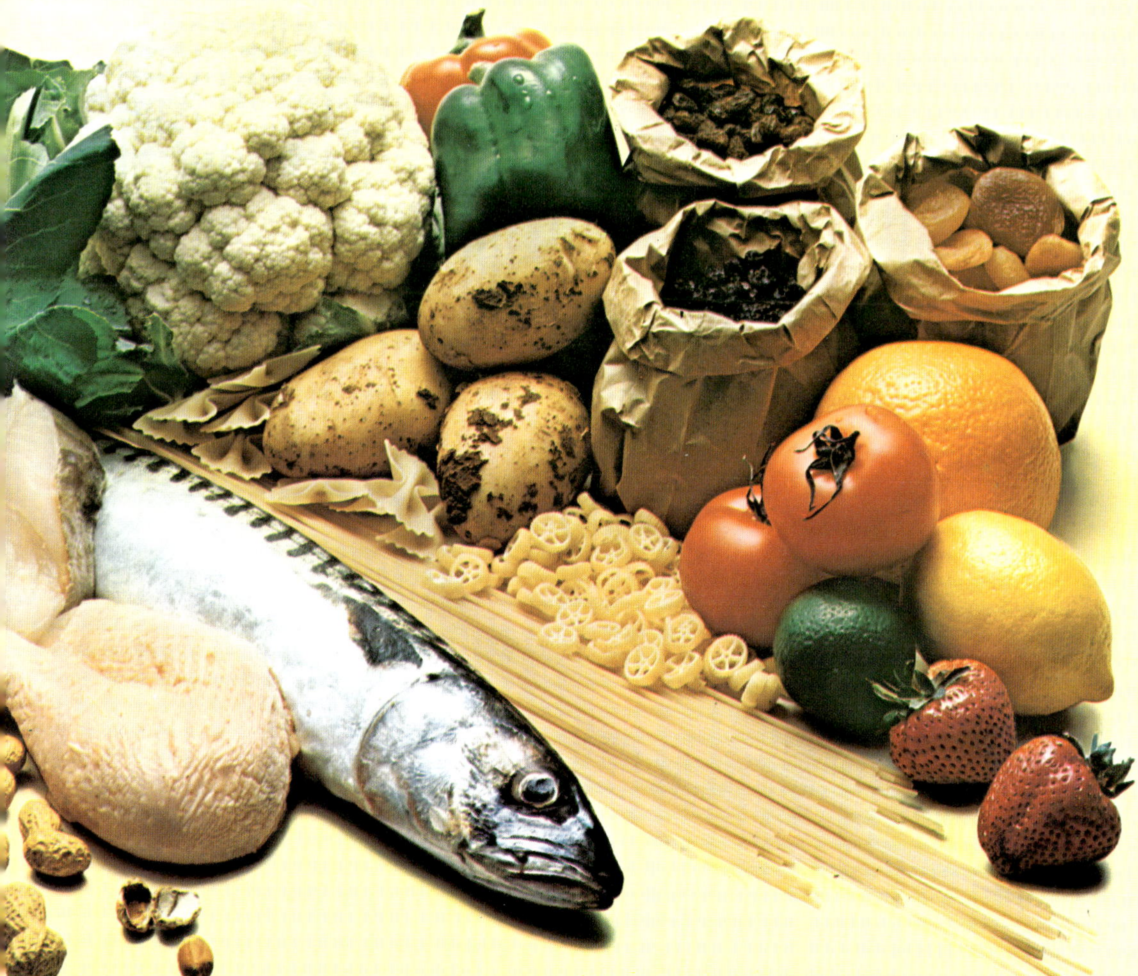

which, unfortunately, may cause gastro-intestinal symptoms as constipation, diarrhea or abdominal discomfort.

Calcium, so vital for the health of teeth and bones, is found in milk and dairy products. One and a half pints of milk contain the mother's daily requirements, but it is important to remember that milk also has a high calorie value. For this reason it may be better to drink only one pint and make up the rest of the daily calcium needs from low-fat dairy products, like yogurt and low-fat milk.

The importance of fiber

The importance of fiber, or roughage, has only recently been realized. Lack of fiber in the diet encourages constipation, hemorrhoids and inflamation of the colon. Fiber is present in all vegetables, fruit, wholewheat bread, bran foods and cereals. It is very important that some of these items should be included in the pregnant woman's daily diet. At this time of life it is more necessary than ever before to maintain a completely balanced diet.

Special diets

Dietary restrictions cause concern only if they reduce the intake of essential foods. Some vegetarian diets are very low in protein, iron, vitamin B12 and folic acid and can lead to poor fetal growth, maternal anemia and the risk of premature labor. It is, of course, quite possible to continue a vegetarian way of life during pregnancy, but it is important to let your doctor know details of your diet.

Changes in the digestive system

It is common knowledge that a pregnant woman sometimes develops a craving for, or a dislike of, particular foods. For instance, some take a sudden aversion to alcohol or coffee, particularly in the first trimester. Later in pregnancy a woman may wish to eat uncommonly large quantities of certain foods. Except in rare cases where the mother is overweight there is no cause for concern. However, when an abnormal craving causes an expectant mother to eat large amounts of things like starch or clay, this is a cause for serious concern (*see* p. 63).

Teeth need extra care in pregnancy and the gums grow a little softer and may need attention. For these reasons it is best for expectant mothers to see a dentist early in pregnancy.

The stomach is affected in various ways by pregnancy: it produces less acid and, because the sphincter muscle is relaxed by progesterone (*see* p. 30), there is a tendency for the acidic contents to be forced back into the esophagus causing heartburn. Antacid tablets may relieve the heartburn. In later pregnancy, heartburn is nearly always eased by sleeping propped up.

Lastly, the intestines move more slowly during pregnancy under the relaxing influence of progesterone. The constipation that is a common problem during pregnancy usually disappears shortly after delivery.

Medications

The health of the mother and the growing fetus are intimately connected but, whereas a healthy diet benefits them both, medications that are good for the mother may not be good for the fetus. Like food and oxygen, drugs can cross the placenta and enter the fetus' bloodstream but not all drugs do so and not all harm the fetus. However, because we know that some drugs are a danger to the fetus, doctors are now careful to prescribe only those medications which are considered safe.

Luckily, most medications used for treatment during pregnancy are known to be safe because they have been used for a long time. Sometimes these drugs may have a minor effect on the fetus and in such cases danger to the fetus must be weighed against the danger to the mother of stopping treatment. This is a decision which has to be made by the doctor who has all the essential information. If you are undergoing any treatment involving a drug or drugs it is vital that your obstetrician know about the treatment as soon as you think you are pregnant.

Severe abnormalities can be caused by taking certain drugs during the early weeks of pregnancy because at this time the fetal organs are still being formed. In particular, hormone preparations should never be used to induce a period when there is any possibility of a pregnancy. Other drugs taken in later pregnancy may, like smoking, merely prevent the baby from being as healthy as it could be.

The three lists opposite have been compiled

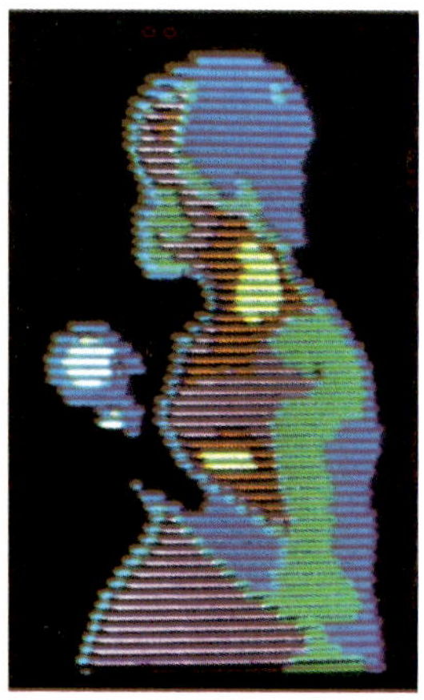

A thermograph (left), which is a heat sensitive picture, shows the warmer parts of the body as red; yellow is cooler and blue cooler still.

A more detailed thermograph (below left).

When the mother smokes, the placenta cools visibly as the blood vessels constrict and blood flow decreases (below), resulting in less nourishment and oxygen for the fetus. The fetal heart beats faster when nicotine enters its circulation.

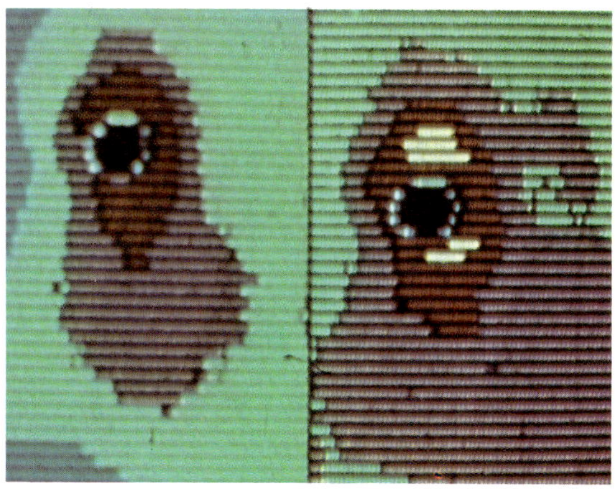

in the light of current medical opinion. They show drugs which should never be used in pregnancy; drugs which are best avoided where possible; and a third group of drugs which are often prescribed for essential treatment with a note on counteractive measures.

Abdominal X rays should never be taken in early pregnancy, or in the second half of the menstrual cycle where the woman may be pregnant because significant irradiation in early pregnancy may cause fetal malformation. Chest X rays may be taken in the middle trimester if the baby is protected by a lead apron. The baby may be X-rayed in the last trimester if this is absolutely essential (*see* pp. 104, 106).

USE OF DRUGS IN PREGNANCY

DRUGS WHICH SHOULD NOT BE USED

Drug	**Use**	**Fetal effect**
Heroin	Drug abuse	Depressed respiration and withdrawal symptoms after birth
Live vaccines, e.g. smallpox, rubella	Immunization	Viral infection
Smoking (nicotine)	Social	Poor fetal growth

DRUGS BETTER AVOIDED

Drug	**Use**	**Fetal effect**
Alcohol	Social	Fetal alcohol syndrome
Streptomycin	Against infection	Possible deafness
Sulfas	Against infection	Anemia (very rare)
Tetracycline	Against infection	Yellow teeth

Note There are substitutes for all of these, such as penicillin and the cephalosporins. Septrin/Bactrim preparations may be used when no other safer antibiotic is effective against infection, but extra folate should be given at the same time.

DRUGS USED FOR ESSENTIAL TREATMENT

Drug	**Use**	**Fetal effect**	**Counteraction**
Anticoagulants	Venous clots	Placental separation Fetal hemorrhage	Good dose control and regular testing
Antithyroids	Thyrotoxicosis	Goiter	Avoided by additional thyroid treatment
Barbiturates	Epilepsy sedation	Withdrawal symptoms after birth (rare)	Baby treated if necessary
Corticosteroids	Various	Cleft palate (unproven)	Surgery after birth
Insulin	Diabetes	Low blood sugar	Good monitoring and dose control. Early testing of fetal blood sugar
Phenytoin	Epilepsy	Fetal abnormalities (infrequent)	Often replaced in pregnancy by phenobarbital
Progesterone derivatives*	Threatened miscarriage	Susceptibility to masculinization in female babies (rare)	Surgery after birth

* Medical opinion is divided on the part these drugs may be able to play in preventing early miscarriage. If such a drug is prescribed the doctor will choose one which he considers as safe as possible.

These lists are a guide to the use of drugs in pregnancy. **If you are undergoing treatment involving any drug, tell your doctor as soon as you suspect you are pregnant.**

Exercise and rest

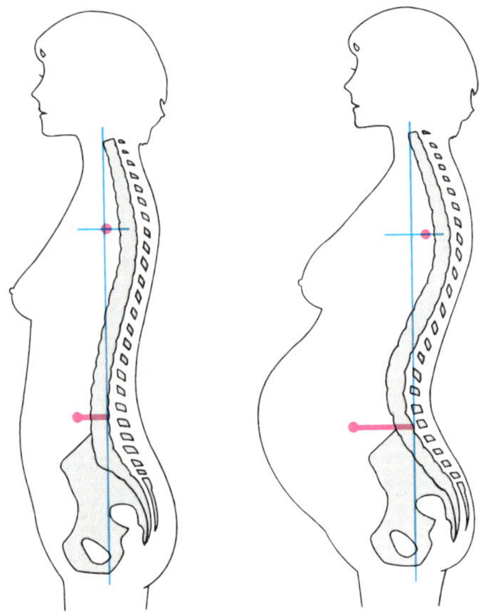

During pregnancy the center of gravity moves further forward away from the spine. There is a compensating tendency to throw the shoulders back and curve the spine, but this causes backache and strain. Keep the back as straight as possible and tighten the abdominal muscles when standing or walking to lessen the protuberance.

Two changes occur during pregnancy affecting posture, the first of which probably depends on the hormones of pregnancy. The ligaments which hold joints together, are made of tissue which is firm and non-elastic in a non-pregnant woman. During pregnancy the ligaments soften and elongate so that moving joints (like the knee) become less stable and fixed joints, especially in the spine and pelvis, like the sacroiliac joints (*see* p. 14), show some signs of separation and movement. As a result additional strain is put on the muscles of the back and backache occurs unless these muscles are strong.

The second factor affecting posture in pregnancy is a change in the woman's center of gravity. This lies just in front of the spine and level with the kidneys in a non-pregnant woman but as the uterus enlarges upward and forward the center of gravity too moves forward, making the woman overbalance. As a result she will be tempted to throw back her shoulders and if this becomes a habit she may strain her back. To prevent this she should strengthen her back muscles and avoid standing for long periods, especially during the last trimester of pregnancy.

Shoes are also important in maintaining good posture. Very high heels and very flat ones are best avoided. A heel of between $\frac{3}{4}$ in and 2 in (2 cm and 5 cm) is best as a slight rise of the heel helps to straighten the spine. If possible pregnant women should alternate between pairs of slightly different heights because this often improves comfort. This also avoids the need to maintain a single rigid, balanced posture which can lead to aching legs.

Getting around

Walking encourages the leg veins to pump blood upward from the feet and serves to guard against a feeling of heaviness in the legs and minor swelling of the ankles. Should swelling occur, however, for whatever reason, it is essential to rest with the feet up and the back well supported (*see* chapter 5).

There is no reason why pregnant women should not take walks, providing they do so in moderation, and they have not been advised against it by their doctor. Walking is healthy; but any prolonged period of standing should be avoided.

Traveling by car and driving are perfectly safe in pregnancy, but pressure from the firm edge of the seat can occlude the leg veins and if

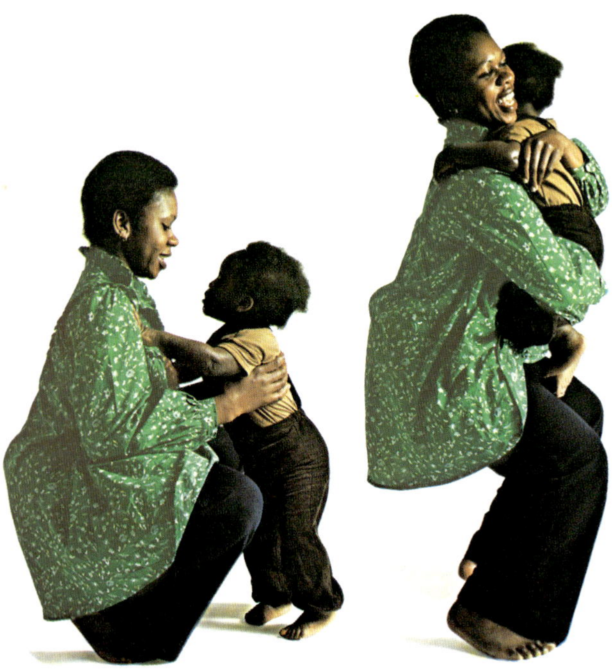

When lifting a child or a heavy object (left), do not lean down. Bend the knees and squat, keeping the back fairly straight.

Working at the kitchen sink (right) often involves awkward bending forward and difficult reaching. Standing with the body turned slightly to one side can be helpful.

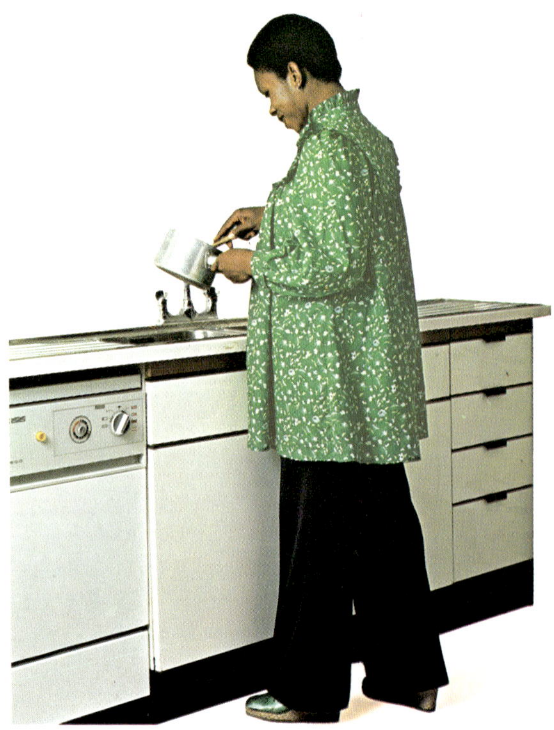

the journey is long may lead to blood clots. Any long car trips should therefore be planned to include a stop every hour so that the pregnant woman can get out and stretch her legs. It is important that seat belts always be worn in such a way as not to chafe the breasts or constrict the abdomen.

For really long journeys it is better to fly because it is then possible to walk around. Long trips of any sort should be avoided after the thirty-sixth week in case labor begins. Airlines in general will not allow a pregnant woman to fly when she is beyond the thirty-second week. This is not because flying has any adverse effect on the mother-to-be, but because aircraft are not equipped to cope with a woman in labor. Pregnant women who wish to fly before that time may require a note from a doctor to confirm that all is normal. Most international airlines have their own medical center at their headquarters and if there is any doubt whether a mother-to-be will be allowed to fly it is best that she seek advice well in advance of her planned traveling time.

No pregnant woman should have a vaccination (*see* p. 39) and for this reason, if you are traveling abroad, it is wise to carry a letter from your doctor certifying pregnancy and claiming exemption.

Rest

Rest and relaxation are essential to a healthy pregnancy. Ideally the expectant mother should set aside a period each day when she can relax completely. The best way to relax is to lie down or to sit with the back well supported and the legs raised (*see* below).

Sleeping and relaxing lying down becomes more difficult in pregnancy and mothers are advised to experiment with different positions until they find the one that suits them best. In general, expectant mothers usually find it is better to lie on their side during the last trimester.

Above all, it is important to learn to relax, whether walking around, sitting or lying down. Simple guidelines to relaxation are given in chapter 5.

Sports

The expectant mother may do moderate exercise or participate in non-contact sports. Those who regularly play such sports as tennis, golf or swimming may continue as long as no complications or excessive fatigue occurs – in fact, it will be beneficial.

Work and leisure

Many expectant mothers are working full-time and some will work almost to the end of pregnancy with no ill effect. When a woman gives up work remains a matter of personal choice, unless she is advised to do so by her doctor. If a woman has had previous miscarriages or periodic bleeding during the pregnancy, for example, it is best for her to leave work at an early date and allow more time to rest. In addition, if the work she does is considered dangerous to pregnant women the expectant mother will be advised to give up her job, although in certain circumstances an employer may try to find pregnant women alternative work. While still working, particularly in the third trimester, the expectant mother should make sure she has enough rest and avoids physical strain. After stopping work she should take the opportunity to have a rest every afternoon. Entertaining, where it is not too tiring or does not go on too late, is fine. But the expectant mother should limit her activities if she discovers that she is becoming too tired.

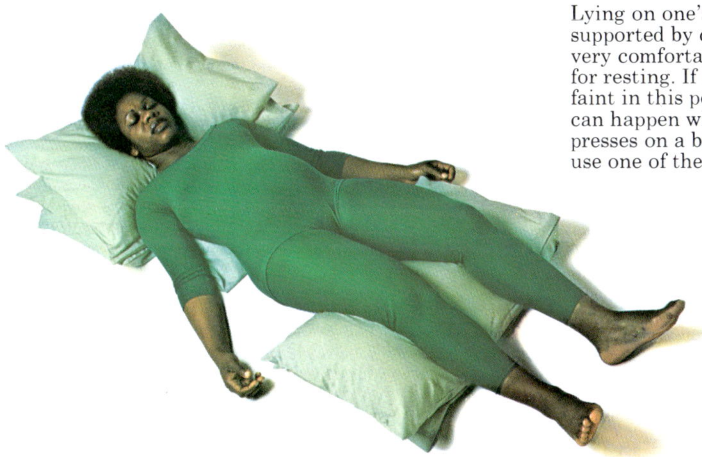

Lying on one's back, well supported by cushions, is a very comfortable position for resting. If you feel faint in this position, as can happen when the baby presses on a blood vessel, use one of the others.

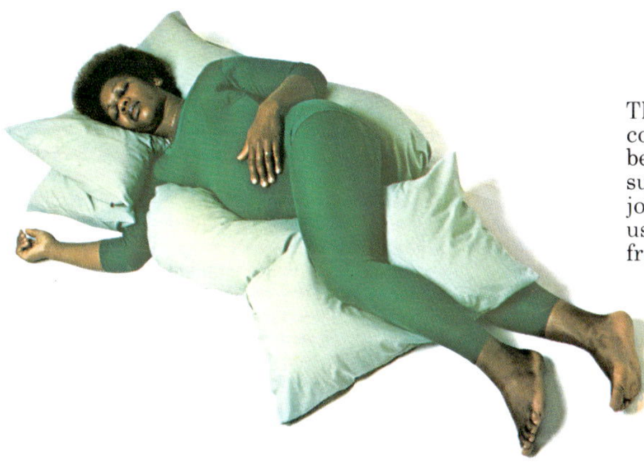

This position is also very comfortable. The cushion between the knees helps support the sacroiliac joint and is especially useful for people suffering from sciatic nerve pain.

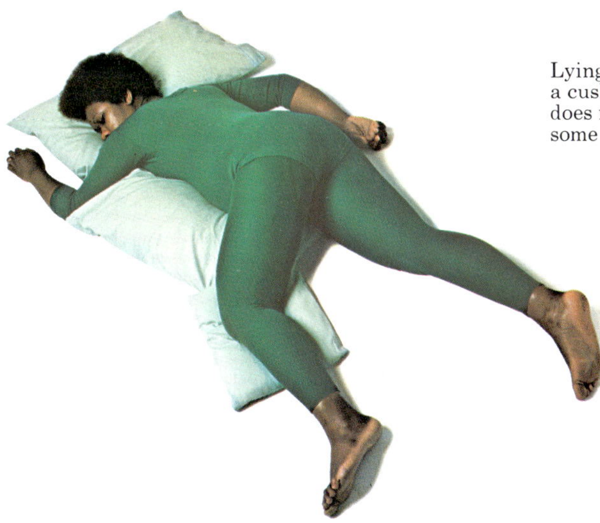

Lying on one's front, with a cushion under the knee, does not harm the baby, as some people fear.

Personal care

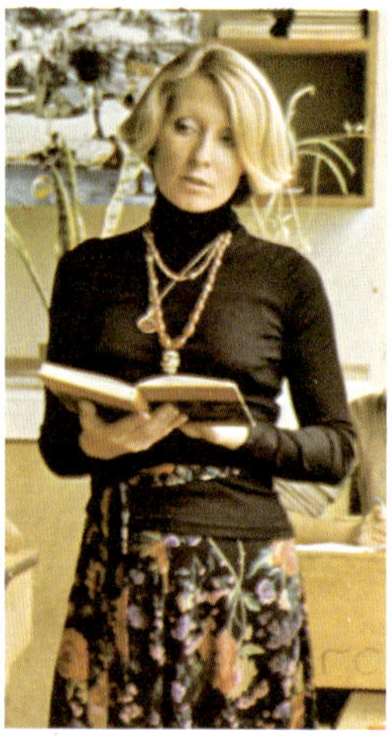

If a pregnant woman is fit and well she can continue working as long as she wants to do so.

Pregnancy frequently enhances a woman's attractiveness. Once any problems of early pregnancy have been overcome she often looks radiantly well. Quite apart from her pleasure at being pregnant there are good, biological reasons for her vitality.

The skin

During pregnancy the texture of the skin can improve so much that those who use makeup may find it unnecessary. The skin is affected by the burst of activity associated with most tissue during pregnancy. The capillaries dilate under the influence of hormones and blood flow increases, raising the temperature and often heightening the color.

At the same time the tissues retain a certain amount of extra fluid. This is especially likely to alter the facial features and even a slight rounding of the contours adds to the impression of health.

Fluid retention and increased blood flow are the result of hormonal influence. Hormones also stimulte the pigmentation cells to produce more melanin, giving the skin a browner tone. This is especially obvious with the darkening of the nipples (*see* p. 34): other areas are also affected. The line down the middle of the abdomen from the umbilicus to the pubic hair darkens and is then known as the "linea nigra" or black line.

Some women, particularly those with fair skin, develop bronze markings on the face known as chloasma or "the mask of pregnancy" (*see* chapter 4). This is more common in dark haired women and depends to some extent on exposure to sunlight. The color change tends to be most prominent on the forehead, cheeks and nose, missing the eye hollows which appear pale by comparison. The phenomenon closely resembles the tanned face of a winter sportsman whose eyes have been protected by goggles. After delivery it slowly fades.

Increased production of sebum in the skin, a higher body temperature and the effort of carrying the pregnancy means that you will perspire more and will be more susceptible to minor infections. When washing it is important to pay special attention to cleansing and drying the area beneath the breasts.

Pregnancy hormones also affect various skin conditions such as acne, eczema and psoriasis, but unpredictably. It can cure them, make them better, worse, or even be the precipitating cause. Avoid heavy makeup if you have a tendency to acne.

Stretch marks may appear on the breasts and low abdomen during pregnancy. Known as *striae*, they are associated not only with pregnancy, but also with obesity, especially when caused by hormonal imbalance. The hormones seem to affect the skin in the area where weight is put on, causing the deep

Antenatal exercise

Exercise during pregnancy is important because it not only helps to maintain your muscle tone, but also to strengthen your muscles generally.

The first exercise shown here strengthens both abdominal and thigh muscles; be sure to tighten your buttocks to keep your pelvis stable. The second exercise stretches out back muscles; go forward only as far as you feel is comfortable. The third exercise strengthens arms as well as back muscles. The fourth strengthens the arms and chest; from six months on, the expectant mother should support her head with a pillow.

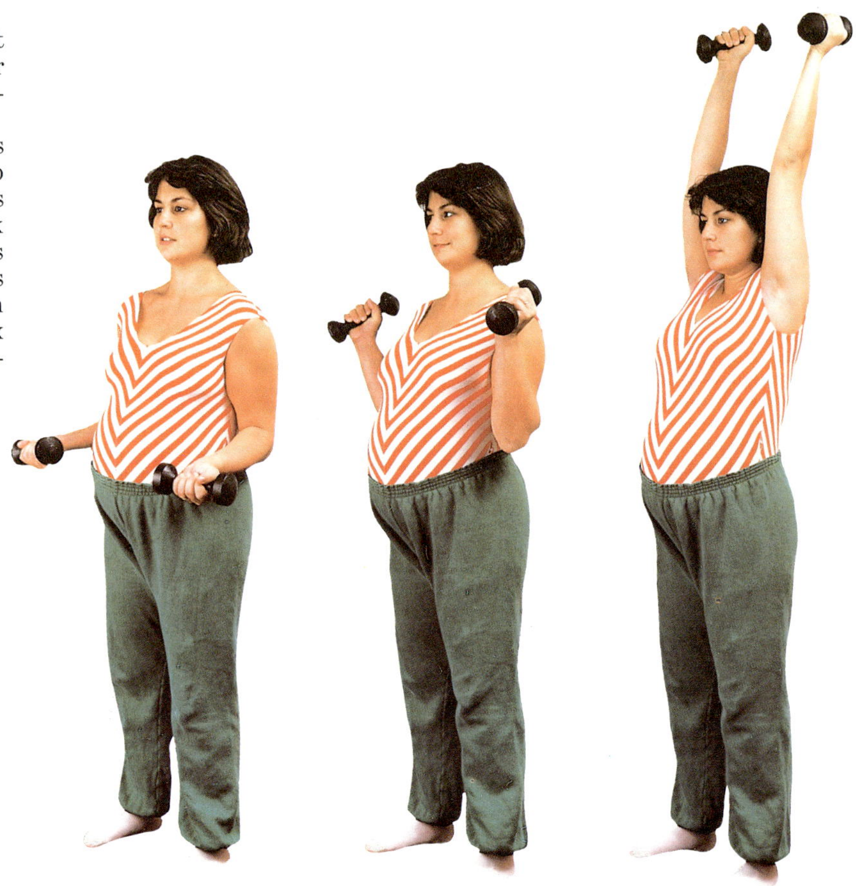

Stand erect, feet comfortably apart. Raise free weights (dumb bells) to shoulders, then over head, back to shoulder level, then down. Repeat.

layers to lose their elasticity. These then separate and the covering skin becomes thinner. At first the stretch marks are red or blue but, after pregnancy, they fade to a silvery white and become much less obvious. They never completely disappear.

Hair

Hair is often thicker during pregnancy because less of it falls out than normally. It is also more oily, so it may be necessary to wash your hair more frequently than usual. After delivery quite a lot of hair may be lost. If this occurs, hair growth returns to normal in six months. During the last trimester and postpartum period, curly hair may become less wavy.

The vagina

With the vaginal and uterine changes that accompany pregnancy (*see* p. 30), the acidity of the cells lining the vagina decreases and this may encourage vaginal infections and discharge (*see* chapter 4). Not all extra discharge, however, is caused by infection. Increased activity of the cervical glands produces extra mucus. Gentle external washing is all that is necessary to cleanse this area.

Clothes

Being pregnant doesn't mean you need to change your whole approach to the clothes that you wear. Providing they are not restrictive many of the things you already have can be worn or adapted for pregnancy. As well as the range of clothes specifically designed as maternity wear, there are many styles in the stores which are perfectly suitable for wearing when you are expecting a baby. Smock styles, with gathers or pleats falling from the neckline are full and easy to wear and they do not accentuate the hips. A loose, hip-length top can be worn over slacks, which can either be special maternity slacks or your usual ones, perhaps held up by suspenders when they can no longer be zipped up in the usual way.

It is generally more comfortable to wear loose-fitting clothes. Avoid tight slacks, especially those in synthetic fabrics, and wear cotton underwear. If you feel your abdominal muscles need some support you can wear a light panty girdle, but this is not essential. It is very important that your bra is comfortable and the cups are large enough to give adequate support. If shields are worn in late pregnancy (*see* p. 35) there will need to be sufficient room to accommodate them. Some women prefer to wear a bra designed for breast-feeding if their breasts grow markedly larger and heavier.

Support hose are a good investment, even if you do not have varicose veins. They need not be unattractively thick and heavy. Maternity hose need not be worn unless you find that ones in available sizes no longer fit.

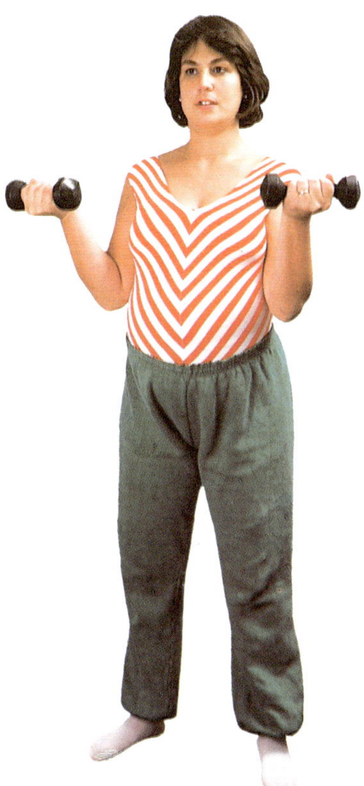

Stand erect, feet comfortably apart, toes straight forward. With arms down at sides, bend elbows, raising weights forward and up to shoulders keeping upper arms at sides. Repeat.

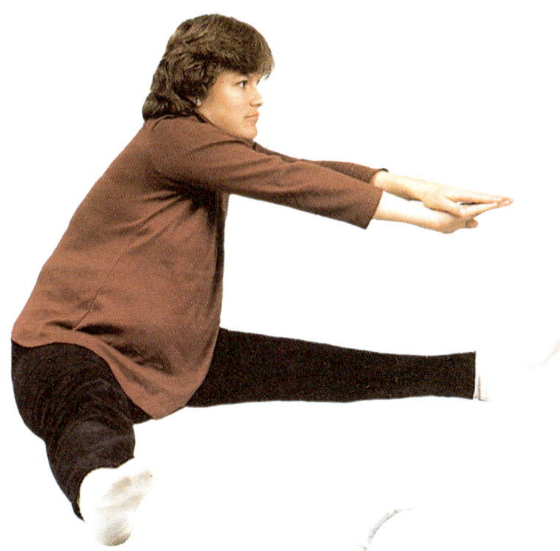

Sitting on floor, legs straight and comfortably spread apart with back straight, raise your arms to shoulder height and stretch forward. Place one hand on top of the other. Bend gently forward over one leg, then the other, reaching out and down toward toes. Repeat.

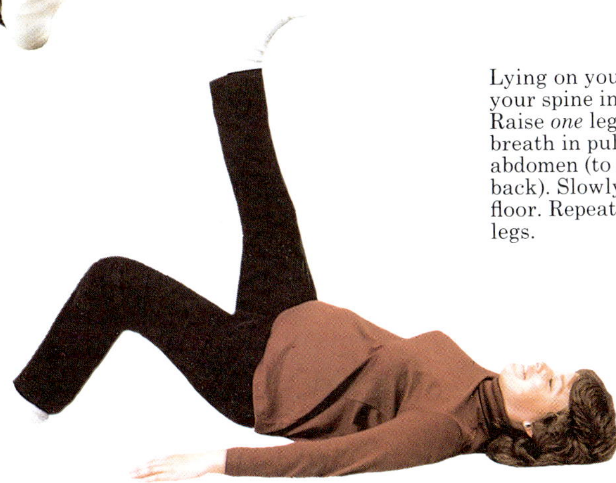

Lying on your back, press your spine into the floor. Raise *one* leg up, take a breath in pulling in abdomen (to support lower back). Slowly lower to floor. Repeat and alternate legs.

The growing fetus

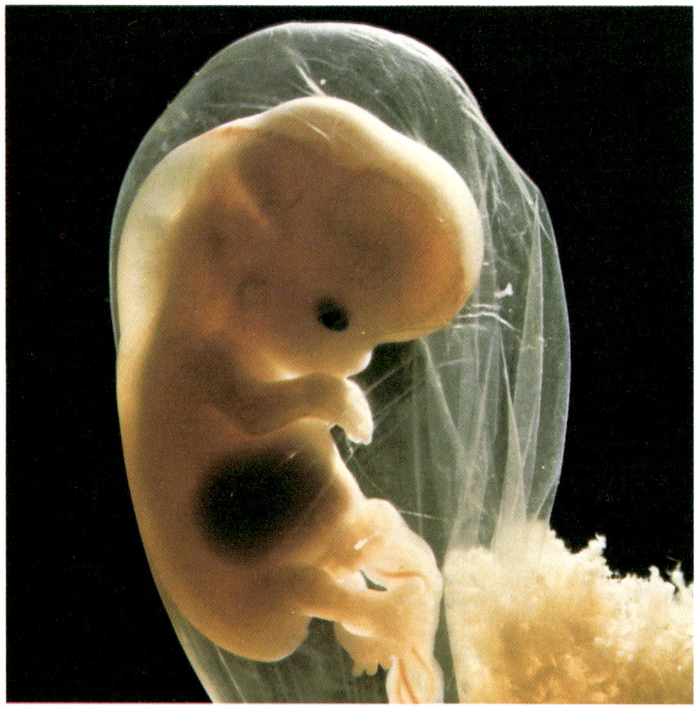

CHAPTER 3

Nourishment and protection

The first trimester

The second and third trimesters

Weight and position

Fetal health

Cross references

See also	Chapter
Breech delivery	7
Causes of abnormality	1
Problems in pregnancy	4
Delivery date	2
Fetal circulation	2, 9
Genetics and inheritance	1
Hormones	1
Premature and postmature babies	4, 9
Smoking and drugs	2
The mother in pregnancy	2

The last chapter concentrated on the physical and psychological changes in the mother during pregnancy and on the measures she can take to improve the outcome of her pregnancy. This chapter deals with the growing life within the uterus starting from the point where we left it in chapter 1.

The journey of the newly fertilized ovum during the seven days between fertilization and implantation is extremely hazardous. The ovum, a microscopic ball of cells which divides rapidly as it travels down the fallopian tube, has no means of propelling itself. It is wafted along by the movement of the hair-like cilia which line the tube; so long as the tube is healthy the ovum should arrive in the uterus by the fourth day after fertilization. It is nourished within the uterine cavity for three days and implantation of the ovum begins on the seventh day. Any delay in transport, caused by a damaged fallopian tube, for example, may cause the ovum to implant in the tube – in this case there will be no chance of a successful pregnancy.

Once the ovum has implanted in the uterus the early development of the baby occurs at an incredibly fast rate and with bewildering diversity when one remembers its origin as a single cell invisible to the naked eye. The word embryo is used to describe the baby during the first eight weeks of life within the uterus. During this time the cells continue to multiply and at the same time develop the characteristics which make it possible for them to form different structures (bone, blood and so on). In medical language this is the stage of embryogenesis.

By the end of the first eight weeks most of the organs that make up a human being are already formed. Throughout the remainder of the pregnancy

A human fetus eight weeks from conception. Although it is only about $1\frac{1}{4}$in (30mm) long, its face and body are becoming defined and almost all the major internal organs have formed.

they become more distinct and mature and increase in size. Under ideal circumstances they will all be working normally for many weeks before birth. The term fetus is used to describe a baby after embryogenesis. This roughly corresponds to the last two trimesters of pregnancy. This chapter focuses on the growth of the fetus.

The findings of medical research and rapidly advancing technology in the field of antenatal care make it possible to tell the story of fetal growth in some detail. Pictures produced by ultrasound scans and the technique of fetoscopy show the live fetus in the uterus. Since the changes that occur in the fetus are greatest early in pregnancy, the development of the fetus is described every week to begin with and then only once every four weeks. Throughout pregnancy, the placenta is the vital link between mother and fetus. A separate section explains the development and functions of the placenta, and of the fluid which surrounds the fetus during its growth.

Pregnancy is divided for convenience into three approximately equal parts known as trimesters. Each trimester lasts about three months or, in the more precise terms preferred by doctors, 13 weeks.

By the end of the twelfth or thirteenth week, the baby can be said to be fully formed. From then onward it simply grows and matures. An important consequence follows from this. Once a fetal organ has been properly formed, it is very unlikely to be malformed no matter what happens to the mother or the fetus. It is only during the first trimester while the organs are still forming that external factors, such as medications taken by the mother, can seriously interfere with the formation of the fetal organs. Congenital malformations – those which are not inherited but which are present at birth – are almost entirely the result of harmful influences during the first trimester. For example, German measles (rubella) acquired during the first trimester can result in severe congenital malformations.

Most babies develop in the uterus without any problems and achieve a healthy birthweight having grown at roughly the correct rate. Checking on the growth rate of the fetus is an important part of routine antenatal care. There are many ways of doing this, from the simple traditional methods (such as measuring the size of the mother's abdomen) to the sophisticated modern techniques of ultrasound.

The final birthweight of a baby depends on a number of factors, some of which are environmental, such as the food the mother eats or the climate she lives in, and some of which are genetic, such as the race or sex of the baby.

Many parents are naturally worried about the possibility of producing a baby which has some defects. Serious abnormalities, whether inherited or congenital, are rare, but parents will appreciate the value of an honest discussion of the risks involved (and the degree to which the dangers are increased by factors such as the mother's age). Beyond routine checks for normal development there are a number of tests which doctors perform to detect abnormalities. These include blood screening tests, amniocentesis, ultrasound and fetoscopy. Where there is any concern that a couple will produce a baby with some abnormality it is always advisable to consult your doctor who will put these fears in perspective and advise you on the best course of action. Occasionally, he will have to refer a couple to a genetics specialist if their situation is very complex.

Nourishment and protection

THE DEVELOPING PLACENTA

a The placenta begins to develop after the outer layer of the blastocyst has burrowed into the wall of the uterus. An inner layer of cells containing fetal blood vessels begins to form fingerlike projections within this outer layer.

By the time of implantation, the fertilized ovum has developed into a ball of cells (the blastocyst). After implantation the ball continues to grow and becomes hollow, while at its center a group of specialized cells soon begins to grow. This group of cells, called the inner cell mass, will ultimately become the fetus but at this stage it is no more than a vague shape protruding into the central cavity of the blastocyst.

The outer cells of the blastocyst are covered with small fingerlike projections called chorionic villi. These burrow into the lining of the uterus seeking nourishment until those which have penetrated deepest erode some of the small uterine blood vessels and become bathed in the mother's blood. At this point the burrowing stops and villi start to multiply and form branches. It is these villi which form the basis of the placenta.

The villi continue to grow in number and develop further branches until a very large surface area is in contact with the maternal blood. It is this which allows the placenta to function as the vital link between the mother and the fetus.

As the placenta develops, blood vessels form in the villi and fuse with neighboring ones until an extensive system of vessels is built up. These vessels are surrounded by layers of special fetal cells which eventually separate the blood of the fetus from that of the mother, allowing food and oxygen to pass from the mother to the fetus, and waste products to pass in the other direction.

At the same time as the blood vessels are forming in the villi, others are forming in the inner cell mass within the blastocyst (called the embryo at this stage). Three blood vessels emerge from the embryo and join with those of the developing placenta. These form the basis of the umbilical cord, which links the embryo to the placenta, and at either end of the cord they divide into smaller and smaller vessels. At this time the primitive heart is also forming, and by the end of the fourth week after fertilization, in other words, two weeks after the first missed period, it begins to beat. At this point the embryo measures less than $\frac{1}{3}$ in (10 mm) – smaller than a dime.

With the passage of time, definite changes occur in the structure of the placenta which are closely related to its function. The villi continue to grow and branch, and this not only increases their surface area but also provides a firm attachment to the wall of the uterus. The layer of cells dividing the fetal blood from the mother's blood becomes thinner, though it is important to remember that under normal circumstances the two circulations never mix.

By the twelfth week of pregnancy, the placenta is a separate organ and the remainder of what was the outer part of the blastocyst has developed into a set of membranes which are loosely attached to the inside of the uterus and which contain the developing fetus and the amniotic fluid – the fluid which surrounds the fetus. At term, the placenta will weigh

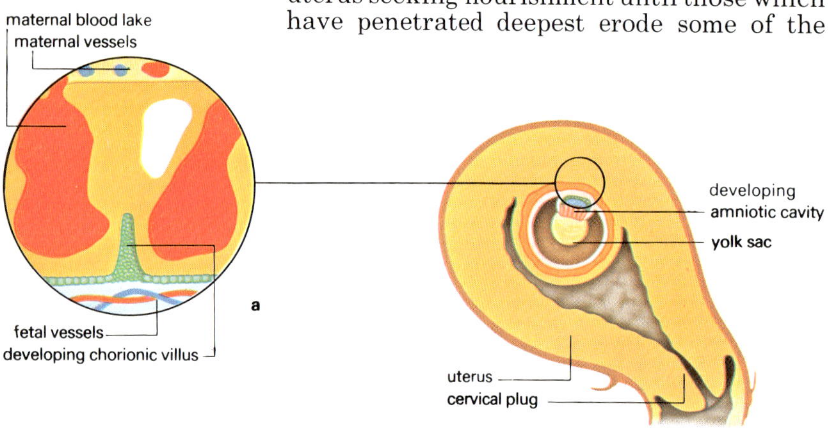

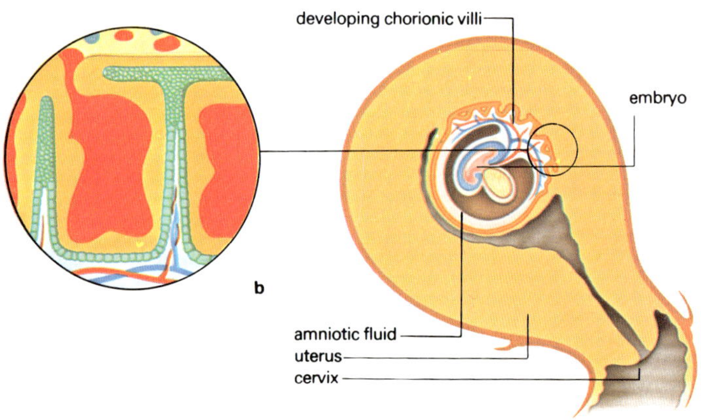

b Some of the mother's blood vessels are eroded by the burrowing activity of the blastocyst, and pools of maternal blood flow into the spaces between the outer layers of the blastocyst. The fingerlike projections containing the fetal blood vessels begin to branch sideways.

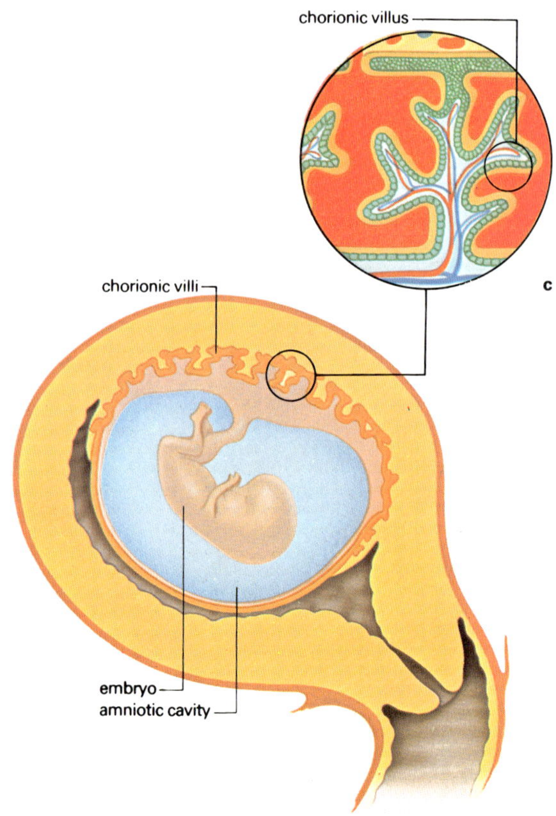

c The projections from the blastocyst (the chorionic villi) branch to form a complex pattern of fetal vessels. The placenta now has a structure similar to the one it will display throughout pregnancy.

approximately one sixth of the total weight of the fetus, or about 1 lb (500 g).

The function of the placenta

The placenta is responsible for the transfer of nourishment to the fetus, and of the waste products it produces to the mother so that they can be excreted (*see* p. 32). This exchange between mother and fetus takes place in the tiny villi of the placenta which lie in a large, constantly changing pool of maternal blood. With each maternal heartbeat, blood loaded with oxygen and nutrients enters this pool and blood loaded with carbon dioxide and waste products leaves. The fetal heart pumps blood containing waste products down the umbilical cord to the placenta, and receives the blood which returns from the placenta along the cord and which is rich in both oxygen and essential nutritional components.

The placenta also acts as a barrier to protect the fetus against potentially harmful substances. Many medications, however, can cross the placenta and harm the fetus. Certain medications should not be taken while pregnant for this reason. Whether any substance will cross the placenta depends on the molecular weight – the size of the smallest particles in it. In general the smaller the molecule, the easier its passage across the placenta. The vast majority of drugs pass the placenta, as they are composed of small molecules. The substances which are mainly prevented from crossing are the larger proteins and the blood cells of the mother. Some medications, however, can be given to the mother with the knowledge that there is no chance that they will reach the fetus.

Among the substances which cross the placenta are some of the mother's antibodies – chemical substances which are found in the blood and which give protection against particular diseases (*see* pp. 33, 52). In this way a degree of immunity from diseases is given to the fetus, and this lasts for about six months after the baby is born, when it is able to start producing its own antibodies.

The placenta produces a large variety of hormones, some of which are believed to help maintain the supply of food to the fetus, while others, like human chorionic gonadotrophin (H.C.G.) are thought to be important in maintaining the pregnancy during the period of early gestation (*see* p. 17).

The amniotic fluid

Throughout pregnancy the fetus is surrounded by a liquid, the amniotic fluid, which is contained within the amniotic sac. It used to be thought that this fluid remained the same throughout pregnancy, but it is now known that there is a continuous turnover.

The amniotic fluid is thought to come largely from the fetus although it also comes from the mother, passing through the amniotic membranes covering the placenta. During the early part of pregnancy the skin of the fetus is porous and the amniotic fluid is thought to pass through it. As the weight of the fetus increases, the volume of fluid increases proportionately. After about 16 weeks the skin of the fetus becomes thicker and impermeable and the kidneys start to produce dilute urine. From mid-pregnancy onward this urine is the main source of the fluid. During the last third of the pregnancy some of the fluid comes from the lungs of the fetus.

Although the volume of the amniotic fluid increases tenfold between the twelfth and fortieth weeks of pregnancy it is also removed in various ways. Some is swallowed by the fetus and some is absorbed through the umbilical cord and the membranes covering the placenta. The amniotic fluid performs a number of important functions: it provides the fetus with a liquid environment of constant temperature in which growth and movement are uninhibited; it allows the excretion of urine; it acts as a buffer against shock – sudden pressure upon the uterus is evenly distributed and is less likely to damage the fetus; it allows the fetal swallowing mechanism to develop fully long before it is needed for taking in food after birth. The liquid environment also enables the fetus to begin moving its chest in breathing-like movements before birth. Finally, the amniotic fluid discourages the growth of certain bacteria, and serves as a guard against infection. Samples of the fluid can be taken and tested to check fetal health.

HOW THE PLACENTA WORKS

d Two layers of cells keep the fetal circulation in the placenta separate from the maternal blood. Through these cells the vital exchange function of the placenta takes place. Carbon dioxide, waste products and hormones pass from the fetus to the mother; oxygen, nutrients and hormones are transferred in the opposite direction. Certain drugs will be able to cross from mother to fetus, while others will not.

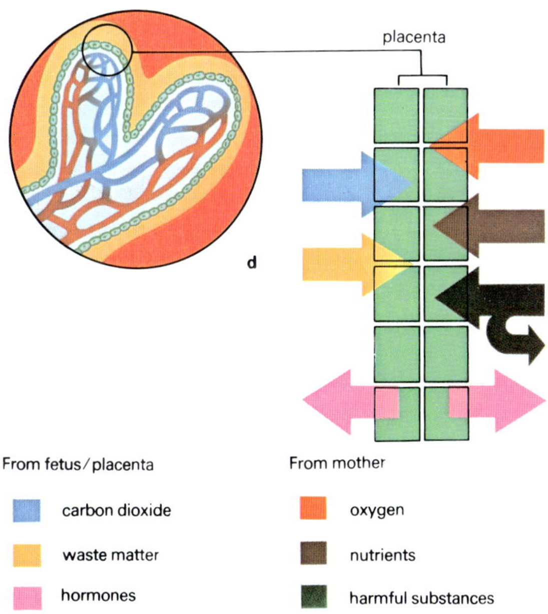

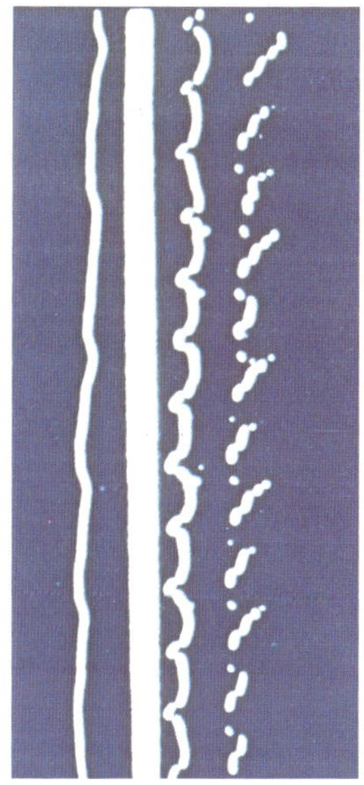

The fetal heartbeat can be detected after about seven weeks of pregnancy. Ultrasound echoes from the fetal heart movement are recorded in waveform. In this readout, the fetal heartbeat is on the right-hand side of the solid white line.

The first trimester

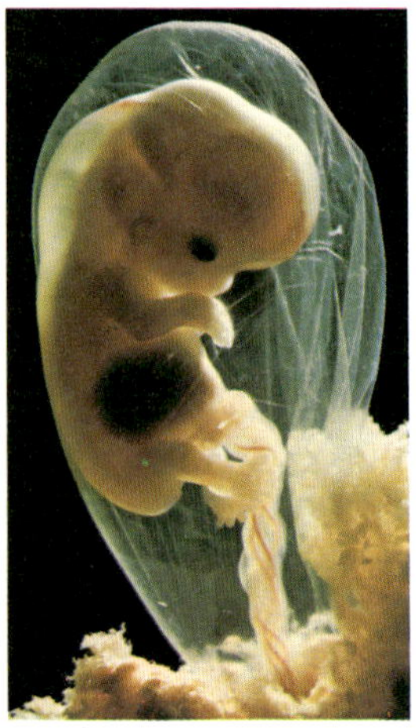

The fetus at 8 weeks with the umbilical cord visible.

The first trimester covers the first thirteen weeks of pregnancy (but since pregnancy is calculated from the date of the last period, and conception takes place about two weeks after a period, this is the first eleven weeks after conception). During this stage we find the most dramatic change of all: from a single cell far too small to be seen by the naked eye to a fetus which is approximately 3 in (75 mm) long and easily recognizable as a small human being, with all the essential organs formed and functioning, although in a primitive way.

3 weeks: In a regular 28-day menstrual cycle, fertilization takes place at the start of the third week and implantation occurs seven days later. Occasionally the process of implantation results in the escape of a few drops of maternal blood from the vagina – the so-called "implantation bleeding".

4 weeks: By the end of the fourth week the embedded pregnancy would be just visible to the naked eye. The embryo is developing and some of the chorionic villi, from which the placenta will develop, have made contact with the maternal blood supply. This primitive placenta has started to produce the human chorionic gonadotrophin (H.C.G.) – a hormone vital to pregnancy as it prevents a menstrual period from occurring (*see* p. 17).

THE DEVELOPMENT OF THE FACE

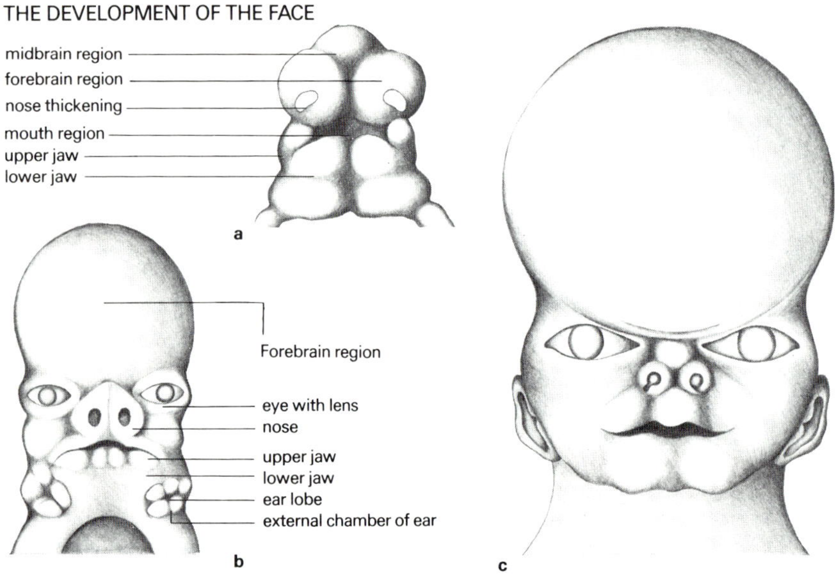

The emergence of a recognizable human face during the first trimester dramatically illustrates the speed at which the fetus develops during the first few weeks of pregnancy:
a the face at $4\frac{1}{2}$ weeks;
b the face at 7 weeks;
c the face at 8 weeks.

5 weeks: During this week a ridge of tissue forms down the length of the embryo. This is the rudimentary nervous system; the large end develops into the brain and the rest forms the spinal cord. In the center of the embryo a blood vessel has formed which will soon become the primitive heart. The amniotic sac is easily identifiable and contains a few milliliters of fluid. At this stage the embryo measures only a fraction over $\frac{1}{10}$ in (2 mm).

6 weeks: The embryo doubles its length to about $\frac{2}{10}$ in (5 mm) and organs begin to form. By the end of the week the spinal cord, brain, ears and eyes have started their development. The tissue from which the lungs form appears as well as the earliest parts of the stomach, liver, pancreas, intestines and kidneys. There are two pairs of limb buds, from which the arms and legs will take shape. The primitive heart starts to beat by the twenty-eighth day following fertilization, although it does not yet look like the heart of a baby.

At this stage the mother may know she is pregnant. Her menstrual period is two weeks "late" and a pregnancy test performed on her urine would usually be positive. She will often have some of the symptoms of early pregnancy – fullness and tingling of the breasts, frequent urination, early morning nausea or even vomiting. If a doctor performed a vaginal examination at this stage he would not be certain that the woman was pregnant but an ultrasound scan would show the pregnancy clearly (*see* p. 54).

7 weeks: The major organs continue to develop during this week. The head is changing very rapidly, and is beginning to look human. The eyes have formed, although the skin covering them – the future eyelids – is still intact. The jaw and mouth are emerging and there are holes for the nostrils although the nose itself is not formed. The head is bent forward over the chest and the whole embryo is C-shaped.

The limb buds have grown and are now clearly identifiable as arms and legs. Small clefts have appeared at their ends which will later separate into fingers and toes. The muscles have started to develop and the earliest bone-forming centers from which the skeleton develops are present.

Blood vessels already extend throughout the body and the heart now has a more complex shape. The intestine is almost com-

The fingers and toes form rapidly during the first trimester. After 13 weeks of pregnancy, the hands and feet already look remarkably similar to those of a mature human although they are still smaller than an adult's fingernail.

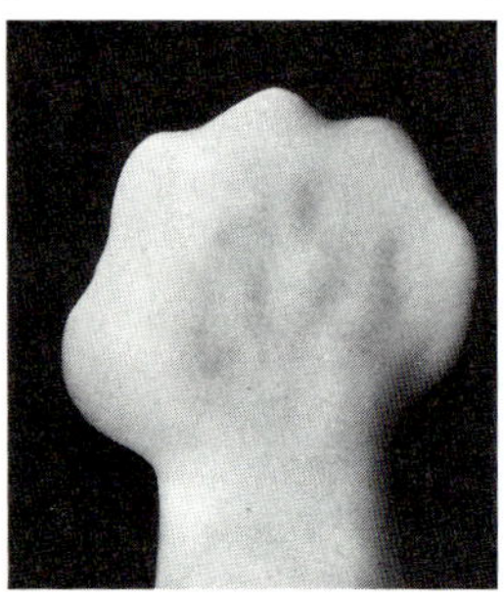

The hand of an embryo at 6 weeks.

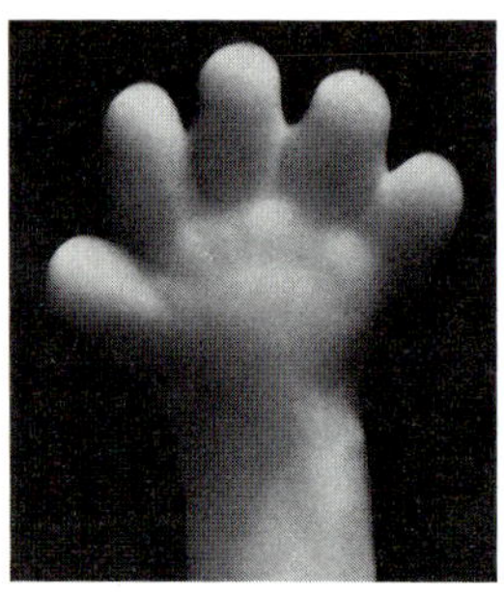

The finger ridges are visible by 7 weeks.

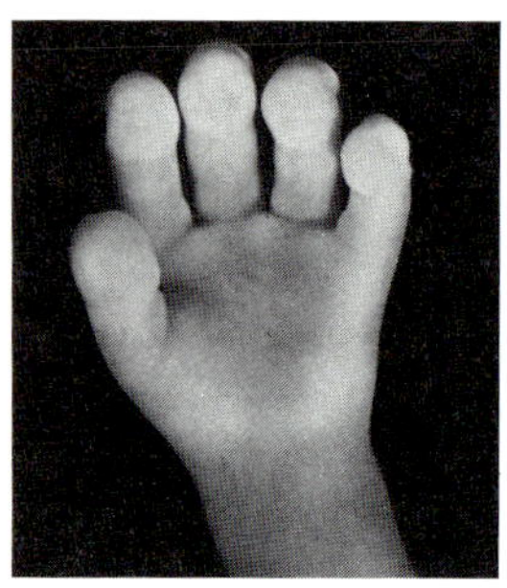

Fingers and thumb with pads seen at 8 weeks.

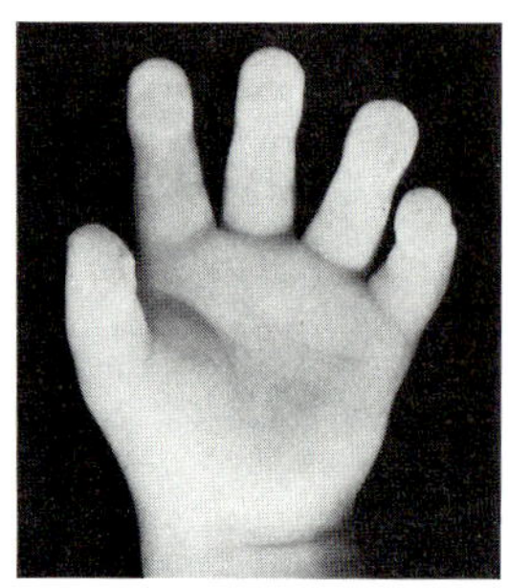

The finger pads have regressed by the 13th week.

plete but is not yet in position; the liver and kidneys have developed but are not functioning. Organs such as the thyroid gland, gall bladder and spleen have started to emerge. The chest is properly formed, though the lungs are still tiny, solid structures. The tissue which will develop into either ovaries or testicles can easily be identified, but it is not possible at this stage to tell the sex of the embryo by examination. An ultrasound scan at the end of the seventh week can show the heart of the embryo beating rapidly at about 160 beats per minute.

8 weeks: By this time almost all the major internal organs have been formed and the finishing touches are being applied to such structures as the spleen and bladder. The heart has been functioning for two weeks, and now some of the other organs begin to function in a primitive way. The eyes already have some coloring and this is the main time for growth of the middle ear – responsible for both hearing and balance. The fold of the external ear has yet to develop.

The head is still very large in proportion to the body but the future neck can already be seen as a groove. The mouth is easily recognizable and the nostrils are beginning to form, although, because of the very rapid growth of the brain at this time, the face occupies a much smaller proportion of the head than it will later. The embryo makes its first small movements at this time and these can be detected by careful ultrasound examination although it will be at least another eight weeks before the mother will be able to feel them.

By the time the second period is missed, the embryo measures some $\frac{6}{10}$ in (17 mm), the pregnancy sac fills about two thirds of the uterine cavity and the uterus itself has grown so that a doctor can readily feel that the mother is pregnant. Henceforth, the embryo is called a fetus. All its parts are present, if not fully formed. From now until the end of pregnancy it will grow larger and the various organs will become more sophisticated and mature until they are capable of sustaining the life functions of the newborn baby.

9–12 weeks: By the end of the tenth week, the inner portion of the ear is complete and the outer part has started to grow. By the end of the twelfth week it will have assumed its adult shape. The muscles develop further and grow so that by the end of this period, the movements of the arms and legs of the fetus are both frequent and purposeful.

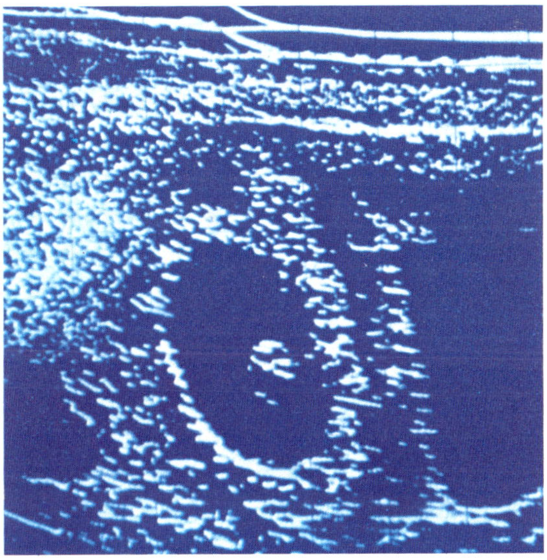

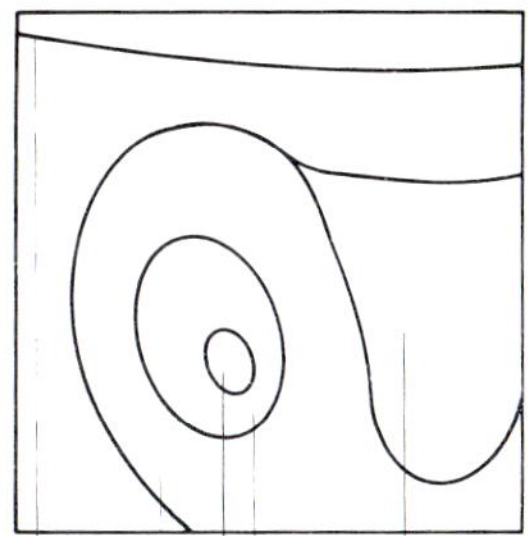

In this photograph of an ultrasound scan, the 8-week-old embryo can be seen as a distinct patch within the cavity of the uterus.

At the end of the twelfth week, the fetus is easily recognizable as a small human being, although the head is still very large in proportion to the body. The various components of the arms and legs can easily be seen but the fingers and toes are still joined together by webbing. The sex of the child was determined at the moment of conception; the ovaries or testicles have now developed within the body but the external genitals are still in that intermediate stage of development where they are neither male nor female.

The heart is completly formed and pumping blood around the fetal body and down the two arteries in the umbilical cord to the placenta, now recognizable as a separate organ.

13 weeks: Though still large in proportion to the body, the head has become erect and the body has started to straighten out. The fingers and toes are now separate digits, and the nail beds, from which the nails will grow, have started to develop. The amniotic sac contains just less than $3\frac{1}{2}$ oz (100 ml) which allows the fetus complete freedom of movement and growth. The uterus has enlarged to the point where it can now be felt as a small, soft swelling just above the pubic bone.

By the end of the first trimester, the fetus is a tiny, but fully formed, human being which weighs 1 oz (30 g) and is 3 in (75 mm) long.

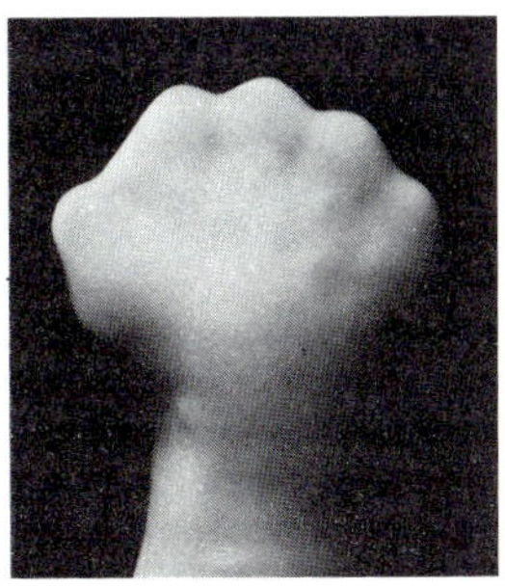

The embryonic foot seen after 7 weeks.

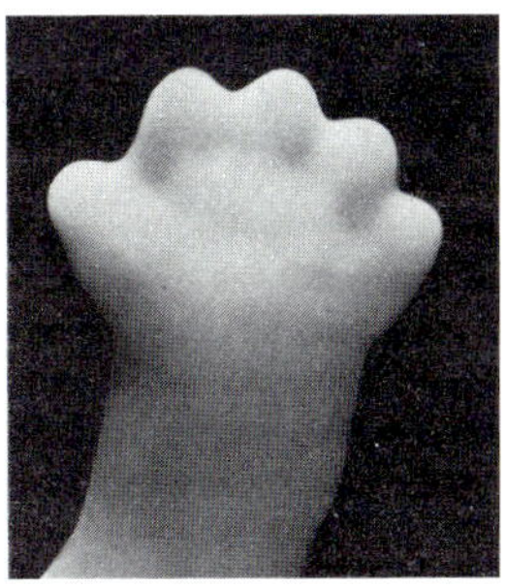

Toe ridges emerge two days later.

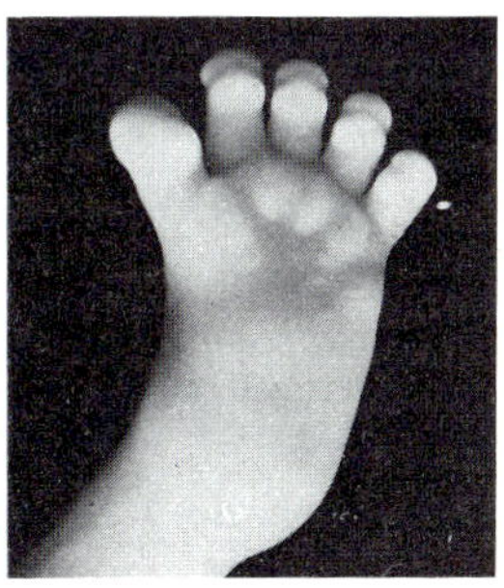

Toe pads and the emerging heel are visible by 9 weeks.

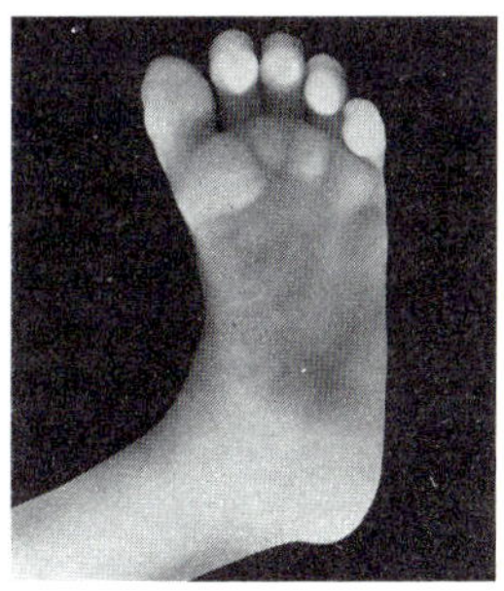

The toe pads have regressed by the 13th week.

The second and third trimesters

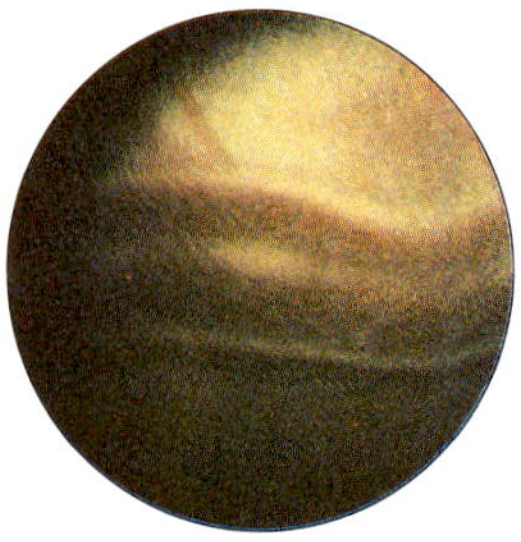

It is now possible, for the first time to see parts of a living fetus within the uterus. This picture shows the umbilical cord. The instrument that makes this feasible is called a fetoscope a slender telescope which can be inserted into the uterus under local anesthetic. The technique has been developed recently, but it has already been used successfully to check aspects of fetal development.

During the last two trimesters of pregnancy all the organs of the fetus increase in size but more important than size or weight are the changes that will enable the baby to accomplish the abrupt change from the fluid environment of the uterus to life in air and to enjoy an existence separate from its mother.

16 weeks: The fetus is now some 6 in (15 cm) long and weighs about 4 oz (120 g). Its tiny body is bright pink as the blood vessels show through the delicate, semi-transparent skin. A fine downy hair is starting to grow over the whole surface of the skin, and the eyebrows and eyelashes are beginning to emerge. All the joints of the limbs can move, the fingers and toes are separate and fully formed, and the fingernails and toenails are in place. The external genital organs have now developed to the point where the sex of the fetus can clearly be distinguished.

The fetus is now making many movements but it is still too early for the mother to feel them. The volume of amniotic fluid has increased to about 8 oz (250 ml) and in this environment, despite the fact that the lungs are very poorly developed, the chest moves from time to time as if the fetus were breathing. These movements will gradually become more frequent and regular but their purpose is not yet understood.

By 18 weeks the fetal heart can be heard with a special stethoscope. Actually, the heartbeat can be visualized as early as seven to eight weeks by using a realtime ultrasound instrument.

Women who are pregnant for the first time usually feel fetal movements at about 19 weeks, whereas those pregnant for the second time tend to sense them some two weeks earlier. The first fetal movements that the mother feels have been variously described as "the fluttering of a butterfly" or "the bursting of tiny bubbles". A week to ten days after first having these feelings the mother is quite sure of their origin and quickly notices their increasing strength.

20 weeks: The weight of the fetus and volume of the amniotic fluid have both doubled between 16 and 20 weeks. The fetus now swallows the amniotic fluid and the kidneys produce fairly large quantities of a still very dilute urine. Scalp hair has started to appear.

The proportions of the different parts of the fetus – head, torso and legs – change dramatically during pregnancy. At this stage, the head accounts for approximately 33 per cent of the total length of the fetus (during the first trimester it was as much as 50 per cent) and the legs take up a similar 33 per cent. By birth, the head will account for 25 per cent and the legs will have increased to 40 per cent.

During the early stage of fetal development the placenta was much larger than the fetus but the two reach equal weights just after the sixteenth week. After that the growth of the placenta is much slower than that of the fetus.

24 weeks: By this stage the fetus weighs about 1 lb 2 oz (500 g). In the U.S. the fetus is now termed viable. If the baby were born it would have little chance of survival, but the birth must be registered whether it lives or dies. The arms and legs have normal amounts of muscle tissue but the body is still thin and the skin a little wrinkled because virtually no fat has formed under the skin. This will occur from now on. The eyelids are no longer fused but remain closed. The glands within the skin start to produce a greasy, cheeselike material known as the vernix. It is thought this acts to prevent any damage to the skin which might result from continuous immersion in the amniotic fluid.

The mother now feels very vigorous fetal

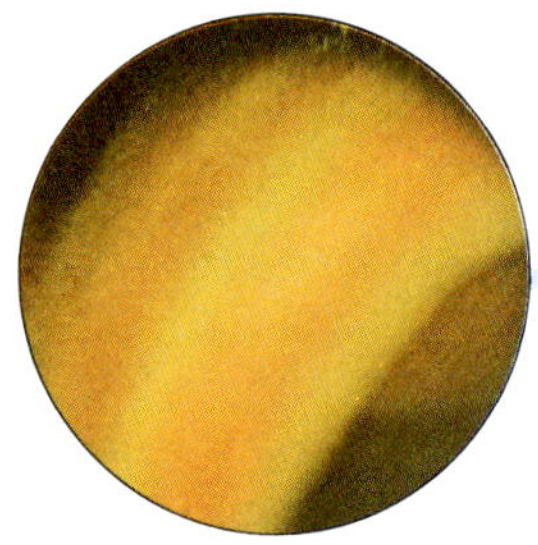

The umbilical cord of a fetus seen through the fetoscope.

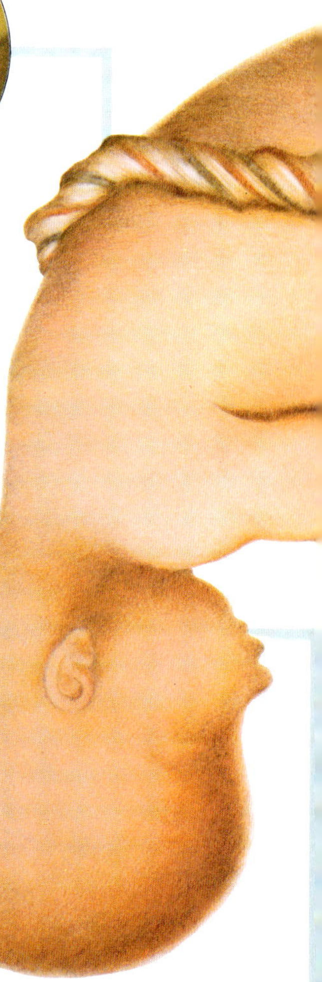

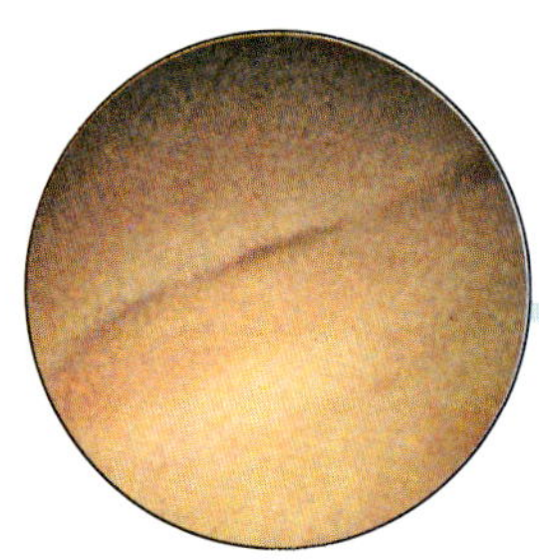

The lips have already formed around the mouth of the fetus by the 17th week.

Photographs can be taken through a fetoscope. Those on this page, including one of a placental blood vessel (above), show parts of a healthy 17–18-week fetus. The absorption of light by the amniotic fluid affects the quality of the photographs, while their color depends on the color of the fluid, which varies from clear to dark yellow. What the doctor sees when looking through the fetoscope is in fact clearer than the photographs suggest.

movements and the uterus has risen to slightly above the level of her navel. Provided the mother is not overweight, an experienced doctor can now feel the position of the fetus in the uterus. Every antenatal examination from now on will include checking the fetal heart and the position of the fetus, although the latter matters little at this stage since the amniotic fluid in which it floats allows the fetus to alter its position at will.

28 weeks: With the laying down of fat under the skin, the body of the fetus starts to grow at a slightly faster rate than the head. By now the whole body is covered with vernix and the fetus weighs approximately 2 lb 3 oz (1000 g). If born at this time, the child would have an 80 per cent chance of survival; it would require intensive neonatal care.

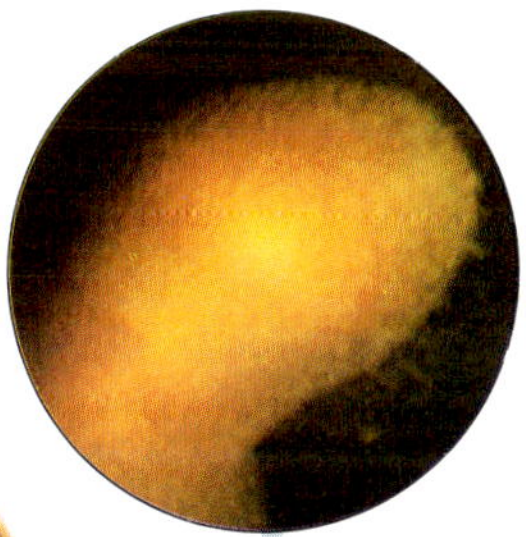

The penis of a healthy 17–18-week fetus.

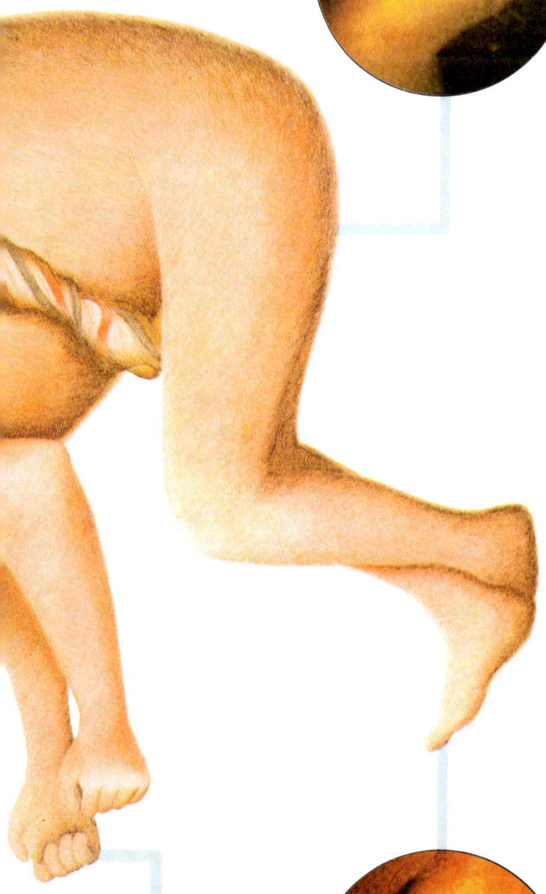

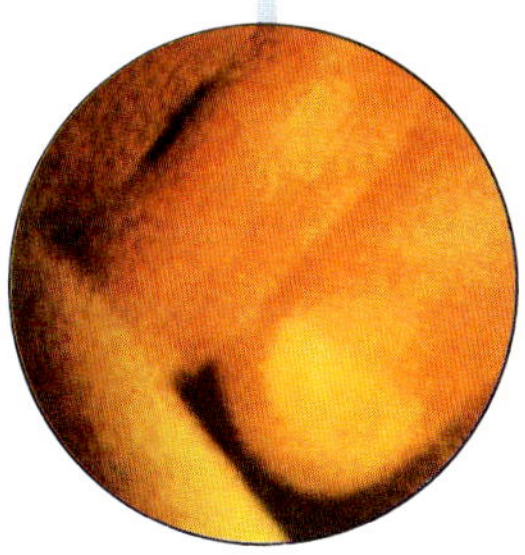

The toes of the fetus are clearly recognizable here.

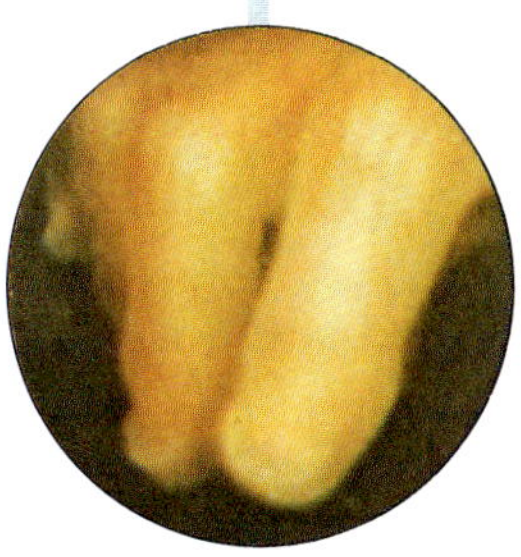

The fetoscope shows that the fetal hands with their nails are developing normally.

Sometimes the mother will feel a gentle rhythmic jarring of her abdomen at intervals of two to three seconds. This is simply the fetus hiccuping, although it is amniotic fluid rather than air which enters and leaves the lung passages. The sensation often lasts for only a short time but it may continue for half an hour or more; it is a normal occurrence and is no cause for alarm.

32 weeks: The four-week interval between the twenty-ninth and thirty-second weeks of pregnancy brings the fetus to the point where, if born prematurely and given good neonatal care, it has a very good chance of living.

The head and body have now almost reached the proportions of a newborn baby. During the last four weeks, the lungs have begun to mature and this process will continue for another four weeks. The fetus now weighs about 4 lb (1800 g) and the placenta just under 1 lb (450 g); the volume of amniotic fluid is approximately $1\frac{1}{2}$ pt (0.7 liter).

36 weeks: Even using the most exact measurements, the head and body are now in the same proportion as those of a newborn baby. A great deal of fat has been laid down. The fetal kidneys are fully mature and the liver is now able to cope with some of the waste products produced. If the fetus is male the testicles have descended into the scrotum. The bones of the skull are still very soft and pliable but this is necessary to allow the head to pass through the birth canal during labor. During the preceding four weeks the lungs have matured considerably and a child born at this time has a better than 95 per cent chance of living.

The fetus now fills the uterus. It is no longer capable of its former weightless acrobatics and usually assumes its final position – in 96 per cent of cases head-down. In approximately half the women having their first baby, the head of the fetus has descended into the pelvis (the medical term is "engaged"), and in the remainder it will do so during the next two weeks (*see* p. 53). In second and subsequent pregnancies, however, this often does not happen until the onset of labor.

40 weeks: As the fetus increases in size and the volume of amnotic fluid decreases the fetus has less space to move about in. The mother often notices this in the last week or two, and at the same time she can often distinguish more easily between arm and leg movements. The fine downy hair has disappeared from most areas of the fetus but is usually still found on the back and shoulders. Throughout the pregnancy as new skin is formed the outermost layer dies and is shed. This process is more pronounced during the last few weeks of intrauterine life, and as the vernix covers the outer layer, it too is shed. As a result, the

Weight and position

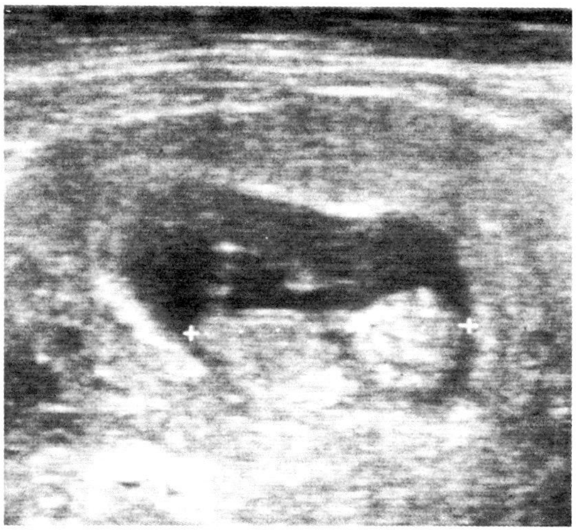

The picture presented by an ultrasound scan is seldom immediately recognizable and requires expert interpretation. In this picture of a fetus 11 weeks and 6 days old, the crosses represent electronic calipers placed at the head (right) and the bottom (left). The "crown rump" measurement, determined by the calipers, will indicate the length of the fetus.

amniotic fluid, formerly clear, becomes milky from the flakes of vernix and skin floating in it. Only a few patches of vernix are still left at birth, usually over the back, in the groin and the armpits.

The average length of human pregnancy is 280 days, or 40 weeks, but, since some fetuses mature faster than others, a full-term pregnancy is usually regarded as one which ends in delivery anywhere between 38 and 42 weeks. Exactly what causes labor to begin is still unknown. It is believed that the fetus itself determines the onset of labor and that it does so when it is mature enough to survive outside the uterus. The birth of premature babies, however, indicates that the fetus, like all humans, is capable of making mistakes. Fortunately these mistakes are rare and seven per cent of babies are born prematurely.

Unlike most members of the animal kingdom, whose young are usually born feet first, all but about four per cent of babies have assumed an upside-down position (i.e. head-down) by the time labor starts. At birth, the average fetus weighs about 7 lb 8 oz (3420 g) but the range of birthweights is quite large, and anything between 5 lb 9 oz (2500 g) and 8 lb 13 oz (4000 g) is regarded as normal. The hair on the scalp at birth varies in length from 0.8 to 1.5 in (2 to 4 cm) and the nails reach to the end of the digits or may even protrude a little. The white part of the eye is fairly white and the iris is nearly always blue because the eye coloring is not fully formed in newborn babies. Exposure to light often changes this color within a few weeks.

During the last trimester the fetus acquires some of its mother's antibodies. These are disease-resisting proteins formed in response to the diseases the mother has had and they give the fetus a temporary immunity to some diseases, like measles, mumps, whooping cough and German measles (rubella), which might otherwise be disastrous to the newborn baby. These antibodies have a short life-span and have usually disappeared by the time the baby is six months old, when he can produce his own antibodies.

The changing weight of the fetus is one important aspect of its development which has been frequently referred to on previous pages. At first the growth is very rapid but during the last few weeks of pregnancy and after birth the rate of growth slows down considerably. This is just as well since, if a baby were to continue growing at the rate of a 34-week fetus, it would weigh about 200 lb (88 kg) at its first birthday.

The weight of the baby at birth is important although it does not necessarily indicate the future health of the child. Birthweight depends on a great variety of factors, over most of which the mother has no control. One such factor is the genes which the child inherits from his or her parents. Sex is determined by the chromosomes which carry the genes (*see* p. 21) and males are generally heavier than females. If born at 40 weeks, male babies are on average 5½ oz (150 g) heavier than female babies. The genetic code is different for each individual and there is at present no way of measuring its exact influence on birthweight. The effect of many other things, including the size of the mother and the situation in which she lives during pregnancy, can, however, be assessed – at least in a broad statistical sense.

Factors affecting birthweight

The old saying that large women have large babies is true enough. Maternal size, including both height and weight, is probably the largest single influence on birthweight. Mothers who eat well, who have enough rest and who pay attention to themselves and to the advice they are given by their doctors also tend to have heavier babies.

Birthweight also tends to increase slightly with each child, so that a second child can be expected to weigh more than the first and a third will usually be heavier still. Twins weigh less than single babies born at the same stage in pregnancy although together they may weigh as much as 13 lb 3 oz (6 kg).

A third factor that affects the weight of the newborn baby is the amount the mother gains herself in pregnancy. We recommend (*see* p. 36) that women gain a maximum of 28 lb (12.5 kg) in pregnancy. Women gaining no weight in pregnancy give birth to babies weighing some 10½–14 oz (300–400 g) less than those gaining 44 lb (20 kg) or more. Women who put on more than 44 lb do little to further increase their babies' weight but, as many have found, they will seldom be able to regain their pre-pregnancy size or shape.

It is, however, difficult to influence the birthweight of an infant consciously by diet during pregnancy. This is because the fetus will generally take what it needs from the mother, even if she can ill afford it. For example, a mother whose diet does not include enough iron may become severely anemic toward the end of pregnancy; yet her baby will not be anemic. In this case the fetus has removed iron from its mother to the detriment of her health. If the mother is severely undernourished fetal growth may be retarded.

EFFECT OF SMOKING
ON FETAL WEIGHT

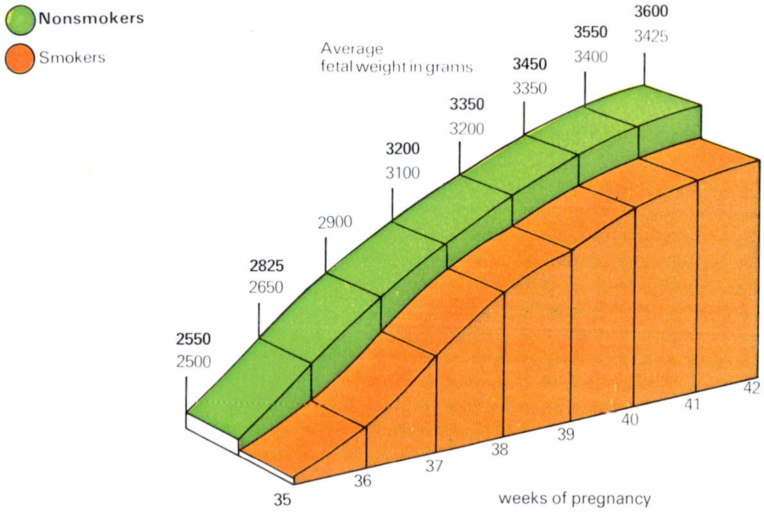

On average babies born to smoking mothers have grown more slowly and have a lower birthweight than those born to non-smokers. They also suffer more long-term ill effects.

Smoking even ten cigarettes a day significantly reduces birthweight. The greater the number of cigarettes smoked during pregnancy, the worse the effect. No pregnant woman should smoke if she wants to give her baby a good start in life. Smoking can be prevented.

Other aspects of maternal health may affect birthweight. For example, inadequately treated diabetes results in an unusually large baby, while raised blood pressure and kidney disease may limit the function of the placenta and therefore result in poor fetal growth and a low birthweight.

Fetal position

During the third trimester, the fetus tends to take up a position in which its spine is parallel to its mother's. As its room for maneuver within the uterus becomes restricted at this time this is the most comfortable position it can adopt.

The majority of babies assume a head-down position toward the end of the third trimester. It is unlikely that this is the most comfortable position for the fetus, as some authors have suggested, but it is certainly the easiest and safest from the point of view of delivery. Since the head is the heaviest part of the fetus it may also be due to gravity. Probably the most important reason is that the space needed for the buttocks and legs is larger than that needed for the head. The upside-down pear-shape of the uterus means that there is more space for the buttocks and legs to be accommodated at the top end.

Once the widest part of the child's head has descended into the pelvic cavity (where the bones of the pelvic girdle surround it), there is unlikely to be any physical obstruction to a normal delivery through the vagina. This descent is known as the engagement of the head. In women who are pregnant for the first time it usually occurs between the thirty-sixth and thirty-eighth week. When this happens, the whole uterus often moves down a little, providing the mother with a sensation of relief; her breathing becomes easier because of the reduction of pressure on her diaphragm and lungs. During second and subsequent pregnancies engagement of the head may not occur until the onset of labor.

Abnormal fetal positions are sometimes the result of an unusual positioning of the placenta or of a multiple birth (*see* chapter 7). It is, however, worth saying something here about the breech presentation which occurs in three to four per cent of births at term. In these cases the fetus fails to settle into the usual head-down position and it is the buttocks (or breech), which are presented for delivery. Breech presentations are particularly common with premature babies and with the second twin. Breech babies have particular problems in labor. If the fetal head is relatively large for the maternal pelvis, difficulty in delivery is likely because the head does not have a chance to mold or change shape. This may cause severe hypoxia and trauma. Therefore, a vaginal delivery is attempted only if all obstetrical conditions are favorable. If a woman has a breech presentation with her first baby, many obstetricians would never deliver her baby through the vagina even if conditions are favorable. This is because the obstetrician does not want to take a chance with an "unproven pelvis". Over half of breech babies are delivered by cesarean section.

The head is engaged when its widest part has passed through the pelvic brim. The lowest portion of the head is then usually at the level of the ischial spines.

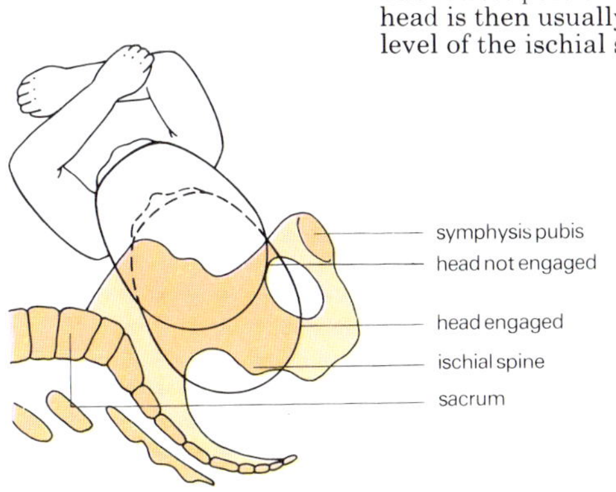

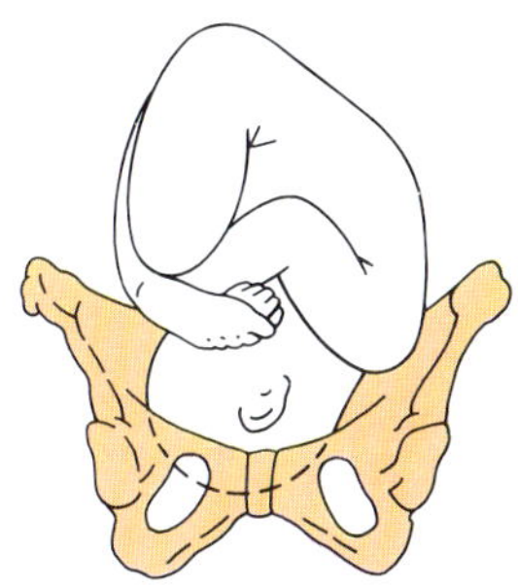

The most common position for the fetus to adopt before birth is shown here, with the head down and facing left.

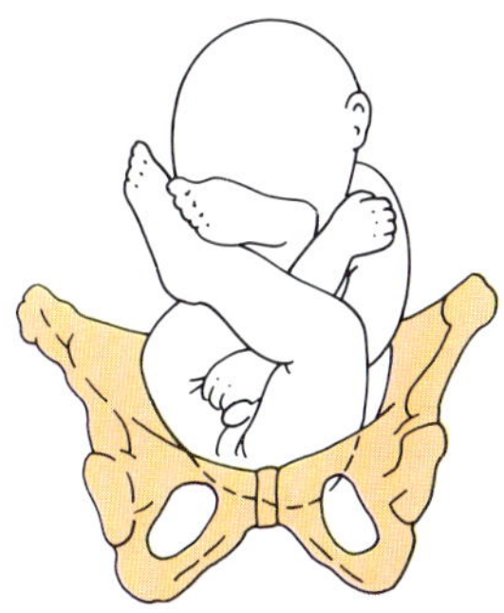

A breech position (above) with the buttocks presented for delivery first, occurs in 3 to 4 per cent of births at term.

Fetal health

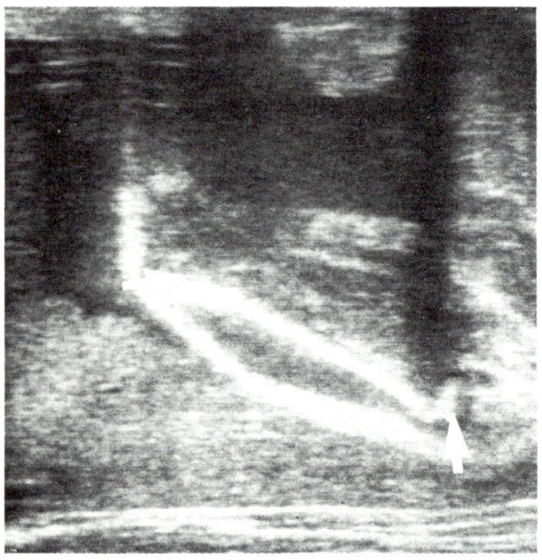

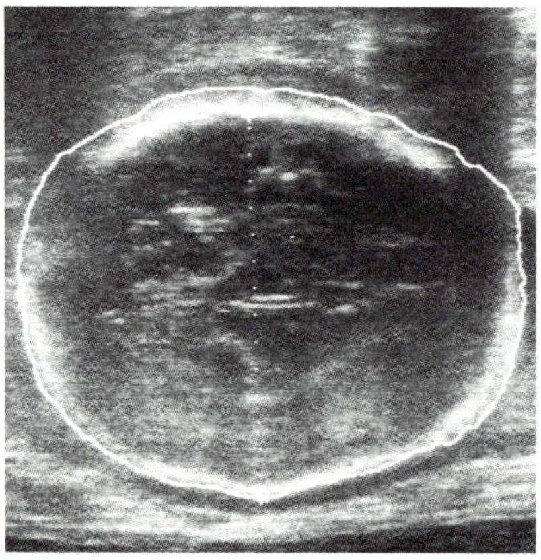

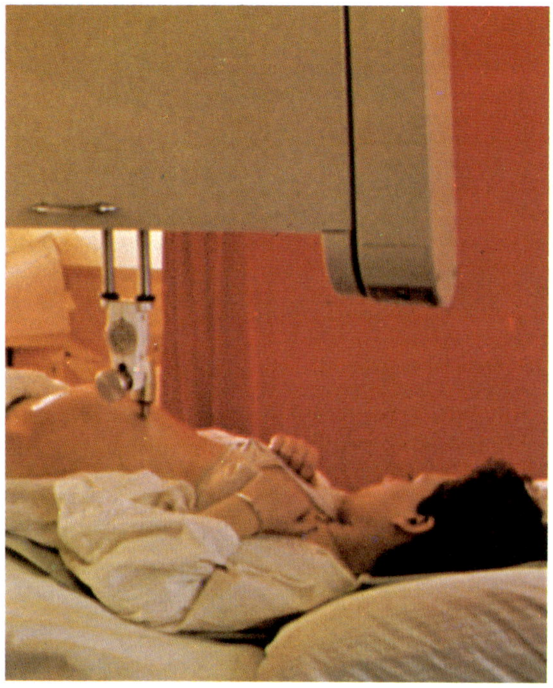

Ultrasound (far right) is a simple, safe and painless procedure which enables the doctor to gauge the development of the fetus. To determine the correct age of the fetus the length of the femur, or thigh bone (above left), and the biparietal diameter of the head (above right) are measured. These measurements are then compared to a table of normal values to determine the age of the fetus. This fetus is 34½ weeks old.

Pregnancy is a healthy process of the body and should not be regarded as a disease. It is, however, a complex process which requires proper antenatal care to ensure that the mother's health does not suffer and that the fetus grows normally. Babies whose intrauterine growth is slow, and who are therefore born smaller than they should be, have a mortality rate four times higher than normal infants. Those that do survive have a significant risk of physical and mental retardation. The first object of antenatal care of the baby is therefore to make sure that the growth of the fetus is progressing well.

Certain mothers, such as those with raised blood pressure and those who smoke – especially heavy smokers – are more likely to have a small baby. Sometimes an obstetrician may suspect that all is not well with the fetus. Vaginal bleeding during the second trimester is associated with poor fetal growth later (although bleeding in the first trimester does not have the same association). Poor maternal weight gain and weight loss (except in the last two weeks of pregnancy) are also associated with poor fetal growth.

Unfortunately, the majority of babies with a low birthweight are born to mothers whose pregnancies are essentially normal. Assessment of fetal growth is therefore one of the most important aspects of antenatal care. The obstetrician has a number of tests for assessing fetal growth; and since growth is a continuous process these assessments will be repeated through pregnancy.

Checking fetal health

At each antenatal visit the pregnant woman is weighed, preferably on the same scales and wearing the same weight of clothing. An experienced doctor can also deduce whether the fetus is growing at the normal rate by carefully feeling the size of the uterus. Some doctors use calipers or a tape measure to get a better record of the growth since the last visit. The heartbeat of the fetus will also be checked simply by using a stethoscope.

It is vital to know as nearly as possible when conception took place. Calculations based on the date of the last menstrual period can be wrong (p. 27). Where doctors are unsure of the length of a pregnancy an ultrasound scan will give a more accurate date.

Ultrasound is now used in nearly all hospitals and it will be worth briefly explaining how it works. The technique, which was first developed during the Second World War to detect enemy submarines, involves transmitting sound waves which are far above the range of human hearing. When these waves strike objects of different densities the returning echoes vary in intensity. The echoes can be shown up as dots of light on a screen.

Ultrasonic examination is a safe procedure which causes no ill effects or discomfort to the patient. The woman lies on a table and her abdomen is coated with an oil which helps to give a clear acoustic picture. As a probe which is attached to the ultrasonic instrument is passed over the woman's abdomen, the doctor interprets the echo picture on the screen to find out the size and position of the fetus.

Ultrasonic measurement of the fetal head circumference and biparietal diameter (width) together with the femur (thigh bone) length, especially early in the second trimester, allows the age of the fetus to be determined accurately. This technique is based on two assumptions: that fetuses do not vary in size much in early pregnancy and that most of the factors responsible for slow fetal growth start at the beginning of the third trimester. Once the age of the fetus has been established, ultrasound can be used to check that the growth rate is normal. It also shows the presence of twins long before either the mother or the doctor suspect they are there.

Fetal health can be indirectly assessed by tests performed on the mother's blood and urine (*see* p. 28). A particular hormone (estriol) is excreted in the mother's urine over a 24-hour period. The level of estriol normally rises in a predictable way as the pregnancy advances. If the level fails to rise, or if it falls, this may mean that there is something wrong with the fetus and/or the placenta. The amount of estriol is not a foolproof indicator of fetal health, since the level can be affected by other factors unassociated with pregnancy. The estriol test has largely been replaced by observing fetal heart rate patterns or examining the fetus with realtime ultrasound.

The pattern of the fetal heartbeat is another indicator of fetal health which is commonly employed and it is called the nonstress test. The fetal heart rate monitor is applied to the mother's abdomen. The acceleration of the fetal heart rate with fetal movement is considered favorable. If such an acceleration does not occur, then the clinician may perform an oxytocin challenge test. An intravenous infusion of dilute oxytocin is started and the heart rate pattern during uterine contractions is studied. Where the mother has three contractions in ten minutes, the fetal heart rate response is evaluated. If there are fetal heart rate decelerations with contractions, this is considered a "positive" test and the fetus may be at risk. The absence of decelerations is a "negative" test which is a favorable result.

One direct method of judging fetal health is for the mother to count the number of fetal movements she feels over a particular timespan, on the assumption that a healthy fetus will move a lot more than one in poor health.

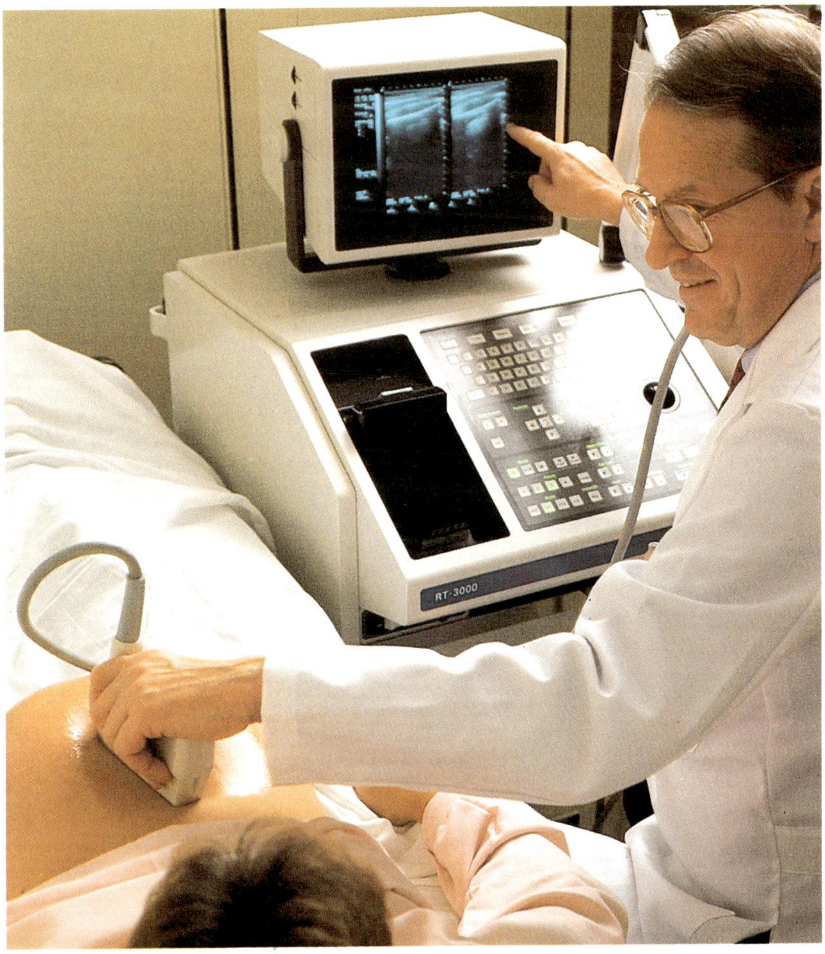

During an ultrasonic examination the mother has the opportunity to see the exact position of the fetus. The doctor will help her to interpret the picture on the screen and explain how the fetus is developing.

Fetal abnormalities

The first question that a mother asks is, "Is my baby all right?" About 95 per cent of the time the doctor is able to say that the baby is fine and healthy but sometimes he or she has to say that something is wrong. This section provides a brief summary of a very complicated topic. Women who wish more information should consult their doctor.

As every baby is unique there can be no definite distinction between what is normal and what is not, but four to five per cent of all births involve some abnormality of the baby. More than half of all abnormalities are slight and require no treatment or can be treated so that the child will not suffer any major handicap. These include such things as birthmarks, extra folds of skin, hernias of the umbilical cord, extra fingers or toes, harelips and minor disorders of the intestine or heart. In two per cent of births an abnormality may be severe.

The causes of abnormality

Fetal abnormalities are divided into two main groups. Inherited problems – which account for less than one in five of all abnormalities – can be traced to one or both parents and may be passed on to the next generation (*see* p. 21). Most congenital abnormalities (that is, abnormalities present at birth) are not inherited from the parents and cannot be passed on to the next generation. They develop after conception because something has interfered with the normal development of the fetus, usually during the first trimester when it is most vulnerable to such influences (*see* p. 47).

Couples who think that there may be an inherited illness or defect on either side of the family should ask their doctor – before starting a pregnancy – to put them in touch with a geneticist (a specialist in the field of heredity). He will inform them whether the defect is inheritable, what the risk factor is in their case, and whether the problem can possibly be diagnosed during pregnancy.

The group of abnormalities not inherited is much larger. The three best-known causes of these abnormalities are infections (e.g. German measles), drugs (e.g. thalidomide), and X rays. These factors cause only a minute proportion of congenital abnormalities, and no cause is known in the vast majority of cases; but if pregnant women observed the following advice, there should be a reduction in the number of congenital defects:

Never take any medications during pregnancy unless they are prescribed by a doctor who is aware that you are pregnant. Avoid people with any infectious disease, especially of the virus type (e.g. influenza). If you are told you need an X ray of the pelvis or abdomen tell the doctor you are pregnant. Wherever possible you should avoid having an X ray during the second half of any menstrual cycle if there is the slightest chance that conception has occurred.

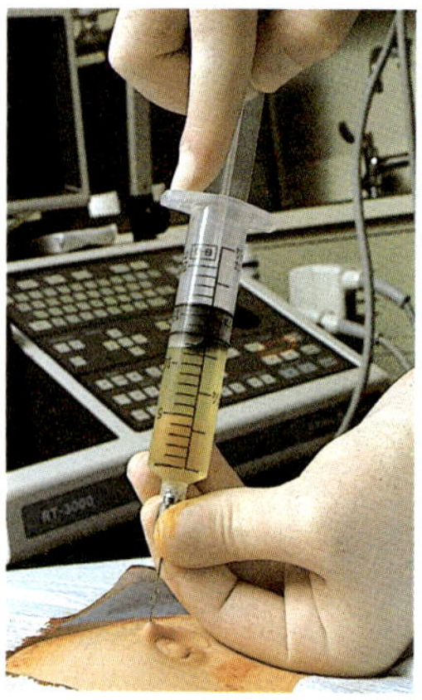

There is no reason why amniocentesis should not be a relaxed procedure (left). The test is carried out by inserting a needle through the mother's abdomen into the amniotic sac (above) to remove a sample of the amniotic fluid.

The mother's age

A woman who has children toward the end of her reproductive years (say, between 35 and 45 years) faces a greater risk of having a child with certain abnormalities than a younger woman. Even so, at the age of 45 she is still very likely to have a perfectly normal child. The risk of having a child with Down's Syndrome (mongolism) increases clearly with the mother's age. Down's Syndrome is caused by the presence of an extra chromosome in each cell (*see* p. 22), which usually causes short stature and slanted eyes (hence the name) and always results in mental handicap. The following table shows how the chance of having a live-born child with Down's Syndrome increases with maternal age. There seems to be a slight link between paternal age and fetal abnormalities.

MATERNAL AGE (inclusive)	33–4	35–6	37–8	39–40	41–2
RISK	1:600	1:350	1:220	1:120	1:60

Other abnormalities caused by chromosomal variations also become more frequent as the mother gets older but the link is less strong and these conditions are all much rarer than Down's Syndrome. None of these risks should prevent an older woman from deciding to have a child but it is certainly sensible for her to take medical advice.

Spina bifida

Spina bifida is a congenital abnormality of the nervous system, called a "neural tube defect", with no known cause. Half of all neural tube defects involve a failure of a major part of the brain and the skull to develop and in these the infant does not survive. In the other half the fetus has a defect somewhere along the spine – hence the name "spina bifida". These babies frequently survive but they may be paralyzed from the waist down. These children may be mentally normal but much more often they tend to be severely mentally handicapped.

In the United States neural tube defects of both kinds occur in 1 out of every 1000 pregnancies. A couple who have produced one child with a neural tube defect are much more likely to have another child with the same defect than a couple who has not had one.

Diagnosis of abnormalities in pregnancy

Most congenital and hereditary abnormalities cannot be diagnosed during pregnancy, and may not be easily diagnosed even at birth. If the condition can be discovered in pregnancy, no form of treatment will undo the damage already done. All that the couple can be offered is the choice between continuing with the pregnancy or terminating it.

Amniocentesis

The chief method of diagnosing abnormalities at present is the amniocentesis, in which a sample of the amniotic fluid is taken for analysis. The test is best performed at about

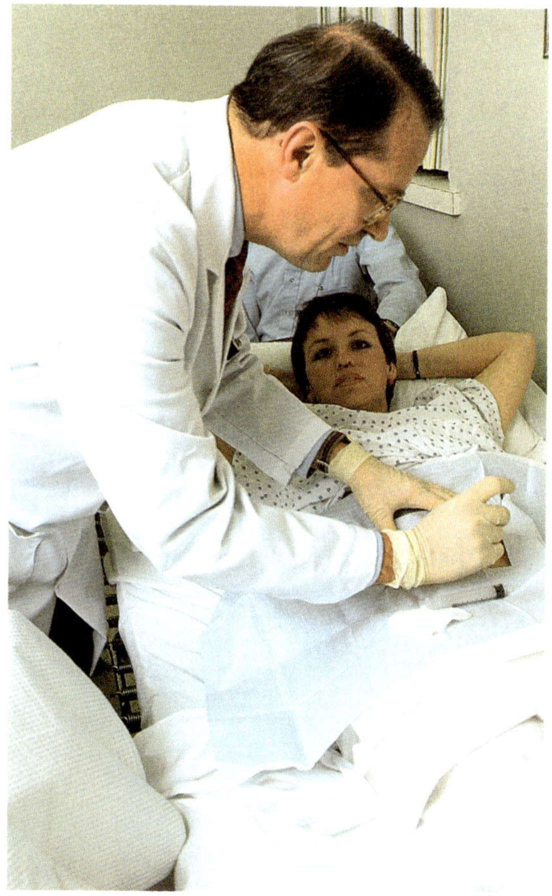

15–17 weeks when the fetus can easily spare the $\frac{7}{10}$ oz (20 ml) usually removed. The technique is fairly simple: a needle is inserted through the mother's abdomen into the amniotic sac. Amniotic fluid is then aspirated.

The amniotic fluid contains cells which have been shed by the growing fetus. Some of these are alive, and can be separated from the liquid in which they float and analyzed for chromosomal abnormalities. Such analysis is highly specialized and the result is often not available for three weeks.

The amniotic fluid, minus its cells, can also be tested for chemicals which are found in abnormal amounts where there are certain congenital abnormalities (for example, spina bifida or anencephaly). With this type of test the answer is usually available within a week.

In the past antenatal diagnosis of this kind was limited to those couples who were very seriously in danger of giving birth to an abnormal child. Now, most doctors offer the choice of amniocentesis to all women over the age of 35 and to those who have a history of a child with spina bifida.

The technique of amniocentesis, however, brings with it some risks which can be reduced by using ultrasound to show the position of the fetus and the placenta before the needle is introduced. Even so, about 1 in every 500 women who have amniocentesis subsequently has a miscarriage. This is important and must be weighed against the risks of giving birth to

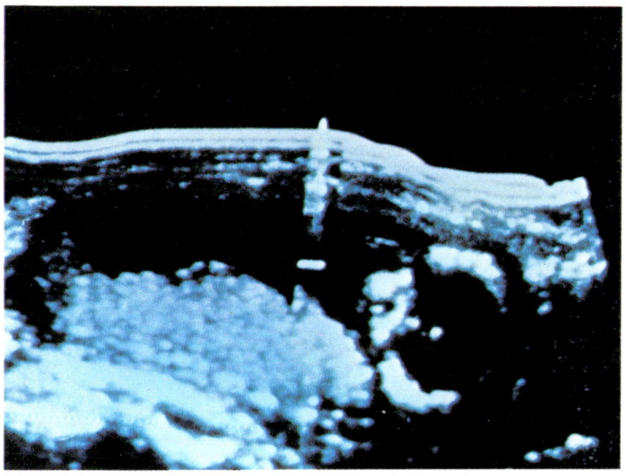

Inserting a needle into the uterus is not without risks as it may be followed by a miscarriage in a very small percentage of cases. The use of an ultrasound scan (above) to establish the position of the fetus and guide the needle does, however, reduce the danger.

The fetoscope is the very latest tool designed to check the health of a fetus. It enables the doctor to look at the fetus directly, through a needle inserted in the uterus (below). Photographs of part of a living fetus taken through a fetoscope can be seen on pages 50 and 51.

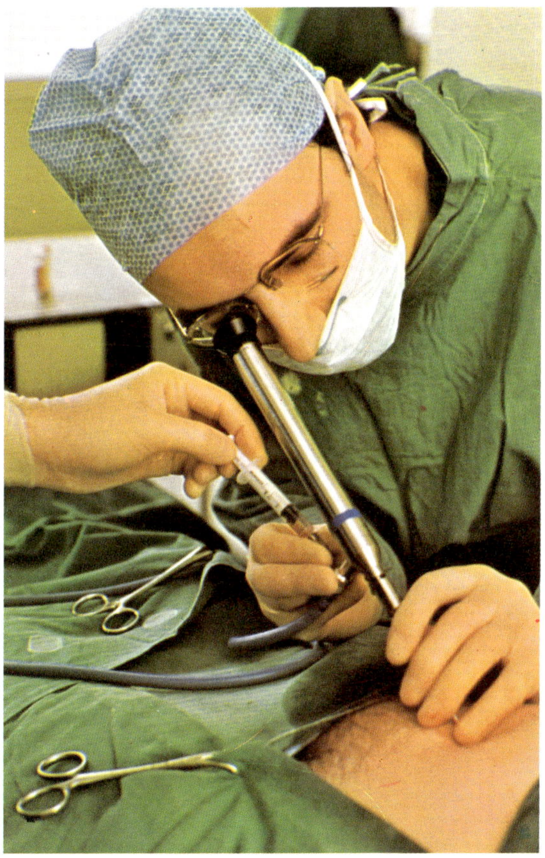

a child with a particular defect. It is therefore vital that the couple should know the numerical risks involved before they decide to have the test. A specialist will be able to advise them about the risks; the final decision to go ahead and have the amniocentesis can only be made by the couple themselves.

Chorionic villus sampling

A new technique for obtaining a sample for genetic diagnosis is called chorionic villus sampling. The main advantages are that the procedure is done earlier in pregnancy, at eight to ten weeks' gestation, and sampling villi allows more rapid diagnosis than genetic amniocentesis in which exfoliated cells from the amniotic fluid have to be grown in culture.

A soft, slender catheter is passed through the cervix under the guidance of ultrasound. A syringe is used to aspirate chorionic villi for genetic studies. Although this procedure has many advantages, it has a higher pregnancy loss than genetic amniocentesis. The best estimates of pregnancy loss range from 1 to 3 per cent.

Other methods of diagnosis

A simple method of screening for all women involves taking a blood sample at about 16 weeks for alpha fetoprotein levels. This can be used to identify possible defects in the nervous system of the fetus (like spina bifida). Although this method of screening is not foolproof it has rapidly become popular in regions where these defects are relatively common and some doctors now use it as a matter of routine. The technique is useful because it makes it possible to determine women who are thought to be at risk. If the result is abnormal the woman is then recommended to have an amniocentesis to confirm whether or not the fetus has an abnormality. Where there is an abnormality the couple are offered the possibility of terminating the pregnancy. It is expected that, by performing selective terminations of affected pregnancies, the number of babies born with defects of the nervous system could be reduced to something like one quarter of the present total. It is important to remember, however, that in all such cases the major decisions – from whether to have an amniocentesis to whether to continue with the pregnancy – are always left with the parents.

Ultrasound, which does not usually show minor fetal malformations, can sometimes show a major abnormality like spina bifida. There is also a new tool which allows the obstetrician to see the fetus in the uterus. This is a very fine telescope, called a fetoscope (*see* p. 50), mounted on a needle, which is passed through the mother's abdomen in the same way as for an amniocentesis. By looking through it the obstetrician can see if the fetus has any external abnormalities. The fetoscope also makes it possible to take samples of fetal blood for analysis.

Chapter 4
Major and minor problems in pregnancy

Almost every pregnant woman will at some time find she has symptoms that she does not usually have. Some complaints, like nausea or backache, are very common, others like skin rashes, are comparatively rare. In this chapter symptoms and complications of pregnancy are described in alphabetical order. In order to avoid repetition, there are many cross references between symptoms and complications or diagnoses. This chapter should be used like a dictionary for looking things up, rather than reading straight through. The chapter is not totally comprehensive, for reasons of space, but all the common and some of the less common complaints in pregnancy are here. For complaints that are left out, your doctor will be able to enlighten you. Each section gives a short explanation of the condition, with the cause, if known, and describes the usual treatment. Sometimes there is more than one available treatment, and different doctors prefer different treatments.

Most complaints in pregnancy are a nuisance, and some are very unpleasant for the woman; but many do not produce any serious risk to her or to the baby. Others are potentially dangerous and require medical advice. If so, this fact is given at the end of the appropriate section. On many occasions a complaint is not dangerous, but medical advice as to treatment is necessary, because many pills that people normally take are not safe in pregnancy. Medications or pills should be obtained only from your doctor and not just taken out of the medicine cabinet.

It is a well-known fact that medical students and nurses think they are suffering from every illness which they are learning about. Similarly pregnant nurses and doctors may worry about all sorts of complications of pregnancy which they know about but haven't got. Some pregnant women reading this chapter may also worry about things they have read. Some people are worriers, others are not. Mothers-to-be who worry should remember that the vast majority of women pass happily through pregnancy with no serious complications at all. The minority of pregnant women who do have complications should remember that modern antenatal care can prevent many problems from ever becoming serious, and that successful treatment is now available for those complications that were once feared.

ABDOMINAL PAIN

There is a very long list of possible causes for pain in the abdomen in pregnancy. Some types of pain are caused by a complication of pregnancy, others are due to a variety of conditions like indigestion which people can have whether they are pregnant or not. It is important to be able to decide which pains mean you should contact your doctor. The ones which require medical advice are listed here.

When to see your doctor:

1. All types of pain which are spasmodic (like period pains) and which come and go at short intervals (15 minutes or less), particularly if they are associated with the loss of any blood or fluid from the vagina. These pains can occur at any stage of pregnancy, and they must be distinguished from Braxton Hicks contractions (*see* below, **premature labor**), which are not painful.
2. Any other pain which is associated with loss of blood or fluid from the vagina.
3. Pain in the abdomen or back associated with fever, feeling ill, vomiting or diarrhea.
4. Any other severe abdominal pain.
5. Any pain which persists for more than one hour.
6. Pains in the chest associated with abdominal pain.

There are other pains which can wait until your doctor's appointment provided they are mild. Examples are mild low back pain, recurrent indigestion or heartburn.

As a general rule it is better not to take pills from the medicine cabinet for any abdominal pain in pregnancy unless you have already checked with your doctor that they are safe.

In most cases of abdominal pain in pregnancy the doctor can make a prompt diagnosis of what is the cause; but sometimes the cause is very obscure. In this situation, and if the pain is persistent, your doctor may recommend a short period of observation in the hospital until the cause is discovered or the pain gets better. The treatment of any abdominal pain depends entirely on its cause.

ACCIDENTAL HEMORRHAGE: **Placental abruption**

Accidental hemorrhage has nothing to do with having an accident. It is a form of vaginal bleeding or **antepartum hemorrhage** which is caused by the separation of some of the placenta from the wall of the uterus before the delivery of the baby. It is a most uncommon occurrence and the cause is unknown. The condition is serious because it interrupts the oxygen supply to the fetus and can lead to serious blood loss in the mother.

The symptoms of this condition are bleeding from the vagina and constant pain in the lower abdomen after 28 weeks and before labor. The amount of blood loss is variable; it may not be very much but is always more than a period. These symptoms require urgent medical advice and hospital treatment because the condition is dangerous for the mother and baby. Quite often some blood collects inside the uterus behind the placenta and drains out very slowly. A woman with this condition may therefore lose more blood from her circulation than is immediately apparent.

If only a small area of the placenta separates and a woman reaches the hospital quickly, the fetus may be found to be alive but distressed from lack of oxygen. In this case rapid delivery, usually by cesarean (*see* pp. 93–5 and 109), can produce a live healthy baby. Unfortunately, in many cases too much of the placenta is damaged and the baby cannot survive. In these circumstances labor is induced and the baby is delivered as quickly as possible. There is often more bleeding as the placenta is delivered, but the blood can be replaced by a blood transfusion if necessary.
See doctor immediately.

ALBUMINURIA *see* Proteinuria

AMNIOTIC FLUID, too little or too much (oligohydramnios and polyhydramnios)

Oligohydramnios is present when there is less amniotic fluid around the baby than normal; and polyhydramnios is present when there is too much amniotic fluid. It can be quite difficult to decide in the doctor's office whether a woman has too much or too little amniotic fluid.

If the uterus is much bigger or smaller than expected, then an abnormal volume of fluid is a possible cause. The amount of fluid cannot be easily measured directly but it can be estimated. If the baby is easily felt with the wall of the uterus touching all around then oligohydramnios may be present. If the uterus is distended and it is only possible to feel part of the baby in it and the baby floats away from the examining hand then polyhydramnios is present. An **ultrasound scan**, will confirm whether there is a lot or a little fluid present.

Oligohydramnios is relatively common in the last two or three weeks of normal pregnancies. The amniotic fluid diminishes and the woman often loses some weight at the same time. This reduction of fluid is more likely to occur in association with a **small-for-dates** baby or **placental insufficiency**, and in such cases it can occur much earlier in the last trimester. Oligohydramnios is also caused by **premature rupture of the membranes** when some of the fluid leaks out. In very rare cases it occurs when the fetal kidneys are not producing normal amounts of urine.

Polyhydramnios is sometimes suspected in the middle trimester in normal pregnancies. In these women no cause is found, and the amount of fluid then seems to become normal as pregnancy progresses. Several problems of fetal or maternal health can also cause polyhydramnios. These are **Rh immunization** (*see* chapter 2); **diabetes** (*see* below) associated with a large baby; **twins**; and, very rarely, certain abnormalities of the fetus such as **spina bifida** or **anencephaly** (*see* chapter 3). Polyhydramnios can also occur if the baby is not swallowing normal amounts of the amniotic fluid.

Polyhydramnios is usually fairly mild and the main problem it causes is discomfort to the mother. Occasionally, however, polyhydramnios is really excessive. In these cases the uterus becomes very distended, tense and uncomfortable, and it may be necessary to rest in the hospital.

The cause, if any, of polyhydramnios can by found by doing urine tests, blood tests and an X ray or an ultrasound scan. The worst cases are usually caused by a rare complication of twins, where the blood circulation of the two babies mixes in part of the placenta, or by some abnormality of the baby.

The treatment depends on the cause. If the baby appears to be normal then it is better for the woman to ease her discomfort by resting in bed. Sometimes some fluid can be removed by doing an **amniocentesis** (*see* p. 56). Labor is induced as soon as the baby is mature or earlier if the distension of the uterus is serious. If the baby is not normal then labor will be induced as soon as possible.

AMNIOCENTESIS *see* p. 56

ANEMIA

A mild degree of anemia is very common in pregnancy. It can be prevented by taking iron and folic acid pills during pregnancy, starting when the nausea of early pregnancy stops (*see* p. 33). Some women find that these pills make them constipated – a nuisance, but usually avoidable, as there are many different types of pills on the market and it should be possible for most women to find one variety that will suit them.

Severe anemia sometimes develops in women who either were anemic before they became pregnant or who have lost blood during the pregnancy. In cases of severe anemia, iron may be given by injection or with the help of an intravenous drip. In the latter case, the mother will need to spend a short time in the hospital.

Certain races and ethnic groups are more prone to anemia than others. These groups include people of Mediterranean background as well as some Blacks. The types of anemia from which they suffer, known as Mediterranean anemia, or Thalassemia, and sickle-cell anemia respectively, are caused by the presence of unusual types of hemoglobin (the red pigment in the blood cells). In these cases the anemia cannot be cured by iron treatment but can usually be improved by taking the vitamin folic acid.

ANTEPARTUM HEMORRHAGE

Bleeding from the uterus after 28 weeks of pregnancy and before labor may take the form of a few spots of blood on the clothes or it may be as heavy as a period. On rare occasions, enough blood may be lost to require a blood transfusion. Women should always get medical advice for any blood loss during pregnancy.

There are several causes of antepartum hemorrhage. Bleeding from the cervix, which has an increased blood supply in pregnancy, sometimes occurs after intercourse. Bleeding can also occur from a **placenta previa** (*see* below) or from placental abruption, sometimes called **accidental hemorrhage** (*see* above). Sometimes no cause for the bleeding is ever found. Antepartum bleeding comes from the mother, rarely from the baby.
See doctor immediately.

ANXIETIES in pregnancy

At the beginning of pregnancy most women are very pleased that they have conceived and that they are fertile. This is a very normal reaction, but the fact of the pregnancy is often associated with all sorts of practical problems which may cause anxiety for the mother-to-be.

For some people living quarters are inadequate for a child, or another child, and the family must move to a larger home or apartment. For some women, a first pregnancy leads to marriage, or changing from a working woman to a full-time mother. For an unfortunate minority of women, although pregnancy may be wanted by them, their social situation makes it impossible for them to bring up a child. These women may have to consider a termination of pregnancy.

For women who have waited several years for a baby, early pregnancy is a time of great happiness, but also there is usually some anxiety that the pregnancy will end unsuccessfully.

Nearly all women are anxious at the beginning of pregnancy that they might miscarry, and most women feel much more relaxed when they reach the middle trimester when the likelihood of a miscarriage is over. They also feel happier because their nausea usually subsides and sleepiness improves at this time. It is a great thrill when the baby can be felt moving in the middle of pregnancy and a relief to know all is well. In the third trimester most women feel well, but find that things take longer to do because of the extra weight! At this stage time is usually spent preparing for the new baby.

Throughout pregnancy there are a number of common anxieties which afflict many pregnant women. Many women worry about pain in labor and whether they can control themselves. It is a good thing to discuss with your doctor what is available for pain relief in labor (*see* also chapter 5). Many women get tremendous help from attending antenatal classes and learning techniques such as psychoprophylaxis for use in labor.

A number of women are very worried about having an abnormal baby. It should be remembered that most abnormal babies are miscarried in the first three months of pregnancy, and that relatively few are actually born. In the middle trimester some abnormalities can be detected by amniocentesis at about 16 weeks of pregnancy when there is still time for a termination. These abnormalities are Down's Syndrome, other abnormalities of the chromosomes, spina bifida and a few other rare conditions. If you are especially worried about any particular abnormality, then discuss it with your doctor early in pregnancy and he will advise you if there is likely to be a risk and whether it would be advantageous to have an amniocentesis performed. Women with a history of Down's Syndrome or spina bifida in their family, and women over 35 years or approaching 35 years of age, are usually recommended to have the test done. There is still a small risk of abnormality which can occur in any pregnancy, but it should be remembered that the vast majority of babies are perfectly normal (*see* chapter 9).

Some women, particularly those who have already lost a baby through stillbirth, worry about their baby surviving. At this moment about 15 out of every 1,000 babies born die just before or after birth. This means that 985 out of 1,000 babies born survive. The chance of losing a baby is extremely small in normal healthy women, but some complications of pregnancy may increase the risk. If a woman has already lost a baby it is usually better if she can find out why it happened so that all precautions can be taken in her next pregnancy to avoid any trouble.

A few women fear they will not survive labor. With modern maternity care, normal healthy women who have regular antenatal check-ups, and take medical advice seriously, need not worry about their own safety.

The maternal mortality in the U.S. is less than 14 in every 100,000 pregnant women. In many cases this tragedy happens when a woman has not had antenatal care or when she has ignored advice to go into the hospital for some complication of pregnancy. Others of these tragic cases are women who have some serious medical condition such as heart disease which increases the risk to them presented by pregnancy. Any woman with any medical condition can always get advice from her doctor as to whether pregnancy might be any risk to her. If she has decided to have a baby, then she should start her antenatal care early in the first trimester. She and her doctor may decide that she should be cared for at a medical center. There are many thousands of women with quite serious medical conditions who have had a successful pregnancy and a safe delivery with proper care.

Other anxieties in pregnancy relate to life after the child is born. Many women worry about their ability to look after a child, some worry about the responsibility and restrictions of their freedom and others worry about relationship to their husband or partner.

Another worry may be child care. It is one of the unfortunate results of small families that many women are unfamiliar with babies. They cannot remember having younger brothers and sisters. Child care is in fact not very difficult and the population explosion has demonstrated that most mothers do very well bringing up their children. The nurses on the postpartum floor make sure before a woman goes home that she is able to feed, bathe, change and care for her baby. Mothers, mothers-in-law, friends and relatives will all help sometimes whether you want it or not. Your pediatrician or a newborn baby clinic is a good place to go for advice about any worries you may have about your baby.

Other worries that people have about pregnancy usually relate to the effects on them and their baby of pregnancy complications. Some pregnancy complications certainly do increase the risk to the baby, but it may only be slight. Information on complications which can affect the baby is given in this chapter. If you are particularly worried about one special problem, then discuss it with your doctor. Most things are not so bad when the facts are known.

Pregnancy complications which are treated by admission to the hospital can cause great worries. There may be problems about arranging care for other children at home. Sometimes a father cannot get time off from work to help. The hospital social workers can be a great help in solving many family and home problems.

BACKACHE

Backache is often a very troublesome complaint in pregnancy. Women who start a pregnancy with any back complaint find it aggravated during pregnancy; other women may get backache either during the pregnancy or after the baby is born.

During pregnancy the joints of the back and pelvis loosen (*see* p. 14). There is also a shift in the center of gravity of the body, because of the increasing weight in the front part of the woman's body. To compensate for this shift a woman has to bend the top half of her body backwards a little, in order to keep her balance (*see* p. 40). Very high-heeled shoes put additional strain on the back and should be avoided during pregnancy.

Backache in pregnancy can be relieved in a number of ways. Women can wear low-heeled shoes and do exercises to strengthen the muscles which support the joints in the back. Advice on which exercises are best and advice on posture can be obtained from a physiotherapist (*see also* p. 76). Since most people spend about eight hours in bed at night this is also an important time for looking after the back. Very soft mattresses allow the body to sag in the middle, causing backache whichever way a woman lies. It is much better to have a good firm mattress and if necessary place a large board under it, allowing the back eight hours in a good position.

Very severe backache sometimes occurs in people who have previously suffered from back conditions such as a slipped disc. Medical advice is desirable in these cases. X rays of the back should be avoided in early pregnancy as they may harm the fetus. Treatment for severe problems is usually rest in the hospital on a very firm orthopedic mattress with boards under it, until the pain goes or until labor starts. If a slipped disc does not respond to treatment, and the baby is mature, labor can be induced.

BACTERURIA *see* Urinary infections.

BLEEDING *see*
- Accidental hemorrhage;
- Antepartum hemorrhage;
- Ectopic pregnancy;
- Evacuation of the uterus;
- Hydatidiform mole;
- Mid-trimester miscarriage;
- Miscarriage;
- Placenta previa;
- Urinary infections.

BLOOD PRESSURE *see*
- Hypertension;
- Edema;
- Proteinuria.

BRAXTON HICKS CONTRACTIONS *see*
- Premature Labor.

BREASTS *see* Leaking breasts;

BREECH

The presenting part of a fetus is the part which is lying over the cervix, so it is the first part of the baby to be born. If the fetus is lying with its bottom downward and head up, this is called a breech presentation or a "breech" for short – the breech being the baby's bottom. The more common position is head-down, and this is called a cephalic (meaning head) or a vertex (meaning top of the head) presentation.

Generally, if your doctor suspects that your fetus is in a breech presentation an ultrasound scan will be done. If you are still in early pregnancy watchful waiting is in order because the fetus may turn spontaneously.

In pregnancy the fetus has plenty of room in the uterus and can lie in any position inside it. Toward the end of the middle trimester many babies are found lying as a breech. During the next few weeks the majority of these babies turn themselves around and lie head-down as a cephalic or vertex presentation. Because of this, very premature babies are often born as a breech, but most term babies are born as a vertex (*see* chapter 7).

A breech delivery is more difficult than a vertex delivery. There are also certain complications sometimes associated with breech babies. First, for the reasons already explained, many premature babies are born as a breech, and although the actual delivery of a premature baby is usually easy because they are so small, the baby may suffer the usual complications of being premature (*see* below, **premature labor**).

The second problem of breech delivery is that the baby's head – the largest part of the baby – is born last, and if there is a tight fit between the baby's head and the mother's pelvis, delay can occur when the baby is already half delivered. In order to avoid any undue delay, which would be dangerous, it is essential to know that the mother's pelvis is a reasonable size before the delivery. For this reason X rays are taken of the mother's pelvis before labor or very early in labor in all women with a full-term breech baby. The size of the pelvis can be measured from the X rays and the baby's head size can also be measured from an **ultrasound scan** (*see* below). If there is likely to be a tight fit between the baby's head and the mother's pelvis it is safer for the baby to be delivered by cesarean section. If there is plenty of room for the baby's head, then a breech delivery should be relatively easy.

The third problem with a breech delivery is that if a mother has any complications such as raised blood pressure, or has a small-for-dates baby (*see* below, **slow fetal growth**), then there is an increased risk to the baby born as a breech. In these cases the doctor may also recommend a cesarean section for a safer delivery.

Because of the problems associated with breech deliveries many doctors recommend turning the baby around, a procedure called "version", during the last few weeks of pregnancy. There is no advantage to be gained from doing a version before 32 weeks, as the majority of babies which are lying as a breech before this time turn themselves around. After 32 weeks many babies still turn around – sometimes just before labor starts – but it is not possible to tell which babies will and which will not be able to turn themselves. Medical opinion differs as to whether it is best to try to do a version on all breech babies after 32 weeks or to leave them alone.

Version can be very easy provided there is plenty of fluid around the baby and the mother's abdominal muscles are fairly relaxed. The doctor places two hands on the mother's abdomen. First, with gentle pressure, the doctor must ease the breech out of the mother's pelvis, then it is slowly pushed up one side of the mother's abdomen with one hand while the other hand guides the baby's head down the other side of the abdomen until it rests over the pelvic brim. If version is not easy, or causes any discomfort to the woman, then it is better not to do it at all, because a difficult version can produce damage to the placenta and this would constitute a potential risk to the baby.

A more detailed discussion of breech delivery can be found in chapter 7.

CALCIUM TABLETS *see* Cramps
CARPAL TUNNEL syndrome *see* Edema
COLOSTRUM *see* Leaking breasts

CONSTIPATION

Constipation is a fairly common complaint in pregnancy. It is important to realize that it is not necessary for a pregnant woman to have a bowel movement every day but, whatever the frequency of her bowel movements, the motion should not be too hard and straining should not be necessary.

The best treatment for constipation is by diet rather than by laxative. Most of the diets recommended for constipation include high fiber foods such as bran – as found in bran varieties of breakfast cereal. Other meals should contain plenty of vegetables. Sometimes iron pills make constipation worse, and it is then best to try another type of iron preparation, as it is usually possible to find one which is less constipating.

If dietary treatment fails, a laxative may be necessary, particularly for women who habitually take one. Not all are safe in pregnancy, so advice on the safe varieties should be obtained from the doctor who might recommend a gentle suppository rather than medication taken by mouth.

CRAMPS

Cramps, mainly in the legs, often occur in late pregnancy. They may be more troublesome in the summer and also at night. One theory states that there is an alteration in the amount of calcium in the muscle of the leg during pregnancy, and doctors who hold this view recommend treating cramps by taking antacids to bind the phosphorous in the intestinal tract, allowing the calcium to be absorbed.

Various other treatments have been tried, such as increasing the intake of salt. This should not be done if the woman suffers from edema (*see* below). Certain tranquillizers, which relax the muscles a little, can sometimes be helpful when cramps are both frequent and severe. But such medication is best avoided in pregnancy. If cramps are not too severe or too frequent, then it is better not to take pills, but to gently move the foot so as to stretch whichever muscle is painful.

CYSTITIS *see* Urinary infection

DATES, wrong dates and maturity

For centuries it has been known that pregnancy lasts for approximately nine months. Accurate calculation shows that the average length of a pregnancy is 280 days or 40 weeks from the start of the last menstrual period. This is only an average time and many pregnancies last for longer or shorter periods – but it becomes obvious that a meticulous record of menstrual dates is important.

Doctors usually calculate the expected date of delivery of the baby by adding one week and subtracting three months from the first day of the last period as this is approximately 40 weeks. This date is also known as term.

It is most important for all concerned to know when the baby was conceived and when it is likely to be born. This makes it possible to know how far advanced the pregnancy is.

Fetal maturity is normally calculated in weeks rather than months from the date of the last period. An accurate knowledge of the fetal maturity is needed to decide whether the uterus and the fetus are growing normally, or whether they are smaller or larger than expected. Knowing the exact age of the fetus also makes it possible to decide whether it is wise to induce a baby. For example, in conditions such as **elevated blood pressure** (*see* below) or **placental insufficiency** (*see* below) it is dangerous for the fetus if pregnancy is prolonged past term, and also if labor is induced too early. For all these reasons it is of great help to the doctor and to the mother and her baby, if she can give a reliable date for her last menstrual period.

Unfortunately it is not always possible to give the date of the last period and, even if it is known, it may not be useful in calculating fetal maturity. Sometimes the date is forgotten; sometimes there was no period because the woman became pregnant immediately after a previous baby. Sometimes a woman does not have periods regularly every month and may have missed one or two periods or a woman who stopped "the pill" may miss a number of periods before becoming pregnant, which serves to confuse the dates. In all these circumstances the normal calculation of the date of delivery gives rise to inaccurate dates.

Other methods must then be used to estimate fetal maturity and the delivery date. A vaginal examination in the first three months of pregnancy is usually enough, but examination after a third month of pregnancy is not very accurate. A clue to fetal maturity is sometimes given by the date when a woman first feels her baby move. This is approximately 18 weeks with a first baby and 16 weeks with subsequent babies.

If there is no sure way of knowing how far advanced a pregnancy is, it may be necessary to do some tests. One or two **ultrasound scans** (*see* below) between 15 and 30 weeks give a very reliable guide to fetal maturity by measuring the size of the fetus. An **amniocentesis** is a very good test to find out if the fetal lungs are mature. This is often done if a pregnancy must be terminated for medical indications like pre-eclamptic toxemia or diabetes mellitus. The amniotic fluid is tested for the presence of a substance which allows the baby's lungs to expand properly.

In at least a third of all pregnant women, there is some uncertainty about the dates. This uncertainty may be worrying but, provided the woman remains well with no complications, and the fetus is growing normally, no intervention is necessary. Nature usually produces the baby when it is mature, which may not be exactly on the expected date.

DEPRESSION *see*
Emotional changes in pregnancy.
DIABETES *see* Sugar in the urine.

DISTURBED VISION
Disturbed vision is uncommon in pregnancy, but occasionally women with otherwise normal vision find a temporary difficulty in focusing or suffer from double vision and wonder if they need glasses. Sometimes visual disturbance is associated with **edema** (*see* below). In some women who have severe pre-eclamptic toxemia (*see* below, **hypertension**) with a very high blood pressure visual disturbance can be much worse. They suffer from double vision, difficulty in focusing and occasionally some loss of part of their field of vision. These changes may be associated with severe headaches. Urgent treatment for the high blood pressure is required. The vision returns to normal within a few hours or days of the blood pressure falling again. This is usually after delivery of the baby.

ECTOPIC PREGNANCY
Ectopic pregnancies are rare. They occur when a newly fertilized ovum is held up in the fallopian tube and embeds there instead of moving into the uterus. The pregnancy soon outgrows the tube, which bursts causing leakage of blood internally. Usually the mother will feel severe pain in the lower abdomen starting one or two weeks after a missed period, and may also have slight vaginal bleeding. Sometimes the woman feels faint. If these symptoms occur it is essential to see a doctor as this condition requires an operation to remove or repair the damaged fallopian tube.
See doctor immediately.

EDEMA
Edema is due to excess water in the body, which causes swelling in certain areas, most commonly the feet and ankles. It is more likely to occur in late pregnancy and in hot weather. Some weight gain is always associated with edema. Women with varicose veins are more likely than others to get swollen ankles. Firm pressure with a finger over the bone in the lower part of the leg for about 20 seconds will leave a small dent in the skin if edema is present. Because of the effect of gravity, which causes the fluid to collect in the legs, the feet are most likely to suffer from edema, but it can also be present in the face, hands and body.

A woman will become aware that her fingers are swollen if her rings become tight. Sometimes very mild swelling of the hands is associated with pins and needles in the fingers. This is usually caused by pressure of the fluid on one of the nerves in front of the wrist, and is called carpal tunnel syndrome.

Mild edema is fairly common in pregnancy. Most women find that it disappears overnight, when they are lying down, but returns later in the day, when they are walking around. If a woman finds her feet or hands are swelling, she should let the doctor know on her next visit to his office. In the majority of women, edema is just a nuisance and is not serious; but, in a few, it may be associated with raised blood pressure and the condition of **pre-eclamptic toxemia** (*see* below), and this requires special treatment.

The treatment of edema on its own is simple. The swelling tends to disappear if you lie down or sit with your feet up as high as possible. Mothers may not, however, be able to rest enough, particularly if there are other children at home, or if they go out to work, but they should rest as much as possible. Raising the foot of the bed on books can reduce the swelling overnight. Some people also find that a low sodium diet helps as salt encourages the body to retain fluid. Avoid all salty foods like bacon and stop adding salt to food.

If these remedies fail and edema remains acute, or is causing symptoms such as pins and needles in the fingers, then your doctor can prescribe diuretic tablets which will remove some of the fluid. Diuretics generally are not used in modern obstetrics because of some unfavorable side effects.

EMOTIONAL CHANGES
Pregnancy is a time of great emotional changes. A woman can be quite unlike her usual self; she may laugh and cry over nothing. She may be forgetful or find she cannot concentrate on anything for very long, even on things she normally likes doing. All sorts of stories she has heard or read in books about pregnancy can produce real worries about possibilities which never occur.

There are all sorts of reasons for an emotional upheaval in pregnancy. For a woman having her first baby the most important reason is that soon she will be a mother, have a baby to care for, then a child to bring up. She is faced with a complete change of lifestyle and a commitment to the child for many years to come. For a woman having a second or later baby there is all the anticipation of another child and perhaps the thought that this one will complete her family. The changing hormone levels in the pregnant woman (*see* chapter 2) also have an effect on her emotions, and can make her either elated or depressed for no apparent cause.

It is perfectly normal for a woman to get a bit depressed or a bit anxious at times during her pregnancy. In a few women, however, depression or anxiety can be severe and last longer than a few hours and these women should see their doctors. Their emotional state can be improved with tranquillizers, some of which are safe in pregnancy. Any tranquillizer should only be taken on prescription and you should make sure that the doctor knows that you are pregnant.

Women who have suffered from "nerves" in the form of anxiety before pregnancy occasionally get a recurrence at this time. They should see their doctors as soon as they feel their emotional state upsetting them. It is better to start treatment early, as improvement is then faster.

Women are not alone in their emotional reactions to pregnancy and childbirth. Faced with "competition" from the new baby and with increased financial responsibility, husbands or partners often participate in what can become an intense emotional atmosphere in the home. Both partners must be aware of each other's worries; a growing abdomen and rising hormone levels do not excuse the pregnant woman from lack of concern for her "pregnant" husband or partner.

EVACUATION OF THE UTERUS
DILATION AND CURETTAGE (D & C)
Evacuation of the uterus is a minor operation in which the remains of a pregnancy, called the products of conception, are removed from the uterus. It is performed in cases of **missed abortion** or **incomplete abortion** (*see* **miscarriage**). Under a general anesthetic a small suction tube is passed through the vagina into the uterus in order to empty it of its contents. Not only does this operation empty the uterus, it also stops the bleeding associated with an incomplete abortion.

FLATUS, FLATULENCE *see*
Gas and gas pains

FAINTING, feeling faint and supine hypotension
During the early part of pregnancy, there is an increase in the amount of blood circulating, associated with changes in the tone of the blood vessels and also changes in distribution of the blood around the body (*see* chapter 2). While these adjustments are occurring some women may feel faint or actually have fainting attacks, because there is a temporary reduction in the blood supply to the head.

Certain situations and actions will encourage a feeling of faintness, including crowded rooms and stuffy atmospheres, standing (not walking) for a long time, any sudden shock or fright and, sometimes, mere fatigue.

The best treatment for feeling faint is to sit down or lie down, preferably in a place where there is some fresh air, for instance by an open window. Situations which bring on attacks should be avoided if at all possible.

In late pregnancy many women feel faint or nauseated if they lie flat on their backs for more than a few minutes. This condition, called **supine hypotension**, occurs because the enlarged uterus rests on, and partially obstructs, the flow of blood in the inferior vena cava, (the main vein which returns blood to the heart from the lower half of the body). As a result the cardiac output decreases, blood pressure falls, and the woman feels faint. Treatment is very simple; if the woman turns to lie on her side or even sits up she will feel better in one or two minutes.

If fainting attacks or blackouts are recurrent in pregnancy then they should be reported to your doctor.

FOOD CRAVINGS

Traditionally pregnancy is a time of food cravings. Women often find they suddenly want to eat a lot of a particular food or that they dislike food they enjoyed before they became pregnant. It is not known quite why this happens. It may be that the body develops a desire for some particular food it needs, for instance, salt. Alternatively, cravings may be caused by changes in the sense of smell brought about by pregnancy (*see* below, **taste and smell**). Women often report that the smell and taste of certain foods is nauseating, especially in the early months of pregnancy.

Well known fads include a craving for acidic foods, like pickles, or salty foods like peanuts. None of this is a cause for concern. Fattening foods eaten to excess, however, will put on more weight than is good for a pregnant woman. Occasionally women want to eat something strange like chalk, coal, starch or mud, which could be harmful.

GLUCOSE tolerance test, Glycosuria *see* Sugar in the urine

GAS AND GAS PAINS

Some women find they are very troubled by gas during pregnancy (**flatulence**). Sometimes people get a lot of gas in the stomach which makes them want to burp (**eructation**), or a lot of gas in the large bowel which they have to pass (**flatus**). Sometimes the gas just rolls around the abdomen causing a pain like cramps and a feeling of being distended.

Most gas is swallowed air. Some people swallow a great deal of air with their food and between meals, usually with no idea at all that it is happening. It is not at all easy to stop swallowing air. Eating slowly can help; antacid pills or liquids are sometimes tried for flatulence but are not always helpful. If you suffer from gas pains, it is important to avoid constipation, which makes them worse (*see* **constipation**). Gas may, however, be troublesome for a short period of time and then lessen without any treatment at all.

HEADACHES

Some people are prone to headaches; others get migraine, which is a particularly severe form of headache. During pregnancy, some headache sufferers find that their headaches improve or come less often; others find they worsen or come more frequently. Women who never normally have headaches may start to get them, although the headaches are often limited to a particular time of pregnancy. The pain may come fairly often in the first trimester and then stop completely; or it may start late in pregnancy. A very severe headache in the last trimester requires urgent medical advice as it can be due to raised blood pressure.

Headaches usually require no treatment. However, if the pain is bad, a doctor will prescribe analgesics. Some migraine pills and other headache pills that contain a substance called ergotamine should not be taken during pregnancy, and it is thus essential to get advice from your doctor.

HEARTBURN and indigestion

All sorts of different aches and pains may be called either "heartburn" or "indigestion". Heartburn is relatively more common in pregnancy than at other times, but indigestion is probably less common. Heartburn is a burning sensation just behind the lower part of the breast bone (or sternum). It is caused by a small amount of acidic stomach juice which enters the lower part of the food pipe (or esophagus), and irritates the lining. Occasionally a little stomach juice comes up as far as the mouth and this juice also tastes acidic.

In pregnancy there is increased pressure on the stomach from the growing uterus and there is some relaxation of the muscle that normally stops stomach juice flowing upward (*see* p. 38). Heartburn is not serious, but it is not very pleasant either. It can be improved by relieving the pressure on the stomach. Avoid tight clothing and physical activities like stooping if possible. If heartburn occurs at night then sleeping half propped up with pillows can help.

Stomach acid can also be neutralized with the help of antacid pills. Some of these pills, however, also contain aspirin, and these should be avoided as they may make the heartburn worse. In pregnancy all antacids should be obtained only on prescription. It may also help to take a quarter of a teaspoon of bicarbonate of soda, dissolve it in a cup of warm water and drink it slowly. This remedy often relieves the pain but may produce some gas.

Indigestion is a dull pain in the upper part of the abdomen usually near the midline. It may be caused by food which has upset the stomach, or by too much acidic stomach juice in the duodenum (this is the piece of intestine which leads from the stomach). Antacid pills can relieve indigestion and milk drinks are sometimes helpful as well, but some pregnant women find milk nauseating and for these women it is better just to take antacid pills.

HEMORRHOIDS

Hemorrhoids are enlarged veins in the rectum. Occasionally they appear for the first time in pregnancy, and women who have hemorrhoids before becoming pregnant often find they get worse during pregnancy. The symptoms associated with them may be itching or soreness or skin tags around the anus. These skin tags form in association with the hemorrhoids. Occasionally they produce a little bleeding. The symptoms can be partially prevented by avoiding **constipation**. Soreness and irritation can be relieved by using creams or suppositories which you can obtain on prescription from your doctor. If bleeding occurs it should be reported to your doctor and you should have a check-up to confirm that it is not vaginal bleeding.

HYDATIDIFORM MOLE

Hydatidiform mole is a very rare complication of early pregnancy, in which the placental tissue grows into small cysts. Sometimes the embryo grows for a short while but it never survives.

This condition is one of the rarer causes of bleeding in early pregnancy. It can be diagnosed by an **ultrasound scan** (*see* below), or from a pregnancy test as the extra placental tissue produces excessive amounts of pregnancy hormones. The mole is easily removed by an operation, **evacuation of the uterus**, or D & C.

After the removal of a mole most women are advised by their doctors to postpone another pregnancy for a year, as these moles occasionally recur and are more likely to do so if a second pregnancy occurs quickly. It is also very important to repeat a blood pregnancy test at intervals during that year so that a recurrent mole can be diagnosed and treated early. If the patient becomes pregnant this valuable test will no longer be helpful.

HYPEREMESIS GRAVIDARUM *see* Nausea and vomiting

HYPERTENSION and pre-eclamptic toxemia

At every visit to the doctor a woman can expect to have her blood pressure taken. It is an important part of antenatal care. A woman's blood pressure in the first trimester is very similar to her normal non-pregnant blood pressure. It drops slightly lower than normal in the middle trimester, but there are no symptoms due to this, and it returns to normal in the last trimester.

In a few women, blood pressure rises above normal limits toward the end of pregnancy. The rise of blood pressure is called hypertension. Hurrying to the doctor's office will often make a woman's blood pressure rise on arrival, but in this case a short rest will bring it down to normal. Mild hypertension on its own is not very serious, although occasionally it causes a slight slowing down of the growth rate of the fetus.

However, a small proportion of women with hypertension also develop protein in their urine (*see* below, **proteinuria**), or **edema** (*see* below). This is the condition of pre-eclamptic toxemia. The condition is usually quite mild, with a slightly raised blood pressure and just a trace of protein in the urine. However, it sometimes becomes severe, with a very high blood pressure, a lot of protein in the urine and marked swelling of the face, hands and lips. If severe pre-eclampsia is not diagnosed or treated properly then it can result in a seizure (known as eclampsia). This is why it is important to have regular blood pressure checks and urine tests in pregnancy. In spite of a lot of research the cause of pre-eclampsia is still unknown.

The treatment of mild hypertension is to rest and to check the blood pressure and test the urine for protein very frequently. Some doctors advise a short period of rest in the hospital, others allow their patients to stay at home and teach them to test their own urine for protein every day. In many women blood pressure soon returns to normal. In others it remains slightly raised but in a few women it continues to rise. If a woman's blood pressure continues to rise, or if she develops proteinuria, then hospitalization is necessary.

In the hospital the mother is usually confined to bed except for visits to the bathroom. She may be given sedatives to help her rest. She may be given a reduced salt diet to discourage edema. Sometimes pills to reduce blood pressure may be helpful. On this type of regimen most women improve and can be allowed up, but in a few the blood pressure does not improve.

Sometimes pre-eclampsia affects the placenta and the nutrition of the fetus suffers, so that it grows more slowly than normal. It is possible to check whether the placenta is working well by measuring placental hormone output in a 24-hour specimen of urine, or measuring the hormone levels in the blood. Any change in the fetal growth rate can be discovered by an **ultrasound scan** (*see* below). If at any time it is thought that the mother's blood pressure is a real risk either to herself or to her fetus, then it becomes necessary to induce labor and deliver the baby early. After delivery the woman's blood pressure usually settles down within a few hours or days. The baby no longer depends on the placenta and can obtain what nourishment it needs in the form of milk.

Essential hypertension. A small number of women start pregnancy with a raised blood pressure. They may or may not know that their usual blood pressure is higher than average. Usually this raised pressure causes no symptoms. This condition is known as essential hypertension. When a woman with essential hypertension becomes pregnant her blood pressure may fall to normal levels in the middle trimester and then rise again in the last few months of pregnancy. If nobody knows what her normal blood pressure is, and it has not been measured very early in pregnancy, then she is usually thought to have pregnancy hypertension. This does not matter as the treatment is very similar. In cases of essential hypertension the blood pressure does not return to normal levels after the baby is born but to the level it was at before pregnancy began.

INCOMPETENT CERVIX *see*

Miscarriage
Premature labor
Premature rupture of the membranes

INEVITABLE ABORTION *see* Miscarriage

INSOMNIA *see* Tiredness

ITCHING of the skin

Itching of the skin occasionally occurs in late pregnancy and can be most unpleasant; if severe it may even interfere with sleep. Sometimes it is associated with a rash caused by a slight alteration in the working of the liver, which is thought to be due to hormone changes. The itching becomes more acute in a hot atmosphere so it is better to keep as cool as possible by wearing lighter clothes particularly at night. Nylon and wool are best avoided next to the skin; cotton is preferable.

Bland skin creams and cooling lotions help some people but their effect does not last long. In most women the itching fluctuates but may not disappear until the baby is born. The doctor may possibly prescribe antihistamines in the most severe of situations.

LEAKAGE OF URINE (stress incontinence)

Toward the end of pregnancy a few women find that coughing or straining causes the loss of one or two drops of urine. This is caused by an alteration in the position of the bladder neck, due to pressure from the uterus. The condition is usually very mild. The loss of urine must be distinguished from loss of amniotic fluid caused by **premature rupture of the membranes** (*see* below). For this reason it is important to consult your doctor. Stress incontinence can be helped by emptying the bladder frequently so it doesn't overfill. Sometimes it may be necessary to wear a sanitary pad. The condition usually corrects itself after the baby is born, but doing postnatal exercises speeds recovery.

LEAKAGE OF FLUID *see*

Miscarriage
Premature rupture of the membranes

LEAKING BREASTS

Toward the end of pregnancy many women notice that their breasts produce a small amount of opaque fluid called colostrum. They may find the secretion on their clothes, particularly on waking in the morning. This leakage is quite normal and is caused by activity in the breasts as they prepare for the new function of producing milk after the baby is born. No treatment is necessary. Women should wash the breasts gently with soap and water and protect their clothing, as colostrum can stain certain fragile fabrics.

MIGRAINE *see* Headaches

MISCARRIAGE, Spontaneous abortion

Miscarriage is the spontaneous loss of a pregnancy that occurs before 20 weeks and most commonly in the first three months. A miscarriage is often called a spontaneous abortion.

Between 10 per cent and 20 per cent of pregnancies end in a miscarriage – a very disappointing event to people who have looked forward to having a baby. Repeat miscarriages are even more disappointing. In a large percentage of early miscarriages, however, the fetus is abnormal and a miscarriage is nature's way of preventing abnormal babies from being born. In these cases it is better to lose a bad pregnancy early and then have a normal baby in the next pregnancy. The first symptom of a miscarriage is usually vaginal bleeding, which is called a threatened abortion.

Threatened abortion

Bleeding from the vagina before 20 weeks of pregnancy is a symptom which always requires medical advice. It may occur as the first sign of a miscarriage, or it may occur for no apparent reason, and the pregnancy can carry on normally to term. Vaginal bleeding may be very slight and less than a period or very heavy with the loss of large clots. Occasionally it is bad enough to require a blood transfusion. The heavier the blood loss the more likely it is that a miscarriage will follow.

Slight bleeding which follows a few days or weeks after a normal period can also be due to a delayed period. It is sometimes very difficult to distinguish a delayed period from bleeding in early pregnancy. Irregular bleeding can lead to difficulty in deciding when a pregnancy actually started and how advanced it is.

Most doctors initially advise rest at home for women who suffer from slight bleeding in early pregnancy. Rest means lying down for as much of the time as possible – something that may be very difficult when there are other children in the family. In many cases, after a few days rest, the bleeding lessens to spotting, then stops, and the pregnancy continues normally. If the bleeding becomes heavy, or if pain occurs, the doctor will probably arrange for admission to the hospital. Some patients who have previously had one or more miscarriages will be advised by their doctors to rest in the hospital if there is any sign of bleeding at all in their next pregnancy.

Missed abortion

Sometimes when vaginal bleeding occurs the embryo dies but miscarriage does not take place at this time. In these cases, known as a missed abortion, the pregnancy test may become negative and if an ultrasound scan is done it will reveal that the embryo has stopped growing. If this happens it is usually best to have the remains of the pregnancy (called the products of conception) removed by a minor operation called an **evacuation of the uterus** (*see* above). If this operation is not done, a miscarriage will eventually occur but there may be more blood loss.

Inevitable abortion

The first symptom of miscarriage is usually bleeding; the second symptom is usually intermittent pain, very similar to period pains. This occurs as the cervix opens up, and once the cervix is open the miscarriage is inevitable. The doctor can see if the cervix has opened by a vaginal examination. Many women are needlessly worried that a vaginal examination should cause a miscarriage; a gentle probing will definitely *not* provoke a miscarriage. Sometimes a vaginal examination is followed by bleeding. This is usually due to loss of blood which has already collected inside the uterus and upper vagina, and is released by the examination.

Once a miscarriage is inevitable the pregnancy sac, or "products of conception" is usually passed quite quickly in a complete abortion. If the sac is not completely expelled or if bleeding is heavy, the doctor will recommend an **evacuation of the uterus** (*see* above). Sometimes a miscarriage occurs at home with surprisingly little bleeding or pain. If this happens call your doctor and keep the pregnancy sac or clots for him to check. He will then be able to tell you whether the miscarriage is complete – or incomplete. In the latter instance, you will need to go into the hospital for a curettage (D & C).

Mid-trimester miscarriage (Late miscarriage)

A miscarriage which occurs in the middle three months of pregnancy (between 13 and 28 weeks) is much less common than an early miscarriage. In some cases miscarriage may occur because the cervix is unable to remain closed and cannot hold the pregnancy in the uterus. This is known as an incompetent cervix, and is frequently caused by damage to the cervix in a previous operation, such as a D & C, or a late termination of pregnancy. This type of miscarriage often starts with the loss of fluid instead of blood.

If a woman has had one mid-trimester miscarriage or if examination of the cervix in mid-pregnancy shows that it is opening up, then a simple stitch around the cervix will keep the cervix closed and allow the pregnancy to continue normally. This stitch is called a cervical, McDonald, or Shirodkar suture. The stitch is inserted under a general anesthetic after 14 weeks of pregnancy. (It does not prevent early, or first-trimester, miscarriages.) The stitch is removed just before the baby is due or earlier if labor starts early.

MONGOLISM *see* Amniocentesis
MONILIA *see* Vaginal Discharge

NAUSEA and vomiting

One of the earliest symptoms of pregnancy is feeling sick. Traditionally nausea occurs in the early morning but it can occur at any time of day or even throughout the day. Sickness is probably caused by rising levels of the hormone estrogen which are produced by the developing placental tissue (*see* chapter 3). Some pregnant women have very little nausea; others are quite sick and vomit. Often a pregnant woman's sense of smell becomes much more acute (*see* below, **taste and smell**), and some odors seem to aggravate nausea.

Hunger can also make the nausea worse. Eating something like a dry cracker with tea first thing in the morning, even before getting up, helps to relieve early morning nausea. Snacks between meals may help daytime nausea but when the nausea is severe it may be necessary to lie down for a short time. Persistent nausea can be improved with anti-emetic medications, but you should only take those medications prescribed by your doctor because this is the time in pregnancy when the embryo is most vulnerable.

Morning sickness pills often make people feel sleepy and it is therefore best to take them at bedtime; they will still be effective the next morning. The best and only thing that can be said about this nausea is that it does stop eventually, usually by the twelfth week of pregnancy; very occasionally it persists into the middle trimester.

Vomiting in pregnancy is even more unpleasant than nausea. Occasional vomiting, perhaps two or three times a week, can be treated in the same way as nausea, with food, rest and antiemetic pills. Vomiting which occurs daily or more than once a day is uncommon but much more serious as it can prevent the woman from getting enough food and liquid for her needs. She will lose weight and may get very thirsty.

If vomiting is frequent, it is very important to call your doctor. Vomiting can cause starvation, and tests will show if this is the case. A specimen of urine can be tested for substances called ketones which appear in cases of starvation. If ketones are present, it will be necessary for the mother to go into the hospital. It is rest which helps, and most women find that the vomiting stops in the hospital as they enjoy almost complete rest. Very rarely a mother will have to be fed through an intravenous drip for one or two days. Vomiting of this kind, called **hyperemesis gravidarum**, does not harm the baby. Once the vomiting ceases and the mother can go home, it is unlikely to recur if she gets enough rest.

OLIGOHYDRAMNIOS *see* Amniotic fluid
PINS AND NEEDLES *see* Edema

PLACENTA PREVIA

In this condition some or all of the placenta is lying in the lower part of the uterus, either close to the cervix or even over it. Placenta previa occurs in between one in 100 and one in 200 births.

When most of the placenta is low-lying, it can cause bleeding in the last 12 weeks of pregnancy (*see* above, **antepartum hemorrhage**). This bleeding is sometimes bad enough to require blood transfusion. The bleeding is painless and usually stops after a few hours of bed rest. It can recommence, however, and patients who have had bleeding from a placenta previa are therefore safer if they rest in the hospital until the baby is safely delivered.

The diagnosis of a placenta previa can be made with an **ultrasound scan** (*see* chapter 4), which gives a picture of the placenta in relation to the cervix. The previa is "total" if the placenta covers the cervix and "partial" if it is adjacent.

A placenta previa also prevents the baby's head from entering the pelvis and prevents normal delivery. The obstruction means that the baby must be delivered by cesarean section (*see* pp. 93–5, 109). This is usually performed early at 38 weeks of pregnancy, as excessive bleeding may be a big problem if the pregnancy is allowed to go into labor at term.

If a placenta previa is suspected but it has not been possible to confirm it during pregnancy, a vaginal examination is carried out at 38 weeks and a cesarean section is done only if the placenta is found lying over the cervix. This vaginal examination is not done earlier as the examination could in itself start more bleeding.

Sometimes only one edge of the placenta is in the lower part of the uterus. In this case it may be drawn up out of the way in labor, permitting a vaginal delivery without any extra blood loss. If it does cause bleeding in labor, however, a cesarean section may be necessary.
See doctor immediately.

PLACENTAL ABRUPTION *see* Antepartum hemorrhage
PLACENTAL FUNCTION tests *see* Slow fetal growth
PLACENTAL INSUFFICIENCY *see* Slow fetal growth
POLYHYDRAMNIOS *see* Amniotic fluid

POSTDATISM and POSTMATURITY

Postdatism means a pregnancy that continues beyond term. Postmaturity is a post-term pregnancy in which the fetus is at risk due to placental insufficiency. The average fetus is mature and ready to thrive outside the uterus by term (40 weeks of pregnancy) which is when labor normally occurs. At term the average placenta supplies both nourishment and oxygen efficiently to the fetus even under the stress of labor. If the pregnancy continues beyond 42 weeks the fetus goes on growing slowly but placental efficiency may not always keep up with fetal growth. The resulting situation is known as relative placental insufficiency. This can be detected by means of a non-stress test (*see* p. 55).

In a normal pregnancy the placenta usually works well up to 42 weeks, but in a pregnancy complicated by conditions like hypertension the placenta may become relatively insufficient soon after 40 weeks. In such cases the risks to the baby increase if the pregnancy is prolonged.

Postmaturity can best be diagnosed if the length of the pregnancy is certain and the woman's dates have been confirmed (*see* above, **dates**). If it is thought that postmaturity is likely to be a risk to the baby then labor will be induced (*see* chapter 7). The postmature baby is often more alert than babies born at term and may have rather dry skin and longer finger- and toenails than a baby born at term.

PRE-ECLAMPSIA *see* Hypertension

PREMATURE LABOR

Premature labor is the occurrence of labor after 24 weeks and before the baby is mature (*see* p. 52). Babies born before 37 weeks of pregnancy usually require special care after birth because of prematurity. Labor starts early in some women for no apparent reason, but sometimes premature labor follows **premature rupture of the membranes** (*see* below).

The uterus normally contracts or tightens at irregular intervals throughout pregnancy in painless motions that are called **Braxton-Hicks contractions**. These become stronger and more frequent as pregnancy progresses, but are not associated with any opening of the cervix or threatened delivery. The contractions of premature labor are regular, stronger and more frequent than Braxton-Hicks contractions and cause the cervix to open. If a woman feels strong regular contractions in late pregnancy she should seek medical advice.

Premature labor can sometimes be caused by an incompetent cervix (*see* above **mid-trimester miscarriage**). If this happens a stitch, known as a MacDonald or Shirodkar suture, can be put in the cervix at the beginning of the next pregnancy to prevent premature labor happening again.

Sometimes the contractions of premature labor begin and then stop after a few hours, and the pregnancy proceeds normally. Often labor continues and the baby is born prematurely. Many premature babies manage very well. Others may suffer from breathing or feeding difficulties, from jaundice or low body temperature (*see* pp. 132–3). In view of these problems doctors usually try to stop premature labor to allow the baby to mature in the uterus. Various substances which suppress uterine contractions can be given to women in premature labor with the aid of an intravenous drip. If this treatment is successful, labor stops completely, or is at least postponed for a few days; if it is unsuccessful, the baby will be born.

The major change that takes place when a baby is born is that he or she starts to breathe. To do this the baby must have mature lungs. Since the lungs mature in the last trimester, breathing difficulties – known as respiratory distress – are the biggest problem that faces premature babies. The more premature the baby, the more likely they are to occur as the organs of the baby will be insufficiently developed.

In recent years, new techniques have been developed to lessen respiratory distress. The lungs of the premature fetus can be induced to mature by giving the mother injections of large doses of one particular hormone. The treatment takes 48 hours to be effective, and if doctors can prevent delivery for at least 48 hours, then the hormone will have enough time to act on the baby's lungs so that they can cope with life outside the uterus without incurring respiratory distress.

After the birth very small premature babies may have to be nursed in an incubator in a special care unit. The baby's mother is welcomed in these units and is encouraged to help care for and feed her baby until he or she is big enough to be ready to go home.

See doctor immediately.

PREMATURE RUPTURE of the membranes

Normally the membranes which line the uterus and surround the fetus remain intact until the onset of labor at term, but occasionally they rupture quite suddenly and for no apparent reason. The only symptom is the leakage of fluid (known as the amniotic fluid) from the vagina. Usually only a small amount is lost, but this symptom always requires medical advice.

It is important to distinguish between the leakage of amniotic fluid and urine, which can also sometimes leak unexpectedly in pregnancy. The fluid and urine smell quite different, and if the water is collected, tests will easily distinguish between them. Leakage of amniotic fluid must also be distinguished from a **vaginal discharge** (*see* below), which may be quite marked in pregnancy.

Sometimes, after a few days rest in the hospital, the hole in the membranes may close and seal, thus stopping the leakage. The amniotic fluid is then quickly replaced by the fetus and the membranes. Leakage may recur later in the pregnancy, but often the pregnancy proceeds normally to full term.

There are two main complications which sometimes follow a rupture of the membranes. These are **miscarriage** or **premature labor** (*see* above), and infection. Where labor starts prematurely treatment can be given to delay it, providing there is no infection. At the same time hormones can be given to prevent the baby suffering from breathing difficulties in the event that it is born early. If the amniotic fluid is infected the mother will have an elevated temperature. In this case a swab will be taken from the vagina, the bacteria identified, and the infection treated with antibiotics. If there is any infection, and labor begins prematurely, it is usual to allow labor to continue and give antibiotics to the baby after it is born if necessary.

Sometimes premature rupture of the membranes is the result of an incompetent cervix (*see* above, **mid-trimester miscarriage**). If this is the case the cervix can be strengthened with a stitch (a MacDonald or Shirodkar suture) in the next pregnancy in order to prevent the condition occurring again.

PROTEINURIA

Proteinuria, sometimes called albuminuria, means that there is some protein in the urine. Normally a woman's urine is tested for protein at every antenatal visit and occasionally in a normal pregnancy a trace of protein is found. More than a trace of protein is abnormal. Proteinuria can be caused by a **vaginal discharge** (*see* below) contaminating the urine, by a **urinary infection** (*see* below) or by **pre-eclamptic toxemia** (*see* above).

It is fairly easy to distinguish between these three conditions. The middle part of a stream of urine must be collected and tested. It will not contain protein if the proteinuria is caused by a vaginal discharge, which affects only the first part of a stream of urine. The specimen can be cultured or grown in the laboratory, and bacteria will be found if the urine is infected. In pre-eclamptic toxemia the proteinuria is always associated with raised blood pressure.

The treatment of proteinuria is that for vaginal discharge, infected urine or pre-eclampsia – whichever is present.

PULMONARY EMBOLISM *see* Thrombosis in the veins

PYELITIS *see* Urinary infection

RECURRENT MISCARRIAGE

Unfortunately some people have more than one miscarriage. Miscarriage may be due to an abnormality of the fetus occurring by chance more than once, or it may be associated with poor hormone production by the developing placenta. Often the reasons for miscarriages are unknown.

Many treatments have been tried to prevent recurrent miscarriage. Resting sometimes helps. Some doctors prescribe hormones to assist the pregnancy, but their value is still unproven. Some doctors recommend abstaining from intercourse from the time the pregnancy test is positive until after 12 weeks. Again, however, the value of abstention is unproven.

In the normal woman who is pregnant and has not had a miscarriage before, it is best to carry on in her usual manner provided she is well; it should not be necessary either to take hormones, or to avoid intercourse, or to take excessive rest. Research shows that in the normal pregnant woman there is an 80–90 per cent chance of carrying a baby past the miscarriage stage. It is also comforting to know that many women have had a completely normal baby even after a series of three or four miscarriages.

RH-DISEASE *see* pp. 33–4

RIB PAINS

Pains in the lower ribs are fairly common toward the end of pregnancy. They are usually due entirely to mechanical factors. Sometimes the pain is due to the fetal head or bottom pressing under the ribs on one side. Every time the fetus moves to try and stretch itself it gives another push to the lower rib cage. Sometimes pain in the lower ribs is due to tension in the muscles and ligaments attached to the ribs, which have to accommodate the upper part of the growing uterus.

Rib pains can be worse in women carrying twins. These pains are uncomfortable but they do not mean that there is something wrong. There is no cure, but it is often possible to relieve the pains by altering your position and perhaps sitting in a different type of chair, or even standing up when they occur.

SALIVATION

Some women find that during pregnancy they produce excessive amounts of saliva, which force them to keep swallowing. This symptom is often, but not invariably, associated with pregnancy nausea or vomiting. If salivation is mild it is better not to take pills, but if it is very severe, anti-nausea pills will dry it up to a certain extent and may be worth trying (*see* above, **nausea and vomiting**).

SKIN RASHES

A wide variety of skin rashes can occur in pregnancy and your doctor's advice should be taken about all of them. If the woman suffers from German measles (Rubella) in early pregnancy, this can cause fetal abnormality (*see* p. 55), but most other rashes have no effect on the fetus. Some but not all rashes cause **itching** (*see* above). Many skin rashes disappear after a few weeks but some persist until the baby is born. Treatment with various creams helps some rashes but not others; in all cases these creams should be obtained by prescription.

SHIRODKAR SUTURES *see*

Miscarriage
Premature labor
Premature rupture of the membranes

SICKLE-CELL ANEMIA *see* Anemia

SLOW FETAL GROWTH, small-for-dates and placental insufficiency

Most babies grow at very similar rates for the first six or seven months of pregnancy. If the fetus appears to be very small for its age (known as small-for-dates) during these months, it is likely that the dates have been wrongly calculated (*see* p. 27). After six or seven months individual growth rates are much more variable, with big babies growing faster and small babies growing more slowly, so that at term a baby's normal weight can be anything from 5½ lb (2.5 kg), or less, to 9 or 10 lb (4 or 4.5 kg), or more. As a general rule, small women have smaller babies and large women have larger babies.

During pregnancy the detection of the small-for-dates baby is most important but not always very easy. It is a great help if the mother's dates are certain and reliable. With this information and regular antenatal visits, it is often possible to detect a slowing of the fetal growth rate by routine examinations of a woman's uterus. In some cases a woman fails to gain any weight for a month or so, or even loses weight, if the fetus is growing slowly. Women who have had a previous small-for-dates baby or who have had a stillborn baby, and women over 35 years of age who are having their first baby, are more likely than others to have a small baby. A woman whose pregnancy is complicated by **pre-eclampsia** (*see* above) is also more likely to have a small baby.

In a small number of cases the baby grows normally at first but its growth rate slows down in the last few weeks of pregnancy. This occurs because the needs of the fetus outstrip what the placenta can supply, and the condition is called **placental insufficiency**.

If retarded fetal growth is suspected, it is possible to perform tests, known as placental function tests, to check that the placenta is working well (*see* pp. 54–5, chapter 3 **fetal growth**). Provided these tests prove normal, slow growth rates are not likely to be any problem for the baby. If the tests show any degree of placental insufficiency, then it may be possible to improve the working of the placenta and accelerate fetal growth by resting in bed. The amount of rest required depends on the degree of placental insufficiency. If this is mild, rest at home will be enough; if severe, it may be necessary to rest in the hospital during the pregnancy.

Often placental insufficiency is very minor – sometimes not even enough to affect the placental function tests. All that happens in these cases is that the fetus stores fewer nutrients in its liver than normal, and develops a bigger appetite after the birth.

Where placental insufficiency is severe, there is marked slowing of growth, and the fetus becomes obviously small for the dates. Doctors will then consider delivering the baby early in order to give it more nourishment in the form of milk. As a general rule, however, provided the fetus does not stop growing completely, it is always better for the fetus to remain inside its mother until at least 38 weeks of pregnancy (i.e. two weeks before term). The fetus is then mature enough not to suffer any of the ill effects of prematurity (*see* above, **premature labor**). Such babies may be quite small when they are born but with frequent feedings they soon put on weight.

If the doctors decide that the risk to the baby from placental insufficiency is greater than the risk of prematurity, it will be necessary to deliver a growth-retarded fetus before 38 weeks. Small-for-dates babies have a slightly increased chance of becoming distressed in labor and all women with such babies should therefore be monitored during labor.

SPINA BIFIDA *see* p. 28

SPONTANEOUS ABORTION *see*

Miscarriage

SUGAR IN THE URINE, Glycosuria

Normally a pregnant woman's urine is tested for sugar at each antenatal visit. Although most women are likely to be concerned if they find that they are passing sugar in their urine, this is quite common and very seldom of any serious significance. During pregnancy a normal woman's kidneys are less efficient in preventing the sugar entering the urine.

This problem is likely to occur at about 32 weeks of pregnancy. Normally the amount is very small. The presence of this small amount of sugar on one or two occasions can normally be ignored. Sometimes, however, sugar is found in nearly every urine specimen tested. This may mean that the sugar level in the blood is raised. A glucose tolerance test, in which sugar is measured after the mother has taken a glucose drink, will show if this is the case. Usually the glucose tolerance test gives a normal result and the pregnancy proceeds without problems.

In a few women the glucose tolerance test shows a raised blood sugar level, and treatment is needed. This takes the form of a diet and, very rarely, injections. If a woman's blood sugar level remains high in pregnancy then her baby is likely to grow faster than normal. This can produce problems at the time of delivery and also after the birth. After delivery of the baby, the woman's blood sugar and urine test both return to normal quickly.

Glycosuria in pregnancy is relatively common. It must not be confused with the condition of glycosuria in the non-pregnant woman, which is called diabetes and is relatively uncommon. When a diabetic woman becomes pregnant she will require very close supervision in order to ensure that her blood sugar remains as close as possible to the normal level.

SUPINE HYPOTENSION *see* Fainting

TASTE AND SMELL

In early pregnancy some women find that their sense of smell becomes more acute than it was previously and that they smell things they had not noticed before. Certain smells may become very annoying – perhaps a scent that the woman previously liked, or something mundane like cooking smells. Change in the sense of smell can persist during pregnancy but usually improves after the first trimester.

The sense of taste is closely linked to the sense of smell and sometimes a woman finds that she has an unusual taste in her mouth for a while. In such cases it is advisable to have a dental check-up, unless one has been done recently. Provided there is no tooth decay, little can be done about abnormal tastes, other than using a mouthwash or drinking tea. This symptom also tends to improve in later pregnancy.

TEETH AND GUMS

There is an old saying that a woman will lose one tooth for each baby she has. This saying is based on the fact that dental decay and gum disease are comparatively common during pregnancy and breast-feeding.

The gums may be slightly swollen and bleed more easily than normal, and the mouth bacteria that cause tooth decay are more active, so that pregnancy is a time when preventive dentistry can be especially important for a woman.

Most dental treatments can safely be carried out in pregnancy, but dental X rays should be delayed until after the first trimester. Certain antibiotics (tetracyclines) that are sometimes given for tooth infections should not be used in pregnancy as they discolor the baby's teeth (*see* chapter 2). As in all cases of medical treatment in pregnancy, a woman should make sure the dentist knows she is pregnant.

THALASSEMIA *see* Anemia
THREATENED ABORTION *see* Miscarriage
THROMBOPHLEBITIS *see* Varicose veins

THROMBOSIS IN THE VEINS

During pregnancy the blood clots more easily. Clotting is likely to occur if the circulation through a blood vessel is poor and stagnates; a similar but milder effect is seen in women on "the pill". Stagnation of the blood sometimes occurs in the veins in the calf of the leg where a clot then forms. This is called thrombosis.

Thrombosis is a very rare complication of pregnancy but is more likely to occur in women who are spending a lot of time lying in bed. Women who have to rest in bed during their pregnancy should therefore make a conscious effort to move their legs around at regular intervals. In the hospital the physiotherapist will recommend a series of exercises in order to maintain good circulation in the legs.

One symptom of a leg vein thrombosis is pain in the calf that worsens when the foot is bent upward, stretching the calf muscles. Sometimes, too, the ankle swells. These symptoms should be reported to the doctor. If examination of the leg confirms that a clot has formed, treatment may take the form of serial injections of heparin (anticoagulant). It is necessary to test the clotting activity of the blood frequently during treatment so that the correct dosage of heparin can be determined. Too many anticoagulants can produce excessive bruising during normal activities; conversely, too few anticoagulants can enlarge the vein clots. These anticoagulants are stopped before labor, to permit normal clotting activity at the time of delivery.

If a deep vein thrombosis is not treated, there is a possibility that a piece of blood clot will break off, enter the circulation and lodge in the lungs where it causes chest pain and is called a **pulmonary embolus**. Women who have had several vein thromboses at any time, and women who have had a pulmonary embolus may possibly need anticoagulant treatment during most of their pregnancy.

TIREDNESS and insomnia

Many women find it very difficult to keep awake during pregnancy, particularly in the early months. They find they need more sleep at night and like to have a rest after their lunch as well. They also have less energy for normal activities and easily become tired, particularly if they are going to work or have other children at home. The only treatment for fatigue and irritability in pregnancy is to slow down and rest when possible while realizing that most people feel much better and more energetic after the first trimester has passed. Toward the end of pregnancy the tiredness may recur, mainly because much more of an effort is required for normal activity.

Insomnia may also be a problem at this time; it can be due to the physical adjustments of pregnancy (baby kicking, backache, increased weight) or to normal emotional anxieties about the changes and new responsibilities the baby will bring. Insomnia can often be improved by having a snack just before going to bed; hot milk also helps. Physical discomfort can be relieved by placing additional pillows under the small of the back or under the stomach if resting on the side (*see* p. 41). If insomnia is persistent your doctor might prescribe sleeping pills, but it is far better not to take sleeping pills in pregnancy, if this can be avoided.

TWINS and multiple births

Twins occur in about one in 80 births, and triplets occur in about one in 5,000 to 10,000 births. Multiple births of more than three babies have until recently been extremely rare; the use of certain fertility drugs has increased their numbers in the last few decades.

Some infertile women can be helped to achieve a pregnancy by fertility drugs. The one given in pill form, called Clomid, usually produces a single baby but occasionally caused twins. Infertility is also treated by injections of pituitary hormones and these may stimulate the ovaries to produce several eggs at once. A few women have had quadruplets or quintuplets as a result. Most women given this treatment however, still usually produce a single baby. This section mainly discusses twins as they are more common than other multiple births.

To a pregnant woman the news that she is going to have twins is usually rather daunting, although twins sometimes run in families, and are almost anticipated. Most couples are quite pleased once they are used to the idea; some are not. Although twins require a tremendous amount of hard work after they are born, some women are very happy to have two children "for the price of one pregnancy".

Twins can also be good company for each other as they grow up. A woman who has decided she wants one more child to complete her family, however, may not be so happy to find that there will be two.

If a woman already has a child or children, coping with twins after they are born may not be too much of a problem. With the assistance of her husband, friends and relatives, most women manage very well. People are often very helpful in lending an extra crib or high chair for the second baby.

It is certainly more difficult if the twins are the first children and the mother has to learn with two, but there are still many people around to help. The nurses in the hospital will make sure a mother is able to care for her babies before she goes home. It is most important that a woman with twins as first children should make use of any offers of help from husband, relatives and friends, who can often be enlisted to feed the babies. Obviously it is most useful to know someone else with twins who can give moral support.

Diagnosing twins can sometimes be very easy and at other times very difficult. If a woman's uterus is found to be consistently larger than expected for her dates then the doctor will suspect that she is carrying twins. Sometimes it is possible to feel the two heads and the two bodies through the abdomen. The outlines can be felt more easily if there is a lot of amniotic fluid, and if the mother has had previous pregnancies. Sometimes the woman herself senses she may be carrying twins because she feels much more movement than in a previous pregnancy.

In some women, however, it is extremely difficult to diagnose twins, as the uterus may not appear to be larger than normal. This is particularly likely if the woman's abdominal muscles are well-developed and tense and if one baby is lying behind the other. In these cases no one may realize that the woman is carrying twins until very late in pregnancy. Rarely, no one suspects twins until one baby is delivered, and, much to everyone's surprise, out comes the second one.

If twins are suspected it is important to find out for sure. An **ultrasound scan** (*see* below) at any time in pregnancy will usually show both fetuses. An X ray can be done instead of an ultrasound scan but should be postponed if possible until after 28 weeks, as it is then safer for the expected baby or babies.

A woman with a twin pregnancy is more likely to become anemic and will be told to take iron pills. Apart from extra iron, however, special food is not normally necessary unless the woman was very undernourished before pregnancy started.

A woman with twins develops a larger abdomen and may find it more difficult to get around and do normal housework toward the end of pregnancy. Help in the home and someone to do the shopping are particularly important. If a woman with twins finds she is getting very uncomfortable, she may need to rest in the hospital for a period of time before delivery.

Women with twins go into labor prematurely more often than women with one baby. Labor may be two or three weeks early, which makes little difference, but it is sometimes as much as a month or two early. This is because the uterus becomes fully distended much earlier than usual. Several methods have been tried to prevent premature labor in twins but their effectiveness is unproven. Some doctors recommend that women with twins be encouraged to rest in bed between the thirty-second and thirty-sixth weeks of pregnancy. After 36 weeks, when there is less risk of the babies being born prematurely, she is allowed to increase her level of activity.

Other doctors will perform a vaginal examination and only recommend bed rest if the cervix is not firmly closed. Still other doctors recommend no special treatment.

Twins are more vulnerable than single babies at the time of birth.

ULTRASOUND SCAN

The ultrasound scan is a technique for obtaining pictures of the fetus and placenta inside the uterus by means of sound waves on a monitor which resembles a television screen. It is safe and produces no discomfort. An ultrasound picture can tell the maturity of the fetus and whether it is growing normally; it also locates the placenta and the amniotic fluid and determines the numbers in a multiple birth.

The scan can be static or show motion as seen with realtime ultrasound. When the latter modality is used the actual fetal motion is observed as it occurs. It is fascinating to see how frequently the fetus moves arms and legs. The mother only perceives about half of the fetal movements. Realtime ultrasound can show fetal respiratory movements in utero. The presence of fetal respiratory movements is interpreted as a sign of fetal well-being. The absence of such movements may mean that the fetus is just asleep. The test may need to be repeated later. The absence of fetal respiratory movements in a high-risk pregnancy can indicate fetal jeopardy. The technique is described in more detail on pp. 54–5.

URINARY FREQUENCY

Passing urine frequently is very common in early pregnancy, and often a woman will need to get up at night to pass urine. Most women find the condition improves after a few weeks, but it may return toward the end of pregnancy, when the baby's head enters the pelvis and presses on the bladder.

Passing extra urine in early and late pregnancy is not usually associated with any pain. Painful urination is usually caused by **urinary infection** (*see* below). In this case, a urine test should be done by the doctor and, if infection is found, it should be treated with antibiotics.

URINARY INFECTION

Infections in the bladder occur more often in pregnant than in non-pregnant women and women who normally suffer from cystitis often find that it recurs in pregnancy. In spite of this, the majority of women pass happily through pregnancy without any urinary complications at all.

Sometimes a mild infection known as **bacteriuria** is present in the bladder without any symptoms at all. Bacteriuria is usually discovered because routine tests at the doctor's office show that there is protein in the urine (*see* above, **proteinuria**). The type of infection can be diagnosed by growing a culture from the infected urine in a laboratory. The infection can then be treated with antibiotics.

Cystitis occurs when a bladder infection is bad enough to cause symptoms, like pain on urinating, urinating very frequently, and occasionally having blood or pus in the urine, making it look very cloudy. All these symptoms require medical advice.

Once the type of infection has been identified the most effective antibiotic can be given. These antibiotics must be obtained by prescription because not all antibiotics are safe to take in pregnancy. It is also helpful to drink a lot of fluid to wash out the bladder. Cystitis symptoms usually clear up within 48 hours of starting treatment but may recur unless the whole course of antibiotics is taken.

Sometimes a mother passes urine frequently late in pregnancy because the baby's head is causing pressure on her bladder. This is not cystitis and is not painful, but it is better to have a urine test done to be absolutely sure there is no possibility of infection.

Pyelitis occurs when infected urine is present in the kidney as well as in the bladder. It usually occurs because some urine and bacteria have run back from the bladder to one of the kidneys. The woman feels ill, has a high temperature, and sweats. Pyelitis also produces pain in the kidney, which may be felt in the back and on one side just below the ribs. These symptoms require medical advice. A specimen of urine must be cultured to identify the infection and appropriate antibiotics can then be prescribed by your doctor.

Again it is important to drink a lot of fluid which helps to wash out the kidney. Pyelitis symptoms usually ease within 24 hours with the right antibiotic, but the whole course of antibiotics should be taken to avoid recurrence. Provided pyelitis is treated promptly by your doctor, it should not affect the pregnancy.

VAGINAL DISCHARGE

Vaginal discharge is very common in pregnancy because the pregnancy hormones increase the vaginal secretions (*see* pp. 30, 42). In addition, the protective mechanisms that normally prevent vaginal infection are reduced so that the possibility of infection is more likely.

The most common vaginal infection is yeast (**monilia**). The fungus which causes monilia is very widespread and is commonly present in the vagina without causing symptoms. In pregnancy it can multiply and probably cause a discharge. The discharge may be either white or yellowish and somewhat thick, and it can cause severe irritations and soreness.

Medical advice is required for any of these symptoms. Usually a swab taken from the vagina can be used to confirm the type of infection and medication can then be prescribed to be inserted into the vagina every day for 3 to 10 days. They are best used at night because they stay inside better. Sometimes the discharge recurs later in the pregnancy and a second treatment will be necessary.

Monilia is the most common cause of vaginal infection in pregnancy but other types of infection, including rarely venereal infections, also occur. All these other infections can be cured very easily in pregnancy provided the right treatment is given and the partner is also treated. It is most important if you suffer from vaginal discharge to treat it before labor occurs. If this is not done monilia can cause an infection of the baby's mouth (thrush) after birth, and other infections can give the baby a "sticky eye".

VARICOSE VEINS

Pregnancy usually makes varicose veins worse, and occasionally varicose veins will appear in pregnancy for the first time. Varicose veins can cause aching legs or swollen ankles and their treatment in pregnancy is not entirely satisfactory.

Many people get relief by wearing elastic stockings. If these are difficult to wear in late pregnancy elastic tights can be worn instead, although the latter are rather hot in the summer. All varieties of supporting hose should be put on before getting out of bed in the morning. The thinner varieties of elastic stockings are fairly attractive but give less support to the legs; thicker and firmer types are less attractive but can always be covered by slacks or a long skirt.

Women with varicose veins should avoid standing; it is much better to walk around to keep the circulation going. When sitting, prop up the feet on a stool or a low chair. If the varicose veins are very troublesome they can safely be injected during pregnancy, but this should be done by a specialist in the technique. After this treatment it is very important to follow all instructions given by your doctor.

Occasionally a varicose vein becomes inflamed in pregnancy and the area of the vein becomes reddened and very tender. This condition is known as **thrombophlebitis** and is treated by wearing some form of support for the varicose veins and a cover of soothing cream, obtainable on prescription. The inflammation starts to settle down within a week, but may take several weeks to disappear. Often the varicose vein that has become inflamed disappears after the inflammation settles down. This inflammation in a vein must be distinguished from **thrombosis** in the calf veins (*see* above), because the treatment is entirely different.

VENEREAL DISEASE *see* Vaginal discharge

VOMITING *see* Nausea and vomiting

Preparing for labor

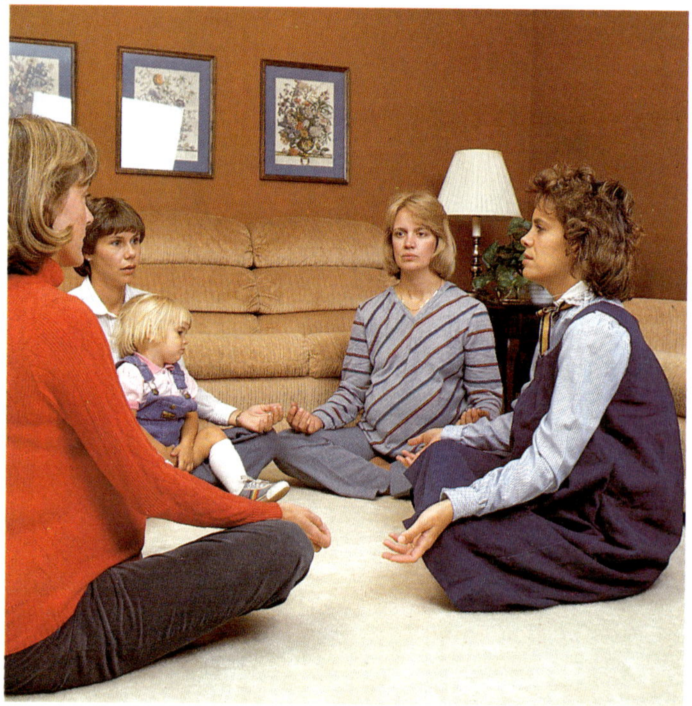

CHAPTER 5

What happens in labor

Relaxation

Breathing in labor

Other aids for labor

Pain relief

Only now, when we are able to produce totally painless labor, have we learned – to our astonishment – that this pain serves a purpose, however indefinable. Certainly it seems to form an important part of the mother's physiological and psychological processes, possibly even increasing her intimate attachment to her baby. And without having undergone labor and birth pains some mothers can actually feel deprived of their experience of childbirth.

We do not, however, understand why there is such a wide spectrum of pain. Five per cent of mothers have very little or none in labor. For most mothers the degree is tolerable, even if severe. But for a relatively small proportion of mothers the level of pain is intolerable and it must be relieved to a greater or lesser extent by medication or conduction anesthesia.

Pain in labor arises from the uterine contractions which produce the opening of the cervix. Between contractions the pain disappears entirely. If the time for the opening of the cervix is relatively short (i.e. four to six hours) most mothers find even a severe level of pain tolerable. During labor, however, no one knows how long this process will take and it is often the length, rather than the severity, of painful contractions that influences the decision to ask for pain relief.

Most of the pain in labor is felt during the first stage (*see* p. 78), which is usually longer for first babies. In subsequent births labor is often shorter and so more tolerable.

The mother's feelings play a very important part in her reaction to pain in labor. It is often a great help to her if she can view each contraction not as another pain but as another effort of the uterus to open the cervix, allowing the baby to enter the world. Once

Cross references

See also	Chapter
Antenatal care	2
Antenatal classes	2
Female sex organs	1
Hormones	1
Illness in pregnancy	4
Labor and birth	6
Preventing complications	7
Rest in pregnancy	2

The ability to relax helps the mother to rest when she is pregnant, and to keep control during the birth. The techniques of yoga, which these women are learning, can be very useful in promoting relaxation.

the cervix has opened she will have an overwhelming urge to bear down and push her baby out. The pain will then disappear.

Pain in labor is a subject frequently neglected in books about childbirth because of the mistaken idea that by discussing pain or preparing her for it the mother-to-be may be frightened. Indeed, for many years the very existence of pain in labor was denied. Dr. Grantly Dick-Read carried out research which led him to believe that pain in labor was caused principally by the "fear-tension-pain" syndrome: "The fear of pain actually produces true pain through the medium of pathological tension." His teaching was that if a woman understood what was happening to her, accepted birth as a natural event and did not expect to suffer pain, she would be completely relaxed during labor and would experience little or no pain. Although Dick-Read's work is acknowledged as a major breakthrough, it was felt by many that it was not the whole answer. The mother's role was still a passive one.

Later the technique known as psychoprophylaxis ("mind-prevention"), based on conditioned reflexes, was developed in Russia. The French doctor, Fernand Lamaze, and his disciple, Dr. Pierre Vellay, were largely responsible for the spread of this method in western Europe and the United States. Psychoprophylaxis demands the active participation of the mother using specific breathing and other techniques. With this method the woman is in complete control, and it works very successfully for many.

Unfortunately, in their efforts to counteract the negative attitudes of the past, some teachers have given women the impression that preparation for labor makes it painless. Many mothers and teachers would now like to see a more balanced approach. Pain is part of labor. Painless labors do occur but the majority of labors are painful to a greater or lesser extent. If this is accepted, preparation can teach women how to cope with pain – not to run away from it but to view it constructively. Such training can enable a woman to go into labor understanding the whole process, confident in herself and what she can do, but able to make use of modern pain relief methods should she need them (*see* pp. 82–3). If this happens she will be prepared whatever pattern her labor takes.

A woman who has decided to have an epidural block may, however, feel that preparing for labor is unnecessary and a waste of time. This is not so. It is still desirable for her to know what happens during labor and to know how to relax. Relaxation and breathing techniques are valuable during the very early stage before she leaves for the hospital. Occasionally, too, an epidural is not completely effective, or it may wear off quite suddenly, and in these circumstances women who have learned breathing and relaxation techniques will be able to employ them for relief.

All the techniques mentioned are best learned in a class. There are many excellent and well-qualified teachers running courses, and methods vary from class to class.

For women who cannot attend a class, the following chapter provides a basic introduction to the principles of relaxation and breathing techniques and gives a simple method which can be learned and practiced at home. There are also details of modern pain relief methods with their advantages and disadvantages.

What happens in labor

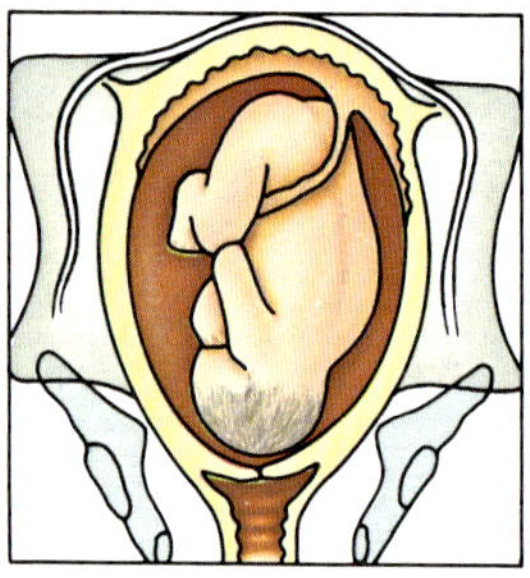

The contracting uterus expels the baby in two stages: in the first, the cervix is effaced (thinned) and dilated, and in the second stage the baby is pushed down the birth canal.

Before a baby can be delivered, two major processes have to occur in the uterus. First the cervix has to be effaced, shortened, and completely dilated (opened up) so that the second process, in which the baby descends through both the pelvis and its muscular floor, can begin to take place.

The process the cervix undergoes is a complex one. The cervix is made of a substance which can change its consistency and thus its shape. Before effacement, it is a rigid structure below the head of the fetus, separating it from the vagina. It forms a canal about 1 in (2.5 cm) long and $\frac{1}{8}$ in (2 or 3 mm) across, sealed with a plug of mucus (*see* p. 15). With effacement the cervix softens and its upper end thins and opens out, allowing the fetal head gently to enter it. Effacement usually occurs before labor with a first baby, but during early labor with subsequent ones.

In many women, especially first-time mothers, the fetal head enters the pelvis (becomes engaged) in the last month of pregnancy. If not, this takes place early in labor.

The first stage

During the first stage of labor, the tiny canal left in the center of the cervix opens up until it is 4 in (10 cm) in diameter – wide enough for the fetal head to pass through. The labor nurse or doctor measures the opening at regular intervals by placing two fingers inside it, touching the baby's head. The dilation is very slow at first (in the latent phase) but accelerates (in the active phase) toward the end of the first stage of labor. Second or subsequent babies almost always arrive in a lot less time than is taken for a first labor.

The dilation of the cervix occurs because of the contractions of the uterus, which is in effect one large hollow muscle, probably the most powerful in a woman's body. Contractions start at the top of the uterus (the fundus) and spread out and weaken by the time they reach the lower segment. With each contraction the muscles in the upper segment of the uterus become tense and shortened; the lower segment and the softened pliable cervix are stretched wider.

After each contraction the muscles of the uterus relax but remain shorter and the cervix therefore remains stretched. This is possible because of a unique property of the muscle fibers in the upper segment of the uterus, known as retraction. Unlike other muscles, the biceps for example, those of the uterus do not resume their original length when they relax but remain a little shorter each time. The result is that the cervix is gradually pulled over the baby's head, like someone slowly pulling on a turtle neck sweater. At the same time as the cervix dilates the space at the top of the uterus gets slightly smaller and the baby is pushed down toward the opening.

When the cervix has been pulled past the head, and forms part of the main body of the uterus, it is said to be fully dilated. This is the end of the first stage of labor. It is also the time when the membranes usually rupture and a small amount of warm clear fluid will trickle

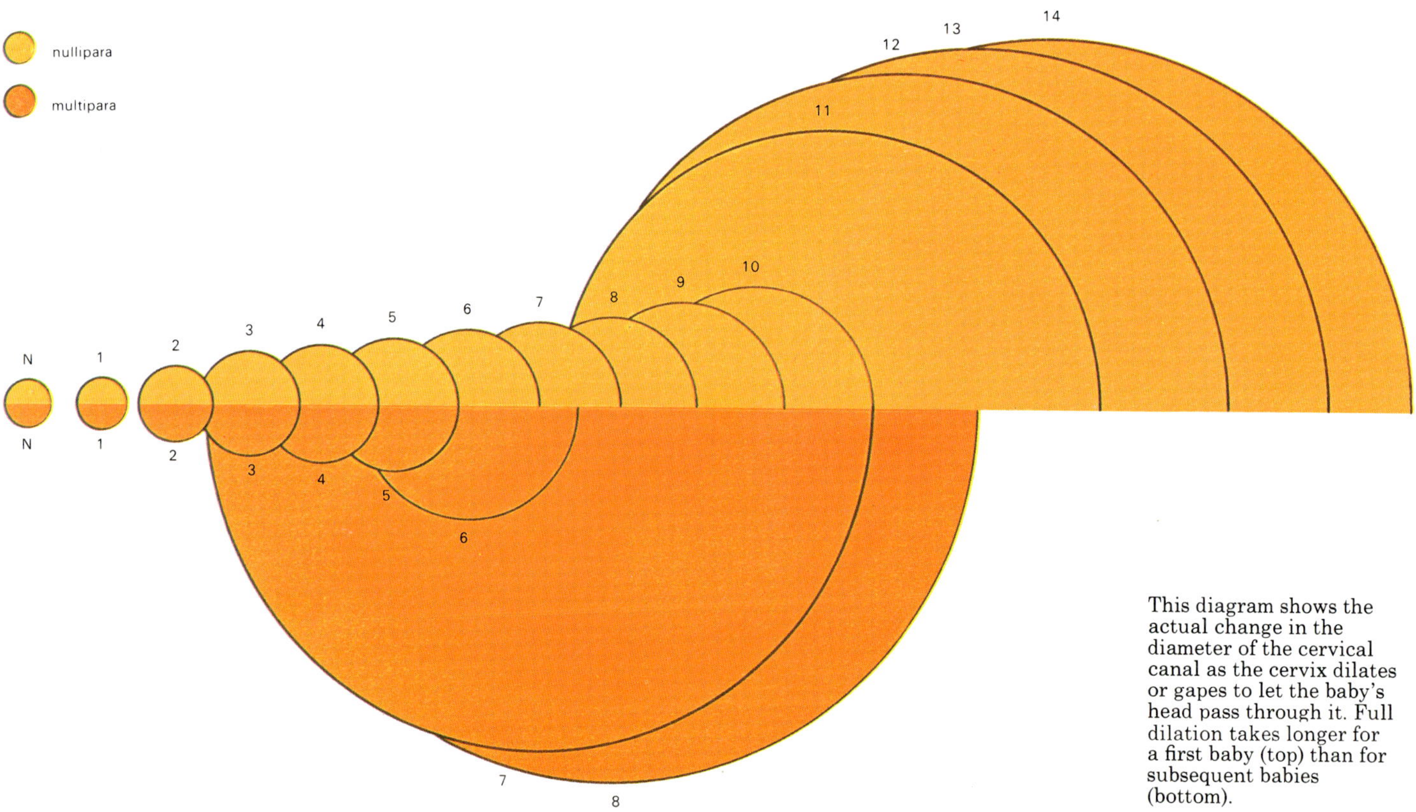

This diagram shows the actual change in the diameter of the cervical canal as the cervix dilates or gapes to let the baby's head pass through it. Full dilation takes longer for a first baby (top) than for subsequent babies (bottom).

out of the vagina. Some doctors, however, puncture the membranes earlier in the first stage to encourage stronger, more frequent contractions, generally speeding up the labor.

The contractions come at regular intervals. They are usually widely spaced at first, and become progressively more frequent, longer and more intense. Early in the first stage the contractions will probably be 15 to 20 minutes apart and by the end of it at 2 to $2\frac{1}{2}$ minute intervals. This may vary.

To the mother the contractions feel rather like waves of pain: the first and last parts of each contraction are painless, and only the most intense part, the crest, is felt. The pain itself resembles cramps but begins more gradually. How sharp the pain is, and where it is felt, will vary, depending on how relaxed the mother is and on her threshold of pain.

The rest periods between the contractions, when relaxation occurs, are vital to both mother and baby since the contractions cut off the blood supply to the baby and the uterine muscle so that neither can receive much oxygen or nourishment. During the relaxation periods the essential blood supply returns.

The second stage

In the second stage of labor the baby completes its descent through the birth canal. This can happen automatically without either the baby's or mother's help, but the process can be speeded up in the lower part of the birth canal by the mother bearing down or pushing, which women feel an instinctive desire to do. This stage usually lasts about one or two hours in a first labor and less than half an hour in subsequent ones. The contractions become stronger and a little less frequent, to allow the baby a good blood supply and the mother time to rest between pushes. At this time the doctor and nurse continue to keep a constant watch on the fetal heart, either listening to it after each contraction or watching a tracing on an electronic fetal monitor (*see* p. 102). The mother's pulse rate will also be monitored and recorded frequently.

With each contraction the head is squeezed further down into the pelvis and then out through its strong muscular floor. Because human beings have such an oddly shaped pelvis the head of the baby has to turn as it descends. The widest measurement of the head

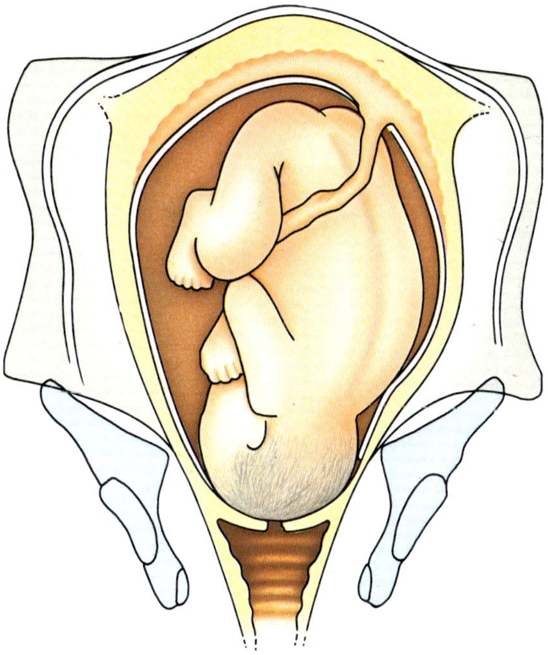

Left: the onset of labor with the cervix already effaced. Below left, late first stage of labor: the cervix is almost fully dilated and the head has rotated to face directly backwards.

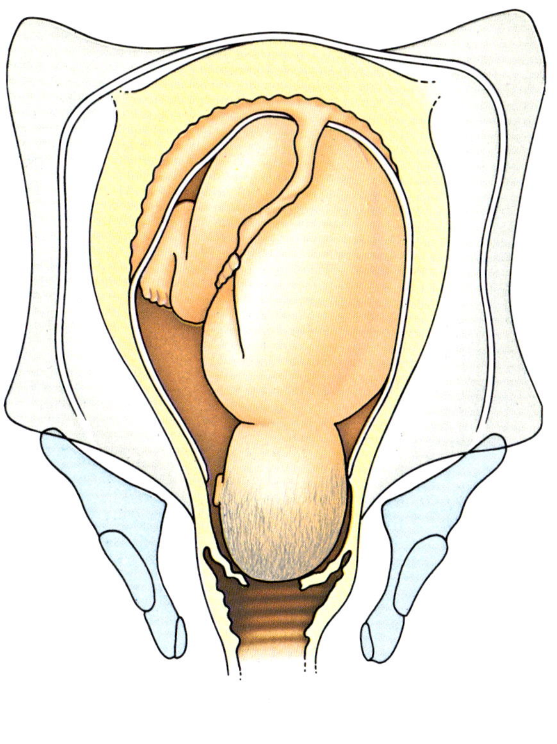

Uterine contractions in early labor, as shown on the tocograph. On the next page is a tocograph trace for contractions in the second stage of labor.

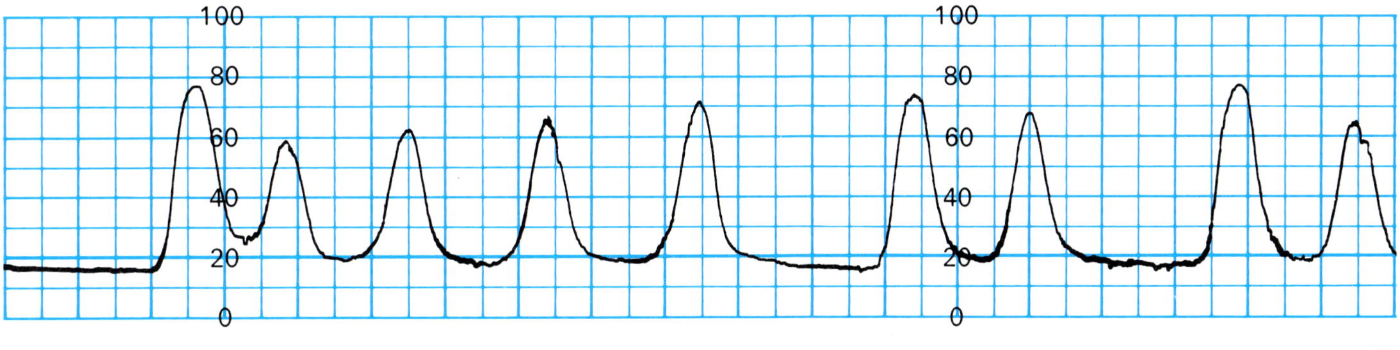

ROTATION OF THE HEAD

Usually at the beginning of labor the baby's head faces to one side. But in the lower part of the mother's pelvis the widest diameter is from front to back, so as the head descends it rotates (right), usually to face the mother's back, though it occasionally turns upward. Another factor which influences the rotation of the head is the smooth concave inner surface of the sacrum. Rotation is usually complete by the time the baby's head reaches the vulva.

Once the head is born, it rotates again to look sideways, in the same direction as before. This is because the shoulders, which are the widest part of the body, are turned into an up-and-down position as they pass through the lower part of the pelvis.

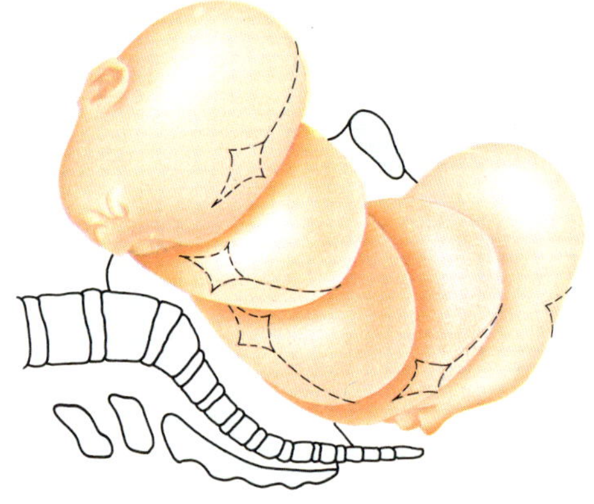

During the second stage of labor, the baby's head rotates. Once the head is born, it rotates again to allow the shoulders to lie from front to back in the pelvic outlet.

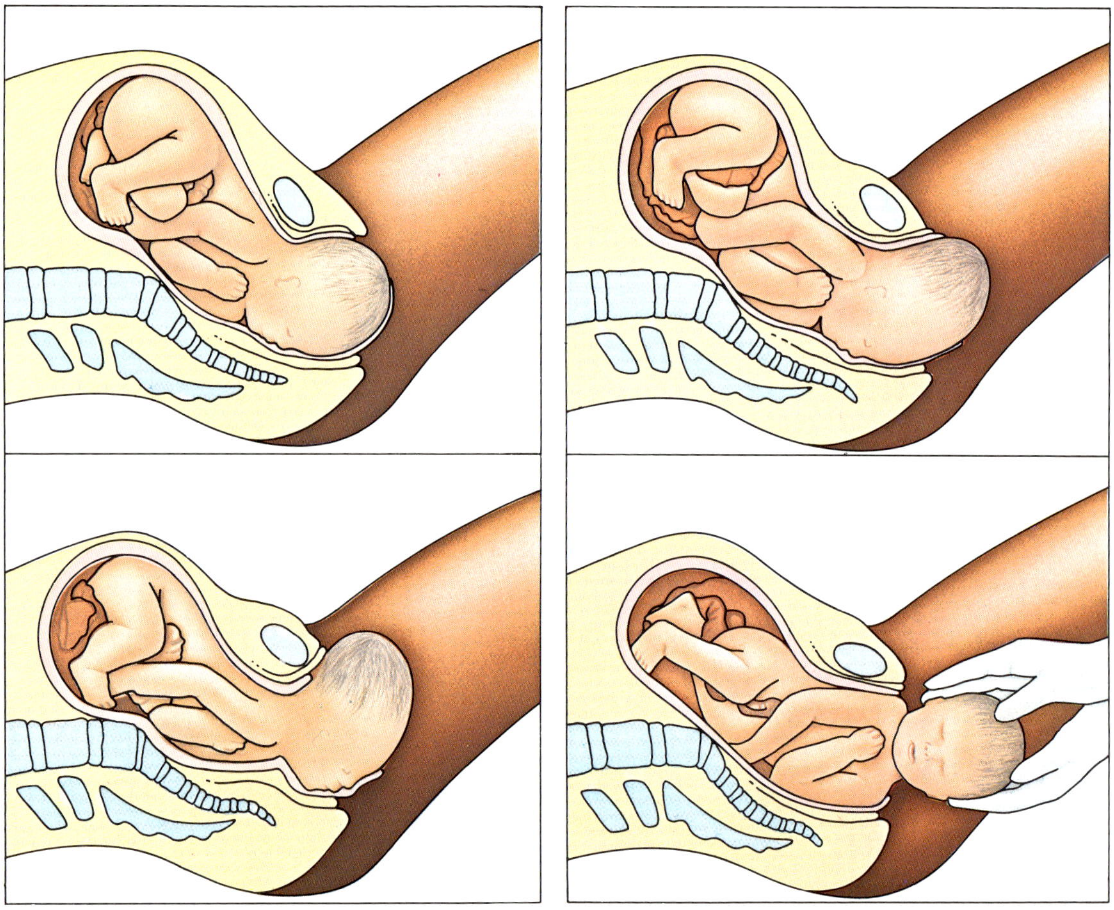

Toward transition from the first to the second stage of labor, contractions are at their most intense, possibly coming every two to three minutes and lasting nearly two minutes.

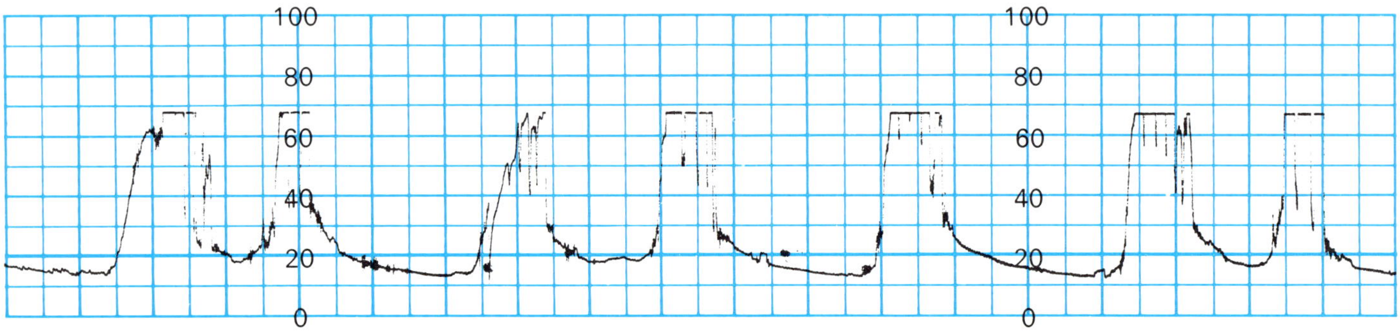

is from front to back and the widest measurement at the brim of the pelvis is from side to side. The baby, therefore, usually begins by facing sideways. But the lower part of the pelvis is diamond-shaped with the widest measurement from back to front. As the head descends, therefore, it turns through an angle of 90° and it nearly always appears looking toward the mother's back (occipito-anterior). Occasionally, however, it is born looking forward, "sunnyside up".

In order to get the widest part of the baby's head through the opening of the vagina, an episiotomy is commonly performed. This is a small cut made, under local anesthetic, in the perineum (which is made up of muscles as well as skin). The value of the episiotomy is to preserve the muscular integrity of the pelvic floor and vaginal outlet. It heals very easily.

While the head is being born, the shoulders, having negotiated the curves of the pelvis, enter the pelvic outlet. In the outlet they lie most easily from front to back, and as they rotate to this position, the head too turns sideways again. With another contraction and another push one shoulder is born, then the other and then the trunk. The rest of the baby slides out easily.

The third stage

As the baby is guided out of the vagina the uterus retracts behind it. The placenta, because it is not made of muscle, does not contract with it and a strain is placed on the layer between the placenta and the wall of the uterus which separate with the next contractions. This layer can be compared to the perforations around a postage stamp in that when a pull is exerted separation occurs. The placenta and its two membranes, the inner amnion and the outer chorion, slide into the vagina. There is always some blood lost at this time. Once in the vagina, the placenta and the empty bag of membranes are carefully pulled down and out, causing no pain to the mother. The placenta itself is immediately examined in detail by the doctor to make sure that it is complete.

As soon as the placenta is squeezed out, the interlacing muscle fibers surrounding the large blood vessels in the uterus contract completely. This seals off the flow of blood as a tourniquet would. When fully contracted the uterus can be felt in the lower abdomen as a hard ball which is approximately the size of a large grapefruit.

Following the delivery of the placenta your doctor may order a medication to decrease blood loss. The medication will be administered intravenously or intramuscularly. Since this works by causing uterine contractions, the mother may be aware of rather strong intermittent contractions. Rarely, the placenta does not separate and the obstetrician must remove it manually. This is necessary in order to avoid excess bleeding. The patient is usually given medicine or anesthesia for pain relief for this procedure.

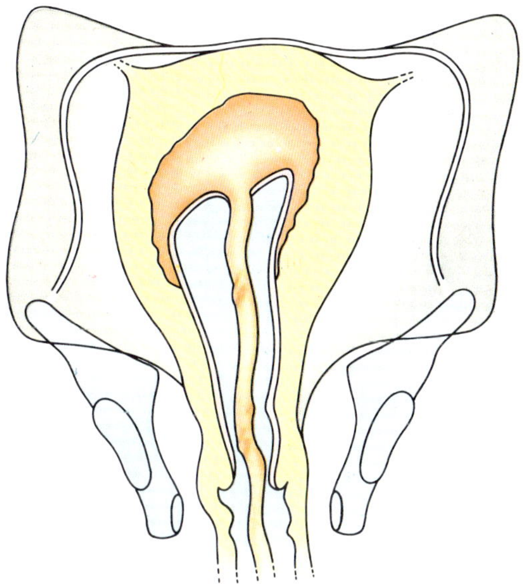

Once the baby has been born, the uterus contracts again and the placenta separates from the uterine wall. The placenta and the empty amniotic sac slide into the vagina and are carefully pulled down and out.

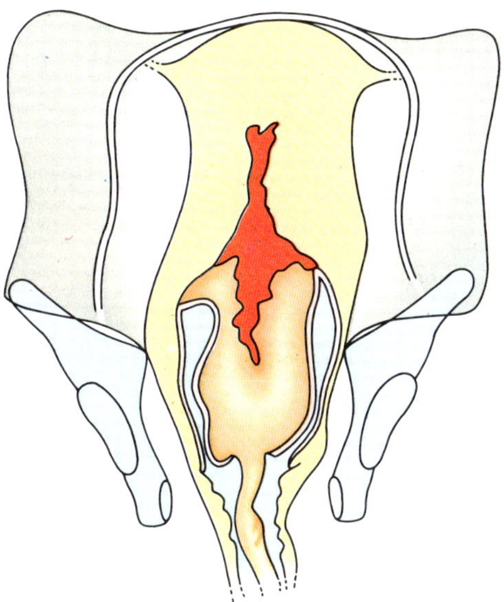

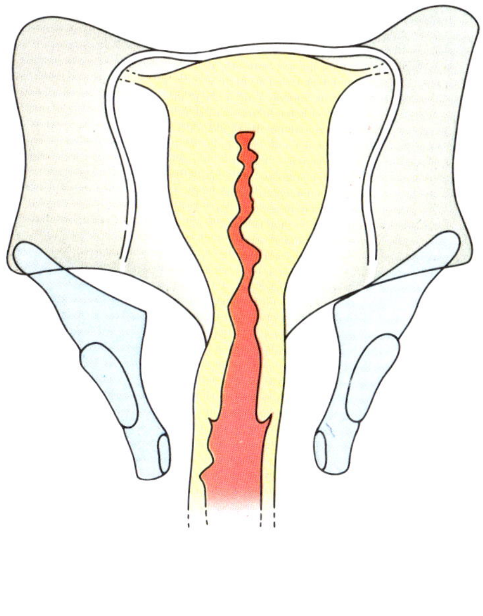

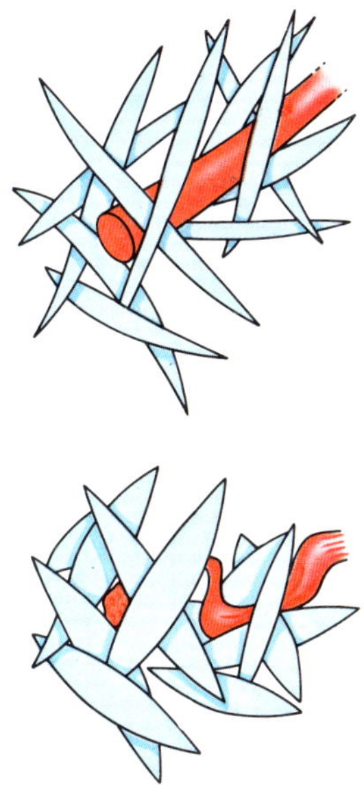

Prevention of excessive bleeding as the placenta separates: the muscle fibers contract and constrict the blood vessels.

Relaxation

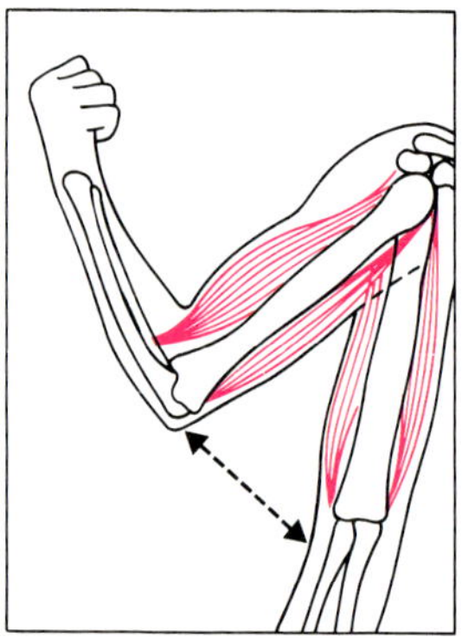

Tensing and relaxing individual muscles is a good way of learning relaxation.

Relaxation and breathing techniques practiced during pregnancy promise a lessening of the pain experienced and a high measure of personal control over labor for the mother – whether she wishes to have a "natural" childbirth or to use some form of pain relief during the delivery (*see* p. 82).

Relaxation is for living, not just childbirth. It is, however, particularly useful throughout pregnancy and during labor, and has great value for both the body and the mind.

Using muscles consumes energy. Tension tightens the muscles and uses up energy needlessly quickly leading to tiredness. Emotional tension follows physical tension. Relaxing the body helps to restore physical energy and a sense of well-being making it easier to handle work, stress or pain. Although total relaxation is only possible when lying down, it is possible to save energy by learning to sit or stand in a relaxed way (*see* below).

All activity uses up energy: the secret of relaxation is to use the correct amount. Standing, for instance, requires a certain amount of muscular tension but it is possible to stand in a tense or a relaxed fashion. To become aware of this, stand with your legs stiffly straight, tense your shoulders and neck muscles and tighten your hands. Then loosen your knees, drop your shoulders, relax your neck muscles and loosen your hands (*see* below).

If you learn to notice when a particular group of muscles is tense and consciously relax them you will gradually come to recognize when you are becoming tense and take measures to counteract it.

Relaxation has a special place during pregnancy since labor is hard work and the more energy the woman has when it starts the better she can cope with it. During labor itself pain seems to be increased by fatigue and tension, and the mother's sense of control reduced. As physical and mental states are closely linked, the less tired a mother is after the birth of her baby, the more relaxed she is likely to be.

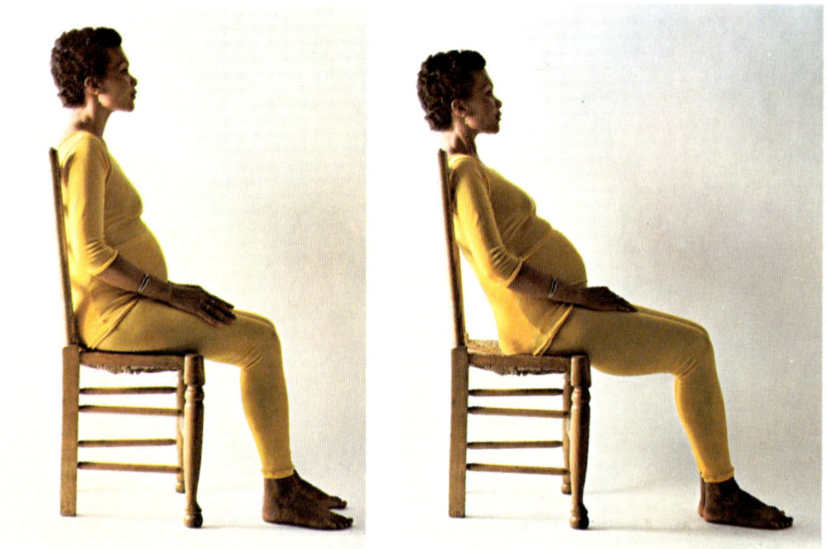

Make a habit of sitting in a relaxed way, but remember good posture is still important. Keep your spine straight and drop your shoulders (above left). Bad posture (above right) is not relaxing and leads to backache.

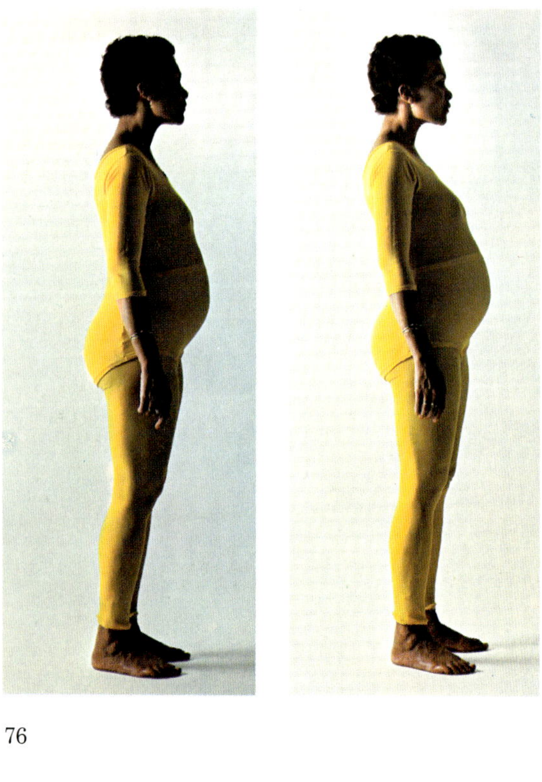

Check the difference between a tense and a relaxed way of standing. First, stand with legs stiff, and tense your shoulders and neck muscles (left). Then loosen your knees, drop your shoulders and relax your neck muscles (far left). Keep your spine as straight as possible.

How to relax

Different instructors have different ways of teaching relaxation. Whatever method you are taught the most important element of all is your mental attitude. Relaxation should not be seen as being lazy or wasting time but rather as a time to restore your body for what it has to do next. Lie down comfortably and give your body permission to let go.

Some people like to relax lying on their backs, well supported by pillows. However, this supine position allows the uterus to press on the vena cava, decreasing the return of blood to the heart and possibly causing faintness. Another position, particularly helpful if you have backache in the lower back, is to lie on the side where there is no pain, again supported by pillows. Relaxing and sleeping on the abdomen is also quite possible and does not harm the baby (*see* p. 41).

One method used to learn relaxation involves tensing a particular group of muscles, say the biceps, at the same time noting how the tendons and muscles feel as they shorten and tighten. Then relax the muscles and notice the changed sensation of slackness and length. Repeat this process with different muscles.

A second method, called disassociation, is particularly useful in preparing for labor. It involves tensing one group of muscles while taking care to keep the rest of the body relaxed. Usually when one group of muscles contracts others contract in sympathy, and this is particularly true in labor when the instinctive response is to tense the whole body each time the uterus contracts. A partner can help the pregnant woman learn this technique by pinching her thigh so hard that it hurts while she concentrates on relaxing the rest of her body. This response should be practiced until it becomes automatic.

Breathing in labor

Breathing techniques for labor vary and some are more complicated than others. The best way to learn is to attend a class and follow the method taught there. If there is no suitable class in your area, the simple, broad-based method described here can be extremely effective.

The value of using a breathing technique in labor is that it gives the mother something to focus on during each contraction, thus taking her mind away from the pain. For these techniques to succeed it is important to take contractions one at a time and to accept the pain as a constructive step towards the birth of the baby. Do not expect a breathing technique to take away the pain of labor. What it can do is raise your pain threshold and enable you to "get above" the pain.

A deliberate pattern of breathing also prevents the mother from becoming tense. A woman who is relaxed and breathing quietly is much less likely to overreact to all the sensations pouring through her. If she is tense neither her body nor her brain works efficiently, and some authorities believe that this can actually affect the smooth functioning of the uterus.

Basic breathing technique

When using a breathing technique some women like to keep their eyes closed and concentrate on the breathing by listening to it or by counting. Others find it more helpful to concentrate their attention on some object in the room (a focal point) and breathe "at" it. The basic breathing technique set out below has three phases, each of which is related to a particular level of pain. Pain levels are subjective, however, and expectant mothers should choose the breathing level which suits them at the time. If the contractions are not too painful at first it is probably sufficient to use just level 1; you can shift to levels 2 and 3 as the first stage progresses.

Level 1: The first breathing technique is probably all that you will need during the early first stage of labor when contractions are often not particularly long or strong.

Start with the lips separated so that the breath comes in and out through the mouth or nose (do not open the mouth wide and consciously breathe in through it, nor close it and breathe in through the nose). This is a relaxed way of breathing which is relatively easy to maintain without taking in too much air.

Give the "out" breath a slight emphasis throughout and allow the air to come back into the lungs of its own accord. If you breathe out too hard you will breathe in too deeply. Similarly, if you emphasize the "in" breath with a gasp you may hold your breath and tense up against a contraction. Breathe rhythmically and gently at lower rib level – just above your "bulge". Work "with" the contraction and aim to soar above it.

Level 2: Second level breathing is useful when contractions get stronger and should follow the "wave" of the contraction. As the contraction builds up, accelerate gradually from level 1, making each breath progressively a little quicker and more shallow. As the contraction subsides, breathe a little more deeply and slow down until you have reached level 1 again. The purpose of this technique is to allow you to rise above each contraction: the shallowest breathing being at the crest or most intense part of the "wave".

Level 3: The third level of breathing, called huffing and puffing, should be regarded as an "extra gear" to use at any time when the contractions are long, strong and painful to a

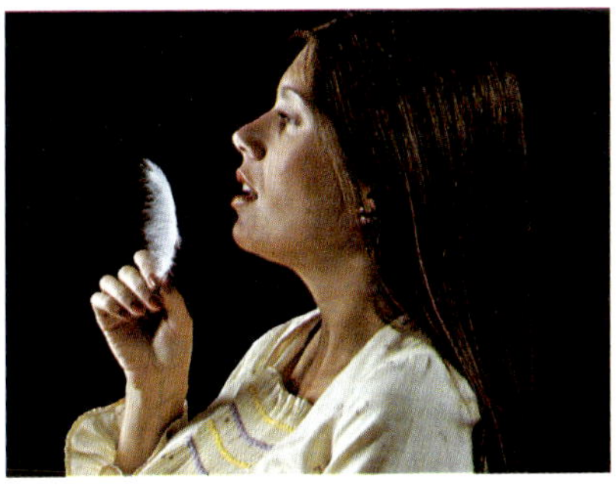

In level 1 breathing, above, the feather is barely ruffled because the mother-to-be is breathing out very gently, in long breaths.

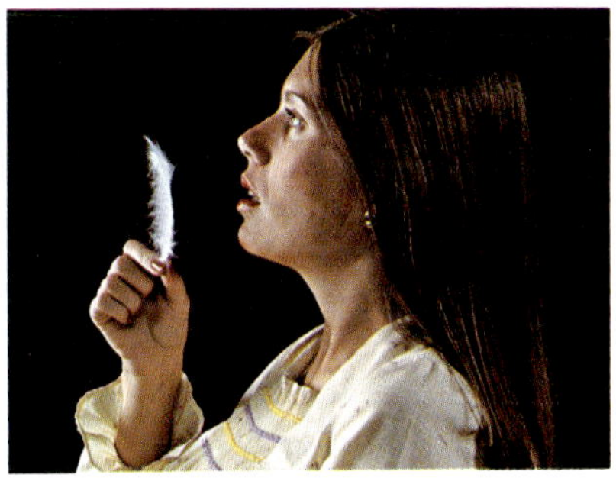

Her breath returns without her consciously drawing it in so that the feather returns to its normal position but does not move toward her.

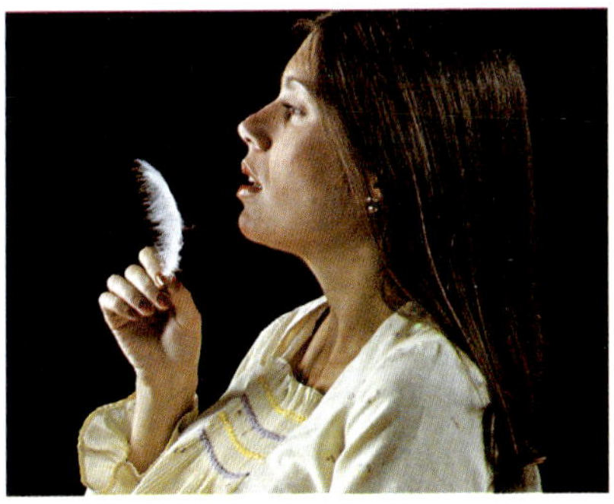

In level 2 breathing, the stronger, shorter outward breaths bend the feather over more.

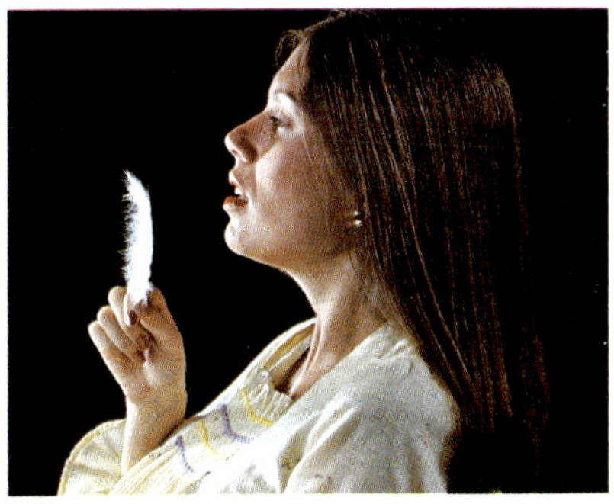

Again the breath is allowed to return naturally, so that the feather is not drawn toward her.

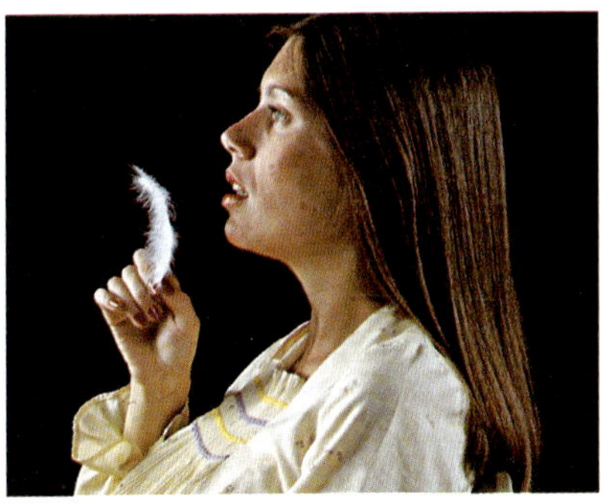

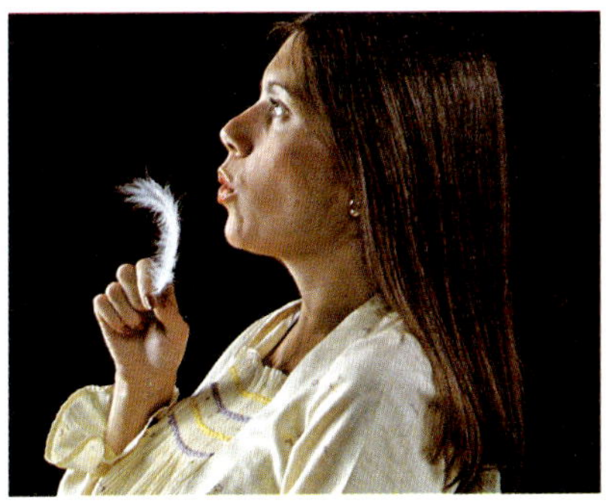

Level 3 – "huffing and puffing" – in which the breaths are stronger and shorter still, starts with two panting breaths (above) left followed by two blowing breaths (above right) with the lips pursed into an O shape. This sequence is repeated, but as in levels one and two, the breath is still allowed to return of its own accord.

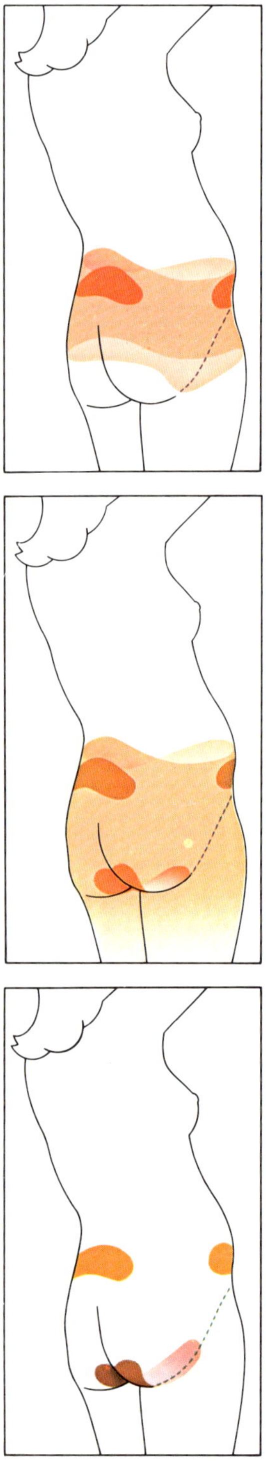

These pictures show the usual distribution and intensity of labor pains, from the first stage (top), through the transition from first to second stage (center), to late second stage and delivery (bottom). The darker the color, the more intense the pain.

point where the other breathing levels seem inadequate.

"Huffing and puffing" is a variation on the shallow breathing of level 2 and develops out of it. Count two very shallow, but controlled, breaths, still emphasizing the "out" breath each time. Then blow out quickly twice, allowing the breath to flow gently back into the lungs each time. The pattern is out-in, out-in, blow-in, blow-in.

Handling labor

The first stage. When contractions start it is a good idea to carry on with normal activities for as long as possible. The first stage can be quite long, especially with a first pregnancy, and if you retire to bed with the first contraction you are more likely to be worried or bored. Another reason for remaining upright is that gravity helps the baby descend toward the cervix. There are some obstetrical reasons why a mother may be advised to go to the hospital from the beginning of labor. For instance, in the case of early rupture of the membranes, the mother should go immediately to the hospital where she will probably be kept in bed.

You may find it is unnecessary to apply the breathing technique with the first few contractions, but as they get stronger, stop what you are doing and breathe with each one. Think of the coming contractions as waves, not sharp, stabbing and sudden pains, but building up, reaching a crest of pain and then subsiding again. Where the contractions are felt varies from woman to woman, depending on the baby's position. They may be felt in the lower abdomen; higher up beneath the breastbone; in a band that stretches from the lower abdomen to the lower back; or only in the back or the legs.

Usually in the early part of the first stage the waves are not very high and pain is not great. As the first stage progresses, the waves get higher, steeper, and more painful and the intervals between them are shorter. Most women will find level 1 breathing adequate at first but it is important to remember that all patterns of labor differ and that thresholds of pain vary from person to person. It may therefore be necessary to use level 2 or 3 breathing as well in the early stages.

The transition stage is the name given to the time between the first and second stages of labor, before the cervix is fully dilated and when the mother may sense an urge to push prematurely. Contractions may be coming so frequently and lasting for so long – perhaps at two minutes intervals and lasting one and a half minutes – that one contraction almost merges into the next. At this time, too, pain is usually at its maximum, and for many women it can be the most difficult part of the whole process of labor.

In the transition stage it is more important than ever to take the contractions one at a time as there is just enough time after each one to prepare for the next contraction. You may find back pressure can be particularly helpful at this stage (*see* p. 80) of labor.

Most women will feel the urge to push during this stage. This is like a compulsive bowel movement and is caused by the baby's head pressing on the rectum. Any such urge should be reported to the doctor who will check to see if the cervix is fully dilated. Until it is seen that this dilation has happened you will be instructed not to push.

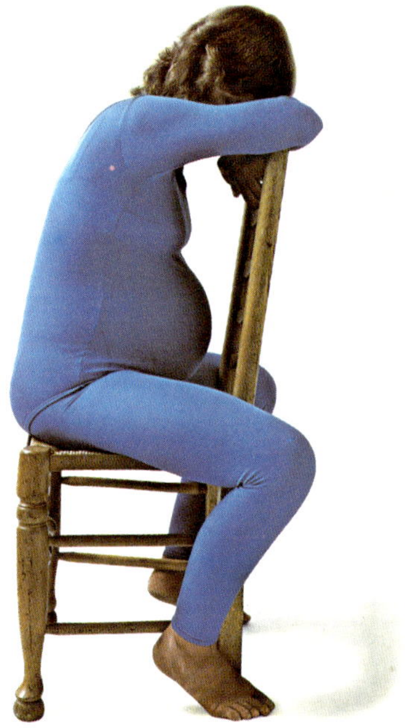

When you feel a contraction starting, stop what you are doing, relax and breathe over it. It is helpful to straddle a chair and rest your arms and head on its back. Alternatively, you can rest against a wall or some other suitable surface.

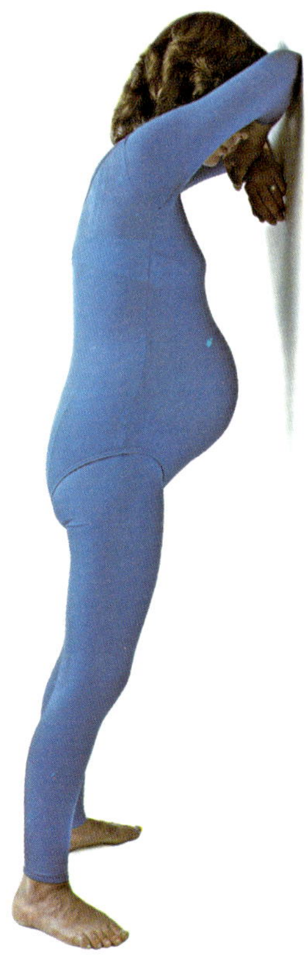

This can be very frustrating and the urge to push may seem overwhelming. "Huff and puff" right through each contraction: this will prevent you holding your breath involuntarily and pushing with it.

Remember at this point that you are nearing your goal. Your partner can help by reminding you of this.

The second stage starts when the cervix is fully dilated and finishes with the delivery of the baby. It is the most exciting and rewarding stage of labor for all concerned – very hard work, but worth all the effort in the end.

Prior to delivery you will have to bear down with your contractions to aid in the descent of

Early first stage contractions can also be eased by pressure on the lower back. Place one hand on top of the other, palms uppermost, on the sacroiliac area (below) and lean back on them against a wall (left).

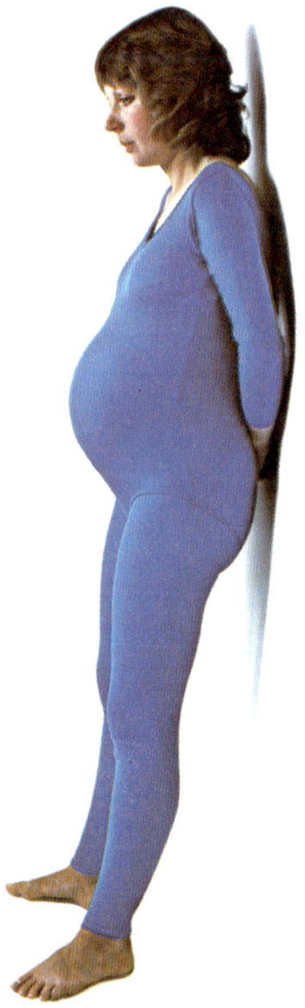

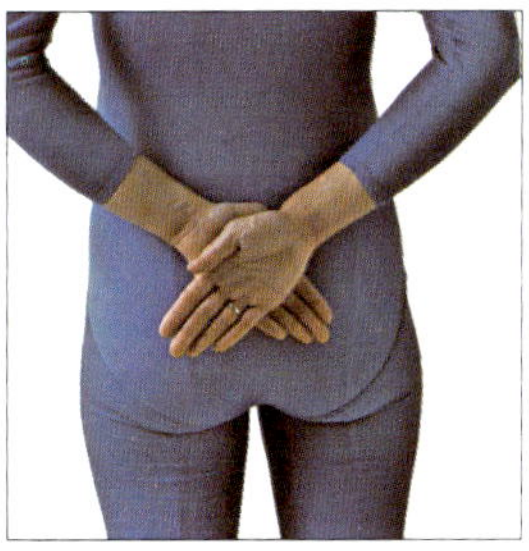

hard" and remember you are pushing out your baby. When you feel you can push no more, make a point of pushing for two more seconds. Then let your breath go with a grunt. If the contraction is still going on, take in another quick breath, tuck down your chin and push again. You might need to give three long pushes for each contraction.

During the contractions a nurse, or perhaps two, will usually hold up your legs although you may prefer to do this yourself. It is very helpful if, when each contraction starts, your partner puts his arms around your shoulders, for support, holds you forward and reminds you to push *long*.

Between contractions lie back and relax and take deep breaths to restore your energy for the next effort. Your partner can help by wiping your face with a damp cloth. During the second stage the baby's head rotates through the pelvis (*see* pp. 74–5).

With a first baby, the doctor will usually wait until the baby's head is visible with a

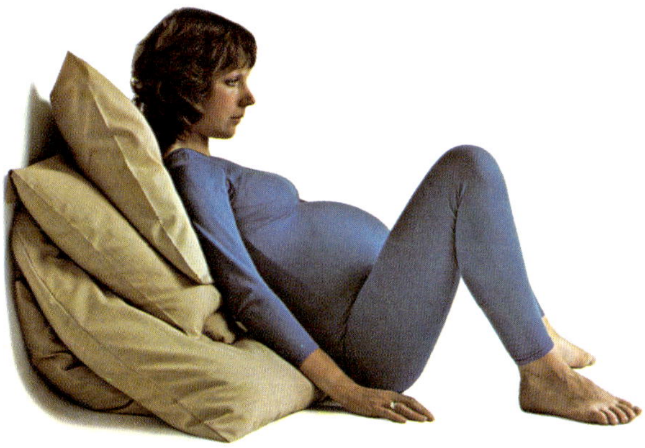

During the second stage of labor make sure you are propped up at an angle of 45 degrees with plenty of pillows. Your partner can help by collecting the pillows together and arranging them in the most comfortable way.

In preparing for labor it is useful to try out the position for pushing. As you push, a nurse will probably hold up your legs. It is comforting if your partner supports your shoulders and back.

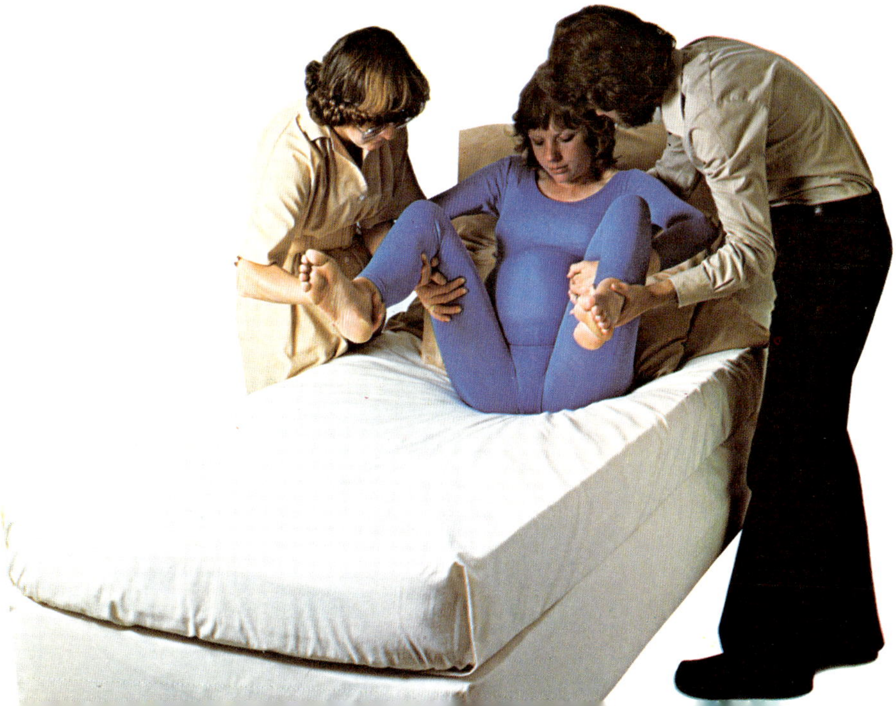

the baby's head. With a first baby, pushing may be required for one to two hours; a shorter second stage is usual with subsequent babies. The best position for pushing before delivery is one with the mother propped up at an angle of 45 degrees. Pushing is much more effective in this position than lying down. If you are not placed in this position you can ask to be. Your knees will be bent and your feet will rest comfortably on the bed.

As each contraction starts, hold your thighs firmly from the outside, pick up your legs, take a big breath in, round your shoulders, tuck down your chin and push. If you bend your elbows forward it will ensure that you round your shoulders, and by opening your legs to the maximum width you will consequently relax your pelvic floor.

Your mental attitude is again important here: think "push long" rather than "push

push before transferring you to the delivery room. With subsequent babies you will probably be transferred to the delivery room at 8 or 9 cm dilation, which is before the baby's head can be visualized. In the delivery room, you will lie on the delivery table with your legs in stirrups, and with your partner positioned slightly behind at your shoulder encouraging you and helping you to concentrate.

Sometimes the size of the baby or its position makes it absolutely impossible for a woman to push the baby out without help. In this case the doctor will use forceps (*see* p. 108).

Once the baby's head has negotiated the pelvis, it appears at the vaginal opening. After only a few more contractions it "crowns" (the widest part passes through the opening of the vulva). At the moment of crowning you may be asked to stop pushing for a while because the doctor does not want the head to be born too quickly. Specific instructions will be given, which will be different for every delivery.

Practicing for labor

Practice the basic breathing techniques each day in the third trimester. Never force the breathing and never try to take shallower breaths than you comfortably can. If you get dizzy or breathless this means that you have been practicing for too long, or trying to impose a pattern too far from your normal breathing rhythm.

It can be useful to tap out the level 3 huffing and puffing as you practice: this is done simply by two taps with the knuckles followed by two taps with the fingers flat.

Once you are familiar with the breathing technique, it is a good idea to use some everyday happening as a "trigger" for an imaginary contraction.

Some women find it impossible to practice the very shallow breathing of level 2: they are only able to manage the steady level 1 breathing and the huffing and puffing. If you find this is so in your own case do not worry. By practicing you will build a sense of purpose and a determination to cope with one contraction at a time (each one a step closer to the birth of your child). You will then find that the breathing will happen almost automatically in labor; your breathing will adapt instinctively to your needs. Some women never use the shallow level 2 breathing, but those who need it find they can do it in labor.

The techniques of disassociation (*see* p. 76) can be practiced with the breathing levels by the mother alone, or with the help of a partner. To practice alone hold an arm or leg stiff, keep the rest of your body relaxed and breathe as if you were experiencing a contraction.

Try out the position for delivery a few times to familiarize yourself with it. If possible pick up your legs as you would to push. There is no need to do this often. During late pregnancy it is an uncomfortable pose but remember that when you reach the second stage in labor the amniotic fluid, which takes up a lot of space, will have gone.

Other aids for labor

There are a number of useful "tools" which can be added to the basic breathing techniques to help a woman through labor. Most call for help and should be practiced with one's partner beforehand.

Back massage. If contractions are felt in the back, firm massage at the bottom of the spine is greatly appreciated by some women. This must be really firm and it is best to use the "heel" of the hand. The woman should be lying on her side and propped up at a slight angle (not lying flat) so that gravity will help the baby move down onto the cervix.

Back pressure may be useful whether contractions are felt in the abdomen or in the back. As the pain starts, the partner should press really hard against the lower part of the back (sacrum area). While pressure is being applied it is beneficial for the woman to hold, or stroke, the lower part of her abdomen. A woman can apply back pressure herself during the early first stage by placing one hand on top of the other, palms uppermost, on the sacral area and leaning against a wall.

Rhythmic stroking can be a valuable aid when contractions become really strong. There are slightly different ways of doing it, two of which are shown here. One can be used by the woman or her partner, whether she is lying on her back or on her side, and the other can be used by the mother alone if she is lying on her back.

With the first method, stroke across the lower half of the abdomen with one hand, describing a semicircle, as shown (fig. 2). For the second method, use both hands and, start-

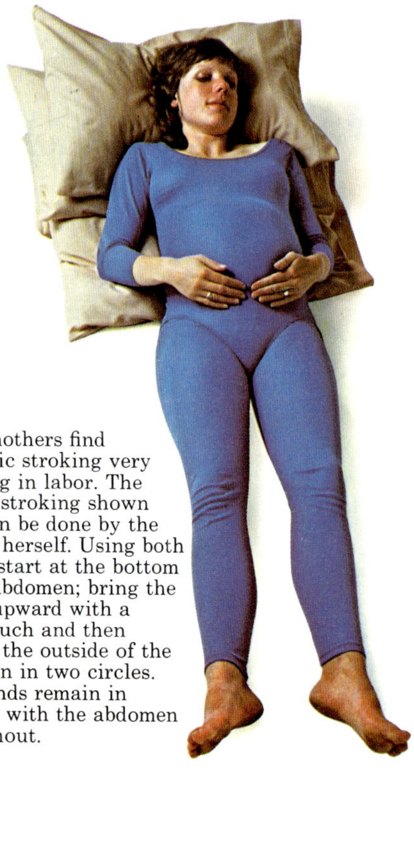

Some mothers find rhythmic stroking very soothing in labor. The type of stroking shown here can be done by the woman herself. Using both hands, start at the bottom of the abdomen; bring the hands upward with a light touch and then around the outside of the abdomen in two circles. The hands remain in contact with the abdomen throughout.

ing at the bottom of the abdomen, bring them upward and then around the outside of the abdomen in two circles, as shown (fig. 1), or in the reverse direction if preferred.

If the partner is doing the stroking it is best used throughout a contraction. If used by the woman herself she may prefer to do it just when the contraction is at its strongest. It is a good idea to sprinkle a little talcum powder on the skin first to stop friction. The rhythmic stroking should be a light movement, but if it is too light it may tickle.

Leg massage can give relief if the contractions are felt in the thighs. Although it is quite possible for a woman to use this technique on herself, it is best performed by her partner who can give really firm pressure Place one palm on the inside of each knee and push firmly along the inside of the thighs to the hips. Bring hands back to the knees again, applying no pressure.

Dealing with cramps. Sometimes during the second stage cramps are felt in the legs, particularly when they are up in stirrups. The answer is to stretch the cramped muscle. If the cramp is felt in the calf, stretch out the leg as much as possible with the heel leading. If the cramp is in the front of the leg, stretch the leg and point the toe.

Contractions felt in the thighs may be relieved by massage. Your partner's help is particularly welcome. He should push firmly along the inside of both thighs from knee to hip, and then bring his hands lightly back to the knees.

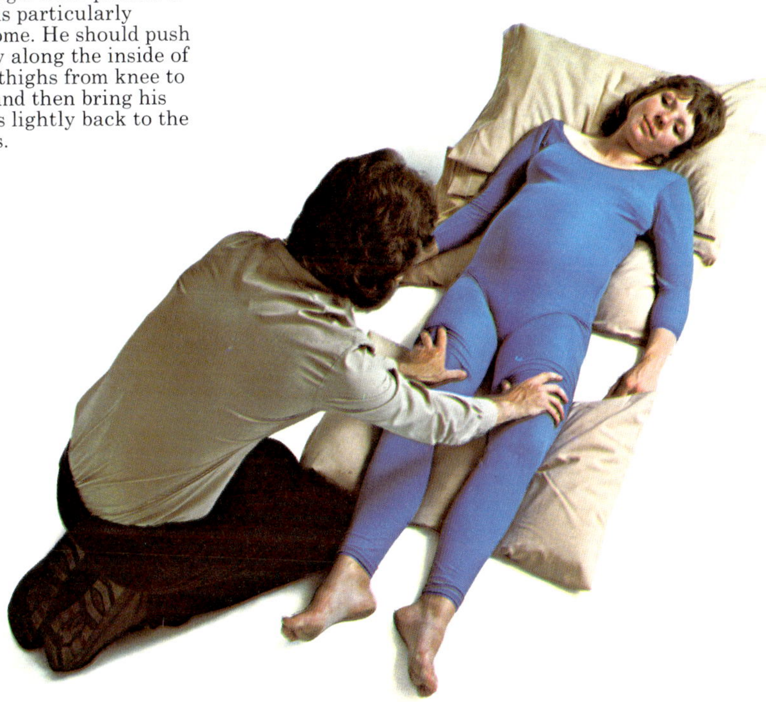

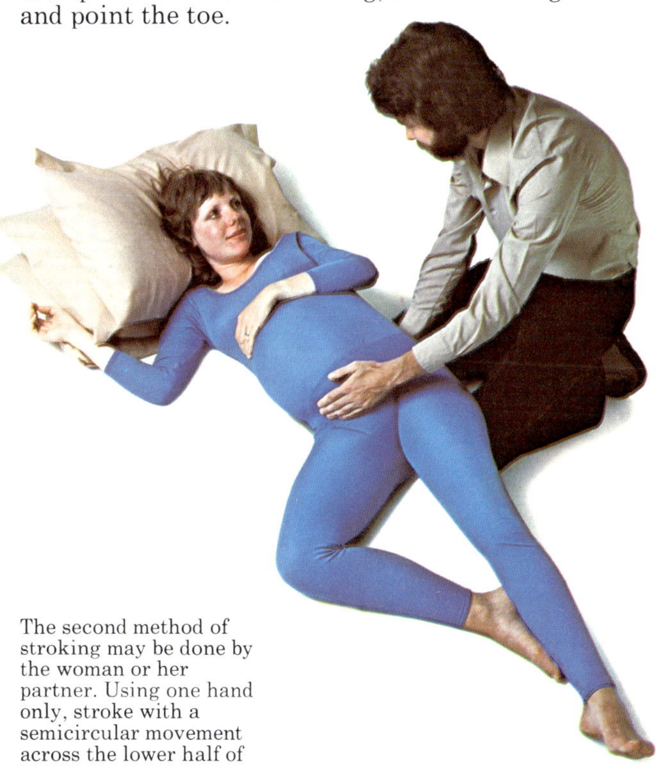

The second method of stroking may be done by the woman or her partner. Using one hand only, stroke with a semicircular movement across the lower half of the abdomen. Lift the hand and go back to the starting position. Or, if you prefer, simply keep the hand still.

Ask your partner to press hard in the sacroiliac area while you gently cradle the abdomen in your hands. Pressure on the lower back can serve to relieve the pain of contractions in a very remarkable way.

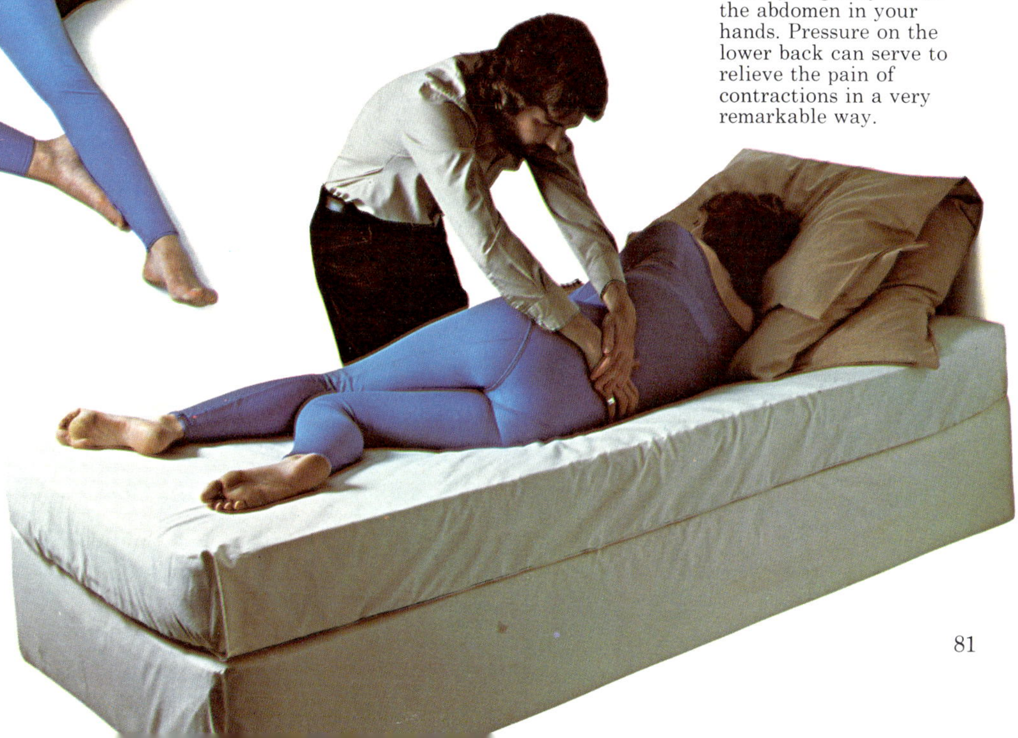

Pain relief

Although some women experience no pain with labor and birth, this is not the usual situation. Generally, patients experience a spectrum from mild discomfort to severe pain. There is no reason for concern, however, because there are many options for pain relief. Whether the mother chooses to use a psychoprophylaxis approach like Lamaze or use medication or conduction anesthesia, she will find a method which suits her well. It is best to discuss your likes and dislikes with your obstetrician well before the onset of labor. Most physicians will discuss this briefly on your first visit to the office.

Because of the wide spectrum of pain in labor all pain-relieving treatments must be left to the personal choice of the mother in concert with her physician. The type of relief she requires and when it is administered can, in normal circumstances, be determined by the laboring mother. She must, therefore, understand about the drugs and techniques used for such relief so that if she requires treatment she can help make a reasonable choice.

There are, however, situations where for sound medical reasons the mother is advised to have a certain form of pain relief which she might not have chosen. Variations in labor such as twins, breech or premature babies, are more safely delivered when the mother has an epidural block.

All drugs that affect the mother affect the baby too. This could become a problem after the baby is born when his own immature systems must remove the drug from his body. Before the mother is given any treatment, therefore, the effect on the newborn baby must be taken into account. Without doubt what is generally best for the baby is no drugs at all but that is not always possible.

Nitrous oxide

This is a mixture of nitrous oxide ("laughing gas") and oxygen which the mother breathes with the help of a hand-held mask or with a mask held by the anesthesiologist. In many hospitals this is not used during the first stage of labor. It may be used on the delivery table during the second stage to help the mother to push effectively.

In many respects this is an ideal pain-relieving drug for labor because it acts quickly. Even quick-acting drugs need time to achieve their effect, however, and at least three inhalations of the gas must be taken before the pain is lessened. Gas is breathed in at the start of a contraction and inhaled during the whole contraction. Between contractions the mother breathes air. Research demonstrates that when nitrous oxide is being used correctly, approximately 70 per cent of women in labor obtain satisfactory pain relief by this method.

Nitrous oxide is beneficial to the baby because in using it the mother breathes a high concentration of oxygen during a period when, because of the contractions, the baby is often short of oxygen.

Even the most ideal drug has disadvantages, however, and although nitrous oxide has no disadvantages in itself, its success is variable and in a certain number of mothers it is ineffective. It can also add to the mother's inclination to feel nauseated while she is in labor.

Centrally acting drugs

Among the drugs that act on the central nervous system the most commonly used is Demerol, which has been well-tried for many years. Demerol is given by injection at the mother's request during the first stage of labor. The doctor may order it to be given intravenously or intramuscularly. Its effect is not to remove all the pain and sensation of labor but to lower the pain to a tolerable level. The main disadvantage of the drug is that it produces a temporary clouding of the consciousness and makes some mothers feel they are losing control of their labors; the experience of delivery is therefore less acute. Demerol can also be given with nitrous oxide if stronger pain relief is required.

Mothers will also want to take into account the fact that the dose and the timing of the drug's administration affect the baby. Large doses given late in labor may cause the baby to be very sleepy and have some difficulty in starting to breathe, but this is usually not a problem as breathing aids are always close at hand. With smaller doses the baby may be only mildly drowsy. This drug may also increase the mother's nausea.

Epidural and other nerve blocks

Local anesthetics act by blocking the nerves that carry the pain impulses. They can be used to give continuous pain relief during labor, generally by means of epidural block, with no long-lasting effect on either the mother or the new baby.

The epidural block is a technique whereby the local anesthetic drug is injected into the epidural space, an area through which the nerves travel from the spinal cord to the uterus and cervix. This space is approached from the mother's back, where the skin is made insensitive with a little local anesthetic. A cannula (hollow) needle is then inserted into the epidural space and a minute tube is threaded through it. The tube is left in place taped to the mother's back until the baby has been delivered, so that repeated doses of the local anesthetic can be injected while, at the same time, causing absolutely no inconvenience to the mother.

The pain of contractions disappears within ten to fifteen minutes of the injection. The mother's feet and legs feel warm and heavy and tingle slightly as if she were suffering pins and needles. Each dose of local anesthetic lasts one-and-a-half hours and then, as the pain starts to return, another dose must be given through the tubing. With this technique an almost totally painless labor can be successfully achieved.

The mother is positioned so that the local anesthetic can flow over the nerves that need to be blocked. Generally she is placed first on one side and then the other. Toward the end of labor she is placed in a sitting position. The epidural block has great advantages in labors with complications (*see* chapter 7); for those mothers who in the past would have had a long and painful labor; and for those who fear labor. Now no mother-to-be need fear that she will be allowed to suffer unduly whatever her labor is like.

The treatment is particularly useful when the mother experiences great pain early in labor and where labor is likely to last a long time. A mother can have an epidural block at any time after labor is established and the cervix is 5–6 cm dilated, but as it takes at least 15 minutes for an epidural block to work it is generally administered earlier rather than later during labor.

It is also ideal in cases where high blood pressure accompanies pregnancy and where other pain-relieving drugs are unsuitable. Epidurals also serve to safeguard the baby in the case of twins, breech babies or premature babies since it ensures that the mother's muscles are relaxed and the baby's head therefore meets less resistance. One of the disadvantages of the block, however, is that the mother may have a decreased urge to push and this may mean that the baby has to be delivered by forceps. On the other hand, should a forceps delivery become necessary it may be carried out at once without the administration of any additional anesthetic.

In a number of hospitals epidural blocks have been used for several years as the primary form of pain relief for normal labors and those with special problems, as it is clearly the most effective treatment and has a good safety record. An epidural block does, however, require a skilled anesthesiologist to administer it. In many hospitals an epidural is available only in exceptional circumstances; this is directly attributable to a shortage of trained anesthesiologists.

Certain safeguards are needed if an epidural block is administered. Firstly, an intravenous drip is set up in case the mother requires extra fluid to prevent any fall in blood pressure occurring once the block has started. The baby's well-being must also be checked constantly. This is best done with electronic monitoring of the fetal heart rate pattern (*see* p. 102). In this way the baby's heart rate can be monitored during each contraction. This is necessary in case the mother has a small fall in blood pressure which would in turn affect the blood flow to the baby via the placenta.

One of the increasingly important uses for epidural and other local blocks is to allow those mothers who need a cesarean section to experience the pleasure of seeing their baby born. With the lower half of her body anesthetized, the mother feels nothing but she is still wide awake. It has been found that the mother who has a cesarean with an epidural block is frequently more satisfied and feels that she has taken a greater part in the birth of her baby than the mother who has a general anesthetic. She, of course, does not see any of the operation which is screened from view, but is able to see her baby immediately on delivery. This is important to her psychologically: it bonds her to the baby. She can discuss her reactions with the anesthesiologist or obstetrician. In most hospitals, the husband is permitted to be present during a cesarean section to offer support to the mother. Lastly, the epidural block is often safer for both the mother and the baby than a general anesthetic.

The disadvantages of epidural blocks are largely emotional, especially for those mothers who desire to experience childbirth in as natural a way as possible. Because she does not feel the contractions or the sense of pushing the mother sometimes feels deprived of the experience of childbirth and subsequently regrets not having all the sensations which accompany labor, including pain. Another effect of this technique is to prolong labor to a certain extent, but with the mother comfortable and in no pain and the baby in a satisfactory state this is not considered a great disadvantage.

A further effect on labor is a 20–30 per cent forceps rate. This is because as well as losing the pain sensation the mother feels little or no urge to bear down toward the end of labor. This sort of forceps delivery does not damage the baby or mother, however, because there is no question of the baby being too large for the mother's pelvis and because the mother is perfectly relaxed and does not require any further anesthetic. The baby is usually born in very good condition. Many doctors let the block partly wear off to make it easier for the mother to push. As a result, the likelihood of a delivery involving the use of forceps is greatly decreased.

Some mothers, however, still feel the high rate of forceps delivery to be a considerable disadvantage, just as they regard the required safeguards needed for an epidural as too great a degree of medical interference in a natural process.

An epidural is not always successful in procuring a totally painless labor. Sometimes the block is not completely effective, leaving a part of the mother's body still with the sensation of pain. A more common problem arises where the mother becomes aware of the returning sensation too late for the following dose to take effect without an intervening period of pain, which often feels that much worse when the labor has hitherto been painless.

Other nerve blocks used in labor include the caudal block which is an epidural block in which the epidural space is reached from lower down the mother's back, and a spinal block which blocks the nerves nearer the spinal cord. The caudal block is used when it is felt that an epidural block would be too slow to take effect.

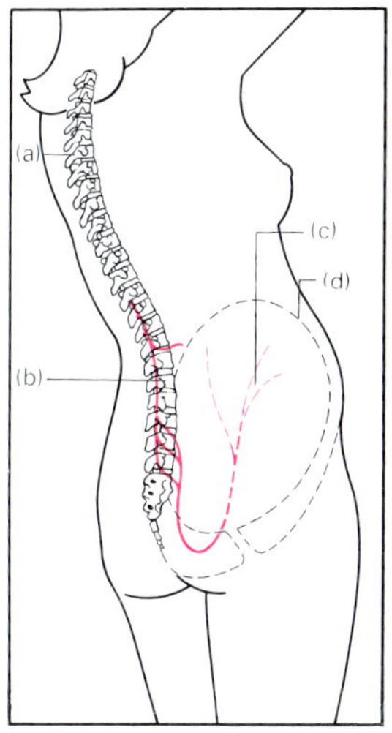

The needle carrying the epidural anesthetic is inserted between two vertebrae of the spine (a) into the epidural space – that is the area between the dura, which protects the spinal cord, and the bone of the vertebrae. The point of entry varies but one possible one is shown at (b). Nerves (c) travel through this space from the spinal cord to the uterus (d) and cervix. The needle (e) carrying the epidural anesthetic is here shown entering the epidural space (f). The spinal cord (g) is shown encased in the dura (h).

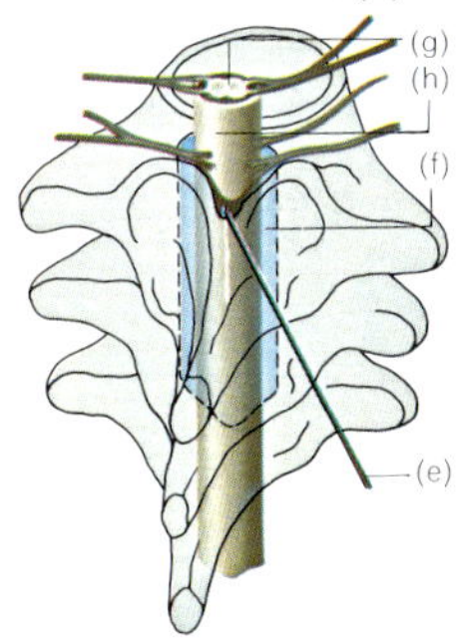

Labor and birth

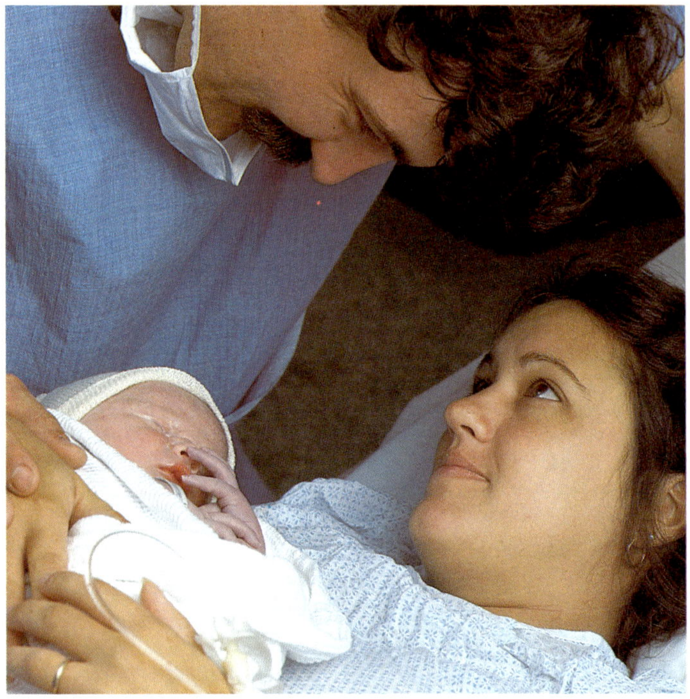

CHAPTER 6

Every mother's experience of childbirth is unique, partly, of course, because every child is unique. But each hospital has different resources, ideas and methods which will also affect her, as will the pattern of each labor, the forms of pain relief used and the amount of medical intervention needed. The involvement of the father or friends and relatives and, above all, the mother's own feelings also play a crucial part.

The physiological processes of labor and birth and the techniques of pain relief were described in the last chapter. This chapter deals with birth as a practical and personal experience, looking at what happens in the hospital, both in the labor room and in the delivery room.

To a large extent, the type of experience you have as a couple will depend upon the amount of preparation you have. This preparation includes reading, going to preparation for childbirth classes, asking questions of your doctor and above all developing a dialogue with other friends who have been through childbirth. As you go through this education process your whole concept of childbirth will develop. Many of the fears and apprehensions will disappear and you will be preparing yourselves for a very positive and rewarding experience.

It is one thing to understand the mechanism of labor, another to recognize the moment at which your own begins. The contractions that indicate the start of labor are not always dramatically different from those which have already occurred in the latter part of pregnancy and their spacing and intensity vary a good deal from woman to woman. This chapter opens with a straightforward account of how to identify the actual onset of labor. *You must remember that no two babies are exactly alike. Not even your own*

Cross references

See also	Chapter
Breathing	5
Complications in labor	7
Labor	5
Premature and postmature babies	9

It is important for both parents to establish contact with their new baby as soon as possible after the birth.

labors will be alike! So when reading this section, use it as a general guide.

This is followed by a section on the practical preparations to be made for a delivery. Something as basic as making sure there is enough gas in the car when the moment to go to the hospital arrives may prove just as important as understanding the process of childbirth. What a mother can expect once she arrives at the hospital will vary but a description is given here of the environment and type of procedures found in one large hospital – from arrival at the reception desk to the well-earned rest in her room.

This chapter describes what will transpire in a normal labor and delivery. Obviously, situations will vary with different hospitals and different doctors. But generally, this description of labor and delivery will pertain to most couples. The circumstances of an actual birth are presented, illustrated by what the birth felt like to a first-time mother.

Then, a discussion of the changing childbirth scene is presented with a special consideration of alternative birthing centers. That hospitals must eliminate senseless, rigid routines and be responsive to patients' feelings and needs is a foregone conclusion. They must be flexible to accommodate patients' psychological needs and, at the same time, provide technological safeguards.

Finally, the Leboyer approach is dicussed. Gentle birth is not really a new technique. After all, doctors haven't been slapping babies' bottoms for decades. But, Dr. Leboyer has put forward an approach that is worthy of consideration. Some of its aspects are beneficial provided the newborn baby is breathing properly and doesn't lose body heat by exposure to room temperature.

Many couples find that they are so caught up in this totally consuming experience of childbirth that the whole thing is over before they realize it. They find themselves looking back and remembering many features of the experience and yet the whole process seemed to come and go without their full realization. This is because the experience is awesome. No matter how sophisticated or experienced a couple may be – the birth of a baby is a moving and emotional event. Even the seasoned obstetrician has been known to have a flow of tears when something particularly touching occurs in the delivery room.

One might think that most babies are delivered at night. Actually this is not so. Most babies are delivered in the day. But since a first labor lasts 12–13 hours obviously some portion of many labors occurs in the night. This portion of the experience seems to be more impressive than the daytime experience.

As you read this chapter and discuss experiences with friends who have been through labor, you will develop your own personal perspective. As a couple, you will learn together and develop a concept of teamwork. The baby – the ultimate reason for all of the planning and effort – will be a product of cooperation. It is not uncommon to hear a new father talking as if he had had the baby. What could be a better way of establishing parent-infant bonding!

In writing this chapter we bear in mind that it is impossible to cover all aspects of labor and birth. Furthermore since every individual's experience will be different we hope that our presentation will be global enough to help you to prepare, as a couple for the magnificent experience. We are convinced that the more information you have the more positive your experience will be.

Birth

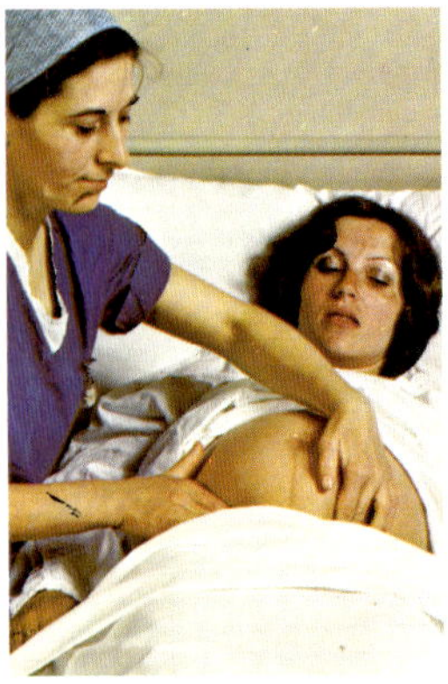

Soon after a woman arrives in the hospital, a nurse will examine her abdomen to find out the position of the baby and to determine whether the head has already engaged.

In contrast to the way it is often portrayed in the media, labor does not begin suddenly. All through pregnancy there have been painless (Braxton Hicks) contractions. Very gradually these become stronger and more frequent and the mother becomes conscious of them as they become uncomfortable. During these contractions a hardening of the uterine muscle can be felt all over the abdomen, making it resistant to the touch. At the same time there is usually a feeling of discomfort or pain in the lower part of the abdomen, or less commonly in the lower back or the legs (*see* p. 78). Any frequent and painful contractions, even if irregular, may indicate that labor has begun.

Labor often starts with the contractions at fairly wide intervals. These vary from one woman to another and may be as far apart as every 30 minutes. Diarrhea may occur as labor starts and the discomfort caused by an early labor is often attributed to it. As the first stage progresses (*see* pp. 72, 78), the contractions become more frequent, and the intervals between each contraction gradually reduce to two or three minutes.

You should contact your doctor as soon as you think you are in labor. The doctor will probably suggest you wait until the contractions are felt regularly at ten-minute intervals or feel uncomfortable. With a first baby, when labor tends to be much longer, there is generally no need to rush.

Sometimes before labor begins a sticky, thick clear blob of mucus streaked with blood comes out of the vagina, often when going to the toilet. Known as "bloody show", this is not necessarily a sign that labor is about to begin since it can appear a few days or so before labor or not until late in labor. Only if the show is heavily bloodstained is it worth contacting your doctor.

If there is a trickle or gush of warm, watery fluid, however, it is important to contact your doctor immediately even if there have been no contractions or show. This may mean that the amniotic sac in which the fetus rests has ruptured ("the waters have broken") and the baby is no longer protected from infection. Another reason for concern if the waters have broken is that it is sometimes possible for a loop of the umbilical cord to slip past the baby along with the gush of liquid. This could result in the cord getting squeezed between the pelvic bones and the baby's head, thus cutting off, or at least reducing, the baby's blood supply. This is fortunately very unusual, but it makes an emergency delivery necessary.

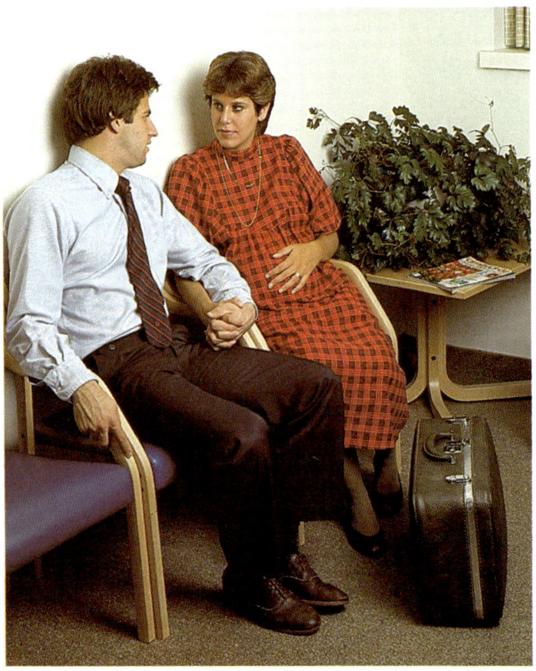

Most hospitals have a day room which the father can use as a base throughout the confinement and where the expectant mother can sit up with him during the latent first stage of labor. A woman giving birth should take with her a suitcase containing everything she is likely to need during her hospital stay.

Practical preparations for a birth

Toward the end of pregnancy there are a number of practical preparations to be made. The basic equipment needed for the new baby in the first month or two should, of course, be organized before the birth. Detailed advice on this is given in chapter 11.

Simple arrangements must also be made for the birth itself. The mother will need to pack a suitcase to take in with her. A list of the minimum requirements is given in the margin of the opposite page.

Arrangements may have to be made for looking after other children during the stay in the hospital. If the trip to the hospital will be by car, remember to keep it in good working order, with sufficient gas in the tank. Find out in advance the best route to the hospital, any parking restrictions in streets next to it and make a practice trip to the hospital. An ambulance or some form of emergency medical service is usually available for emergency transportation, but you should make sure you know how to call an ambulance just in case the need should arise.

If the father is going to be with the mother during the birth, there are certain things he will need. Since he may have to wait a long time he should make sure he has enough food (chocolate is useful), as well as a book or magazine to keep himself occupied. (If he has to leave the hospital during labor he may miss the birth.) In most hospitals he will be able to buy food in the cafeteria but whatever he eats he should never give any food to the mother during labor. He may also need plenty of small change for calling relatives or friends from a pay phone after the birth. Hospital corridors and waiting rooms will be comfortable and cooler than the delivery room, which will be very warm and in which he will be obliged to wear a hospital gown, cap and mask. A thin shirt to wear in the delivery room, and a sweater or jacket to put on outside it are the most sensible clothing.

Always call your doctor before you go to the hospital. Your doctor will then call the hospital so that the staff will be prepared and have your antenatal records ready. This is very important as, if there are any particular problems, they can be quickly noted and the details of your antenatal course and laboratory values can be checked. If you believe you are in labor stop eating or drinking because the digestive process slows down during labor. As a result, food will remain undigested in the stomach; or you could vomit and aspirate the vomitus into your lungs.

What to expect in the hospital

Hospital procedures sometimes seem confusing and unnecessary and for this reason it is well to know in advance what will happen during your hospital stay. A description based on one particular hospital is given here, rather than a general vague account. Procedures differ from hospital to hospital.

First, you meet an aide at the reception desk who will record your arrival, collect files containing your antenatal records and then show you into your labor room.

Once inside the labor room, the admitting nurse will give you a hospital gown and then ask you to lie down on your bed where she will observe contractions and ask you routine questions about the onset, frequency and strength of your contractions, whether the waters have broken and whether there has been any blood or green staining of the amniotic fluid.

Occasionally, an expectant mother appears so near to delivery that these questions are asked immediately and a vaginal examination is done to determine if the patient should be moved to the delivery room.

After the patient is comfortable in bed, the nurse or doctor will feel the quality and frequency of contractions and observe the fetal heart rate with a fetoscope. It is common practice to apply external electronic fetal monitoring to patients in active labor. If this is done, two bands are applied around your waist. One instrument measures uterine contractions and the other measures the frequency of the fetal heartbeat. Once it is determined that everything is going well, attention will then probably be turned to the prep. The pubic hair on the perineum might be trimmed or shaved. Following this many patients are given a suppository or an enema to empty the intestinal tract so that there is less chance of contamination during delivery and to act as a stimulant of labor. The patient then rests in bed during her labor. If she is found to be in very early labor it is possible for her to be out of bed. If her membranes are ruptured she will be told to remain in bed during labor.

In some patients the membranes rupture prior to the onset of labor. In most patients, this will occur during the first stage of labor. When this happens the mother will feel warm fluid running down her legs.

The father is generally with the mother in the labor room offering her emotional and physical support, frequently helping her concentrate on her breathing techniques. When delivery is imminent the expectant mother will be transferred to the delivery room where she will lie on the delivery table with her legs positioned in padded stirrups. The perineal area will be scrubbed with antiseptic solution. Drapes will be put on the mother's legs and abdomen to decrease the chance of infection. The father may then join the mother.

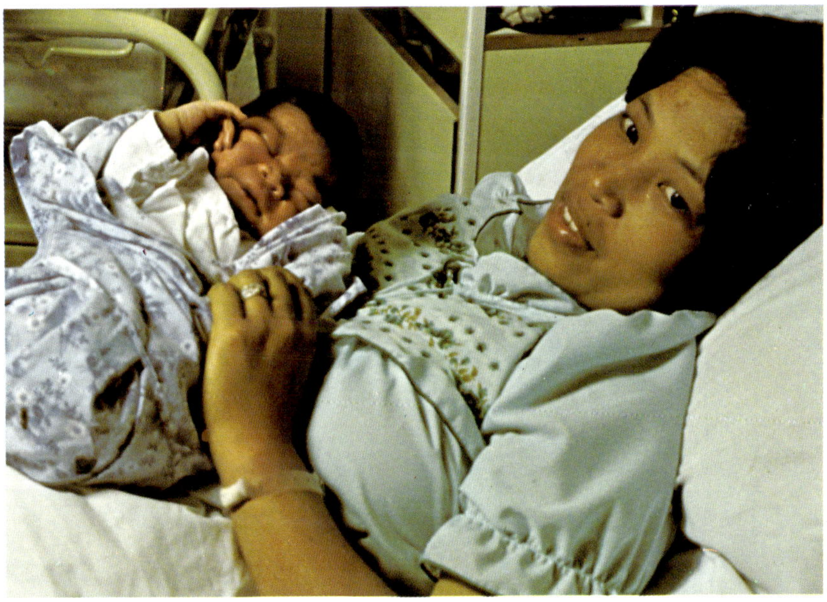

After the birth, the mother will be taken to her room, where she can have a much needed sleep after the exertions of labor.

Throughout labor, your blood pressure, the fetal heart rate and the strength, duration and frequency of contractions are recorded at regular intervals. The two latter might be done by listening through a stethoscope and by placing a hand on the abdomen, or with the help of electronic fetal monitoring. Additional vaginal examinations might be made to check progress. You will be asked to empty your bladder as often as possible during labor and you will probably be given antacid drinks to avoid any ill effects of vomiting in labor.

After the baby's birth, the placenta is delivered and the episiotomy stitched up if one has been performed. You will remain in the delivery room for at least an hour while the amount of bleeding and the degree of contraction of the uterus will be recorded (*see* p. 75). During this time you will have a chance to cuddle the baby and, if you wish, put him or her to the breast.

After your delivery, you will usually be given an opportunity to visit with your baby. During this time the baby may be put to the breast or just held. This is an excellent time to develop maternal-infant bonding. The baby must be kept warm because exposure to room air could allow the newborn's temperature to drop rapidly. Eventually, the baby will be taken to the Newborn Nursery for close observation. After this period, the baby may be brought out to you numerous times during the day for feeding. If you are planning to have rooming-in, the baby will either be in your room continuously or during the majority of the day and be cared for at night in an adjacent nursery. All hospitals have different policies but most modern hospitals afford some form of rooming-in accommodation so that the mother and baby can be together as much as possible.

WHAT YOU NEED TO PACK FOR THE HOSPITAL:

nightgowns (front-opening if nursing)
bathrobe
slippers
several pairs of panties
3 nursing or support bras
toilet articles
reading material
change for the phone

The mother's going home outfit and the baby's clothes can be brought when you arrive in labor. If storage space is limited, the family may bring these in the night before the mother's discharge from the hospital.

The first stage of labor

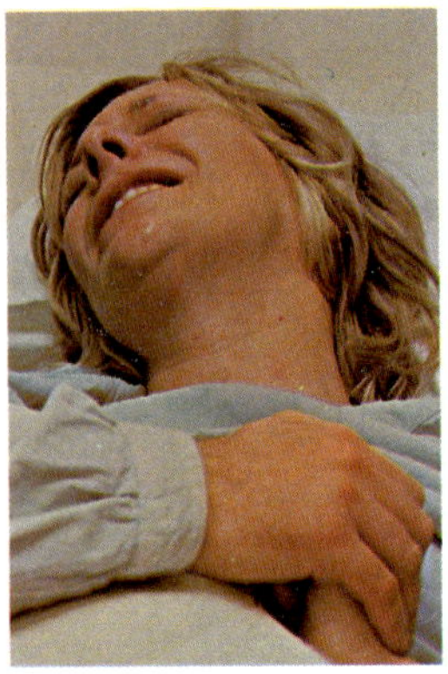

Labor is a time of great concentration for the mother. Training in relaxation helps her to resist the tension which accompanies intense contractions.

The techniques learned in preparation for childbirth classes can be helpful at all stages of a normal labor. They give the mother a better sense of control and make it easier for the father to help her during labor. Jan and Paul both attended antenatal classes and were well-prepared for the birth. Jan found the breathing exercises invaluable.

Jan: *The first contractions came at 2 o'clock in the morning and they took me by surprise. I had expected them to feel like intense Braxton Hicks contractions – a tightening and shrinking of the abdomen – but these were more like menstrual cramps: waves of dull discomfort. They weren't particularly intense and I fell asleep until 5 o'clock when a much stronger contraction woke me up. I went to the bathroom and found a show of blood – now I knew it had really started.*

Paul: *Jan woke me and we timed the contractions. They were coming at 13-minute intervals and lasting 55 seconds. We contacted the doctor. He told us to plan to come to the hospital within an hour.*

Jan: *At first I felt excited and happy. Then, just for a moment, I got the shakes. Paul had to reassure me, and by the time we left for the hospital my nerves had gone. When we were ready to go into the delivery room I was feeling relaxed, cheerful and confident.*

The doctor then ruptured the membranes to release the amniotic fluid.

Jan: *The doctor broke the bag by inserting an instrument into my vagina. It was like a rather long internal examination – not painful but unpleasant. Afterward I could feel the fluid pouring out. It felt rather like passing urine without being in control.*

Jan entered the labor room at 9 am. She was dressed in a green gown and laid on her bed. Two electrodes were placed on her abdomen. These were attached to a machine which measured the baby's heartbeat and the mother's contractions, and traced them on a simultaneous graph.

The contractions now became longer and

"The breathing exercises were invaluable. I depended on Paul to keep me going. Once or twice, when he went out of the room, I felt I was losing control and I had to fight to regain it."

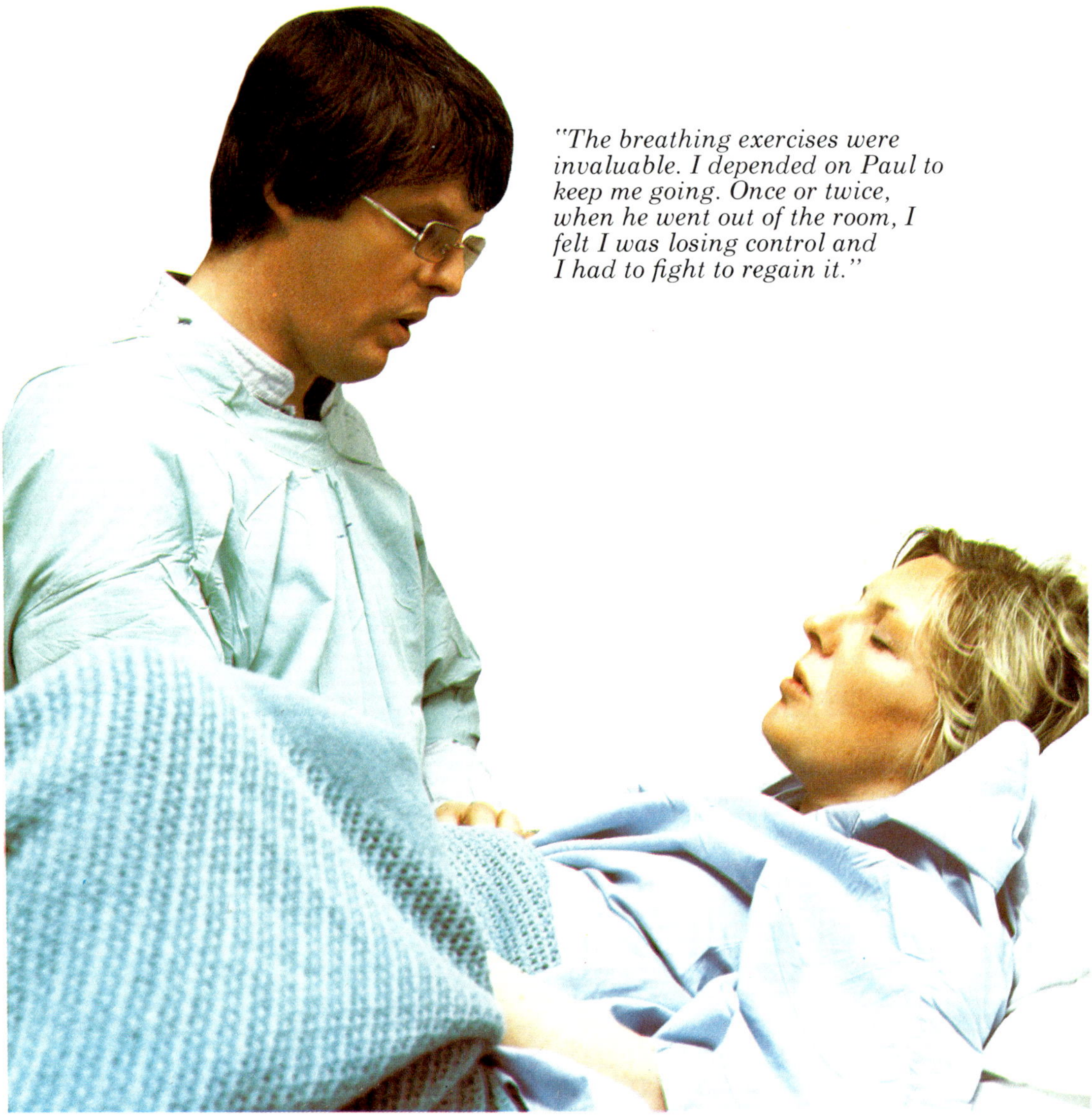

The father's presence in the labor room need not be that of passive observer. He can give reassurance in unfamiliar surroundings, and guide the woman through her contractions if she is using relaxation techniques. Working as a team (right), Paul helps Jan tap out the rhythm of a song as the cervix reaches full dilation.

closer together. By 10 o'clock each one was lasting up to one minute, with two or three minutes in between.

Jan: *Each one was like a wave. At its height it would feel like a tight, squeezing machine was at work inside, and I'd have a dull ache at the base of my abdomen. The sensation was still very much like a menstrual cramp. I was now using the breathing exercises I had learned.*

Each contraction brought with it a desire to tense up. I knew from the classes that that is just what you mustn't do – it dissipates the energy needed later on for pushing and it makes the pain worse. The breathing exercises were invaluable here. I depended on Paul to keep me going. He would time me, counting each breath and slapping out the rhythm on the palm of my hand. If he saw me tensing up he'd remind me to relax, sometimes slapping my arm or thigh muscles. Once or twice, when he went out of the room, I felt I was losing control and I had to fight to regain it.

Paul: *I was able to monitor Jan's contractions on the graph. I could see for myself when a contraction was starting, and guide Jan to the right level of breathing. It helped us to work together.*

During this time the contractions were dilating the cervix to give room for the baby's head to pass into the birth canal, opening a fraction of a centimeter with each contraction. By 11 am Jan was approaching transition from first to second stage of labor. The contractions were at their height, lasting one and a half minutes each, at two-minute intervals.

Jan: *There was no time to relax between contractions. I'd just come down from one and – whoosh! – I'd be into the next. I had developed a backache.*

I was starting to feel tired. I found it very difficult to change position on the bed, and every so often I'd slip down and the nurses would have to come and help me back up into a semi-sitting position. I'd abandoned the low breathing levels, now, the contractions were rising too sharply. The nurse asked me if I'd like medication and I said I would have it if the pain got worse. But, rather to my surprise, it didn't.

Jan's training stood her in good stead. She was one of the fortunate women who can manage labor without any analgesic whatsoever.

Paul: *As each contraction started, I'd gently stroke the base of Jan's abdomen, or rub the small of her back.*

Jan: *The effect of that was marvelous! It soothed and seemed to take away some of the pain. The contractions were really strong now, and I'd started Level 3 breathing. Soon even that wasn't enough to tide me over the contractions. I started tapping my song. We'd chosen 'Roll me over in the clover'. Paul had taught me all ten verses just in case I had a particularly long contraction.*

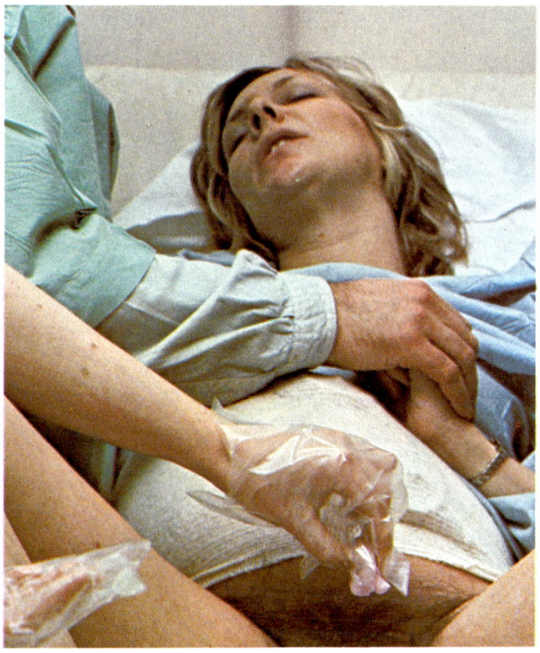

As transition from first to second stage approaches (above), the mother lies down in the birth position, on her back, propped up and with her knees apart. Electrodes measuring the fetal heart rate and uterine contractions are held in place on the abdomen by a wide band.

Relaxation techniques sometimes include tapping out the rhythm of a song at the height of the strongest contractions, and this was a technique which Jan used. Paul was able to help Jan by tapping out the rhythm of their song with her to help her concentrate.

Paul: *In fact we never got past verse six. Jan was meant just to tap it out, and mouth it silently. But toward the end we found we were singing out loud.*

At noon a nurse performed an internal examination in order to measure the opening of the cervix. It was 9.5 cm – just half a centimeter short of full dilation.

Jan: *About this time things suddenly changed. I felt a sudden, overwhelming desire to start pushing. It felt as though every muscle in my body was compelling me to bear down – a strange, heavy feeling centered in my pelvis. This was a feeling I'd never experienced before. But I knew I wasn't fully dilated, and until I was I had to prevent myself from pushing.*

This was the most difficult time of all. I started the panting exercise, designed to stop the diaphragm from pushing down. But I found it difficult to keep up the rhythm. Paul had to guide me. We did it together, panting at each other like crazy. All the time I was fighting this mad compulsion to push. It seemed to last forever.

This difficult period lasted for half an hour. By 12:30 the cervix was fully dilated. The first stage was over and the second stage could begin. Now, at last, she could bear down with her contractions.

The cervix undergoes several changes during labor:
(a) In early labor, where effacement has occurred and the cervix is starting to dilate.
(b) The continuation of dilatation of the cervix.
(c) Approaching full dilatation of the cervix.

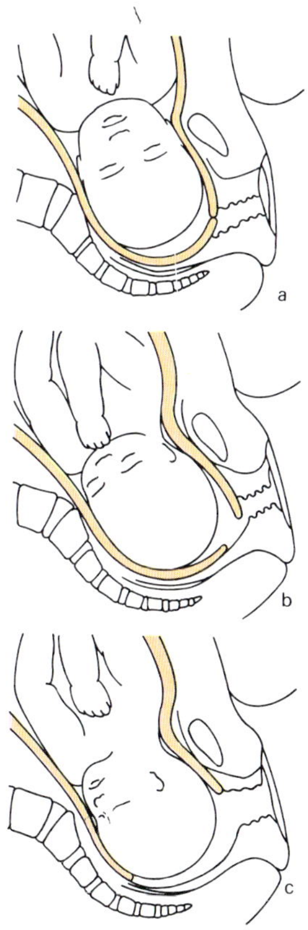

The second stage of labor

The second stage of labor:
Face down, the baby's head is pressed against the perineum, which gradually stretches, widening the vaginal opening.

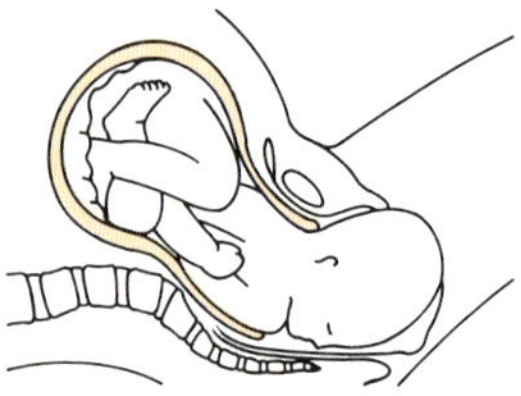

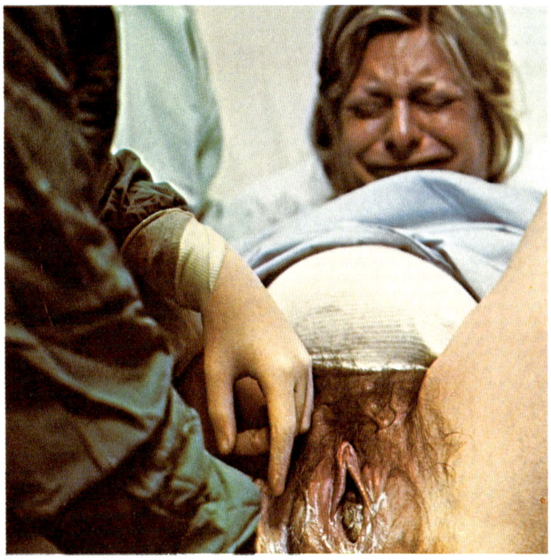

The baby's skull extends as it sweeps up over the perineum. The top of the skull and then the brow emerge first.

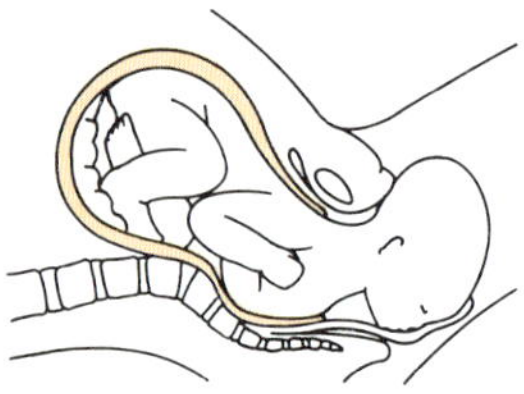

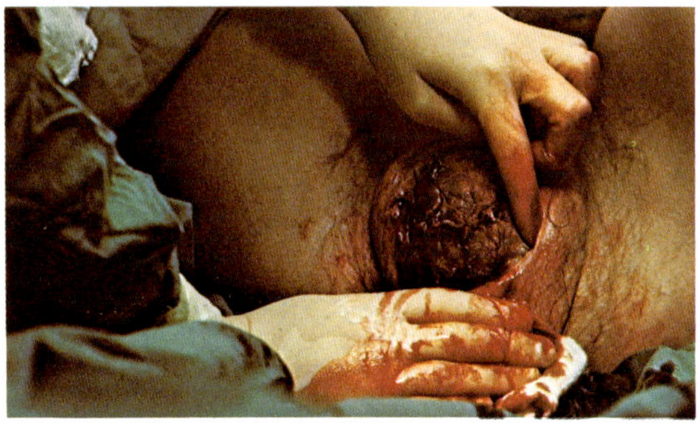

Once the head is born the shoulders rotate in the pelvis, turning the head to left or right.

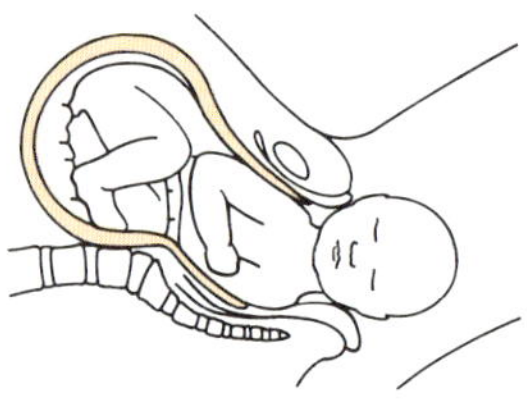

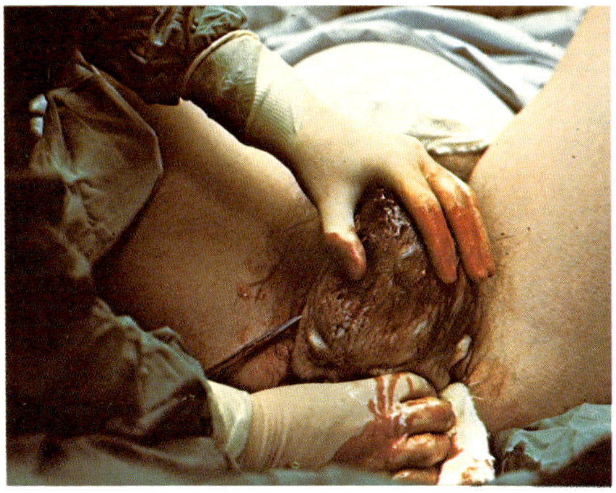

The top shoulder is born first, after which the rest of the body slides out easily.

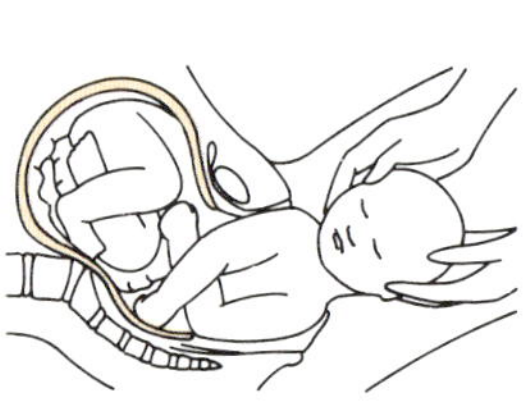

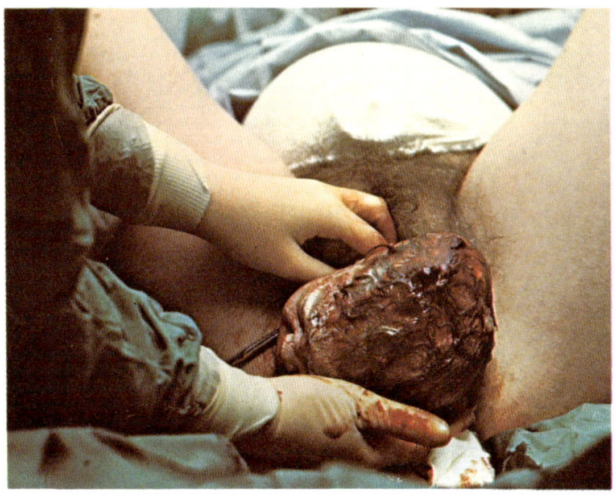

Jan got into the birth position – the knees drawn up and apart. From this point on the compulsion to push does not have to be resisted any longer.

Jan: *The first time I was told to push I felt a great surge of relief – at last I could do what I wanted to do! I gave an almighty push down, and fell back exhausted, only to hear the nurse saying, 'Go on, give another push!' Each contraction seemed to last a long time. I'd take a couple of deep breaths at the beginning of each one, then as the desire to push came on I'd hold my breath and bear down. In the photos it looks as though I'm in agony, but in fact I'm just screwing up my face with the effort.*

In some ways this was the best time. I felt I was achieving something with each push – and Paul and the doctors and nurses were giving enormous encouragement.

After the fifth pushing contraction, the doctor was able to see the head inching down and told Jan her baby had brown hair.

Jan: *From that moment on he became a real individual . . . all I could think of was how much I wanted to see him! The thought gave me the energy to push harder and soon I could feel his head tightening the skin of my vagina.*

This tight feeling is caused by the baby's head pressing on the muscles of the pelvic floor (the perineum), and gradually dilating the vagina. The doctor now administered a local anesthetic to numb the skin around the vagina.

Jan: *I felt the prick of the needle, but I was far too busy to worry about that!*

The doctor then performed an episiotomy, making a cut into the perineum, to enlarge the vaginal opening.

Jan: *The anesthetic had taken away all feeling but I could hear the cut being made.*

The tight, stretching feeling eased a little, I got ready for the final push.

Paul: *It was the only bit that I hated watching and I was pleased Jan couldn't see it.*

On the ninth pushing contraction, the baby's head was eased out, followed by his shoulders. The second stage was complete.

Jan: *I could feel the tightness relax as his head slipped out. I stopped pushing and looked down to watch as he was eased out . . . his little oval head, all sticky . . . and then his tiny wriggling shoulders.*

The doctor told me it was a boy, and then he was held up, all blue and pink . . . and beautiful.

The hospital where Jan had her baby practices a modified form of the Leboyer "gentle birth" technique. The lights in the delivery room were dimmed during the birth and those in-

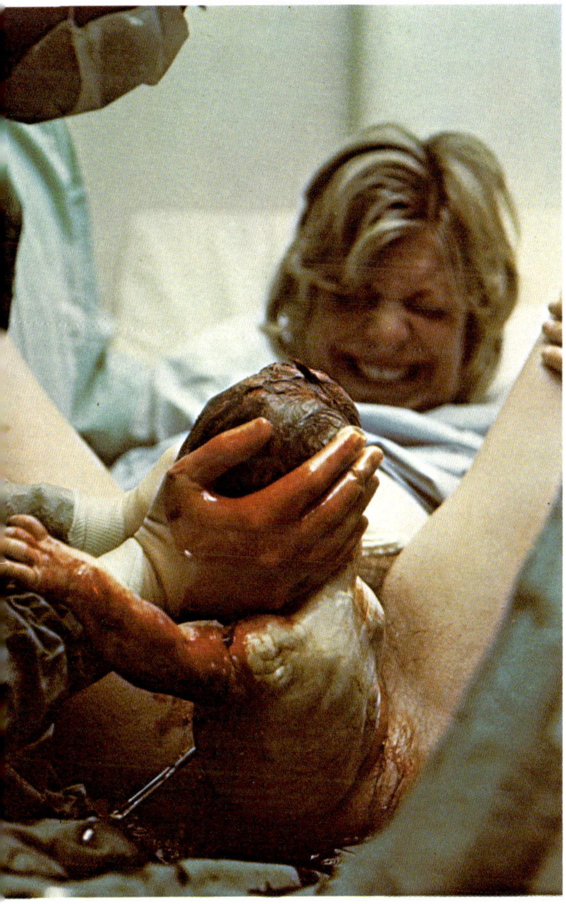

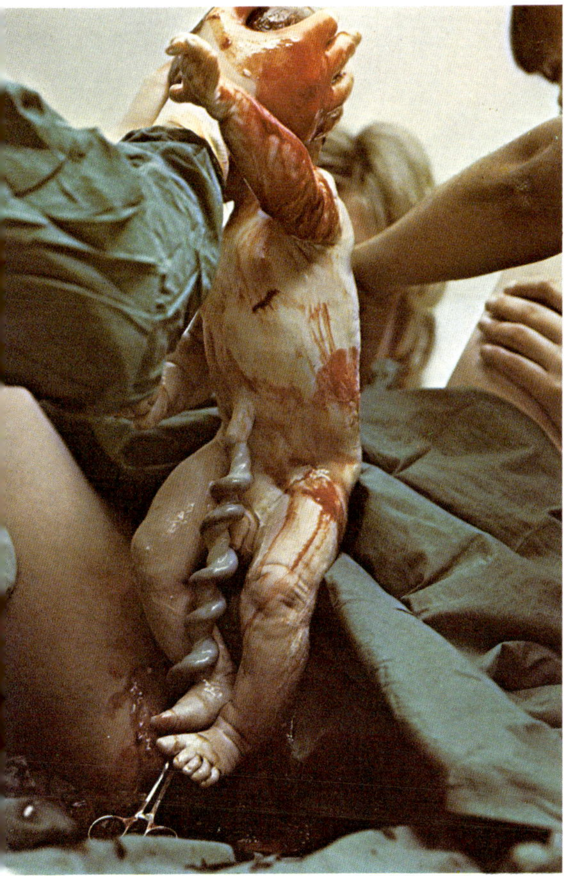

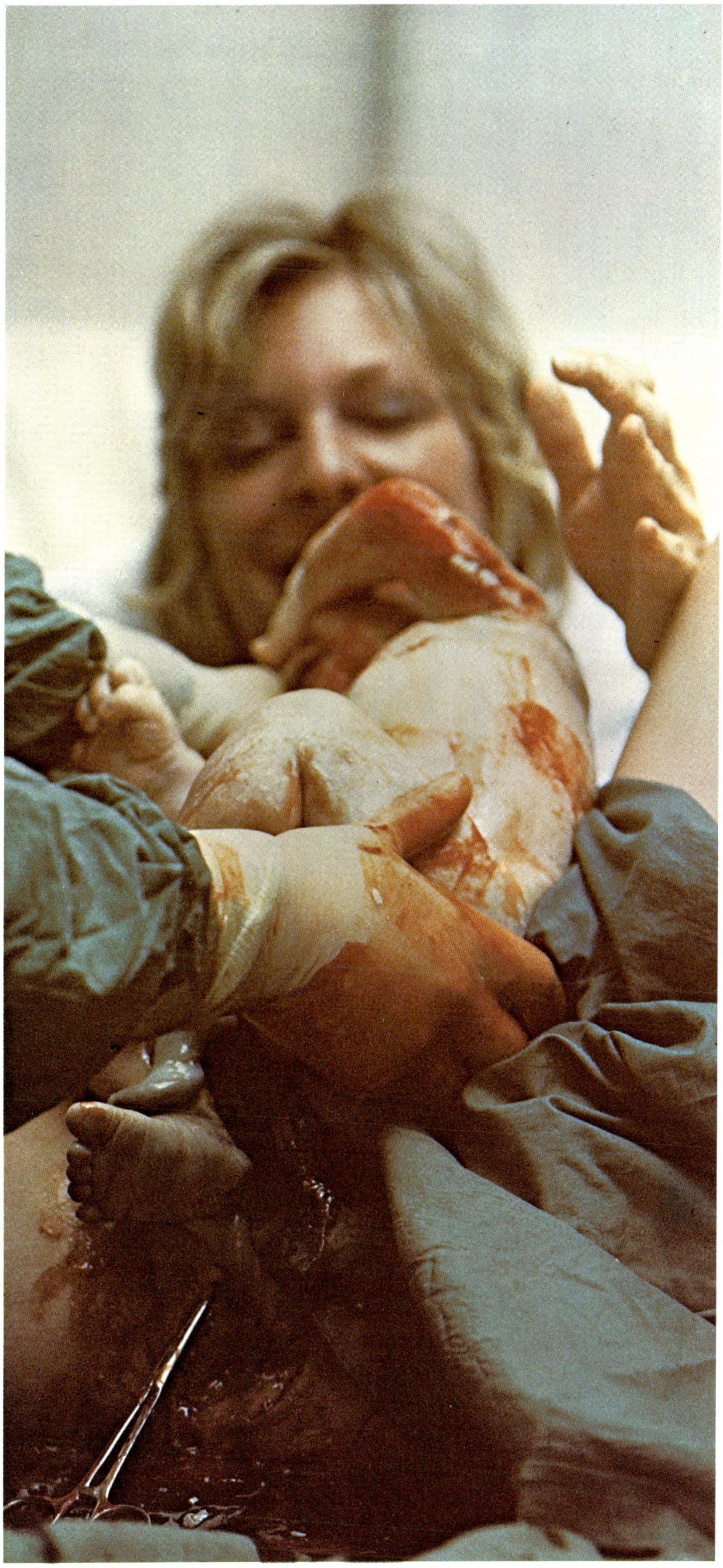

The third stage of labor

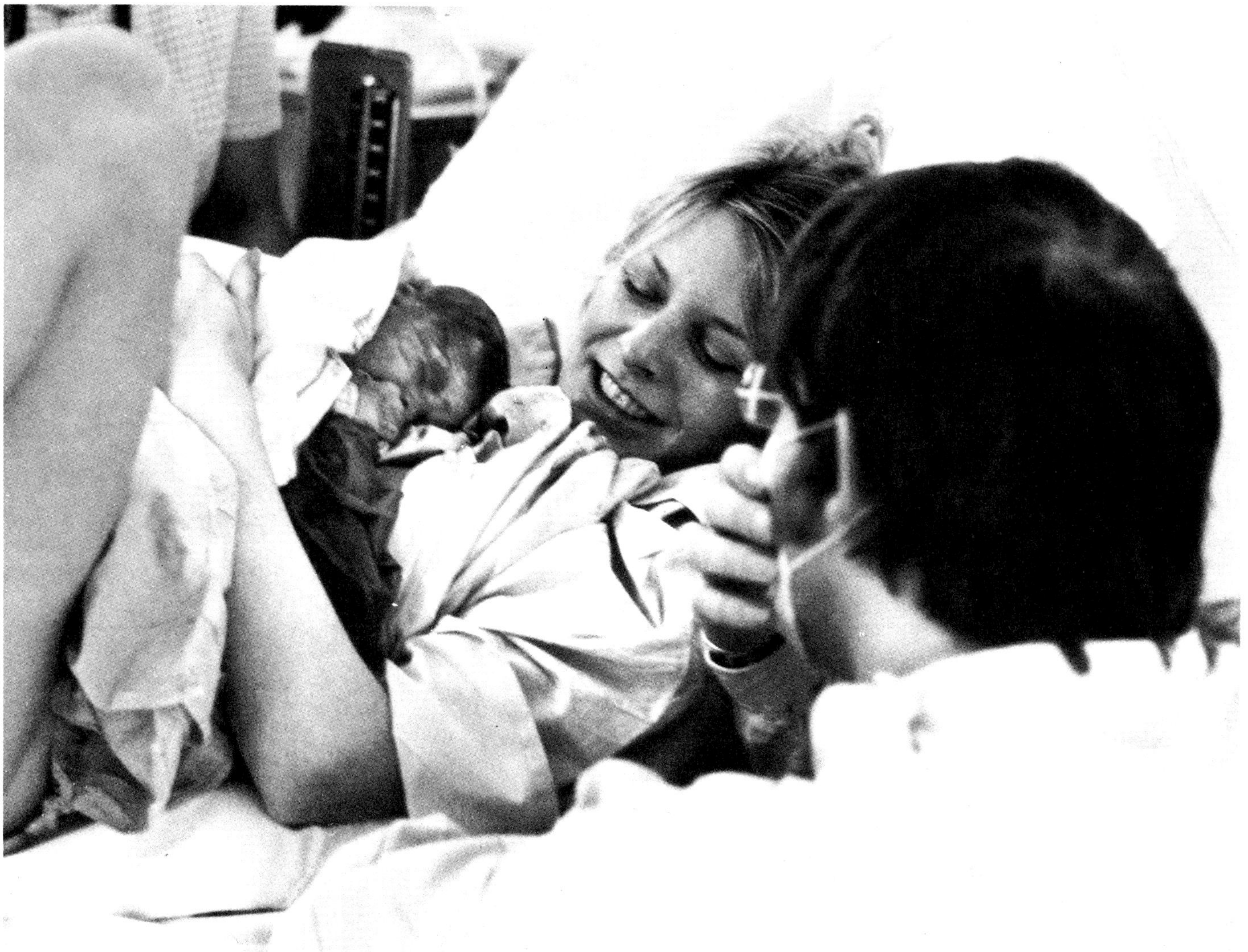

For the father, too, it is important to have a chance to enjoy the moments of quiet triumph that follow the birth.

volved moved and spoke as quietly and calmly as possible. By keeping both light and noise at a low level, the Leboyer approach is designed to ease any trauma for the baby. He also recommends putting the baby on the mother's naked abdomen immediately after birth.

Jan: *I'd expected to burst into tears when I first saw my baby, but all I felt was a marvelous, calm happiness. The doctor held him up and cleared his mouth – he gave a gurgle and a little cry but he didn't yell out. Then he was placed on my abdomen. I can't describe how he felt – warm, and heavy and sticky. The cord was still pulsing a little, and the doctor clamped it a few inches from the navel. The doctor gave him the standard tests for normal responses. Then I drew up the gown I was wearing under my chin, and he was placed onto my breast. I didn't expect him to suck immediately – but he did, and it was a wonderful feeling.*

As well as bringing the mother and baby close to each other, suckling at this stage helps to stimulate the delivery of the placenta, the third stage of labor.

Jan: *While I had the baby at my breast, the placenta came out. I didn't feel it – if there was a contraction it must have been very weak, and the nurse told me not to push. The placenta just slipped out, like a piece of liver.*

I kept the baby with me for nearly 20 minutes, then he was taken away to be weighed. Meanwhile the doctor sewed up the episiotomy. That seemed to take a long time, but I didn't feel anything because the anesthetic was still doing its job. Soon after that I started to doze off. The nurse checked my blood pressure and now and then I would feel just a slight echo of the earlier contractions as the uterus rearranged itself after the birth.

By the next morning I felt perfectly well. My abdomen had shrunk to the size it was when I was about four months pregnant. I was rather sore around the vagina from the stitches, but apart from that there were no unpleasant physical aftereffects. I had slight vaginal bleeding and occasional cramps. But, overall, I felt exhilarated – really excited and proud of what Paul and I had done. I just couldn't wait until he could come back to the hospital so that we could talk together about the birth.

Cesarean birth

Cesarean birth (also known as cesarean section) is the delivery of a baby through the abdominal wall after making an incision in the abdomen and uterus. It can safely facilitate a delivery that would be dangerous or impossible through the vagina.

Cesarean births are done for a variety of maternal and/or fetal reasons. Some of the indications for cesarean section include cephalopelvic disproportion (when the baby's head is too large for the pelvis); previous scars on the uterus including previous cesarean sections or a myomectomy (removal of a benign tumor of the uterus); abnormal presentation of the fetus, for example breech (rear end first); transverse lie (longitudinally across the maternal abdomen) or presenting with a shoulder (instead of a head); placenta previa (placenta covering the cervix); and fulminating preeclampsia (toxemia). Fetal indications include fetal distress, usually hypoxia due to compression or prolapse of the umbilical cord; severe Rh isoimmunization; maternal diabetes mellitus; and extreme prematurity. Some other indications include severe bleeding due to separation of the placenta, active herpes infection and a pelvic tumor obstructing a normal delivery.

Usually, the indications are compelling; that is, they require a cesarean section in order to prevent harm to the fetus or even to avoid fetal death. In some instances cesarean sections are performed to prevent predictable complications to the mother that occur with a hemorrhage or a previous scar on the uterus.

About the procedure

Since cesarean sections are major surgery, they are always done in the operating room with a team of doctors and nurses to make the birth safe. Your obstetrician performs the operation with two physicians assisting. An anesthesiologist administers and monitors the anesthetic. A scrub nurse passes instruments to the doctors. A circulating nurse is present to make certain the cesarean birth goes smoothly. In addition, there is usually a pediatrician and a nurse from the nursery to care for the newborn.

Most cesarean sections are not done as emergencies. They may be performed after a long labor or may be scheduled as "repeat" cesarean sections. A small percentage must be done immediately due to an emergency, such as fetal distress, rupture of the uterus or obstetrical hemorrhage. In such instances, every minute counts. There may not be much time for discussion of the situation with the mother and father, therefore it is important to become familiar with the procedure.

Generally, cesarean sections are classified into three types: low transverse cervical cesarean section; "classical" or vertical cesarean section; and cesarean hysterectomy.

The low transverse cervical section is the best general purpose operation and is used in over 90 per cent of cases. Occasionally, the uterine incision can be made vertically, but in all instances the uterine incision is made in the lower portion of the cervix which is usually thinned out during pregnancy and is not a contractile portion of the uterus. The "classical" or vertical cesarean section is usually employed for extreme emergencies when time is the major factor, for instance, with severe fetal distress. It is also employed for mechanical reasons, for instance with a fetus in a transverse lie. The vertical incision is made in the contractile portion of the uterus increasing the risk of uterine rupture in future pregnancies. The cesarean hysterectomy is rarely used, but can be lifesaving if there is a severely infected uterus, a ruptured uterus, or placenta accreta (when the placenta grows into the wall of the uterus and cannot be separated).

Anesthesia for cesarean births generally consists of an epidural (injection of anesthesia outside spinal canal) or spinal anesthesia when the procedure is not being done as an emergency. But if time is critical, for instance with prolapse of the umbilical cord or severe hemorrhage, general anesthesia is used to put the mother to sleep. Sodium pentothal is injected into intravenous tubing to cause the mother to drift off to sleep. Then a general anesthetic is administered by inhalation technique through a tube placed down the mother's trachea (airway). This technique facilitates a very quick operation. Such anesthesia can be administered in 2 to 3 minutes, and the surgical removal of the baby can be accomplished in 3 to 4 minutes.

Epidural and spinal anesthesia are slower in onset but allow the mother to be awake during the cesarean birth. These wear off in a few hours. The mother can remain comfortable by receiving intramuscular or intravenous injections of pain medication such as Demerol.

The father can be present at a cesarean delivery when it is not an emergency. He sits at the head of the operating table so he can give support to the mother. When the baby is delivered the doctor aspirates mucus and fluid out of the nose and pharynx, then clamps and cuts the umbilical cord. The baby is then shown to the parents. Usually this viewing is very brief because the pediatrician and nursery nurse want to make sure that the baby is breathing normally and has no medical problems. They place the baby in a heated crib where careful evaluation is performed. Following this, the baby may be shown again to the parents.

During this time the doctors have removed the placenta and started to repair the uterine incision and to close the abdominal wall incision. When this is finished the mother usually is transferred back to a room for recovery. She has an intravenous tube running fluid into her vein and Foley catheter to drain urine from the bladder. The intravenous fluids which may prevent dehydration may be maintained for one or two days. The Foley catheter may be removed the next day.

The recovery from a cesarean section is generally rapid for several reasons. First, the

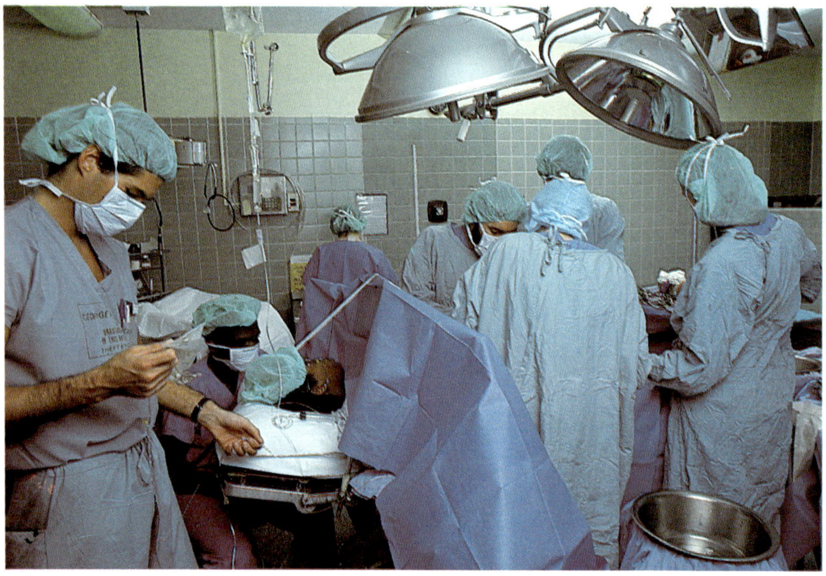

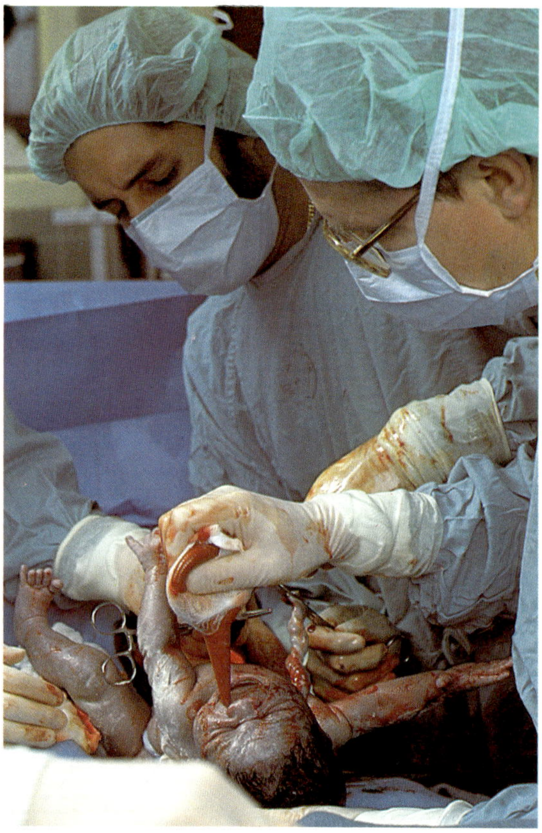

A team of doctors and nurses must be present during a cesarean birth to ensure the safe delivery of the baby (above). In most cases the father is present; he sits beside the mother where he can give the same support and encouragement as in a normal delivery.

Immediately following the birth, and before the cord is cut, the baby's nose and throat are suctioned out to clear the air passages of mucus and fluid (above right).

mother is young and healthy. Second, the abdominal wall has been stretched by the presence of a fetus so that following the operation, the abdominal wall is lax and causes less pain. Finally, cesarean section is a relatively short operation, lasting 30 to 60 minutes, permitting a quick recovery.

As the anesthesia wears off the mother may require some pain medication. If the cesarean section is done after a long labor usually the mother is exhausted and sleeps. But, if the cesarean section is a scheduled or repeat operation, the mother often feels well enough later that day to sit up and nurse her baby. The nurses will help the mother hold and position her baby for nursing. A cesarean birth does not prevent successful breast feeding; the first day may be somewhat difficult because of pain or fatigue, but perseverance will generally be rewarded with success.

Increase in cesarean delivers

At the turn of the century, cesarean section was a dangerous operation. In recent decades, major advances in surgical technique, blood transfusion, anesthesia, and antibiotic therapy have markedly improved the safety. Today, several thousand consecutive cesarean sections can be performed without a single maternal death. Because the procedure has become so safe, it is being used increasingly as an alternative to vaginal delivery. This has resulted in a tripling of the cesarean section rate over the last decade.

In 1980 the National Institutes of Health held a Consensus Development Conference to review the use of cesarean section in the United States because they were concerned about the large increase in the number of cesarean sections. The change in cesarean section rate was found to be:

	All	*Repeats*
1970	5.7%	2.1%
1978	14.7%	4.6%

Today the rate is even higher, but has stabilized. Current estimates indicate that there are an overall 18 per cent, including 7 per cent repeat cesarean sections.

Although between 1970 and 1978 there was marked improvement in perinatal mortality and morbidity, not all of this could be attributed to cesarean sections. There was concern that this trend to an increasing number of cesarean sections was dangerous to maternal health, due to a slight increase in mortality risk from cesarean section versus vaginal delivery. Additionally, it increased the morbidity to the mother, and obviously increased the hospital cost.

The Consensus Development report indicated that the reasons for the increase in cesarean sections were: dystocia (30 per cent); repeat cesarean section (27 per cent); breech (14 per cent); fetal distress (14 per cent); and other (15 per cent).

Dystocia means there is failure to progress in labor, including situations in which the uterus does not function efficiently as a muscular organ to expel the fetus, or in which the fetus is actually too large to be delivered through the pelvis. Repeat cesarean sections are usually performed because of concern that the uterus might rupture during labor. In breech presentations cesarean sections are used because of the concern over the difficulty in delivering the head. When fetal distress is suspected, cesarean section may minimize fetal hypoxia (oxygen deprivation) and potential brain damage.

The maternal morbidity due to cesarean

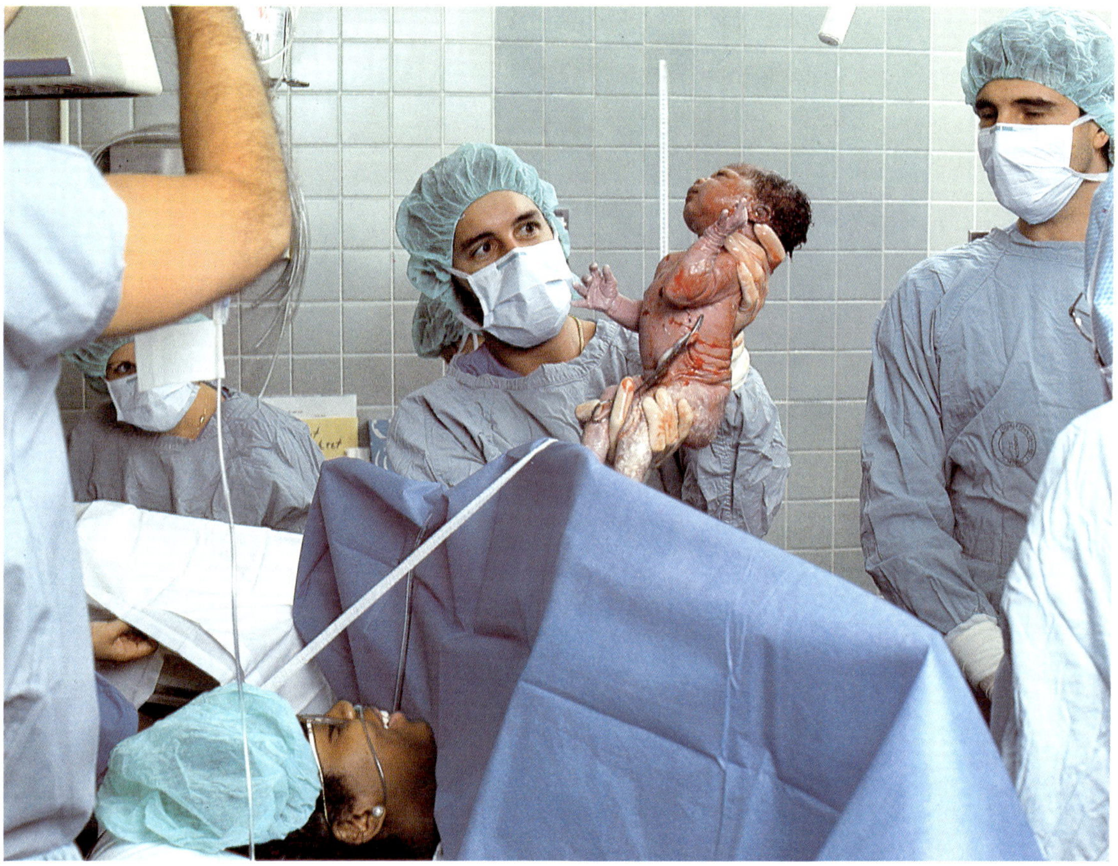

The mother is able to see her baby a few minutes after its delivery and share the joy of its birth with the father and staff. The baby is then placed in a heated crib where the doctor and nursery nurse give it a thorough examination.

Once the examination is complete the mother can see her baby again, and can now establish contact with it and continue the bonding process.

section includes a number of problems. Compared to vaginal delivery, there is a higher incidence of infection such as endometritis (infection of the uterus), urinary tract infection and wound infection. The bladder may take a day or two to return to normal function. The abdomen may become distended and it may be two or three days before the mother has a bowel movement. Additionally, a cesarean section increases the length of hospital stay by two to five days increasing the cost considerably.

From the standpoint of mortality, it is clear that a cesarean birth is a safe procedure. Comparing the maternal mortality statistics from 1960 to 1975 in California, there were 2.6 maternal deaths per 10,000 deliveries, whereas the vaginal deliveries had only 1 per 10,000 deliveries. Obviously, the cesarean birth group included mothers who had conditions that were a threat to their lives, for instance hemorrhage or infection. A more accurate analysis of the risks of cesarean birth can be made by considering the incidence of maternal mortality in repeat cesarean births, since they are not usually accompanied by other problems. In a study which embraced 654 hospitals, there were 18 maternal deaths per 100,000 cesarean sections, or 1.8 per 10,000. So, if one looks carefully at the real figures the incidence of maternal deaths for repeat cesarean deliveries is only slightly higher than they would be for vaginal deliveries.

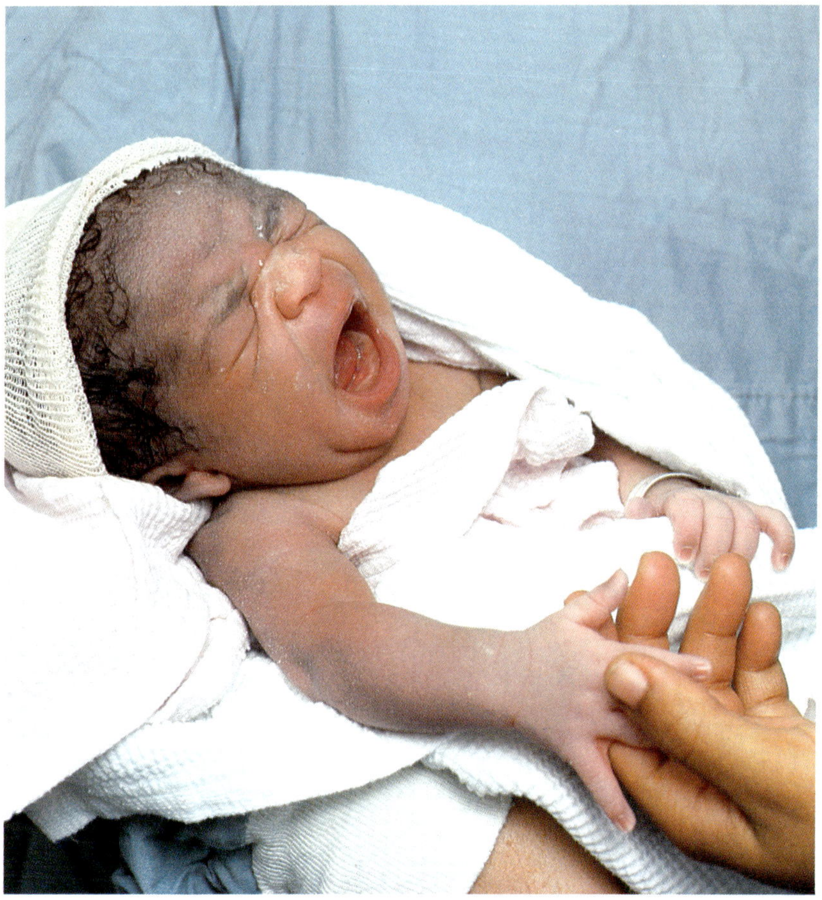

Changing childbirth scene

Approximately three decades ago expectant mothers and fathers began to shape the future of maternity care. This consumer movement played a very positive role in improving the delivery of obstetrical care. Expectant mothers began having meetings and exchanging ideas. They sought out physicians who were willing to be more flexible in their approach to childbirth and who would allow the husband to participate in the processes of labor and delivery.

At this time three separate consumer organizations were formed. The International Childbirth Education Association (ICEA) is an organization which oversees all maternity education programs. The American Society for Psychoprophylaxis in Obstetrics (ASPO) is an organization promoting antenatal, or prenatal, education and psychoprophylactic training for labor so that the patient may need little or no medication. The La Leche League is an organization of women helping others in the art of breast-feeding. These organizations led the evolution in delivery of maternity care. At times their individual members were aggressive and militant but, on balance, over the years these advocates have been constructive and goal oriented.

Approximately thirty years ago the La Maze method of psychoprophylaxis began to be practiced in a few cities around the United States. Over the next few years, numerous organizations were developed to teach prepared childbirth to expectant parents. The vital role of the father was gradually recognized. Today, in most hospitals the father is part of the team, supporting the mother in labor and accompanying her into the delivery room. Most hospitals now allow the father to be present in the operating room for first-time and repeat cesarean sections. Liberalized visiting hours, sibling visitation and rooming-in have all contributed toward improving the psychological environment surrounding childbirth.

These changes did not come easily. Doctors, nurses and hospital administrators resisted change. Indeed, in some areas of the country no change occurred at all. However, in most hospitals the participation of both expectant mother and father has become the rule rather than the exception.

Approximately a decade and a half ago fetal monitoring appeared on the scene. Initially, it was available in teaching hospitals and then it spread to many of the community hospitals. To some, this represented an encroachment upon the comfort and ease with which one could go through childbirth. Some patients felt that the wires and cables encumbered the full participation in childbirth. Additionally, the many routines and rituals that had to be performed by hospital personnel were also viewed as intrusions into the childbirth process. After all, they reasoned, having a baby is a normal process. An expectant mother is not ill. Why should there be so many intrusions and interferences?

The question of home births

A small, but strong movement for home delivery began as a reaction to the technological rather than personal approach to childbirth in the United States. Proponents quote statistics supporting the safety of home deliveries. However, the statistics are often distorted by enthusiasm. They cite England, for example, where home deliveries have been performed for decades. In these arguments, however, they never pointed out that home deliveries are not always done by choice in England and that when they do take place, there is a backup of a "flying squad" of trained professionals able to intervene effectively in a wide variety of perinatal complications.

It has already been well estabished that home delivery bears an unacceptably high risk of maternal and fetal mortality and morbidity. Between the years 1973 and 1976, in New York State 1,488 deliveries took place at home. The neonatal mortality rate in this group was 37/1,000 compared to 11/1,000 in the population delivered in the hospital. Data from Hawaii, Oregon, Michigan, West Virginia, Wyoming, Colorado and Virginia indicate that out-of-hospital births are associated with a risk of neonatal mortality double to quadruple that of in-hospital births. The perinatal mortality rates for Iowa, California, Oklahoma and Kansas ranged from 18.4 to 22.3/1,000 for hospital deliveries, compared to 42.3 to 103.7/1,000 for out-of-hospital deliveries in the same states.

In the United States every patient has access to a hospital delivery. Indeed, by the late 1960s practically all births in the United States occurred in hospitals. The medical profession has become increasingly aware of the possibility of the uncomplicated obstetrical patient suddenly becoming complicated as manifest by fetal distress. Therefore, it is generally believed all deliveries should take place in a hospital setting where electronic fetal monitoring and appropriate therapeutic measures are available, even if not used.

Alternative birthing center

Since home deliveries had been frequently accompanied by very poor statistics from the standpoint of newborn mortality and morbidity, it was felt that reinstituting home deliveries would be a step backwards. There had to be some other way! After careful consideration, it appeared that alternative birthing centers would be the answer. These delivery units can be located in or next to hospitals, with blood banks, operating rooms and all the skilled medical personnel available. But the atmosphere and the attitudes of the modern birthing center are all directed toward a homelike family oriented center.

In the United States, there are freestanding birthing centers, that is ones not adjacent to or in a hospital. Although this is not ideal, by careful patient selection these centers have been able to compile excellent records of safety. Obviously, the ideal setting is to have a birthing unit at a hospital so that all of the resources are available if a problem occurs. After all, if fetal distress or maternal hemorrhage occurs, this is no time to transfer a patient by ambulance. *Obstetrics is one speciality where time is critical if we are to minimize a hypoxic episode to the fetus.*

The patient labors in the birthing room which appears like a bedroom rather than a sterile delivery room. She may have her husband and/or other members of her family present with her. When the time comes for delivery, she is not taken out of the room to a delivery room unless there is a problem. The bed that she labors in is used for the delivery. The baby may be put to her breast immediately. The conduct of labor and delivery is much the way it would be if the process were taking place in the patient's own home.

This seems to be a logical compromise between those who are fighting for home deliveries versus hospital deliveries. The alternate birth center enables the individual to have the comforts and unregimented atmosphere of a home delivery but provides the safety of a full hospital setting, if the need should arise.

Since the patients have comprehensive prenatal care, most risk factors can be identified. If the pregnancy is uncomplicated and the couple can reasonably expect a favorable outcome to pregnancy, then they may be candidates for such a childbirth experience.

The patient enters the birthing room when she arrives at the hospital. The nurse performs the important observations of the mother's temperature, pulse and blood pressure and the fetal heart rate. Generally, the doctor will check the progress of labor, noting the character of contractions, the dilation of the cervix and the descent of the fetal head.

The mother may labor in a hospital gown or her own nightgown. She may receive an enema or not depending upon her arrangement with her doctor. She may bring her favorite pillows from home. She may have her mother, sister or anyone in addition to her husband who will help and support her. Often a couple will have their children present so the whole family can be there at the birth. Obviously there must be a limit to the number of people she can have present if sterile technique is to be maintained. Most commonly a couple and a son or daughter are present.

The personnel is not usually much different than present for a routine labor and delivery. A nurse admits you to the room and follows your progress in labor. The doctor will visit periodically to check on the progress of labor, and make sure you and the baby are doing well. When it comes time for delivery, generally your doctor and one or two nurses are the medical personnel present. Normally there is no anesthesiologist or other medical personnel. Actually the room usually wouldn't accommodate more people anyway.

Generally, no intravenous infusion and no electronic fetal monitoring are used because her pregnancy is uncomplicated. But, to receive standard care the fetal heart rate must be checked every 15 minutes in the first stage and every five minutes in the second, or subsequent, stage of labor.

The husband participates actively in physical and psychological support. He may help by rubbing her back, aiding her in breathing exercises and encouraging her. As labor progresses his encouragement becomes invaluable. The couple has been through a training course together. They may even bring their class notes with them as a handy reference during the labor process.

Sometimes, in spite of meticulous education and preparation, the labor just doesn't seem to resemble what is in your notes. Usually the nurses who work in birthing rooms are very interested in childbirth education and support. Many of them teach preparation for childbirth classes. They are excellent sources of information and encouragement. If such a nurse attends you throughout your labor and delivery you will have a very positive experience. But bear in mind that the average first labor is 12–13 hours and nurses work eight hour shifts. It is not uncommon to have a change of nursing personnel before the baby is born. Don't let this disturb you, because the next nurse will probably be just as supportive and instructive.

As labor progresses the mother enters the transition stage. She is encouraged not to bear down because the cervix is not yet fully dilated. When she is fully dilated, she is told she can bear down to push the baby out. The initial feeling is often uncomfortable. But with some coaching the mother quickly learns to fill her lungs and bear down hard which gives a definite sense of relief. She may push 30 minutes to two hours before her baby is delivered. When the baby is ready for delivery, the back portion (occiput) of his head becomes visible in the vagina. The perineum is prepped with antiseptic solution. The mother is instructed to bear down several times as the baby's head is guided out of the vagina. The nose and pharynx are suctioned out with a bulb syringe to remove mucus and amniotic fluid. The doctor immediately checks to be sure there is no umbilical cord around the baby's neck. The baby's anterior shoulder is delivered, then the posterior shoulder and finally the whole body.

Once the baby is born, the nose and pharynx are again suctioned. The baby may be placed on the mother's abdomen where she may hold him while the doctor clamps and cuts the cord. *It is crucial to keep the newborn baby warm so he doesn't lose any body heat.* The baby may be put to the mother's breast. It is amazing how he knows instantly what to do. As the mother nurses her new baby she spontaneously starts talking to him. The father often reaches out and touches the baby. The parents develop eye contact with the baby and the all important bonding process is off to a good start.

This is a time of joy, pride and excitement.

Many emotions impact at this moment. It is one of the most meaningful experiences in a lifetime. The mother and father joined to create the pregnancy and join again to greet the new life. The mother's sense of well being and accomplishment is exceeded only by this new life she has never seen before but knows she already loves.

Proper preparation

The modern couple usually goes to some form of childbirth education classes. Since other couples are present there is an excellent chance for a good exchange of information. Occasionally, either due to an overzealous instructor or grim determination on the part of one of the expectant parents, the concept develops that if medication is used in labor the couple have failed somehow.

It is a plain fact that some mothers have babies easily and others have a difficult and painful labor. The factors which are operational are the mother's pain threshold, the strength of contractions, the size of the baby, the size of her pelvis and the psychological environment surrounding the labor. It is absolutely unfair to tell or imply to expectant parents that "to take medication in labor is to fail". Proper preparation for childbirth must embrace the fact that some babies just don't fit through their mothers pelvises for a number of reasons. If this occurs, it is likely that pain medication will be helpful to aid you through a trying, long labor. Additionally an epidural anesthesia may also be necessary so that a forceps delivery can be performed. Finally, in a small percentage of instances a cesarean section might need to be done. This couple certainly has not failed. Indeed they have gone through many hours of strong labor before the decision to do a cesarean section was made. If their preparation didn't include this possibility in a constructive manner, they will be upset, disappointed and feel that they have been unsuccessful.

Some mothers will have cesarean sections for other reasons. Sometimes they won't even go into labor. For instance, a mother's first baby in the breech presentation may be delivered by cesarean section before the onset of labor. Is a preparation for childbirth important for such a couple? Certainly, because a well organized course will give the couple all they need to know about the experience with cesarean sections. The course will prepare you psychologically and physically for childbirth. It should also give you a good idea of what you should expect to experience.

Although the vast majority of babies are normal, problems do arise. The possibility of prematurity or bleeding in the third trimester must be considered. The development of a pregnancy-related problem like pre-eclampsia or a labor-related problem like fetal distress should be covered. Finally the problem of a congenital malformation or a baby with a problem with respiration should be mentioned. This is by no means to dwell on the pessimistic side; but if a couple is aware that such problems exist they may be better able to cope if such a problem should arise.

Expectancy is extremely important. For instance, couples with a condition like the Rh-problem know before delivery that their baby could have difficulties and require intensive neonatal management. But, because they realize this ahead of time, they generally handle this remarkably well from the emotional standpoint. The couple who have an uncomplicated pregnancy but whose baby is born with a congenital malformation incompatible with life have to contend with shock, because it was unexpected, as well as grief.

A course should provide preparation for understanding what tests or what aspects of monitoring are important in labor. If everything has been normal in the antenatal course, many doctors don't believe electronic fetal monitoring is essential for the whole labor. If there is any doubt about whether to use it or not, it is better to use it. It is virtually impossible for a nurse to monitor the fetus continuously with a fetoscope. If your pregnancy has a high risk element then electronic fetal monitoring will almost automatically be employed in labor. Generally, instructors cover this aspect of labor fairly well in childbirth education courses.

If your childbirth course is taught at a hospital, you may be fortunate to have your instructor visit you during your labor. This can be very helpful and reassuring. After the labor is over you may be asked as a couple to attend a class and relate your experiences to other expectant parents. This sort of exchange is invaluable for everyone.

The Lamaze method

Many preparation for childbirth courses advocate some form of the Lamaze technique for psychoprophylaxis in labor. This method employs active participation of the father and the mother. It is the most widely used and successful method for providing pain relief in labor and delivery. Once a mother learns to employ her breathing exercises she has a means for relaxation and pain relief which can be used for any labor situations.

This technique has been used successfully for literally millions of births. It makes it possible to go through even difficult labors without taking pain medication. Even though the first stage of labor can be long (perhaps exhausting) the mother gets relief during the second stage by bearing down with contractions. In spite of the overwhelming amount of physical energy expended, the mother seems to endure very well. At the time of delivery, the doctor will probably administer a local anesthetic for the episiotomy. This avoids much unnecessary pain. So, other than the local medication the mother often receives no medications during labor. In some instances, the labor is very long or the patient's pain threshold is low and a small amount of Demerol is helpful to take the edge off the pain and allow some relaxation. This does *not* mean the patient has failed! Furthermore, she has still used the bona fide Lamaze technique. She has just made her very difficult situation slightly better with the aid of some pain medication. On average some patients don't require medication and most doctors don't order medication in labor without first discussing it with the patient. A few doctors have routines for administering pain medication. You should be able to learn if your doctor does this prior to labor. It is important to make sure your doctor knows what your desires are concerning pain medication.

The Leboyer method

Procedures for the management of labor and the handling of a newborn baby are usually based on minimizing the risk of physical harm to mother and child, while using the limited time of the medical staff as efficiently as possible. The mother's views about how she would like to experience childbirth are also to be considered. The feelings of the baby itself do not often play an important part, since these are difficult to determine and concern for his or her physical health comes first.

Delivery rooms in most hospitals have fairly bright lighting to ensure that doctors and nurses have no difficulty in seeing what is going on and steps are taken to make quite certain that the baby is breathing immediately after the birth. The baby's airway is cleared with a mucus extractor. The umbilical cord is soon clamped, and the newborn baby is placed in a bassinet with a radiant heater.

These procedures have been challenged by Frederick Leboyer, a French obstetrician. He argued that the treatment of the newborn baby at birth is bound to influence his or her abilities and happiness throughout life. From psychoanalysis – including his own – Leboyer concluded that birth is a disturbing event because it marks an abrupt change from the safe world of the womb to the unknown and frightening world outside. He saw the baby's first cries as anguished sobs expressing panic at the shock of birth and fear of the new and strange environment.

Leboyer's method therefore seeks to ease the transition from life in the womb to life outside it by prolonging some of the sensations the fetus feels in the uterus and by introducing the baby to the new sensations of the outside world in a gradual way. With his "gentle birth" approach, light and noise in the delivery room are kept at a low level. The umbilical cord is not cut immediately after the birth since, Leboyer argues, this enables the baby to experience "two ways of breathing" (receiving oxygen from the placenta as well as the air) until the cord stops pulsating about two to five minutes after birth. Care is taken to handle the baby very gently.

Leboyer also uses procedures designed to let the baby's sense of touch adjust gradually to the new environment. He claims that contact with clothes is, for the newborn baby, like being scorched, and for this reason he places the baby naked on his mother's naked abdomen, while mother, father and doctor put their hands on his back to recreate the feeling of being held tight in the uterus. Next he bathes the baby in a bath in water just above body temperature for three to six minutes, in the hope that this will evoke the sensations of floating in the amniotic fluid. Only then does he dry the baby and wrap him loosely in soft cotton cloth.

Criticisms of Leboyer's approach

Some of Leboyer's practices conflict with the standard medical principle: that nothing should be done to increase by even a fraction the risk of physical harm to mother or child. Many doctors would say that if you lower the lights at all you are bound to increase the chances that something will be missed and a mistake made; that if the staff talk in whispers they might misunderstand each other; and that by not using a mucus extractor or stimulating the baby's crying he or she might take longer to breathe. This is perhaps an extreme response, but some of Leboyer's practices have been criticized even by those obstetricians who are sympathetic to his general approach to the whole process of birth.

Many obstetricians think the claim that the baby receives oxygen from both the placenta and the air until the umbilical cord stops pulsating is simply untrue and that the blood can actually run back into the placenta if the cord is not clamped immediately and the baby is lying at a level above the placenta. This is a subject for debate.

Doctors are also concerned that bathing the baby immediately after the birth will lower his or her temperature, and they would therefore advise against it. Whether babies like this bath is uncertain anyway: many cry when they are separated from their mothers to be put into it, though Leboyer would say that this is because they are handled too roughly.

We do not know if the benefits of a "gentle birth" will extend through infancy and beyond, making the child more responsive and secure, any more than we know whether the baby's cries at birth are caused by pain and shock. But this should not obscure the simple truth that Leboyer states: treat the senses of a newborn baby gently and he or she will be free to perceive and respond to the environment and the people present (especially the baby's parents). Handle those senses roughly – even with the best and safest intentions – and the baby will cry, with the result that communication temporarily ends.

A modified form of Leboyer's practices makes sense and is used in many hospitals. While the value of bathing the baby remains doubtful, the newborn baby can certainly be placed in skin-to-skin contact with his or her mother and gently held and stroked. Some form of cover – a sheet, for example – will serve to prevent heat loss. To treat the baby gently and take his feelings seriously is admirable.

Complications in labor

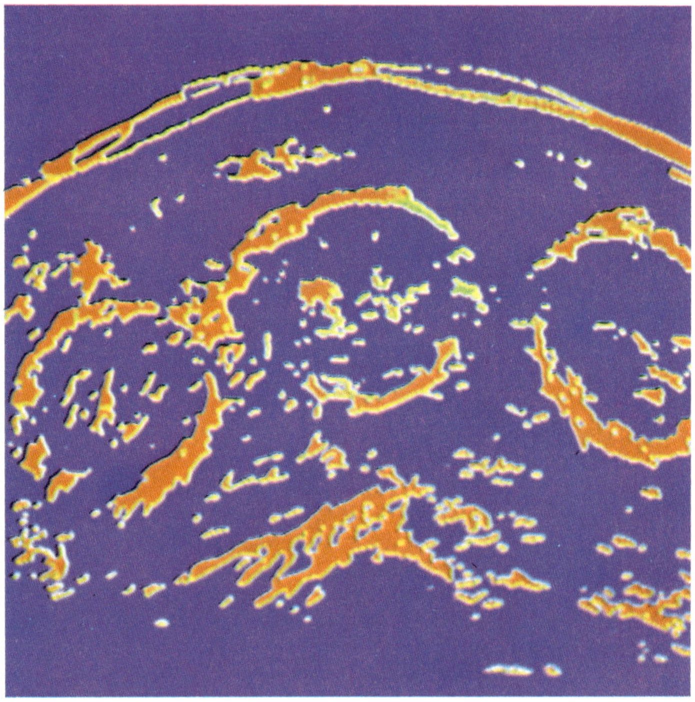

CHAPTER 7

Monitoring

Induction

Delays in labor

Breech babies and twins

Instrumental deliveries

Variations in labor

As has been shown in the previous chapter, "normal" labor includes a wide range of different childbirth experiences. How and when labor begins, its length and the need for pain relief – as well as for other forms of medical help – vary enormously. In this chapter, certain complications which can arise during labor are described, but it should be stressed that there can be no hard and fast distinction between these and variations within "normal" labor.

There is a large number of factors which may, singly or in combination, give rise to unusually complicated or "abnormal" labor. These will be covered in detail in individual sections of the chapter, but they can be briefly listed here. The mother's uterus may not contract efficiently: it may contract too soon or too strongly or, conversely, it may not contract enough. The woman's pelvis may be particularly small or of an unusual shape, making it difficult or impossible for the baby's head to get through. The fetus may be in an unusual position, with the head at the wrong angle or "upside down" in the breech position.

Several problems can arise with the placenta. It sometimes fails to develop sufficiently during the third trimester or it may cease to function efficiently because of "aging" in a longer-than-normal pregnancy. These failings of the placenta can prevent the fetus getting an adequate supply of oxygen during labor. Sometimes the placenta is positioned over the lower segment of the uterus (known as placenta previa, *see* p. 65), which may result in bleeding. If the mother suffers from certain conditions, such as high blood pressure, diabetes, a serious kidney, pulmonary or heart condition, extra precautions will need to be taken during labor. Finally, the mother may be

Cross references

A sonograph establishes the number of babies that can be expected in a multiple birth. The three heads of triplets are clearly visible here.

expecting twins, triplets or even quadruplets. Multiple births often create no problems, but they require careful monitoring.

These, then, are the main factors liable to result in "abnormal" labor. Modern obstetric practice aims to anticipate the effects of these factors and prevent any of them causing harm to the mother or baby.

Doctors must have accurate information about how labor is progressing if they want to know what action, if any, to take. First of all they will need a record of the heart rate of the fetus and of the intensity and timing of uterine contractions. During a "normal" labor, the nurses regularly check the fetal heart rate by listening through a simple fetal stethoscope and they will time the contractions by placing a hand on the mother's abdomen. If there are complications, a more accurate and continuous reading can be obtained of both the heart rate and contractions by using an electronic fetal monitoring device. It is also possible to check whether the fetus is receiving enough oxygen by taking a sample of fetal blood from the scalp of the fetus.

If anything is going wrong with a pregnancy, it may be necessary to start labor artificially, a process known as induction. Induced labor is, in fact, used by doctors even in relatively normal situations, though this practice has been strongly criticized and is now becoming less common. But there can be little doubt that induction is desirable in certain medical circumstances. One method of starting labor artificially is to rupture the amniotic sac at any early stage. This is known as artificial rupture of the membranes, or AROM. Other methods involve administering a hormone which encourages the uterus to contract. A synthetic hormone can be injected into the mother's bloodstream by means of an intravenous infusion, or "drip". This method can also be used to augment, or speed up, a slow labor which has started naturally. The techniques, and the circumstances in which they may become necessary, will be described in great detail in this chapter.

In the second stage of labor, various forms of instrumental assistance may be employed to deliver the baby more quickly. Forceps are sometimes used to help to deliver the baby and they are also occasionally used to change the position of the baby's head prior to delivery to ease descent in the birth canal. The vacuum extractor is another simple piece of equipment which can be used to assist vaginal delivery.

Finally, a cesarean section is sometimes required. The operation, in which the baby is lifted directly from the uterus through an incision made in the abdomen and uterus, may be planned before labor begins, because a normal delivery is thought likely to bring serious complications. It may, however, become necessary if progress in labor stops (e.g. the cervix fails to dilate completely), fetal distress occurs, or if other forms of assisted vaginal delivery (forceps, vacuum extractor) fail or are inappropriate for the clinical situation. Cesarean delivery may be performed for many other reasons besides these.

All the procedures described in this chapter are essentially aspects of preventive medicine, designed to avoid harm to mother or child during labor. Performed in the setting of a well-equipped modern hospital, there is no reason why these deliveries should not go just as smoothly as normal births. There is, therefore, no need to worry if they should become necessary.

Monitoring

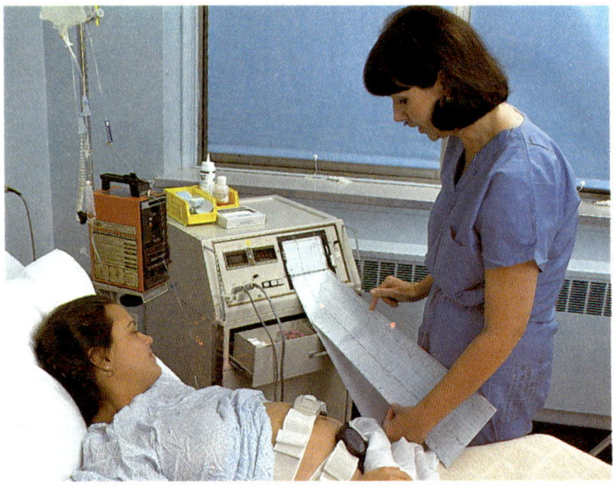

Wires attached to straps around the mother's abdomen are connected to the electronic monitoring equipment which gives a continuous read-out of information about the fetal heartbeat and the strength and duration of contractions.

The fetal heart rate pattern and the quality of uterine contractions are the two basic pieces of information needed to assess whether labor is progressing satisfactorily. Checking these at regular intervals with a stethoscope and by placing a hand on the abdomen is part of the normal management of any labor. The modern electronic methods of monitoring described here may be used in normal or complicated labor. There is still debate whether such monitoring is necessary in normal labors. The use of monitoring in complicated pregnancies is definitely beneficial.

Electronic monitoring methods

Monitoring machines provide a continuous record of the fetal heart rate, using one of two methods. An ultrasound echo signal can be generated and received from a small unit strapped to the mother's abdomen. Alternatively, the minute electrical changes occurring with each fetal heartbeat are detected by attaching a small spiral electrode to the presenting part of the baby, usually its scalp. The first method is simple; it can be used before the membranes have been ruptured and without an internal examination. The second method requires an internal examination and can only be used if the membranes are ruptured, but it usually produces a tracing of better quality.

If the former method is used, then the uterine contractions can be monitored at the same time by using a smaller sensor which is also strapped quite firmly on the abdomen above the upper part of the uterus. If the latter method is employed, then it is possible to monitor the mother's contractions by inserting a fine plastic tube past the side of the baby's head and into the cavity of the uterus. In this case contractions are measured by recording the degree of pressure exerted on the fluid in the tube.

What doctors are looking for in monitoring the fetal heart is any indication that the fetus is not getting enough oxygen. The heart rate in fact normally alters from moment to moment and when this "beat-to-beat" variation is absent this may be an early sign of fetal distress. (It may, however, be due to the effect of drugs given to the mother and is then no cause for alarm.)

Perfectly normal changes in the fetal heart rate also occur because of the stress of labor. The fetal heart rate may slow during each contraction. The placenta is squeezed and the blood flow to the fetus usually diminishes temporarily. This is unlikely to cause problems so long as the uterine muscles relax for long enough in between the contractions. A sign which does need careful attention is when the heart rate slows during a contraction and there is then a delay before it returns to normal. This may mean that the uterus is contracting too vigorously or the fetus is not receiving enough oxygen.

The fetal heart usually beats between 120 and 160 times a minute. Higher rates are often associated with a raised maternal pulse or fever. Rates above 180 or below 110 are unusual and definite warning signals.

Where abnormal traces appear on the read-out from the monitoring device, there are three possibilities for the further management of labor. The baby can be delivered immediately by a cesarean operation or, if the second stage of labor has already begun, the baby can be delivered with the help of forceps or a vacuum extractor (*see* pp. 108–109). Alternatively, a fetal blood sample can be taken to show more precisely how much oxygen is getting to the fetus.

Fetal blood sampling

When taking a sample of fetal blood, the doctor first performs an internal examination and then pierces the fetal scalp with a small blade. This causes a few drops of blood to flow and these are caught in a narrow glass tube. The pressure of the cervix on the fetal scalp prevents further bleeding.

The acidity of the blood is then measured. If it is normal, this shows that the fetus is getting enough oxygen and no immediate action is required, though the fetal heart rate will still be carefully monitored and further blood samples may be taken. If the acidity is increasing, then the fetus must be receiving less and less oxygen. Labor may be allowed to continue if delivery is anticipated soon; otherwise cesarean delivery is indicated.

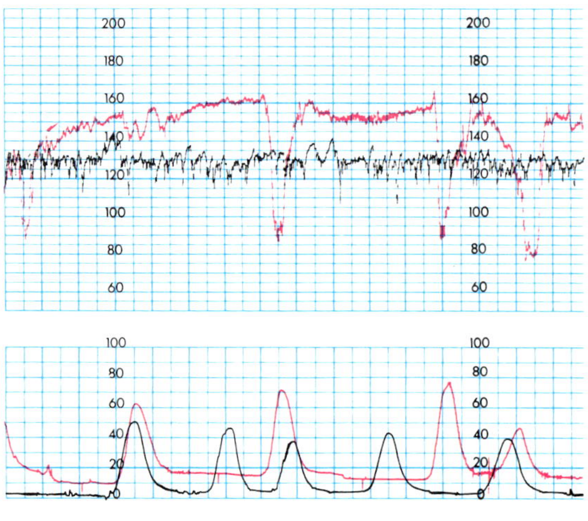

The cardiotocograph trace shows the fetal heartbeat, above, and the mother's contractions, below. Here two sets of traces have been superimposed. Those in black show a fetal heart rate of 130 per minute, with no change during contractions. Those in red show a fetal heart rate of 150 per minute, with a slowing of the rate during each contraction, but a quick recovery. This suggests that the umbilical cord is being compressed during contractions.

Induction

When labor has begun but is very weak, it may be strengthened by artificial means. This augmentation of labor should not, however, be confused with induction, a process by which labor is started by artificial means because of a risk to the health of the mother or the fetus. Labor may be induced for a variety of reasons but in each case it is essential that the dates of pregnancy be accurately known and preferably checked by ultrasonic measurements.

It is common to induce labor if the baby is more than two weeks overdue, so long as the pregnancy dates are certain. Very overdue babies are subject to increased risks during delivery, partly because, as the weeks pass, the fetus keeps growing and the skull becomes less pliable, but, more important, because the placenta ages and becomes less efficient. It may therefore be unable to support the fetus during the stresses of labor. Indeed, where tests show that the placenta is not working well, it may be safer for the baby to be born early and to grow in the nursery.

Heavy smoking during pregnancy, bleeding in the second or third trimester and pre-eclampsia (*see* p. 66) may cause the placenta to work less efficiently. Placental insufficiency can also occur of its own accord and lead to a small-for-dates baby.

When the Rh blood group of the mother is "negative" and the fetus' is "positive", and when the mother's blood has formed antibodies (*see* p. 33), it is also usual to deliver the baby before it is due. This may be anywhere up to eight weeks before the calculated date, if the condition of the fetus is deteriorating sufficiently. Intrauterine transfusions may be administered in the very premature fetus as an alternative to delivery. If the fetus is very severely affected induction of labor may be judged too risky and cesarean section may be employed.

When there is a previous history of unexplained fetal death in late pregnancy, an obstetrician is unlikely to allow labor to occur later than term. Insulin-dependent diabetic mothers are usually induced early – about the thirty-eighth week – as their fetuses are at risk in the last few weeks of pregnancy. Frequently induction is also recommended for mothers with high blood pressure or with kidney disease. Finally, if the mother has had several children and her labors are very short, an induction may be considered, provided she is at term.

Before labor is induced, the state of the cervix is carefully assessed to calculate how much stimulation will be necessary and efforts are made to predict any possible disproportion between the size of the fetus's head and the size of the birth canal. Methods for inducing labor include the simple but often ineffective and now rare practice of giving purgatives and enemas. Much more reliable is the use of artificial hormones, either oxytocin or prostaglandins. Prostaglandin inductions have wide use in Europe. The medicine has not been approved yet by the Food and Drug Administration for use in inductions of live babies in the United States. Prostaglandins have the advantage of softening the cervix in addition to initiating and maintaining contractions. Prostaglandin vaginal suppositories are approved to induce labor with stillborn fetuses earlier in pregnancy.

Oxytocin is a hormone which plays a role in normal labor and which is produced by the pituitary gland. It can now be synthesized but, since synthetic oxytocin is highly potent, a carefully controlled dose must be given. This is achieved by an intravenous infusion, or "drip". A fine plastic tube is inserted into a vein in the forearm or wrist and a sterile solution of oxytocin flows or is pumped directly into the mother's circulation.

It is also possible to induce labor by the simple method of artificial rupture of the membranes (AROM). The doctor punctures the amniotic sac and some fluid drains off. This procedure may cause some discomfort, though little more than would an internal examination. The stretching of the cervix which is involved does feel odd, but it is necessary since it probably stimulates the natural release of prostaglandins.

AROM is normally used together with hormones. Oxytocin may be administered after AROM, following a short pause to see if this method is adequate to start labor by itself. The oxytocin should be administered intravenously with an infusion pump in order to infuse the drug in a precise manner. The infusion pump may be separate from the electronic fetal monitor or integrated into it.

The infusion of oxytocin must be supervised carefully. One of the risks is that the mother's uterus may be very sensitive to the oxytocin. If so, or if too high a dose is administered, a prolonged contraction (tetanic contraction) may occur. This can be harmful because oxygenation to the fetus can be decreased during such a contraction. Usually inductions are performed without complications by carefully adjusting the dose of oxytocin.

Monitoring is carried out continuously during labor and may be used as part of the normal routine. However it is most useful and beneficial when complications arise.

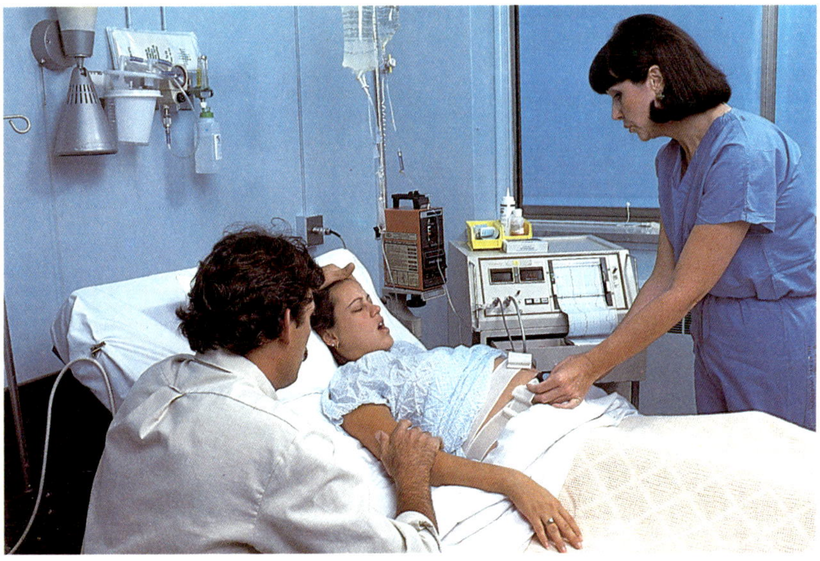

Delays in labor

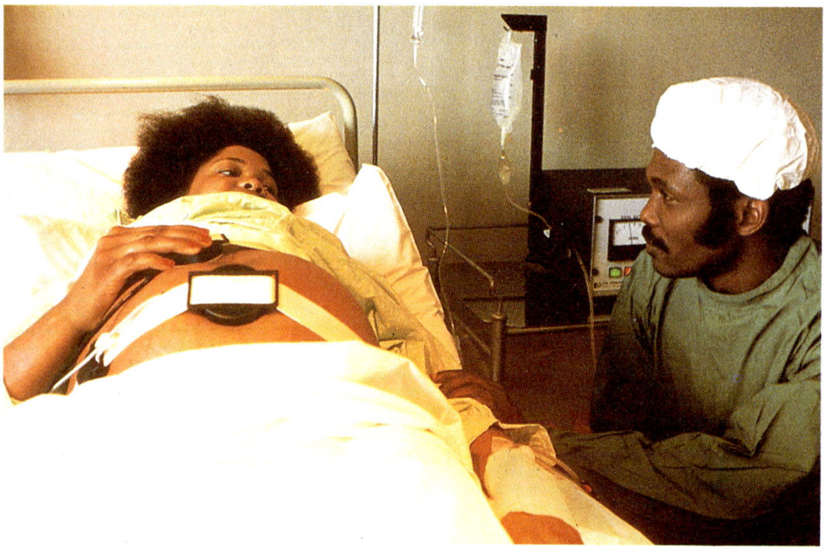

Where doctors suspect labor is not progressing "normally", the information provided by electronic monitoring enables them to decide what action to take.

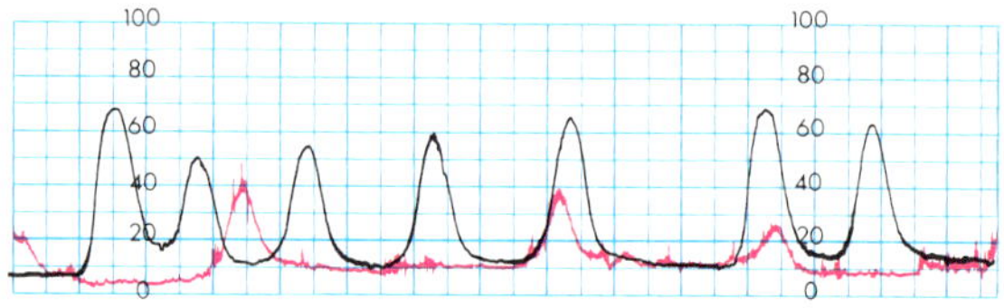

One reason for slow progress in labor can be inadequate contractions. Here two tocograph traces are superimposed. The black trace shows strong contractions occurring every 2 to 3 minutes. The red trace shows weaker contractions occurring only every 4 to 5 minutes.

Slow progress in labor or difficulty in the second stage is often due to a combination of inefficient contractions, incorrect positioning of the fetus's head and a tight fit in the birth canal.

The uterus normally contracts in response to a number of hormones produced by the mother and fetus. But the uterus may not work efficiently, either because the contractions are weak or because they are poorly synchronized. This is more likely in a first pregnancy when, if there is any obstruction to delivery, the uterus tends to stop contracting and the mother goes out of labor.

In labor the fetus should ideally present its head in a well-flexed attitude, that is with the chin tucked into the chest like a sprinter at the start of a race. This ensures that the smallest circumference passes through the mother's pelvis. If the head is poorly flexed, with the forehead leading, a relatively large circumference has to pass through the pelvis. If the uterine contractions are weak, the fetal head often remains unflexed and there will then be a combination of inadequate contractions and an unusually large head diameter to deliver. Progress in this situation is bound to be slow.

The size of the pelvis plays an important part in allowing a normal vaginal delivery. It must be large enough to let the baby's head pass through. In general, tall mothers usually have a pelvis which is large enough, but those who are less than 4 feet 11 inches are more likely to have a problem. Women tend to have slightly larger babies with each succeeding pregnancy and can sometimes have problems with a very large third baby after two uneventful pregnancies.

Problems often occur with a small woman whose bone structure has not developed to its true potential, as when a teenager carries a large baby. This also occurs in women who have come from underdeveloped countries and who bear relatively large babies as a result of both an improved Western diet and a better standard of living.

The shape of the pelvis is also important. A normal pelvis has an inlet which is a wide rounded shape. This poses no problem, because it allows easy rotation of the baby's head and gives plenty of room for the baby's birth. The other extremes, where the pelvis is a triangular or a flat oval shape, can lead to difficulties and prevent easy rotation and descent of the baby.

Antenatal detection of problems

During the first pregnancy, the head of the fetus should engage in the last two weeks before delivery. This simply means that the largest part of the head has passed into the pelvic cavity. Once this has happened, it is clear that there is no disproportion between the size of the head and the pelvic inlet.

X-ray pelvimetry is rarely used in modern obstetrics. It may be indicated when there is probably disproportion between the maternal pelvic and fetal size in order to avoid a long and fruitless labor; it may be performed if the mother has a history of pelvic fracture or if the fetus is breech to determine the adequacy of the pelvic dimensions. It is uncommon to have cesarean section performed without a trial of labor in the absence of significant disproportion. Generally, the physician will allow labor to occur with the knowledge that a cesarean delivery can be performed if progress in labor stops.

Ultrasound scans are helpful to detect the fetus which is very large. Measurements of the head, chest, abdomen and femurs indicate fetal size accurately. Additionally, ultrasound

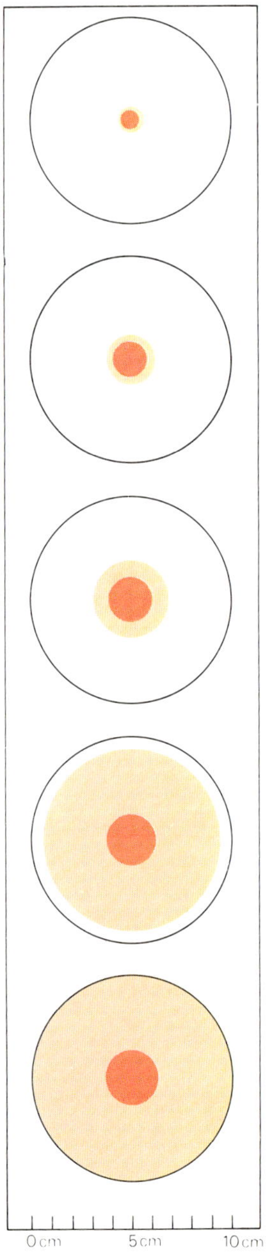

DILATION OF THE CERVIX

Poor progress in labor shows itself in slow dilation of the cervix. If the cervix is dilating less than 1 cm an hour due to inadequate uterine contractions, the membranes may be ruptured artificially if they are still intact. If this does not improve progress, oxytocin may be given. Here normal and delayed dilation are shown at 8, 10, 12 and 14 hours after the onset of labor.

normal

delayed

scans detect other problems which cause problems with labor and delivery such as placenta previa (placenta over the cervix) or fetal malformations that may obstruct a delivery.

Problems in labor

The usual method of assessing progress once labor has actually begun is to measure the cervical dilation at appropriate intervals. The rate of dilation is plotted on a graph and is compared with the curve for normal labor. (The correct rate will, of course, be different for the first birth and for subsequent births, *see* p. 72.) If the rate of progress is slow, then the cause of the delay must be diagnosed immediately and dealt with accordingly.

The problems may be weak or infrequent uterine contractions with a poorly flexed head and a slightly narrow pelvis. In most cases augmentation of labor by an oxytocin "drip" or rupture of the membranes should solve the problem. (These methods have been described on the previous page.) If the reason for the delay is a serious disproportion between the size of the fetal head and that of the pelvis, then a cesarean section will be required. Inadequate contractions usually become apparent early in labor, but disproportion often does not become a problem until later.

Complications of the third stage of labor

In a small number of mothers the placenta does not separate during the uterine contraction which follows delivery of the baby. Provided there is no bleeding, it is safe to wait a little while for the uterus to relax and contract again – this second contraction may release the placenta. The process is often helped by emptying the mother's bladder with a catheter. If the placenta is not delivered after 15–20 minutes it is removed manually by the obstetrician.

If heavy bleeding occurs with the placenta undelivered it means that partial separation of the placenta has occurred. In this case an injection of oxytocic drug is given intravenously and the placenta is removed manually as soon as possible.

Manual removal of the placenta is painless, if a general or an epidural anesthetic is used. The doctor inserts a hand into the uterus through the vagina and gently separates the placenta from the uterus. The placenta is inspected to make sure that none has been left behind. Retained placenta can occur in later pregnancies so mothers who have had this problem previously must be sure their doctors are aware of it, in order that special care may be taken.

Postpartum hemorrhage (P.P.H.) is an excessive blood loss after delivery. If the bleeding is due to poor contractions of the uterus, intravenous or intramuscular ergotrate or oxytocin is given to contract the uterus. If bleeding still occurs after the delivery of the placenta, an oxytocin drip is given to maintain contraction of the uterus; if necessary blood will also be given. If excessive bleeding happens because of a vaginal or cervical tear, simply stitching up the tear itself will automatically stop any bleeding.

Inverted uterus, caused by attempts to deliver the placenta by pulling on the cord when the uterus was not contracting properly, is now extremely rare.

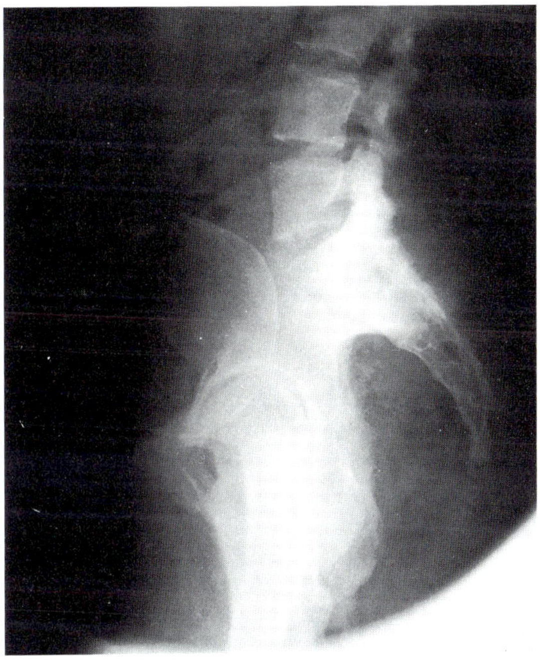

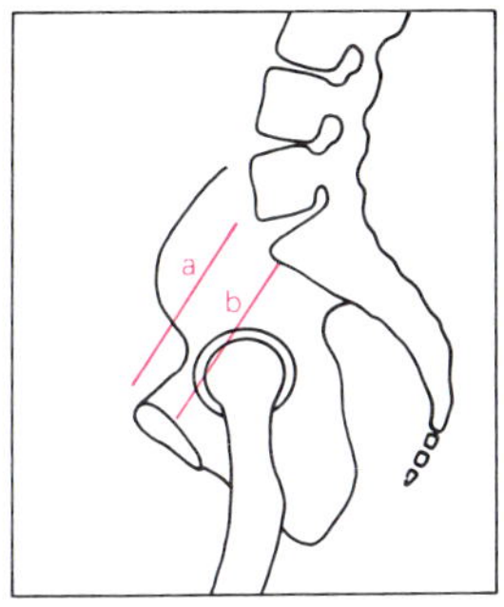

The baby shown in this X-ray photograph cannot be born in the ordinary way because the width of its head (line a) is too large to pass through the pelvic brim (line b) into the pelvis. As a result delivery must be by cesarean section.

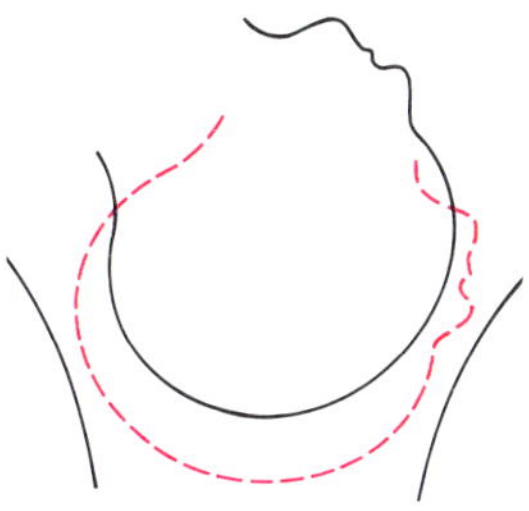

POSITION OF FETAL HEAD
The baby's chin is usually tucked in at the beginning of labor. If the neck is extended and the head back, the diameter of the presenting part is larger and the fit tighter.

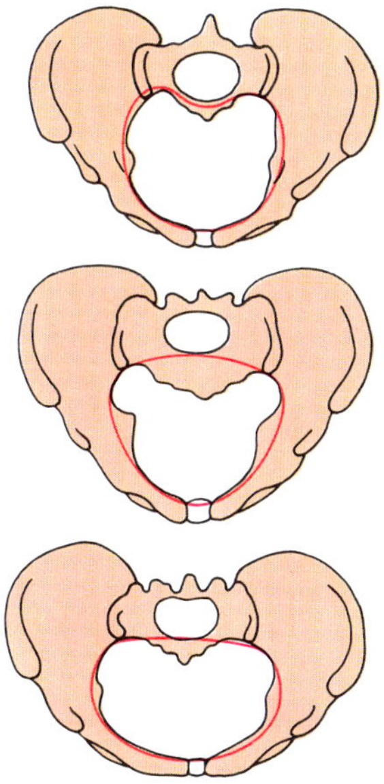

TYPES OF PELVIS
The three types of female pelvis shown have a rounded inlet (top), a more triangular inlet (center) and a narrow or flat inlet (bottom). The first is ideal for childbearing, as it allows easy rotation of the baby's head. The other shapes may cause problems.

Breech babies and twins

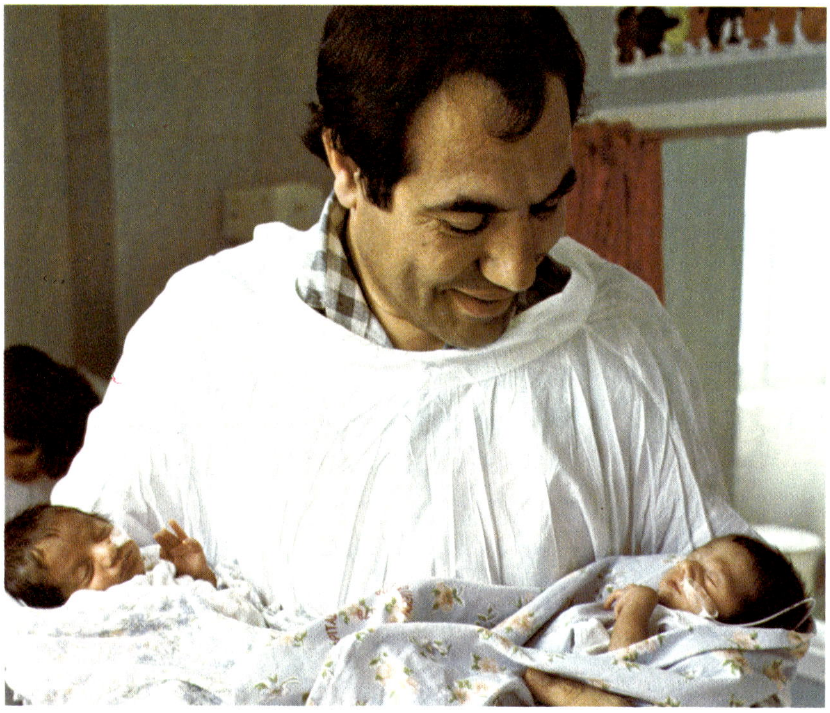

Twins occur in about 1 in 80 births and triplets in about 1 in 5,000 to 10,000 births.

The birth of twins or of a baby in the breech position need not be any more difficult than a normal birth, provided they both present head first. Since, however, these types of birth share some peculiarities, and in a high percentage of twins one of the babies is a breech baby, they are described together.

Twins

When a mother is carrying twins, the uterus reaches the size of a normal full-term pregnancy much earlier. The average duration of twin pregnancies is therefore 37 weeks and premature delivery (before 37 weeks) is also common. At the onset of labor the uterus is stretched more than usual and the strength of contractions may be reduced. As a result labor may last longer than for a single baby.

Ideally the heartbeat of both fetuses should be checked during labor, with the help of an electrode attached to the scalp of the fetus which is to be born first and an external monitor attached to the mother's abdomen to give a separate reading for the second twin. There are many possibilities in the lie and presentation of twins, but the most common is the simplest, with both babies presenting head first. Where one or both of the babies is in a breech position, extra care is taken by the obstetrician (*see* above).

A twin pregnancy with both twins in the head-down position. This is the most common presentation for twins and the birth should be a fairly simple procedure if no other complications arise.

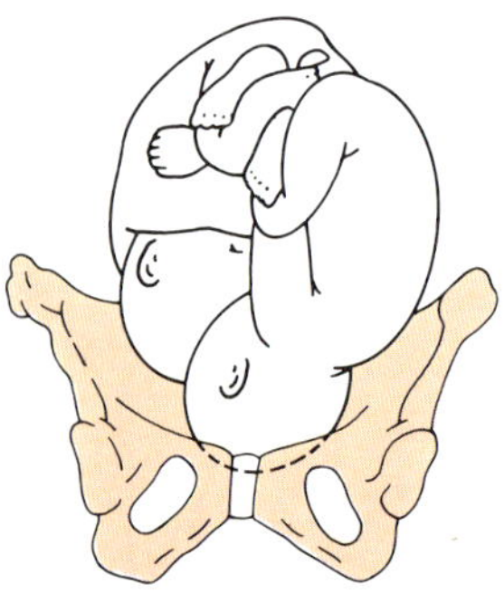

During labor, an oxytocin "drip" will usually be available to counteract any delay. Pain relief may be provided by Demerol or with an epidural block which will allow obstetrical maneuvers to be carried out without the risk of having suddenly to administer a general anesthetic to the patient.

After delivery of the first twin, the uterus would naturally rest for 15 to 20 minutes. The second twin could, however, be at risk during this time since its placenta may have begun to separate. It is therefore usual to have an oxytocin infusion available to reduce the delay and encourage prompt delivery of the second twin. The doctor checks the position of the second twin and, if it is transverse (i.e. lying across the uterus), turns the baby around by massaging the mother's abdomen. He will then rupture the amniotic sac surrounding the second twin and, with good contractions, it should be born spontaneously. If there is any delay, then forceps can be used.

The combination of a large double placenta and an overstretched uterus means that the mother's blood loss after delivery is likely to be greater with twins. As a result the drug ergotrate or oxytocin is often given intravenously to encourage the uterus to contract well. With careful preparation and proper supervision during labor, the delivery of twins need not present any serious problem.

Breech

The birth of a baby in the breech position, that is with the buttocks coming first, should always take place only after careful obstetric evaluation. A vaginal delivery is allowed only after the mother's pelvis has been measured by X ray and the size of the baby's head has been assessed – preferably by ultrasound – to make sure the birth canal is wide enough. If there is any doubt about the safety of a vaginal delivery, or if there are any complicating factors, such as prematurity or a history of obstetric difficulties, then a delivery by cesarean section is best.

The mother goes to the hospital with the onset of labor. But if the membranes rupture before the onset of labor she should go directly to the hospital because the possibility of the umbilical cord prolapsing into the vagina is increased in certain breech presentations.

Labour should progress at the same rate as in a normal delivery; if it is not doing so, the contractions may be stimulated by using an oxytocin "drip". The monitoring devices will be the same as those used in a head-first delivery, except that the spiral electrode, which allows the doctor to record the heart rate of the fetus, would be attached to the buttocks rather than to the head. It is probably best to have epidural analgesia during a breech delivery as forceps are usually used to protect the baby's head; an epidural avoids the need for any local anesthetic. The second stage of labor is considered to have begun when the cervix is opened wide enough to allow the buttocks through, but the mother is not ready for actual delivery until her lower vagina has been completely stretched by the baby's buttocks.

Breech deliveries are ideally conducted by two doctors with a nurse assisting and often with an anesthesiologist and pediatrician also present. During the birth, the mother is in the lithotomy position, that is on her back with her legs bent and her feet held in stirrups, as this enables the doctor to handle the baby

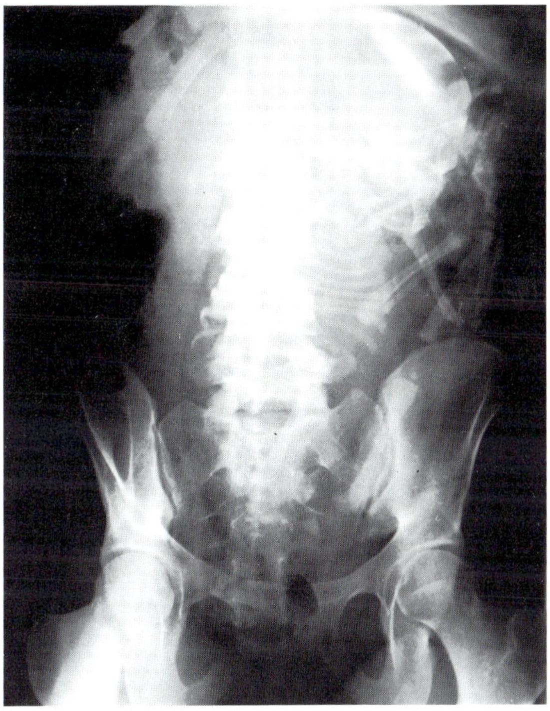

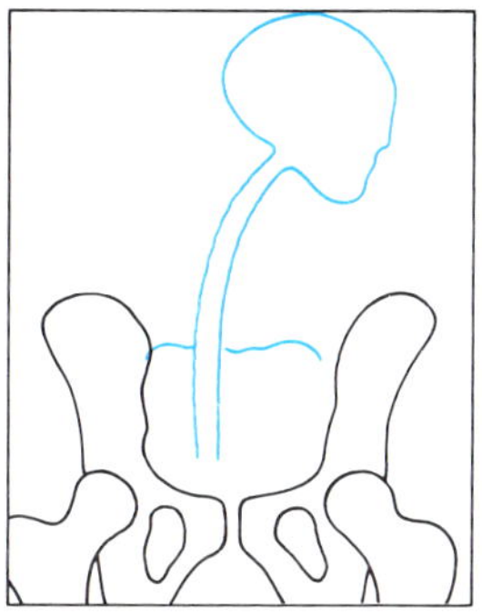

In this X ray the head and backbone of the fetus in the breech position can be clearly seen. The ribs, and extended legs, are also visible.

most easily. An episiotomy will generally be performed in these cases.

Which part of a breech baby is delivered first depends on the exact position of the baby in the uterus. The baby's feet may be delivered before the buttocks if the legs are bent (a complete breech), or after the buttocks if the knees are straight and the legs extend upwards (a frank breech). Once the buttocks and feet have been born, the next contraction delivers the baby as far as the umbilical cord and a loop of cord can be gently pulled down so that the baby's pulse can be counted. With the next contraction, the shoulder blades appear and the baby's arms are then born.

All that remains is the head. This is usually delivered with Piper forceps, with the rest of the baby held upward out of the way in a warm towel. The forceps prevent sudden compression of the head in the birth canal or, worse still, rapid decompression after delivery, either of which might rupture the fragile blood vessels in the head and cause dangerous problems for the newborn baby. When delivering the head, the doctor can control the process by using both hands, instead of forceps. One hand is placed behind the head, one on the baby's face, and the rest of the baby's body supported on the forearm.

Careful breech delivery by experienced doctors normally involves no greater risk to the baby than any other delivery, provided all obstetric factors are favorable. There is an increased risk with older mothers and also if there is an inefficient placenta. Sometimes problems arise because the breech presentation is not discovered until after labor has begun, or because a vaginal delivery proves more difficult than expected, or because the baby is premature as well as being in the breech position. Breech presentation is, in fact, much more common in premature babies (up to 25 per cent at 30 weeks, compared with 3.5 per cent at term) and the complications of prematurity are taken into account when evaluating the risks involved in allowing a breech baby to be born through the vagina. Good obstetrical judgment is critical.

BREECH DELIVERY
In most breech deliveries the doctor assists delivery by manipulating the baby's body, once the trunk and legs are born. Pictures 1 and 2 show the top shoulder being born, then rotation through 180° (with the back uppermost) to release the other shoulder. The body is then allowed to hang down, which increases flexion of the head (3). Once the hairline and nape of the neck emerge, the body is raised so that the face appears, and the rest of the head is born slowly, usually with the help of forceps.

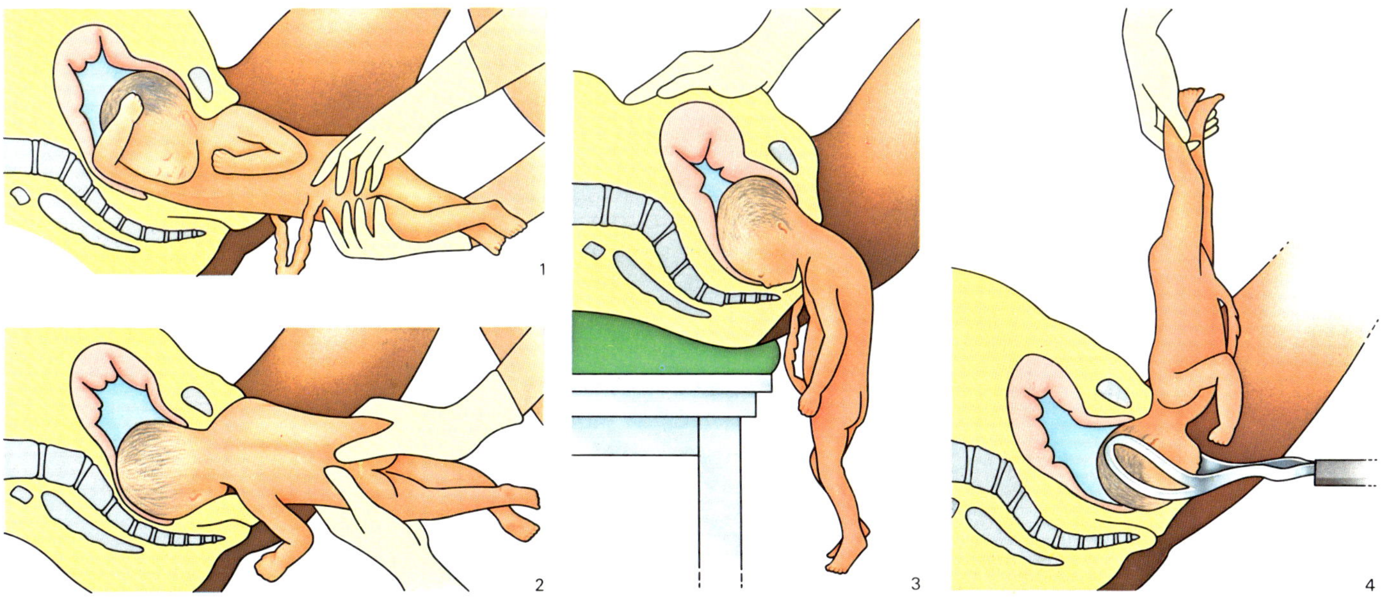

Instrumental deliveries

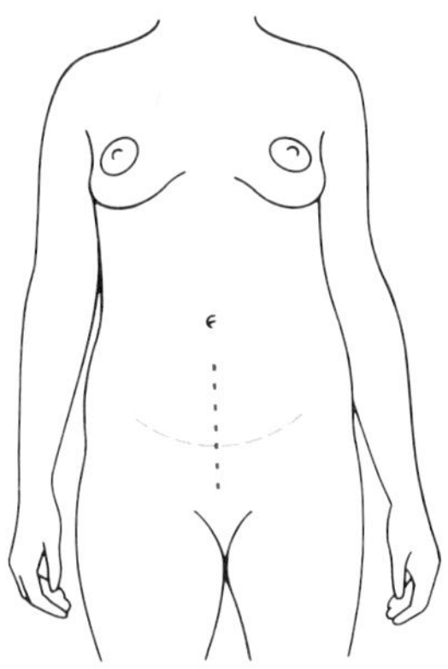

The incision for a cesarean delivery can be vertical or horizontal. Its exact position may depend on medical considerations.

The first successful obstetrical forceps were introduced by the Chamberlen family who then kept their discovery secret for commercial reasons throughout the sixteenth and seventeenth centuries. Modern forceps have been carefully designed to fit the baby's head accurately and to allow a safe delivery. They are used to help draw the baby out during delivery, to rotate his head from an unfavorable position and to protect the head during a breech delivery.

The reasons for forceps deliveries

The most common reason for a forceps delivery is slow progress in the second stage of labor. During the second stage, the baby is increasingly deprived of oxygen as the mother's efforts and the uterine contractions reduce the blood flow from the placenta. Although the fetus can withstand a moderate lack of oxygen for a time, it may begin to suffer after one and a half to two hours. For this reason, it is usual to allow the mother to push for up to two hours in the second stage and then to intervene. The cause of the delay may be the mother's exhaustion, a big baby or malposition of the baby's head.

Doctors may decide to use forceps if it becomes clear that the fetus is in distress because its heart rate slows and then only recovers slowly after each contraction (*see* p. 104). In this situation, if the fetus is not born soon, he may die from lack of oxygen. Forceps are also sometimes used to ease the strain if the woman has a severe heart or lung disease or high blood pressure.

During a breech delivery the fetal head comes fairly rapidly into the pelvis and is born within minutes. The head is compressed as it enters the pelvis and is decompressed as it is born. When this happens too rapidly, it may damage the blood vessels in the brain. This can be avoided by using forceps to protect and deliver the head. At the start of labor the baby's head usually faces to the side, and as it descends it rotates so that the face looks toward the mother's back. If the head does not rotate fully during labor, this gives a large diameter to deliver and produces difficulties in the second stage of labor. Following rotation the head can usually be delivered with ease.

In this situation, it is therefore usual to rotate the head to make the delivery easier. Rotation may be performed by hand, by using a vacuum extractor (*see* below), or by means of the special Kiellands forceps. These have features which allow the baby's head to be rotated without damaging the mother.

Forceps deliveries

Good pain relief is essential during a forceps delivery and can be provided either by an epidural block, which is ideal, or by a local pelvic nerve block (a pudendal block). Occasionally a general anesthetic is necessary but the risks to the mother are greater than with local anesthesia. The woman rests her feet in stirrups and the obstetrician cleans around the entrance to the vagina with antiseptic solution and puts sterile drapes over the legs and abdomen. The bladder is emptied with a catheter to avoid damage. The position of the baby's head is checked and the appropriate forceps are selected and carefully applied. If the forceps are being used to draw the baby's head out, then the pulling is done during contractions so that the forceps and the uterus work in cooperation.

After the delivery of the baby's head the forceps are removed and the rest of the delivery continues as usual. Babies born with the help of forceps may have pressure marks

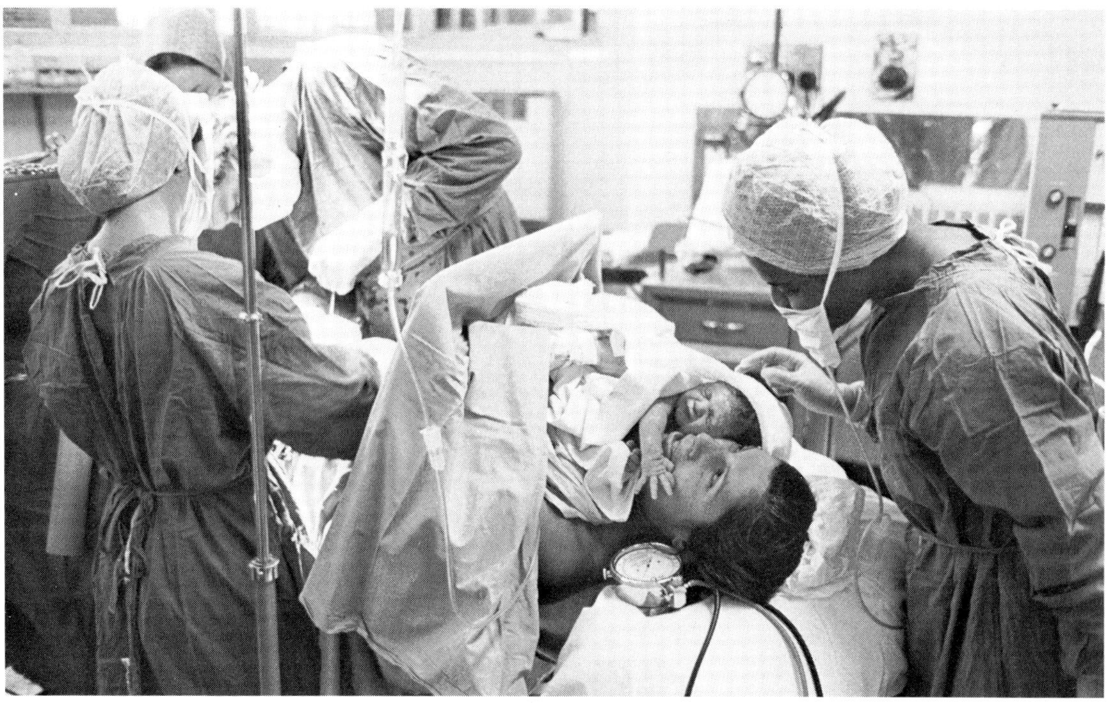

This mother has had a cesarean delivery with an epidural block. She has been given the baby to hold soon after birth, while the uterus and abdomen are being stitched up.

from the blades left on the face, but these unsightly marks are temporary and usually disappear in a day or two.

The vacuum extractor

Although the principle has been known for many years, it was only in the 1950s that a successful vacuum extraction device for aiding delivery was developed. The device consists of a plastic cup which is attached by suction to the baby's scalp. Gentle pulling on the head from the plastic cup is synchronized with the contractions of the uterus. This provides downward traction coordinated with uterine contractions to assist in vaginal delivery. Additionally, the vacuum extractor can assist in rotation of the fetal head to achieve proper alignment for delivery.

Considerable care, patience, and cooperation from the mother are needed to operate the vacuum extractor. One of the advantages it has over forceps is that the head rotates of its own accord during delivery. One disadvantage is that the cup can only be left in place for 20 minutes or damage to the scalp may occur. If the cup pulls off more than once, then this method is abandoned and forceps are used or a cesarean delivery is performed depending on circumstances.

Cesarean delivery

With modern developments in anesthetics and blood transfusion, delivery by cesarean section has become a safe alternative to vaginal delivery and is increasingly used when a normal delivery would present problems. In this operation, an incision is made in the abdomen and uterus, the baby is lifted out and the mother's uterus and abdominal wall are repaired. Sometimes the operation is planned before the woman goes into labor. Doctors advise it if there is placenta previa (*see* p. 65), a dangerously small pelvis, a potentially difficult breech delivery or if the mother has already had a cesarean birth. Other women require a cesarean delivery when problems leading to slow progress or fetal distress arise unexpectedly during the course of labor and thus a vaginal delivery therefore becomes risky or impossible.

A cesarean operation can be performed with a general anesthetic or an epidural block, depending on medical opinion and the woman's wishes as well as on the equipment available. In preparing a mother for the operation, a nurse will empty the bladder and leave in an indwelling catheter, clean the abdomen with an antiseptic solution and place sterile drapes over her abdomen. The woman feels no pain and the incision in the skin is usually low and horizontal. Such a scar heals well and looks unobtrusive: it is known as a "bikini scar". Sometimes, however, the incision has to be made lengthwise on the abdomen for medical reasons.

The baby is usually born within three to five minutes of beginning the cesarean operation and it takes another half hour or so to repair the uterus and abdomen. The skin is closed either with absorbable stitches, which do not need to be removed, or with staples which are removed after about five days. The mother may be able to get up the day of the operation. For the first few days she will be put on a light diet. Following a cesarean delivery the mother may experience varying amounts of abdominal wall pain. But, since the abdomen is generally lax postpartum, the pain is usually not severe. The doctor will order pain medication for the first few days. She should be able to go home within seven days.

The scar should give no problems during the next pregnancy. If the reason for the cesarean delivery persists – a small pelvis, for example – then another cesarean will obviously be performed. If, however, the first operation was because of fetal distress or placenta previa, a vaginal delivery may be possible in subsequent pregnancies. Very rarely, the scar in the uterus may open up during the subsequent labor. If it does, a repeat cesarean will immediately become necessary. After two cesarean deliveries, further births should always be cesarean and women in this situation are normally advised to limit the number of their pregnancies to four or five.

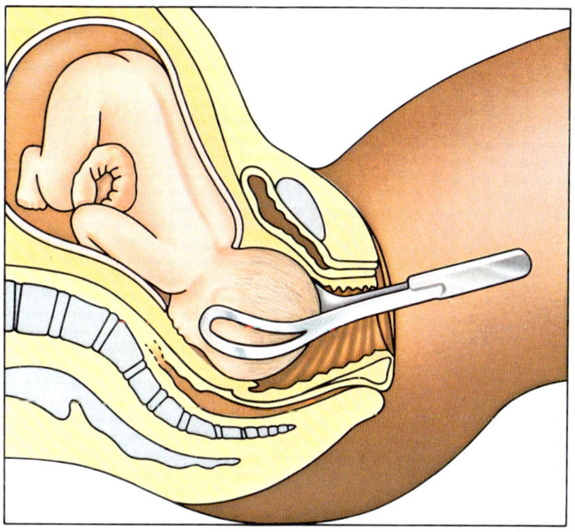

Forceps delivery. The operator's hands are not shown.

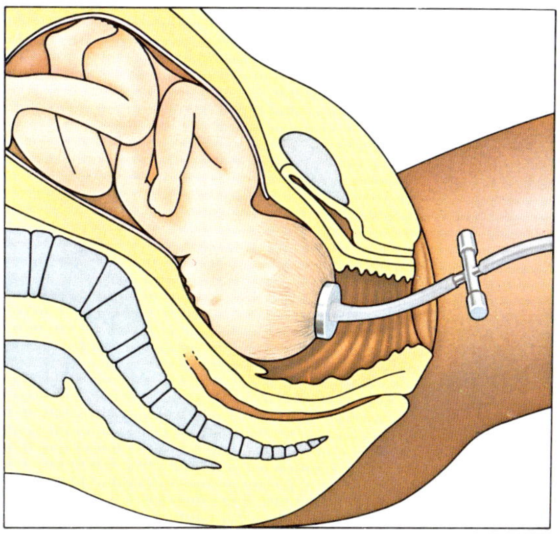

The vacuum extractor or suction cup.

The normal puerperium

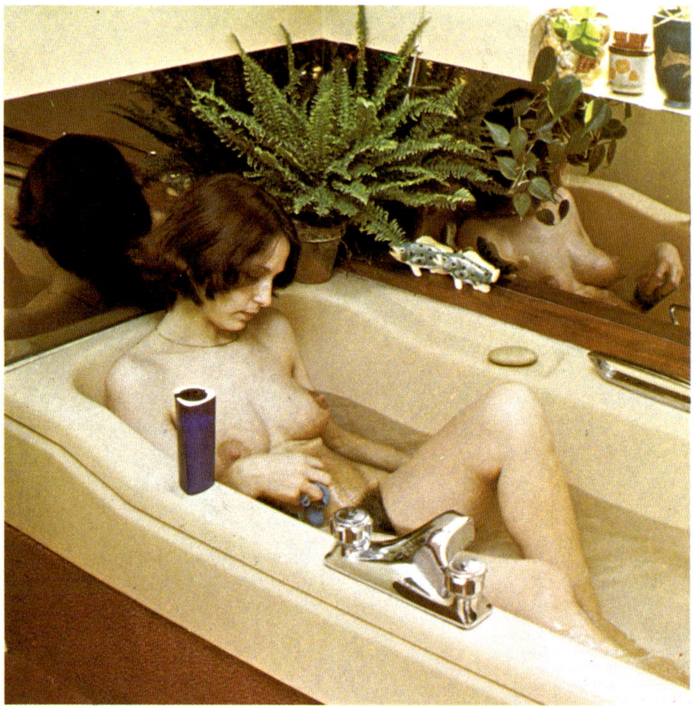

CHAPTER 8

Cross references

See also	Chapter
The new baby at home	11
The child and the family	15
Feeding the newborn baby	10

The puerperium, the six weeks following the birth of the baby, is a very active time for a woman from every point of view.

The puerperium begins immediately after the birth when, with the delivery of the placenta, the uterus begins to return to its non-pregnant state (*see* p. 75). All the changes in the mother's body brought about by pregnancy and labor with one exception are now reversed. The exception is the changes in the breasts that prepare them for breast-feeding. Breast-feeding – discussed in detail in chapter 10 – is established in this period (unless, of course, the mother has decided to bottle feed). At the same time the new mother has to undertake all the day-to-day care of a very demanding tiny baby, in addition to her usual household duties of looking after a home, a husband, and perhaps other children. As if this were not enough, many mothers return to either part-time or full-time employment within a few weeks of birth.

After the initial happiness and relief that follow a successful birth, a mother will want to hold her new baby and to reassure herself that he or she is normal. The doctor first examines him to make sure all is well and then puts him in his mother's arms.

In some hospitals the child is put to his mother's breast within a few minutes of delivery, and many babies are able to suck for a few minutes. Putting the baby to the breast immediately also has advantages for the mother, for it helps to stimulate the contraction of the uterus.

If there is a small tear at the lower end of the vagina, or if an episiotomy has been necessary – which is very common with first babies or with a forceps delivery (*see* p. 108) – the doctor will stitch up the mother soon after delivery. This is usually a

The new mother needs plenty of rest to recover from the hard work of labor. Relaxing in a warm bath will also help to soothe any discomfort from episiotomy stitches.

painless procedure. First some local anesthetic is injected around the area to be repaired, although sometimes this is not necessary as the local anesthetic given before the episiotomy was cut will still be effective. When the area is numb, the edges of the incision are stitched together.

The vagina is usually repaired with catgut which dissolves after about a week. Catgut stitches dissolve, but it is not unusual for the knots, which are on the outside, to drop out in the bath one or two weeks after the area is stitched.

After the baby has been settled in his bassinet and the episiotomy has been stitched, the nurse will check that the maternal pulse, temperature and blood pressure are normal. She feels the uterus which is now in the lower part of the abdomen to check that it is well contracted. She looks at the sanitary pad to see that there has been a normal amount of blood loss after the delivery.

It is usual at this stage for the mother to attempt to empty her bladder. This can be surprisingly difficult, especially if she is sitting on a bedpan. If she is not successful, the nurse will check that the bladder is not overfull. Providing it is not, emptying the bladder can be left until later (*see* p. 123). The mother will then be made comfortable and given a bath and a change of clothes.

For a few hours after the delivery and while the mother rests, the baby is usually kept in the nursery, under the watchful eye of the nurse. Many modern hospitals provide rooming-in facilities, which allow the baby to stay in the mother's hospital room almost constantly so the two can get to know each other and continue the bonding relationship.

The mother should expect some discomfort after the birth while her body readjusts. A certain amount of blood and debris – called the lochia – drains from the uterus after delivery. It is usually a bit heavier than a period for the first 24 hours, then slowly decreases in amount. It may last for two or three or even as long as six to eight weeks. The lochia is bright red for up to a week and then becomes red-brown. The mother will need to wear sanitary pads during this time. Any heavy loss which soaks a pad within a few minutes, or large clots, should be reported to the nurse or doctor. Pads should always be changed regularly as this helps to keep the vulva as clean as possible.

There is no doubt that sitting on stitches is uncomfortable at best, and painful at worst, for at least the first two to three days. This discomfort can be somewhat relieved by taking mild pain-killing pills and by sitting on a cushion or rubber ring. Taking sitz baths once or twice a day can also provide comfort for the new mother.

Feeling depressed and tearful after delivery – known as "the blues" is so common as to be almost a normal event of the puerperium and usually lasts only a few hours or a day. The mother needs the sympathetic ear of the doctor, nurses and family to realize this will pass. If depression persists, or interferes with a woman caring for her child, it is most important to call the doctor as treatment may be needed. If she has help, she may prefer just to cuddle and feed her baby for the first few days. Then she may start to change and bathe him. Gradually she will manage all her baby's needs. Other mothers may not be fortunate enough to have someone to help and must assume all of the responsibility for the child's needs from the outset by herself.

Physical changes

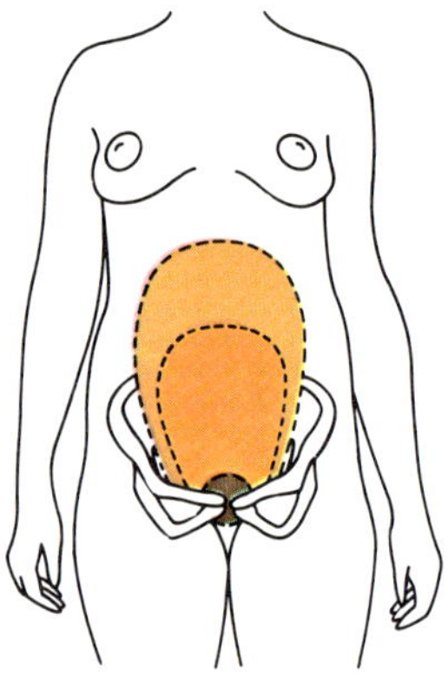

The uterus returns to its non-pregnant size remarkably quickly. The above diagram shows its size at term, immediately after delivery, and six weeks later.

It is the delivery of the placenta, not the delivery of the baby, which causes the mother's body to return to normal. The hormones produced by the placenta maintain most of the physiological (bodily) changes of pregnancy and these hormones disappear from the mother's body within a short time of its delivery. The most dramatic changes of the puerperium occur in the uterus and the breasts but, as well as these, all the other changes that took place during pregnancy and were described in chapter 2 are reversed. The puerperium usually takes about six weeks but it can take longer.

Changes in the uterus

The uterus decreases in size and weight from about 2 lb (1 kilogram) to about 2 oz (50 to 60 grams) in a few weeks. Immediately after delivery the uterus can be felt just below the umbilicus. It is firmly contracted and feels rather like a baseball. The uterus contracts and relaxes at irregular intervals after delivery. These contractions cause after-pains, which are similar to period pains and are most obvious in the first few days after delivery. They may also occur in the following weeks, while the mother is breast-feeding, and even between feedings. These contractions serve to squeeze out any blood which has collected inside the uterus and this blood is passed out of the vagina as the lochia (*see* above).

The uterus gets smaller day by day, and 10 to 14 days after the birth it sinks back into the pelvis and can no longer be felt in the abdomen. It usually takes about six weeks to return to normal size.

The decrease in size of the uterus is called involution. It is due to the gradual breakdown of the excess muscle protein in the walls of the uterus into amino acids which then pass into the bloodstream. From there some of these amino acids are used to build up protein in the breasts to make milk, some are used by the mother's own body, and some are broken down and lost in the urine.

Inside the uterus the lining, or decidua, built up during pregnancy breaks down and is shed in a similar manner to the shedding of the endometrium during a period (*see* p. 16). Endometrium then grows up from the underlying cells and within three weeks it lines most of the uterus except the area where the placenta was attached. It can take from six to eight weeks to cover this area.

Menstruation

The time the first period occurs is very variable. It may start before the lochia has completely ceased or it may be delayed for many months, particularly if the woman is breast-feeding.

With the delivery of the placenta at the time of the birth there is a sudden decrease in the blood levels of the placental hormones estrogen and progesterone. The level of the hormone H.C.G., which has maintained the corpus luteum during pregnancy, falls also. When the level of H.C.G. falls, a series of hormonal activites will begin to occur. The fall in the levels of estrogen and progesterone in the blood once more permits the hypothalamus to trigger the production of F.S.H. and L.H. by the pituitary gland (*see* p. 16). This results in the start of the first menstrual cycle.

The earliest time that ovulation can occur is four weeks after delivery. It is not possible for a woman to become pregnant during this time but it is possible for pregnancy to occur after this without an intervening period because the ovum usually ripens two weeks *before* the first period. Often, however, the first period occurs without an ovum ripening (known as an anovulatory cycle). Menstrual cramps are sometimes, but not always, improved after pregnancy.

In women who are breast-feeding the milk hormone prolactin interferes with the menstrual cycle, and periods are often irregular or missed until breast-feeding stops. This does

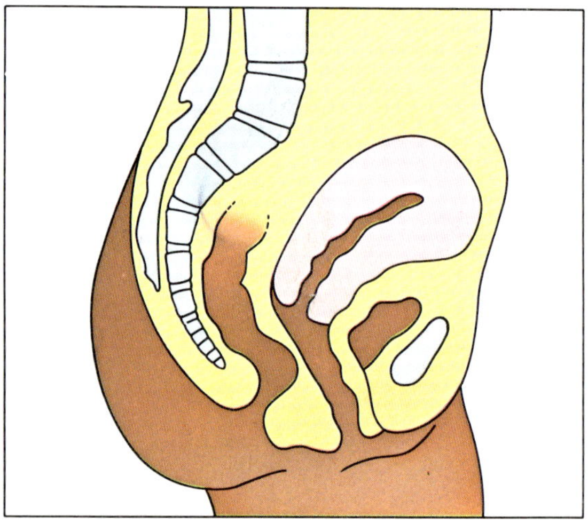

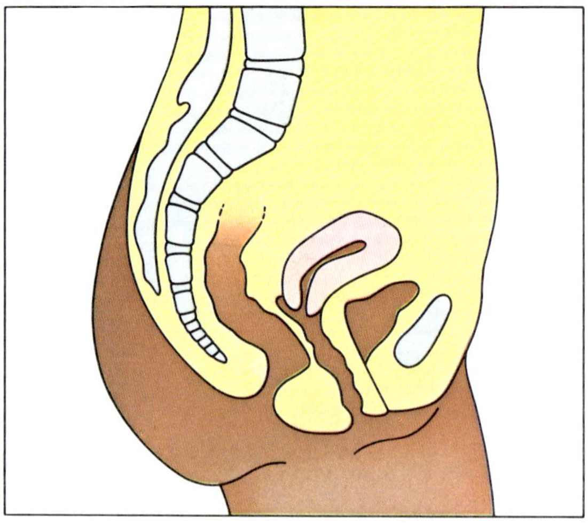

Immediately after the birth, the uterus can be felt just below the umbilicus. At this stage the uterus weighs about 2 lb (0.9 kg) and is about 7 in (1795 cm) long.

The uterus gets smaller day by day until, by about six weeks or so, it has returned to its non-pregnant size: it weighs only about 2 oz (60 g) and is about 3 in (7.5 cm) long.

not always happen, however, and periods can occur during successful breast-feeding. As a general rule, women are less fertile during breast-feeding than they would otherwise be, but conception can still occur.

The cervix
The cervix, which is soft and stretched after delivery, soon starts to return to its normal size and closes down at the level of the internal os between one and two weeks later. The external os often remains open for some time.

Frequently the type of cells which normally make the "skin" of the cervix are damaged by the birth and are rather slow to grow over it once more. A temporary cover of cells from inside the cervix is formed instead. This is known as a cervical erosion, and although it may last for several weeks it does not usually cause any symptoms and does not require any treatment at all.

The vagina
The passage of the baby through the vagina stretches and smooths out the vaginal wall. After a few days the vagina returns to its normal capacity. Tears and episiotomies usually heal quite quickly within the first week and, provided there is no infection, they should be completely healed by two to three weeks after the actual delivery.

Actually, an infected episiotomy is quite rare considering it is nearly impossible to prevent contamination of the area because of its proximity to the rectum. Any infection is usually secondary to the development of a hematoma due to hemorrhage into this tissue.

The breasts
During pregnancy the breasts increase in size and occasionally produce a little clear fluid, called colostrum, under the influence of the pituitary hormone prolactin and the placental hormones estrogen and progesterone. At the same time actual milk production is prevented by the high levels of estrogen circulating in the mother's bloodstream.

After the birth of the baby and the delivery of the placenta the estrogen level falls, and milk production starts, usually becoming established by the third day.

The level of prolactin in the blood, which is very high by the end of pregnancy, also falls slowly, but every time the baby is put to the breast it increases very sharply once more. This means that prolactin, and with it the supply of breast milk, can be increased by frequent suckling.

The release of oxytocin from the pituitary gland, which brings about contractions of the uterus during and after labor, also causes some of the muscle cells in the breasts to contract, squeezing milk from the outer part of each breast into the ducts under the nipple. The mother will feel the milk coming toward the nipple, and this effect is called "let down" of the milk. Mothers will notice that when they hear their hungry baby crying, milk sometimes leaks from the breasts before they have picked the baby up. This, too, is caused by oxytocin, which can be produced in response to the baby's cry.

For women who wish to bottle feed it is often a problem to prevent milk coming. All sorts of remedies were tried in the past, none of them very successful. At one time women were given estrogen tablets or injections for this, but these are now rarely used as they can predispose to leg vein thrombosis (*see* p. 123).

Supporting the breasts and leaving them alone may slow down the milk supply, at least in women who do not have a lot of milk. They may feel some discomfort on the third day after the birth, but this can be relieved by any mild analgesic, for example, aspirin.

Some women, however, experience a great deal of discomfort and leakage of milk, which may persist for several days. They may then be tempted to express the milk (*see* p. 142), but it is important to remember that emptying the breasts by *any* method encourages more milk to form. After a week or two the leakage of milk is usually reduced of its own accord although it may take some time for this leakage to stop entirely.

The blood and tissue fluid
Although some blood is lost when the uterus contracts to expel the placenta, most of the blood circulating through the blood vessels of the uterus is expelled back into the general circulation, which temporarily expands to accommodate it.

The total blood volume, which increases in pregnancy (*see* p. 32), returns to normal over two or three days. This is brought about by loss of extra fluid through the kidneys into the urine. In these few days, therefore, a woman can expect to pass a lot more urine than can be accounted for by the amount she drinks.

The renal system
In pregnancy, the kidney pelvises and the ureters, which lead to the bladder, expand. Within two or three weeks of delivery these begin to resume their normal size and have usually done so within two or three months.

Sometimes, if the delivery has been difficult, or labor prolonged, there is a little bruising of the base of the bladder and the urethra – the tube leading from it. This bruising may make passing urine difficult in the first 24 hours after the birth, but it usually improves very rapidly. Passing urine can also be difficult for an hour or two after an epidural anesthesia, as this numbs the nerves of the bladder as well as those of the uterus. But again the effect wears off quickly. All other systems return to normal. Skin pigment disappears, stretch marks fade considerably, but do not disappear entirely. The digestive system recovers and symptoms of heartburn, constipation and hemorrhoids improve. Diseases or complications of pregnancy such as raised blood pressure, pre-eclampsia and sugar in the urine, all usually disappear in the puerperium.

Postnatal check-ups

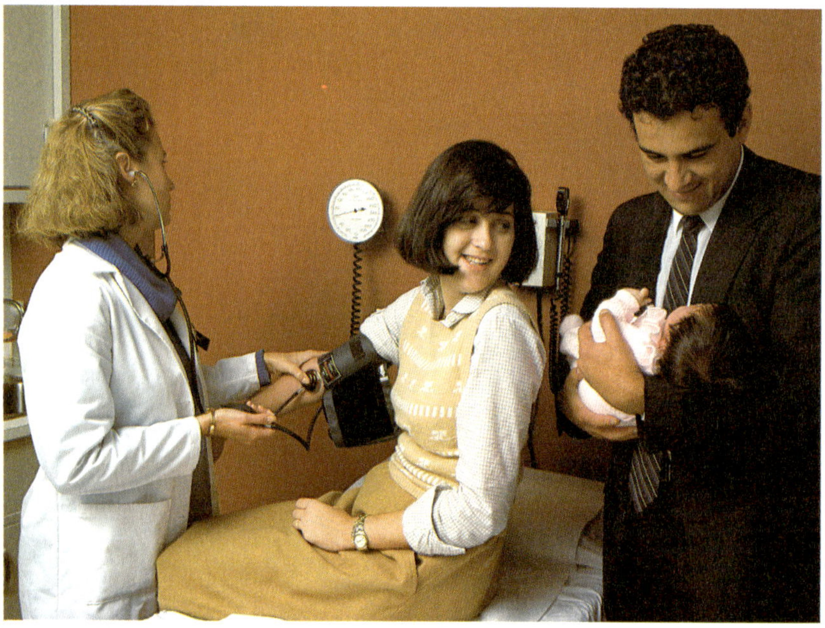

The postnatal check-up, usually about six weeks after delivery, provides an opportunity to discuss any worries you may have, and will reassure you that everything is back to normal after your pregnancy.

Each mother should have a physical examination about six weeks after delivery. It is important to have this examination, as it allows you to discuss any symptoms or worries you have, and allows the doctor to make sure that there are no long-term ill effects from the pregnancy and that your body has returned almost completely to normal.

The doctor is likely to inquire about your general health; whether you are breast-feeding; if your breasts are comfortable; whether the lochia has stopped; and if you have had a period.

Your blood pressure and weight will be checked and a urine specimen obtained. The doctor will usually examine your breasts to make sure that they are back to normal if you are bottle feeding or, if you are breast-feeding, that there are no problems. He will then examine your abdomen to make sure that the muscles are back to their usual strength and that all is well.

Next he will perform an internal examination. This tells the doctor whether or not the uterus is back to its pre-pregnant size and that the ovaries are normal. He will look at the lower end of the vagina to see that any stitches are healed and that the vagina is neither too tight nor too lax (*see* p. 123). Lastly he will probably look at the cervix by passing a metal speculum into the vagina.

After the examination you will have the opportunity to discuss your plans for contraception. Most doctors give family planning advice and will prescribe whatever is required during this consultation.

Intercourse

Often women prefer not to have intercourse until after their postnatal check-up, but this delay is not essential. Intercourse is perfectly safe once any stitches are soundly healed, the cervix is closed and the lochia has dwindled, perhaps about three weeks after delivery. If intercourse is uncomfortable, however, it is better to wait and try again a few days later.

It is not unusual for a woman to feel less desire for some time after her baby is born, but provided the mother's lack of desire is new there is every probability that she will feel better within a few months (*see* p. 123).

Contraception

Ovulation does not usually occur until four weeks after delivery and it is therefore most unlikely that a woman could become pregnant in this time. Contraceptive precautions should be used from four weeks onward, unless another pregnancy is desired immediately.

The contraceptive pill can be taken three to four weeks after delivery. Women who are breast-feeding should not take oral contraceptives. An intrauterine contraceptive device may be inserted during the puerperium but there is a slightly increased risk of it not staying in place and regular checks are therefore important. A diaphragm and cream can be used, but all diaphragms need refitting after a delivery as the vagina can change shape so that the original diaphragm no longer fits properly. Vaginal foam or condoms may be used as an alternative.

On the whole it is better to use a method of contraception which you have previously found satisfactory as the reliability of each method depends on its being used correctly and consistently. The contraceptive pill is over 99 per cent effective in theory; in practice, this falls to 90–99 per cent, depending on the user. For other methods the figures are: intrauterine device, 98 (95) per cent; condom, 97 (90) per cent; diaphragm plus spermicide 97 (83) per cent.

If you and your partner decide that your family will be complete with this baby, it is worthwhile considering whether one or other of you wishes to be sterilized. If you do, you should discuss it fully with your doctor before the baby is born.

If a husband has had a vasectomy operation during his wife's pregnancy, contraception is not needed after the birth, providing at least three months have elapsed to allow his sperm count to drop.

If a wife wishes to have an operation for tubal ligation, this can be performed either immediately after the delivery or two or three days after delivery if there is a question of whether the baby is doing well. If a cesarean is necessary at the time of birth, sterilization can be carried out at the same time.

Parents should remember, however, that all these procedures for sterilization are usually irreversible and it is therefore most important to wait until they are certain they wish it before taking this major step. Recent studies have indicated that some tubal ligations and vasectomies can be reversed by surgery. But, since this is by no means a procedure with a high level of success, no couple should approach sterilization as if it were reversible.

ALTERNATIVE METHODS OF CONTRACEPTION

Unless another pregnancy is desired immediately, contraceptive precautions should be taken within four weeks after delivery. You should discuss the alternatives with your doctor.

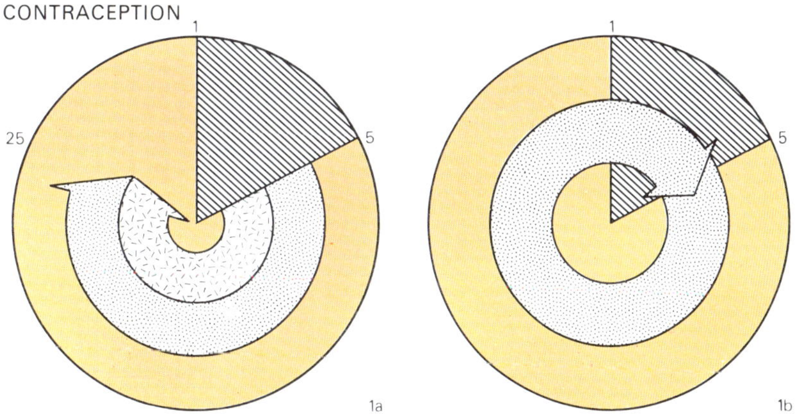

The Contraceptive Pill.
1a Combination Pill. One standard pill, combining estrogen and progesterone, is taken each day for 21 days, starting on the fifth day after menstruation and ending on the 25th day. There is a gap during which no hormone is taken, and menstruation occurs.

1b Continuous Pill. There are 28 pills, containing progesterone only, in each pack. One is taken every day, even during menstruation.

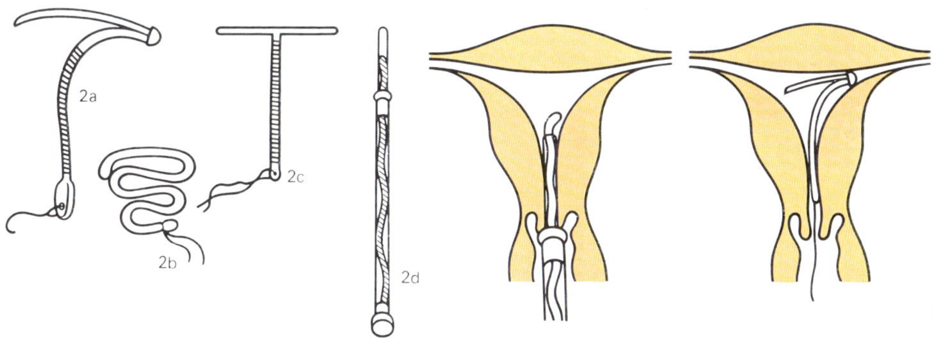

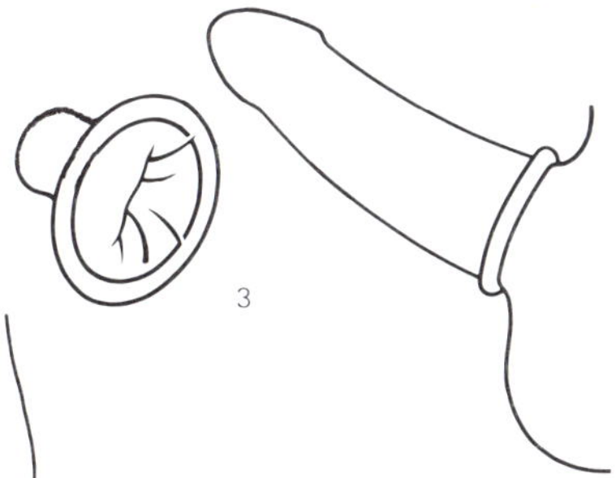

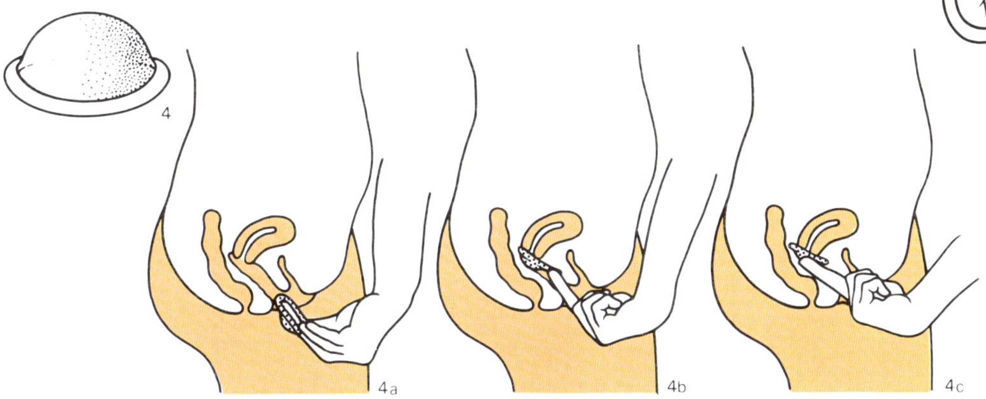

2. The intrauterine device (IUD).
2a Copper 7
2b Lippes loop
2c Copper T
2d Inserting the IUD, by means of a special plastic inserter, should be carried out by a doctor.

3. The condom, or prophylactic, is still very widely used as it can be used without any medical supervision.

4. The diaphragm. After an initial fitting by a doctor the diaphragm can easily be put in place by the woman herself.
4a Diaphragm being inserted into vagina.
4b Placing diaphragm over the cervix.
4c Checking the diaphragm.

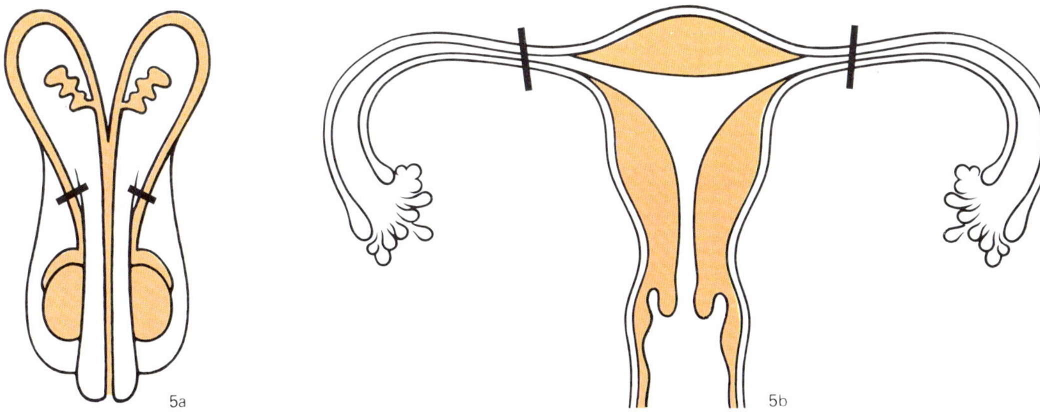

5a Vasectomy. Each vas deferens is cut and tied.
5b Female sterilization. The fallopian tubes are cut and tied.

Activity and postnatal exercises: convalescence

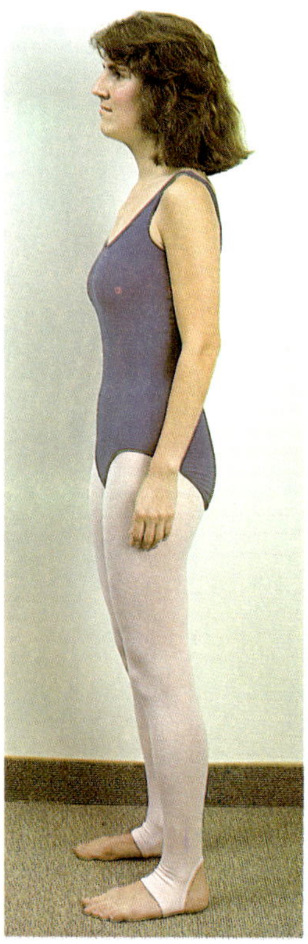

It will take a little time to become accustomed to your non-pregnant shape and weight. Correct posture adds to your appearance and may help to avoid back stress.

Convalescence always seems to suggest recovery after an illness. Pregnancy and labor, for fit women, are usually events to which the body adapts very satisfactorily: they are not illnesses and unless there has been some complication requiring a cesarean section, convalescence as such is not necessary.

What is most needed at first is adequate rest and sleep to allow the body to recover from the extremely "athletic" event of labor. Later, mothers will need to keep themselves fit to cope with the hard physical work of caring for a small baby and learning new skills.

Rest

Fatigue is extremely common in the puerperium. Most women having a first baby cannot imagine just how busy they will be after the birth. A mother goes into the hospital with a pile of books to read and returns home several days later without having opened one of them. She has either been too busy or too exhausted to read. Sleep and rest are essential for the body to readjust to the new state of not being pregnant. Inadequate sleep or rest can interfere with the milk supply of a woman who is breast-feeding, and without rest it is very difficult to cope with a demanding new baby and impossible to enjoy the experience.

Immediately after the birth a good sleep or rest is essential. During the next few days the mother requires more rest than normal, although the baby needs feeding or attention for a large part of the day and night.

In the hospital, if a mother is very tired, the baby can be taken to the nursery at night and given one feeding by a nurse to allow the mother more rest.

When the new mother goes home she can benefit by a relative or friend helping to care for the new baby and the household chores. Today, the husband often assumes many of these responsibilities.

Nights of broken sleep can be very tiring. Avoid sedatives if possible if you are breast-feeding. Drugs can be passed on to the baby in the milk, and any mother who is partly sedated by drugs may not be able to cope with her child properly. A better solution is the old fashioned remedy of a hot milky drink, possibly spiked with a little alcohol at night and a nap in the daytime when the baby sleeps, whether the housework is done or not. A relaxed mother is more important than a spotless house.

Posture

Maintain correct posture. Stand with the feet parallel and slightly apart. Straighten the knees and take the weight of the body on the front of the feet. Correct the pelvic tilt by drawing in the abdomen and tightening the seat muscles. Raise the ribs, lengthen the back of the neck and try to "grow taller". Breathe easily and walk in the corrected position.

Activity and exercise

Most women are able to get out of bed a few hours after delivery, to move their legs and perhaps go to the toilet. This "early ambulation", as it is called, is extremely important. It helps prevent leg vein thrombosis (*see* p. 123) and prevents the muscle wasting and weakness which used to occur when women were kept in bed for days after childbirth.

Exercise is necessary to get the muscles of the abdomen and of the pelvic floor back to normal as quickly as possible. After delivery the center of gravity moves backwards abruptly and, in addition, the new mother has to do a lot of bending, lifting and carrying of the baby. Postnatal exercises have been specially designed to help the body return to normal. They should be practiced conscientiously; often they are neglected once the mother returns home. Housework certainly provides a great deal of general exercise for a mother, but it does not lead to cardiovascular fitness or real strength. The pelvic tilt exercise helps to restore the tone of the abdominal and pelvic floor muscles as well as strengthening the back muscles. It is important that this exercise be done on a regular basis for a minimum of six weeks.

Examples of six useful postnatal exercises are given here. Practice them in bed for the first four or five days after delivery. Later try to set aside at least half an hour each day for a few exercises, followed by complete relaxation to rest the whole body. Remember to keep a good posture and take a short walk each day in the fresh air – this provides the added benefits of a break of routine and time simply to "get away from it all". Finally, do some deep breathing exercises.

1. Pelvic floor: If practiced carefully and frequently throughout the day, this exercise will help tone up the stretched muscles of the pelvic floor.

Lie on your back and contract the muscles of the pelvic floor by drawing in the muscles which close the bowels and the vagina. This movement can be reinforced by tightening up the buttock muscles and pressing the knees together. Tighten the muscles for a count of five, then relax slowly. This exercise may also be done standing up.

2. Pelvic tilt: This exercise strengthens the lower back muscles.

Lie on your back with knees slightly bent and the soles of your feet on the floor. Tighten the buttock muscles and at the same time firmly smooth out the abdomen, drawing in the muscles of the lower abdominal wall, and pressing the hollow of the back on to the floor. Then relax both groups of muscles, allowing the back to hollow slightly.

3. Head raising: Lie on your back with both knees bent, then draw in your chin and raise your head off the floor.

4. Feet and legs: Practice this exercise lying on the floor with legs out straight.

Bend and stretch the ankles fully by pointing the foot down then up. Bend and stretch the toes. Circle the feet inward. Then tighten the muscles above the knees by pressing the backs of the knees down on to the floor.

5. Deep breathing: Place the hands lightly on the lower ribs, gently compress the chest and breathe out slowly, emptying the lungs as completely as possible. Then take a deep breath in through the nose, expanding the lower part of the lungs by pushing the ribs out against the hands.

Clothing

It is much easier if all clothes worn by the mother immediately after delivery are easily washable. Several nightgowns are needed in the hospital, and they are much more comfortable if made of cotton or a cotton mixture rather than nylon. It is a great help if a friend or relative launders them regularly during your stay as it is almost inevitable that the occasional leakage of milk or, in the early days, a little lochia, will stain them. If a mother has decided to breast-feed, the nightgowns should open down the front. The same thing applies to clothing later on: it is impossible to breast-feed wearing a dress which zips up at the back!

Many women find that clothes which they wore before pregnancy are too tight and it is often better to continue to wear fairly loose clothes at least for a short time after the birth. Although it's good for morale to be able to go out and buy new clothes at this stage, it is better to wait until your shape has returned to normal. This generally requires a well structured exercise program. But remember it also requires time!

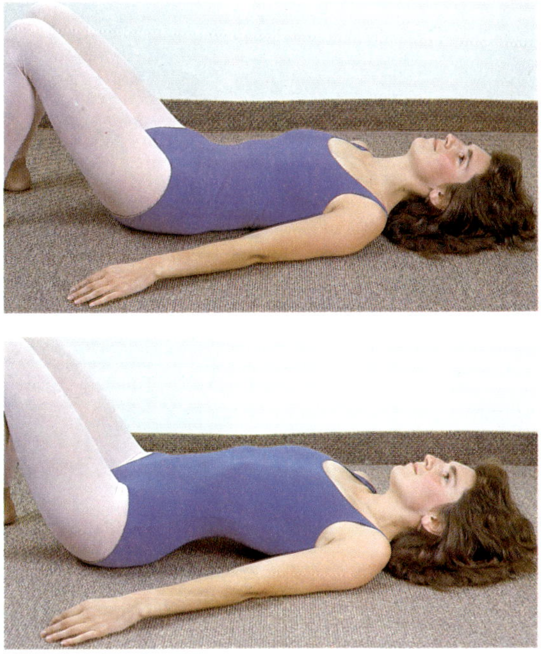

2. Pelvic tilt

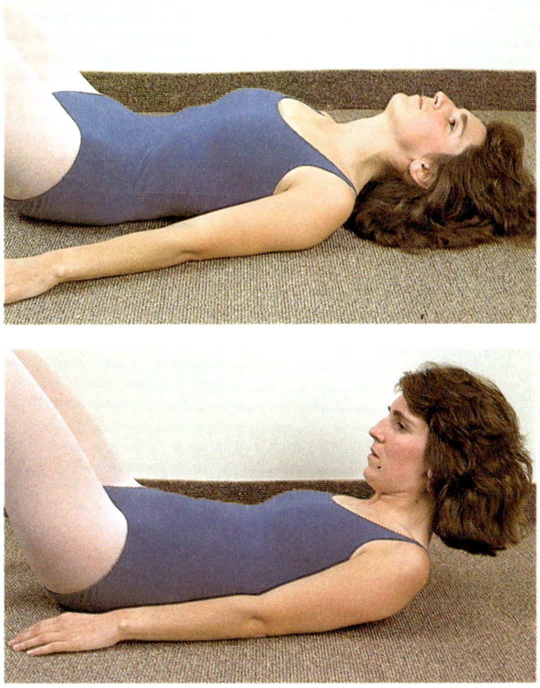

3. Head raising

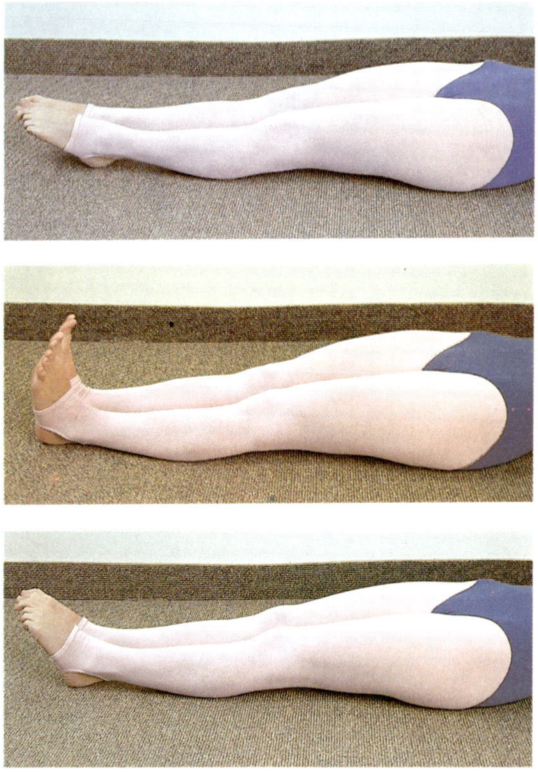

4. Feet and legs

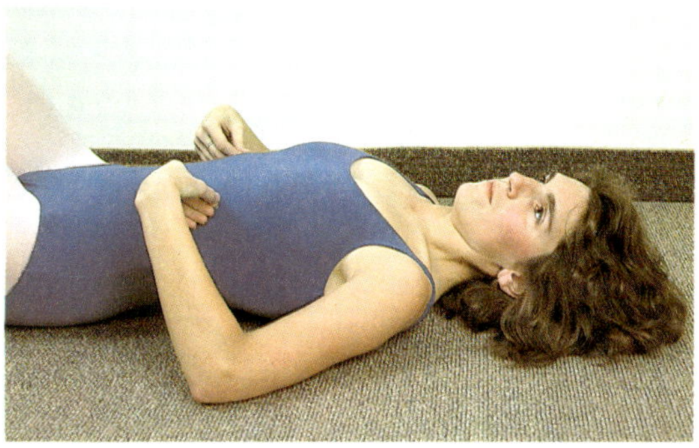

5. Deep breathing

1. Lie on your back, one leg bent, the other straight. Keep the bent leg still. Shorten straight leg, by drawing up from hip and waist. Then lengthen it by stretching down. Repeat with other leg.

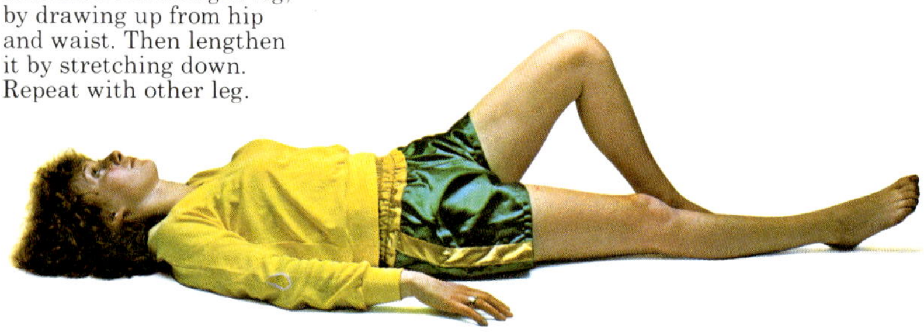

Exercise

As well as postnatal exercises, you may want to practice certain exercises which will encourage your body to return to its normal pre-pregnant shape. Strenuous exercises should not, however, be attempted for at least six weeks after you have given birth.

Four exercises are suggested here, each of which is aimed at a particular part of the body. The first is directed at the waistline, the second at both waist and hips, and the third is designed to tone up the abdominal muscles.

2a Lie on your back, knees bent, arms outstretched sideways. Keep feet and shoulders still, and knees together.

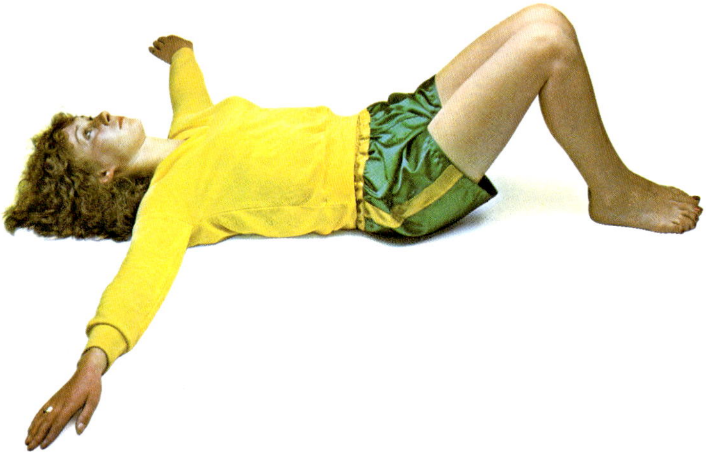

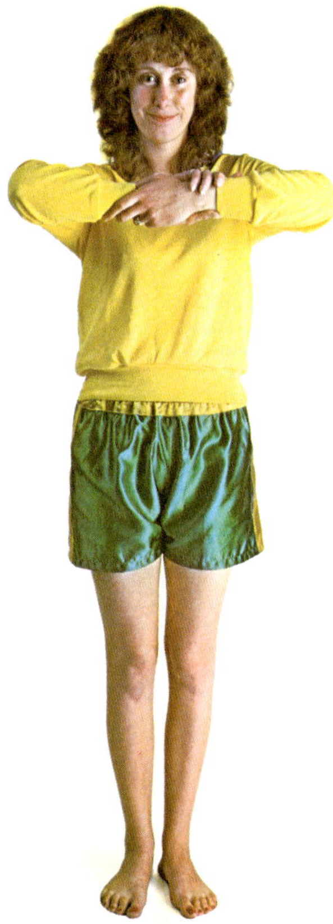

2b Twisting from the waist, swing both knees over to touch the floor on right, while left hip turns toward ceiling. Then swing knees over to touch on the left, while right hip turns toward ceiling. Repeat.

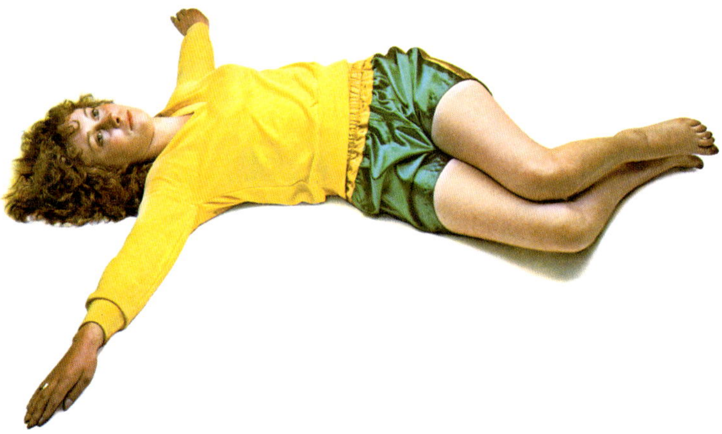

4. Stand erect. Grasp wrists with the opposite hands. Lift both arms until elbows are at shoulder level, and keep them there. Grip hard, and try to push the bones of your wrists toward you elbows. Relax. Repeat.

3. Lie on back, knees bent, feet flat. Tighten abdominal muscles and pull in. Press waist downward hard to round spine. Keeping waist in contact with the floor, lift hips off it slightly by contracting buttocks. Repeat.

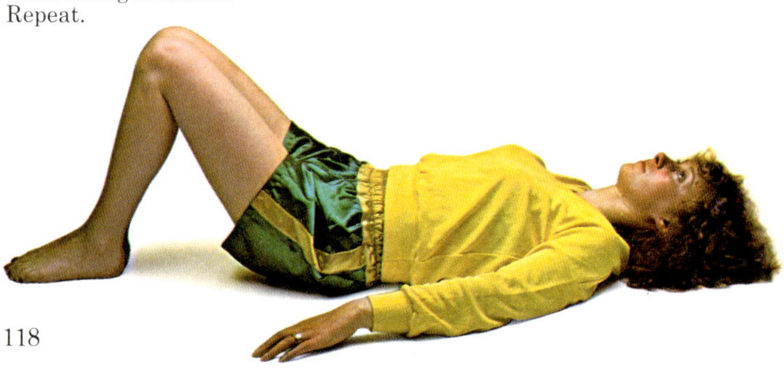

The last will help to firm up the bust, and is important for both breast- and bottle-feeding mothers. Be sensible when practicing these exercises: a few minutes each day, followed by a period of relaxation is more effective than one exhausting session once a week. To strengthen any muscle it is necessary to contract that muscle against resistance. The lifting of free weights or use of a rowing machine will help strengthen your muscles.

Weight and diet

Most women will weigh more right after their babies are born than they did before pregnancy. Sometimes this extra weight is as much as 15 lb (6.82 kilograms) but usually it is much less. A few women never lose this excess weight, and find themselves a little fatter and heavier after each pregnancy. It is important to avoid this because obesity is associated with many of the diseases of later life and you will regret the loss of your figure.

At delivery the weight of the baby, the amniotic fluid and the placenta is lost – a total of between 7 lb (3 kilograms) and 12 lb (5.4 kilograms). In the following two or three days excess fluid is lost from the tissues and circulation, accounting for between approximately 2 lb to 3 lb (1 kilogram and 1.36 kilograms).

In the next four to six weeks the weight of the uterus is reduced from about 2 lb (1 kilogram) to 2 oz (50 grams or 60 grams). Some of the breakdown products (amino acids) produced by this process will be retained by the body and used by it.

The rest of the weight gained in pregnancy is accounted for by fat. In mothers who are breast-feeding much of this fat and the amino acids are used in the production of milk. Judicious food intake and a regular exercise routine should control your weight adequately. Aerobic exercises not only lead to cardiovascular fitness and strength, they appear to promote weight loss as well. After the early post-partum period, try brisk walking, running or riding a stationary bicycle. Aerobic dancing, swimming and cross-country skiing are very effective types of aerobic exercise.

DESIRABLE WEIGHT IN POUNDS AND KILOGRAMS*

HEIGHT (IN SHOES)	SMALL FRAME	MEDIUM FRAME	LARGE FRAME
4′ 10″ 147.3 cm	92– 98 lb 41.7–44.5 kg	96–107 lb 43.5–48.5 kg	104–119 lb 47.2–54.0 kg
4′ 11″ 149.9 cm	94–101 lb 42.6–45.8 kg	98–110 lb 44.5–49.9 kg	106–122 lb 48.1–55.3 kg
5′ 0″ 152.4 cm	96–104 lb 43.5–47.2 kg	101–113 lb 45.8–51.3 kg	109–125 lb 49.4–56.7 kg
5′ 1″ 154.9 cm	99–107 lb 44.9–48.5 kg	104–116 lb 47.2–52.6 kg	112–128 lb 50.8–58.1 kg
5′ 2″ 157.5 cm	102–110 lb 46.3–49.9 kg	107–119 lb 48.5–54.0 kg	115–131 lb 52.2–59.4 kg
5′ 3″ 160.0 cm	105–113 lb 47.6–51.3 kg	110–122 lb 49.9–55.3 kg	118–134 lb 53.5–60.8 kg
5′ 4″ 162.6 cm	108–116 lb 49.0–52.6 kg	113–126 lb 51.3–57.2 kg	121–138 lb 54.9–62.6 kg
5′ 5″ 165.1 cm	111–119 lb 50.3–54.0 kg	116–130 lb 49.0–59.0 kg	124–142 lb 56.7–64.4 kg
5′ 6″ 167.6 cm	114–123 lb 51.7–55.8 kg	120–135 lb 54.4–61.2 kg	129–146 lb 58.5–66.2 kg
5′ 7″ 170.2 cm	118–127 lb 53.5–57.6 kg	124–139 lb 56.2–63.0 kg	133–150 lb 60.3–68.0 kg
5′ 8″ 172.7 cm	122–131 lb 55.3–59.4 kg	128–143 lb 58.1–64.9 kg	137–154 lb 62.1–69.9 kg
5′ 9″ 175.3 cm	126–135 lb 57.2–61.2 kg	132–147 lb 59.9–66.7 kg	141–158 lb 64.0–71.7 kg
5′ 10″ 177.8 cm	130–140 lb 59.0–63.5 kg	136–151 lb 61.7–68.5 kg	145–163 lb 65.8–73.9 kg
5′ 11″ 180.3 cm	134–144 lb 60.8–65.3 kg	140–155 lb 63.5–70.3 kg	149–168 lb 67.6–76.2 kg
6′ 0″ 182.9 cm	138–148 lb 62.6–67.1 kg	144–159 lb 65.3–72.1 kg	153–173 lb 69.4–78.5 kg

*(In indoor clothing), age 25 and over.
Note: For women between 18 and 25, subtract 1 pound for each year under 25.

Diet

From this it can be seen that most women will lose weight slowly in the days or weeks following delivery. Appetite is usually a good guide to the body's needs; it is therefore rarely necessary either to diet or to count calories. Stand on the scales once a week to make sure there is no weight gain, or excessive loss. If necessary adjust your diet accordingly. There is no need "to eat for two", even if you are breast-feeding. This leads to obesity.

There is an ideal weight for everyone; the weight at which they are healthiest. It depends on height, age and build. Every woman should try to regain and keep her ideal weight after her baby is born. This may take some weeks or even months.

Women who are normally overweight because their appetite is greater than their food requirement, and women who are grossly overweight after delivery, particularly if they are not breast-feeding, need to think about how much they should eat. So should women who are underweight. A woman who is breast-feeding needs about 2,000 to 2,500 calories a day as against 1,500 to 2,000 calories for women who are not breast-feeding.

Crash diets after a baby is born should be avoided. A new mother has so much extra to do that she will be much more energetic if she loses only ½ lb-1 lb (225 grams–450 grams) a week and takes several weeks to return to her correct weight. As in pregnancy what is eaten is more important than how much. (General advice on the various types of food that make up a balanced diet is given in chapter 2.)

Never miss breakfast even if you only eat cereal and fruit. It is not necessary to spend a lot of time cooking so long as a proper balanced diet is maintained. Ready-to-serve desserts such as yogurt, fresh fruit, cheese or ice-cream are very nourishing. A woman who is breast-feeding may find she needs a cracker or cookie between meals.

Provided a variety of foods are eaten, including dairy produce, meat or fish, vegetables and fruit, it is not necessary to take any extra vitamins, although women who are found to be anemic will have iron pills prescribed by their doctor. A strict vegetarian should also check with her doctor to make sure that her diet is adequate. If the baby is thought to require extra vitamins these should be given directly to him or her.

Mothers who are breast-feeding are sometimes advised to drink a pint of milk a day. This is fine if you like milk and are not overweight. If you dislike milk, and are on a normal mixed diet, there is no need to drink it as the body can easily convert the food you eat into milk. If you are overweight remember that a pint of milk contains 400 calories.

Often a nursing mother finds that some items of her diet upsets her baby and gives him or her diarrhea. This item may be anything from onions to red wine. If this happens, stop eating the offending items until breast-feeding is over.

Many mothers who breast-feed find they become extremely thirsty, especially during a feeding, so extra drinks of any sort should be taken at frequent intervals during the day. Alcohol, however, can pass to the baby in the milk and large amounts should be avoided.

Check your weight once a week to make sure there is no gain or excessive loss. If necessary, adjust your diet accordingly.

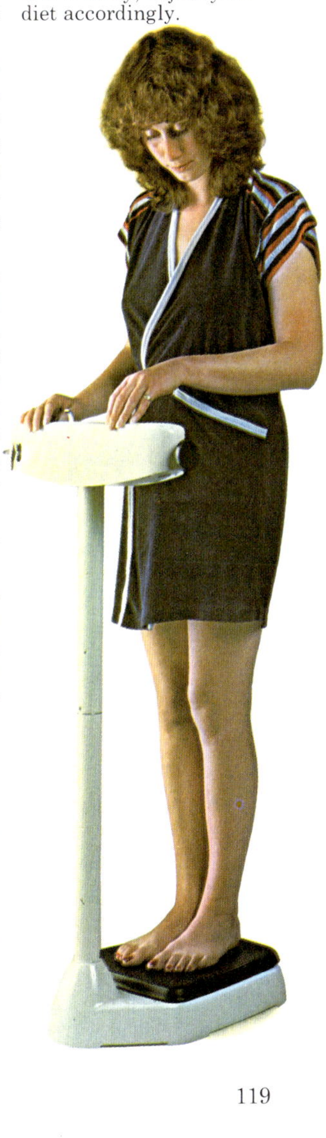

Complications of the puerperium

Complications of the puerperium occur at a time when a new mother has her whole time taken up getting to know and care for her new baby, and she really needs to be in the peak of health. A mother's health at this time is extremely important and she should never ignore her own symptoms because she is "too busy" with the new baby.

Although most complications of the puerperium are not dangerous, a few of them are, and others can lead to prolonged ill health if neglected. Even minor complications cause discomfort and worry, and slow a mother's return to normal activities, and some complications may even result in a delay to her return home from the hospital.

Most problems in the puerperium are easily treated provided that the doctor's advice is followed carefully. This section on puerperal complaints is in alphabetical order. It should not be read straight through but used for reference.

A few extremely common "complaints" of the puerperium, such as painful episiotomy and backache, have been covered in the preceding section on the normal puerperium. Other general complaints are covered in this section.

ANEMIA

Most hospitals check every mother's hemoglobin level a few days after delivery. If the hemoglobin level is too low then anemia is present. Anemia in the puerperium is usually due either to a low hemoglobin level before delivery or to a greater than normal blood loss at delivery. Anemia during pregnancy is best avoided or treated before labor (*see* chapter 4). Excessive blood loss occasionally occurs when the placenta is delivered but in most mothers it can be prevented by the injection of ergotrate after delivery of the baby (*see* p. 105). This injection makes the uterus contract well and also prevents excessive bleeding.

If puerperal anemia is present it can make a mother feel more tired than normal and can also predispose her to infection or to the slow healing of an episiotomy. The anemia is usually treated by taking a further supply of the antenatal iron pills for about a month. In cases of severe anemia an intravenous iron drip may be required (*see* chapter 4).

ANKLES, SWOLLEN *see* Swollen ankles
ANXIETY *see* Postpartum depression

BACKACHE

This is such a common problem of the puerperium that advice on how to avoid it has been given in the section on the normal puerperium under "exercise". Persistent backache may occur for several weeks after delivery, especially in women who have had previous back complaints. There are several methods of easing it. First, posture is important. Avoid bending forward; bend at the knees when picking up the baby; change him at table height instead of bending down. Second, sleep on a hard mattress, or put a bedboard under a softer one. Third, spend a little time night and morning lying on your front. Fourth, exercise the back. Exercises to strengthen the back muscles can be obtained from your doctor or a physiotherapist.

BLEEDING

The normal amount of blood which is lost in the lochia is very variable, but it is usually a bit heavier than a period for the first two or three days, and small clots may be passed. These are often associated with after pains. If, however, large clots are passed, or if the pad is soaked within a few minutes, then this should be reported to your doctor. Sometimes the lochia is normal for a few days and there is then a sudden loss of a variable amount of fresh, bright red blood with clots. This can occur up to a month after delivery. Such blood loss is called **heavy lochia** if mild, and **secondary postpartum hemorrhage**, if severe. The secondary distinguishes this bleeding from primary postpartum hemorrhage which occurs immediately after delivery and is a complication of the third stage of labor.

There are two main causes of this bleeding. First, there may be a small piece of membrane or placenta stuck inside the uterus which didn't come out in the normal manner at delivery; or, second, there may be some infection inside the uterus. Sometimes there is both a retained piece of placenta and some infection.

If the hospital has an ultrasound machine, it is possible to see whether the uterus is empty or not by doing an ultrasound scan. If a piece of retained placenta is seen or if the bleeding is very heavy then it is necessary to perform an evacuation of the uterus (*see* chapter 4). This is done using a general anesthetic and is a very simple procedure. Afterward the lochia usually returns to normal.

If heavy lochia is present but is not severe, and if it is thought that there is nothing substantial inside the uterus, then ergotrate pills are sometimes prescribed. These pills make the uterus contract firmly and this will expel any blood clot from inside and help prevent further bleeding. If the ergotrate pills fail to reduce the heavy lochia or bleeding then evacuation of the uterus may be necessary.

If it is thought that any infection is present either because a woman has a temperature or because the lochia smells infected, then a vaginal swab is cultured in the laboratory to determine the cause of the infection and the most suitable antibiotic is prescribed.

BREAST ABSCESS

If a breast infection is not treated promptly or if it does not respond to antibiotics an abscess can form. This is an uncommon problem which does not usually occur earlier than 10 to 14 days after delivery.

Once an abscess forms, pus is present deep in the breast tissue. The woman feels very ill and may have a high temperature. The breast is usually very tender, but if a lot of antibiotics have been given this tenderness may not be very marked. The treatment in this condition is to have the abscess drained, which involves going into the hospital and having a short general anesthetic. An incision is then made over the abscess to let out the pus. Usually a tiny tube is left in the breast for two or three days to allow complete drainage of all infected matter.

After the operation the wound needs to be dressed frequently until it is healed, so this will probably necessitate several visits to the doctor's office until healing is complete. After an abscess has formed, most people would recommend a change to bottle feeding, but breast-feeding can be continued from the normal breast if the mother is determined to do so as long as the milk from the infected breast is removed with a hand pump and discarded.

BREAST ENGORGEMENT

A common problem in the puerperium is breast engorgement. It usually occurs on the third or fourth day. The breasts become swollen, tender and hot and they feel hard. The condition is caused by a sudden increase in the blood supply to the breasts and an increase in the milk supply. A hungry baby may be able to take most of the milk, but sometimes the breasts are so firm and swollen that he may not be able to suck well. In this situation it is best to squeeze the areola gently between two fingers and express a little milk from the breasts first; then it will be easier for the baby to take hold of the breast well.

If there is a lot of milk left in the breasts after giving a feeding and they are still hard, then they should be emptied either by hand or by a breast pump. Your doctor will give instructions on how this is done. The discomfort of the engorged breasts may be temporarily relieved by covering them with a damp cloth wrung out in cold water or one containing crushed ice, which will cool them. After one or two days the problem of engorgement usually gets better as the blood supply and milk supply adjust to the baby's requirements; the breasts are then much more comfortable between feedings.

Women who are bottle feeding should not empty their breasts as this encourages more milk to form.

BREAST INFECTION (MASTITIS)

Breast infection is uncommon provided care is taken to keep the breasts clean and free from damage, such as cracked nipples, and so long as the breasts are emptied properly at each feeding. If infection does occur the affected breast becomes painful and hot and an area of inflammation can be seen on it. This commonly takes the form of a wedge shaped area with the point of the wedge on the nipple. What has happened is that the milk in one breast lobule is infected and is not draining properly due to blockage of the duct.

A woman with mastitis usually also has a temperature and feels sick. Laboratory tests can be done on the infected milk to determine the cause of the infection. Antibiotic treatment must be given as soon as possible and continued for five days or until all signs of infection have disappeared.

The pain can be partly relieved by holding a wet cloth containing crushed ice, over the breast to cool it. The baby can be put to the healthy breast, but while the other breast is acutely infected, emptying it manually may be recommended by your doctor. The baby can nurse on the affected breast, with no ill effects, particularly after antibiotics are started or after the infection begins to improve.

BRUISED NIPPLES

Bruising around the nipples can occur if the baby is allowed to suck on the nipple instead of taking the areola into his mouth (*see* chapter 10). This bruising makes the nipples feel tender, but it will disappear provided care is taken to see that the baby takes the breast properly and also that on removing the nipple from the baby's mouth he doesn't pull on it. Slip your finger inside the baby's mouth before removing him in order to break the vacuum.

CONSTIPATION

Constipation is quite common in the puerperium when it is usually caused by reduced general activity in the few days following childbirth. It is best treated by a high fiber diet which contains foods such as bran cereal, wholegrain bread and vegetables. Laxatives are rarely necessary, and women who are breast-feeding should not take them as they can give the baby diarrhea. If the constipation does not respond to dietary measures it can be treated with glycerine suppositories. Women who are bottle feeding can take a mild laxative such as a senna preparation if necessary.

CRACKED NIPPLES

A tiny crack in the nipple may occur in the early days of breast-feeding. These cracks are painful especially when the baby starts to suck on the breast. The problem is best prevented by applying a cream such as Mammol to the nipples between feedings for a few days to heal them. The cream must be washed off before the next feed. Care must also be taken to make sure the baby takes the areola into his mouth – not just the nipple – when feeding (*see* chapter 10); the baby must not be allowed to pull on the nipple when taking him off the breast afterward.

Once a crack has formed, it is important to prevent it becoming infected by regular careful washing of the breasts with soap and water. The crack will heal if a cream is used between feedings. If feeding is too painful on the cracked side, then the breast should be temporarily emptied manually, or by a breast pump, and the milk given to the baby in a bottle until the crack is healed.

DROP FOOT

Drop foot is a very rare complaint that can follow labor. It is due to temporary weakness of the muscles on the outside of the leg which pull the foot upward. Because of the weakness of these muscles the foot cannot be held in the normal position at right angles to the leg and so it tends to flop downward.

The muscle weakness occurs because of damage to its nerve supply. The nerves which control these muscles pass through the pelvis and they can occasionally be damaged either by pressure of the baby's head during labor or by pressure from forceps where these are used during delivery. This damage is so rare that it probably only occurs in women whose nerves are particularly vulnerable to pressure from inside the pelvis.

The treatment given is to support the foot in a splint so that it cannot fall below a right angle. Then physiotherapy is necessary to strengthen the muscles while the nerves recover. At first walking is difficult and it may be necessary to use crutches or a walking aid for a few days, and then progress to a cane until muscle strength returns. Recovery is usually complete but it may take a few weeks.

EMOTIONAL CHANGES

Feeling depressed shortly after delivery is so common that it can hardly be termed a complication of the puerperium, and has many names, such as "the blues". A mother often feels on top of the world for the first few days after the birth, then one morning becomes very upset over things which she would normally accept without worry. This is a most trying time for a new mother but it usually lasts only a few hours or a day or two. The best treatment is the sympathetic ear of the doctor and family, and the knowledge that it will all blow over soon. It is really not at all surprising that this should happen. Pregnancy and giving birth are both very powerful experiences. The early puerperium is a physically tiring time and, in addition, there has been an abrupt alteration in the body chemistry, hormone levels, fluid balance and other functions. Any one of these experiences can be emotionally upsetting, particularly when one considers how the much slighter changes in chemical balance during the normal monthly cycle can cause many women to become tense, moody or easily upset.

The point to remember about "the blues" is that they are short-lived and easily accounted for. If depression persists, or if it interferes with a woman caring for her baby, it is most important to have medical advice as soon as possible, as she could be suffering from postpartum depression (*see* p. 122) which will require treatment by a doctor.

EPISIOTOMY BREAKDOWN

Occasionally an episiotomy or tear, which has been stitched up after delivery does not heal immediately and may be very painful. This is more likely to happen if there has been a lot of bruising during a difficult delivery, or if the episiotomy becomes infected. The symptoms of this condition are that the area around the stitches is more painful than usual and on inspection the area looks swollen and inflamed. Sometimes the catgut stitches dissolve before the cut has healed and a gap in the skin can be seen. Sometimes the doctor decides to cut the stitches before healing has taken place in order to allow infection to escape as a discharge, and this will also leave a gap in the skin.

Although all of this sounds terrible, it is surprising how quickly and efficiently the area heals up on its own as soon as the inflammation settles down. The best treatment is to take regular baths twice a day to keep the area clean, and to change sanitary pads frequently. Some doctors also recommend the application of antiseptic solutions to the area but this is not essential. Healing usually occurs without any further stitches and within ten days to two weeks.

During this time, a mother can be up and looking after her baby. For a few days it is helpful to sit on a pillow or rubber ring, and a mild painkiller can be taken if the area is very sore, but the discomfort will usually begin to improve as soon as the inflammation settles down.

Occasionally a small area of the episiotomy does not heal completely for some weeks, and remains uncomfortable. If this should happen then you should visit your doctor for treatment.

HEMORRHOIDS

Hemorrhoids are common in pregnancy and in the puerperium and are discussed on p. 63.

HYPERTENSION

Women who normally suffer from essential hypertension (high blood pressure) will usually find that their blood pressure rises even more during pregnancy. During the puerperium this will slowly return to their normal pre-pregnancy level.

Women who suffer from **pre-eclamptic toxemia** during pregnancy (*see* chapter 4), however, may have elevated blood pressure for a few days after delivery, but their blood pressure usually falls to normal levels within two weeks. In a few women who have had severe pre-eclampsia during pregnancy their blood pressure may take up to three months in order to return to normal levels.

On very rare occasions a woman who has normal blood pressure during pregnancy develops raised blood pressure within a short time of delivery together with protein in her urine and edema. These are the signs of postpartum pre-eclampsia. If the blood pressure rises only slightly then a sedative is usually prescribed. Occasionally the blood pressure rises dramatically and in these cases rest and further treatment are necessary. Medication will be prescribed to lower the blood pressure, to reduce the fluid in the body (through urination), and to sedate the mother (*see* chapter 4). Postpartum pre-eclampsia usually improves within 48 hours, but the blood pressure may remain slightly raised for a period of time up to three months.

INCONTINENCE
Retention of urine or leakage of urine can occur briefly soon after delivery, especially after an epidural, because the nerves which control the bladder are temporarily out of action. This problem corrects itself as soon as the epidural wears off.

A few women suffer from a more prolonged problem of bladder control called stress incontinence. They find that they lose a few drops of urine whenever they strain, cough or make a sudden physical effort. This is due to a weakness of the mechanism which closes the neck of the bladder. In many cases this weakness starts during pregnancy and before delivery (*see* chapter 4), and some women will have already experienced the same problem after a previous pregnancy. If you find this symptom is present it should be reported to your doctor as soon as possible so that he can begin treatment.

In all these cases the first priority is to strengthen the pelvic floor muscles which support the bladder neck by doing pelvic floor exercises repeatedly each day for several weeks (*see* p. 116). These exercises can be taught to you by your doctor if he believes they are appropriate to your particular case.

Occasionally the symptom is not cured by physiotherapy and then an operation will be needed to tighten the neck of the bladder. This is done by putting some stitches around it.

A more severe form of incontinence following childbirth, in which leakage occurs all the time, day and night, is extremely rare in this country but relatively common in parts of the world where maternity care is inadequate. In these cases, incontinence is usually associated with a lengthy labor and a difficult delivery. Prolonged pressure of the baby's head on the bladder wall, which lies in front of the vagina, or damage to this area during delivery, can produce an abnormal opening between the bladder and vagina which causes this distressing disorder. The initial treatment is to leave a catheter attached to a bag to collect the urine in the bladder for several days. This stops the leakage and often enables the damaged area of the bladder to heal up completely without further treatment. If the bladder does not heal then an operation will be necessary to repair both the bladder and the vagina.

INVERTED NIPPLES *see*
Retracted nipples

INVERTED UTERUS
A very rare complication of the third stage of labor, discussed on p. 105.

LOCHIA *see* Bleeding
MASTITIS *see* Breast infection
NERVOUS BREAKDOWN *see*
Postpartum depression
NIPPLES, BRUISED *see* Bruised nipples
NIPPLES, CRACKED *see* Cracked nipples
PAINFUL INTERCOURSE *see*
Sexual problems

"PILES" *see* Hemorrhoids

POSTPARTUM DEPRESSION
This problem sometimes occurs in women who have previously had a nervous breakdown or suffered acute depression following an earlier stressful situation in their life. It may, however, also occur in women who have not had any kind of nervous problems before.

Postpartum depression must be distinguished from a common event called "the blues" which has been described above in the section on **emotional changes** (p. 121). With "the blues", depression and tearfulness may last a few hours or a day or two, but in postpartum depression the problem lasts much longer and the symptoms are more severe.

Several different symptoms may indicate that the woman is threatened with a nervous breakdown at this time. Sometimes the woman herself realizes that something is very wrong; sometimes it is her husband or family or the doctor who can see the problem but the woman herself cannot. The symptoms include insomnia, which can result in almost no sleep at all, and very severe anxiety. The woman may be very afraid for no reason, or she may be afraid that she cannot manage her baby or that she may hurt her baby. Lastly she may suffer from acute depression, which persists for several days and results in her being unable to look after her baby or herself, and may even lead to thoughts of suicide. All these things a woman may notice herself. In other cases someone else notices that the new mother is behaving bizarrely, or perhaps that she is saying or doing things which appear unrelated to what is going on around her.

All these symptoms are very serious and medical advice should be obtained as a matter of urgency. If treatment is given promptly recovery is usually quicker. Treatment usually involves giving medication either as pills or in the form of injections. These can have a dramatic effect and stop the symptoms in a matter of hours. Further treatment with drugs and visits to either a psychiatrist or a psychiatric social worker are sometimes necessary for a few weeks. Many women recover quickly and are well able to manage their new role as mother very soon afterward.

In a few women the symptoms do not respond quickly to treatment and they may be recommended to be admitted as a patient to a hospital for appropriate care. Today, with effective antidepression medication and psychotherapy recovery is usually rapid.

POSTPARTUM HEMORRHAGE *see*
Bleeding
POSTPARTUM PRE-ECLAMPSIA *see*
Hypertension

PRIMARY POSTPARTUM hemorrhage
Excessive bleeding following the third stage of labor, due to various causes. It is discussed on p. 105.

PUERPERAL FEVER
Before antibiotics were discovered puerperal fever – a high temperature after delivery – was a dreaded and dangerous complication of childbirth and was extremely serious. Today, a temperature after delivery is no longer either dreaded or dangerous, but it is still taken seriously, and medical advice should always be sought. There are a number of reasons why a mother may have a fever at this time. The most common is urinary infection or uterine infection, but a high temperature can also be caused by breast engorgement, or breast infection, or by any infection such as flu or a sore throat.

A simple medical check-up will usually show the cause of the fever. In addition the doctor may take a specimen of urine and a vaginal swab and send them to the laboratory for analysis. If an infection is found and the woman is still in the hospital, she may be transferred with her baby to an isolation room. In this way other patients are protected. What treatment she will be given depends on the cause of the fever. Antibiotics are given for infection in the bladder, vagina or breast, and laboratory tests usually indicate which particular antibiotic is likely to be most effective.

A slightly elevated temperature in the puerperium is more common in women who have had a cesarean delivery or ruptured membranes for 24 hours or longer. And in these women their temperature often returns to normal within one or two days. Some of these patients will require antibiotic treatment, depending on the severity of the fever.

PULMONARY EMBOLISM *see*
Thrombosis
RAISED BLOOD PRESSURE *see*
Hypertension

RETAINED PLACENTA

A complication of the third stage of labor, when delivery of the placenta is delayed. It is discussed on p. 105.

RETENTION OF URINE

Soon after delivery it may be impossible for a woman to empty her bladder. This is usually due to swelling or bruising around the urethra (the opening of the bladder). The problem may last a few hours or a few days. Immediately after the birth the nurse or doctor will examine the bladder in the lower part of the abdomen. If she finds that it is very full, and there is difficulty passing water, she will pass a catheter into the bladder through the urethra and empty it. This is not a difficult procedure. If the bladder is not full, then the woman can wait a few hours and will often be able to pass urine successfully.

Occasionally a woman finds that she cannot pass urine for several days after delivery or that she passes only a small amount and her bladder remains nearly full. In these circumstances the catheter is left inside her bladder and attached to a bag to collect urine or it is inserted every few hours until the bladder begins to work normally again. Bladder function always returns although occasionally it takes a few days. Antibiotics may be given to prevent infection of the urine if repeated use of a catheter is necessary. Retention of urine is slightly more common following an epidural but in these cases it only lasts a few hours.

RETRACTED OR INVERTED NIPPLES

This has been discussed in chapter 3 under antenatal care of the breasts. Retracted nipples can sometimes be encouraged to protrude by gentle pressure with finger and thumb on the areola to push them out. This can be done during pregnancy. After delivery the baby will not be able to suck properly if the nipples are still retracted. Sucking is made possible and the nipples encouraged to come out by using nipple shields with an artificial nipple attached to cover the breasts during feeding. The milk is sucked from the breasts through the artificial nipple. Sometimes trying to feed the baby with retracted nipples is a real problem, then it is better to bottle feed for the sake of both mother and baby.

SEXUAL PROBLEMS

A number of factors can contribute to a "loss of libido" on the part of the new mother. Sometimes it would seem that her sexual desires are submerged by her new maternal instincts. Other women find that they are simply very tired from looking after a demanding tiny baby. Some are afraid that they will become pregnant again, and yet others may be afraid that intercourse will damage their stitched vagina.

Adequate rest and help with the baby, a postnatal check-up of the internal organs and vagina, and a discussion with the gynecologist to remove worries about another pregnancy may be all that is necessary for a cure.

Occasionally, however, the new mother's lack of desire persists and can become a source of tension between her partner and herself. It is important to keep the lines of communication open and, where necessary, to seek the advice and help of a sympathetic doctor or marriage guidance counselor. Sometimes there is a physical reason for dissatisfaction or discomfort in intercourse which in itself can lead to a loss of libido.

Vagina, too tight or too lax

A few women find that when their vagina has healed up after being stitched the opening has contracted and seems to be smaller than before they became pregnant. As a result intercourse is difficult or impossible. There are two main causes of this condition. First, many women are concerned either that the stitched vagina may be damaged by intercourse or that they may become pregnant again. As a result they unconsciously contract all the vaginal muscles to protect themselves. The second cause is that the skin itself really has healed up too tightly.

If a woman finds that intercourse is painful or very difficult then she should go to her doctor and mention the problem at her postnatal check-up. The doctor will be able to see easily whether the stitches are soundly healed and whether the vaginal opening is too tight.

Provided the vagina is healed, a tight opening can be enlarged by gently stretching it with a finger or a glass dilator at home. If this is inadequate it is an easy matter to have the opening enlarged by a small cut which is stitched up in such a way as to leave the vagina larger. This small operation means going into the hospital for about two days. If the vaginal problem is associated with worry about another pregnancy contraception can be prescribed.

A vagina which is too lax can result from excessive stretching during delivery or from poor healing of an episiotomy or tear. In this case a woman may find that bath water can get into the vagina and come out again when she stands up. The vaginal entrance may also be too lax for her partner at intercourse. People often do not like to mention this problem to their doctor but they should do so as treatment is available. Sometimes intensive postnatal pelvic floor exercises will alleviate it, but if these fail a minor operation will be needed to open up the healed episiotomy and stitch it up more tightly. This entails spending about two or three days in the hospital.

SWOLLEN ANKLES

Swollen ankles are relatively common during pregnancy (*see* chapter 4), but in most women the swelling disappears without treatment within one or two days of delivery. In a few women, particularly those with varicose veins, swollen ankles may persist for several days after delivery. Occasionally women who have had no trouble during pregnancy develop severe swollen ankles and sometimes swollen legs as well in the puerperium. The swelling tends to be worse in the evenings. Swollen legs or ankles which start in the puerperium should be reported to the doctor.

The swelling is caused by excess fluid (edema) in the tissues. In pregnancy the edema is usually caused by **pre-eclampsia** (*see* chapter 4), by the retention of fluid due to the effect of the pregnancy hormones, or to varicose veins. In the puerperium, pre-eclampsia is most unlikely, and in most women blood pressure is usually normal.

Hormonal fluid retention normally improves in the puerperium but occasionally it persists or even starts at this time for reasons unknown. It can be quite severe and may last for a week or two after delivery. Varicose veins usually improve in the puerperium but they may also take a few weeks to do so.

One other possible cause of swollen legs is **leg vein thrombosis** (*see* below). This is potentially serious and requires medical advice. In these cases the swelling is usually associated with a pain in the calf and is usually worse on one side.

The treatment of swollen ankles depends on the cause. Pre-eclampsia requires rest, drugs to lower the blood pressure, diuretics to increase fluid loss from the kidneys, and sedatives. "Hormonal" fluid retention can be improved by rest with the legs up and diurectics. Varicose veins can be improved by elastic stockings; leg vein thrombosis requires anticoagulants.

TEETH

Teeth decay as often in the puerperium as they do in pregnancy (*see* chapter 4).

Tooth decay is not the result of calcium being taken away from the teeth as is commonly thought. It is impossible to remove calcium from a tooth once it is formed. Tooth decay occurs because changes in the mouth and gums brought about by the hormonal changes of pregnancy encourage dental caries.

THROMBOPHLEBITIS

This can occur both during pregnancy and in the puerperium (*see* chapter 4).

THROMBOSIS IN THE VEINS AND PULMONARY EMBOLISM

This has already been discussed in chapter 4, as it can occur both in pregnancy and in the puerperium. In the puerperium it is more common in certain groups of mothers: women who have previously suffered from thrombosis; women who have had a delivery by cesarean section; and women who have taken estrogen pills to suppress their milk. Puerperal vein thrombosis tends to occur about ten days after delivery.

URINE LEAKAGE *see* Incontinence

VAGINA, *see* Sexual problems

The newborn baby

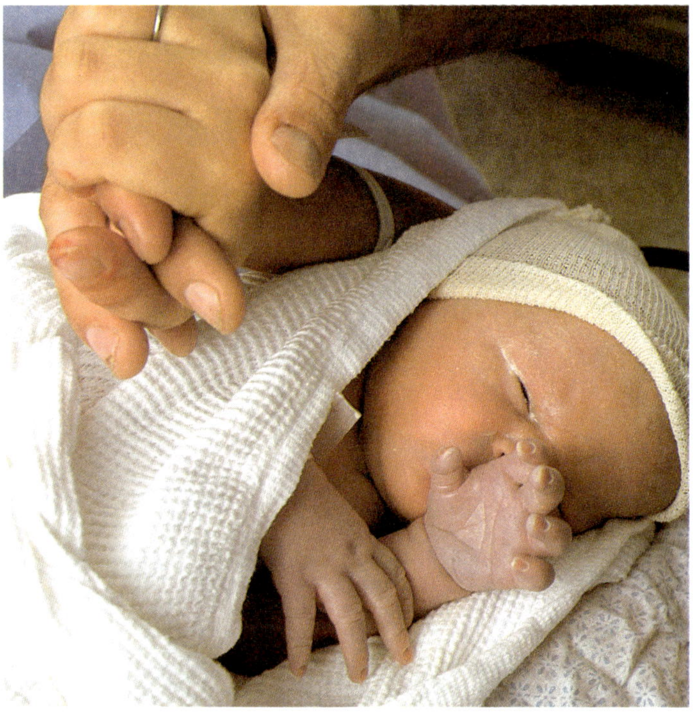

CHAPTER 9

The effects of labor

The baby's appearance

Examining the newborn

Premature and small-for-dates babies

Postdatism and postmaturity

Twins

Birth itself and the first few days of life can be very hazardous for the baby but, as medical knowledge has increased, so the dangers have decreased. Today the vast majority of babies are delivered safely.

The mother and her newborn both require care and attention after the birth. Recently, now that the mother's health during pregnancy and childbirth is so much more secure, a great deal of medical attention has centered on the baby. The "baby doctor" or pediatrician is now an accepted member of the delivery team. In some hospitals he or she is in charge of the medical supervision of every baby from the moment of birth, in others the obstetrician may perform the initial exam in the delivery room. But, soon thereafter, the pediatrician will examine the newborn baby and reassure the mother that everything is all right. He will be more closely involved in looking after any baby who needs special care.

Most recently, concern has centered on the psychological well-being of both mother and baby, which many feel has suffered as the result of an exclusively physical emphasis. The first few days of life are important in many ways for mother and child. During this time they begin to get to know each other and very close ties of affection develop. This relationship, known as "bonding", can develop most effectively if mother and baby are both physically well, are free of stress and are able to be with each other without unnecessary interruption. There is some evidence that the earlier bonding begins, the more effective it is likely to be, and this has influenced medical practice, encouraging in particular the policy of not separating mother and baby unless it is essential to do so. On the other hand, you should not imagine that a problem during the first few days

Cross references

See also	Chapter
Common complaints	12
Growth and development	14
Labor and birth	5, 6

Those first few moments after the birth when the parents hold their new baby are precious, and mark the beginning of the bonding process.

is going permanently to prevent you developing a good relationship with your child. It is also important for the rest of the family to spend some time with the baby during his first few days of life.

The actual experience of birth will have had a profound effect on the newborn baby. It is impossible to measure the psychological impact, and the controversy which surrounds this subject is discussed elsewhere in the book, in the section on "gentle birth" (*see* p. 99). The physical effects of birth are more straightforward. For instance, the baby's head is molded as it passes down the birth canal. The most important change associated with birth is, however, the start of breathing. The baby's first cry often coincides with the first breath. With that breath, the baby becomes a separate being, losing its dependence on the placenta, with all the changes in its circulation that involves.

Some people have an idealized picture of what a healthy newborn baby should look like: pink, clean, chubby and smiling. The reality is a lot more messy and less pretty, though no less beautiful for all that. The newborn baby's general appearance is therefore described in some detail. Actually, words and pictures cannot do justice to a baby's individuality and, although some of the unexpected things (such as the fact that your baby may be covered with white greasy vernix at birth) can be described, it always takes time to get used to a baby's unique looks and individual ways. Birthmarks and rashes are also discussed here. These are not uncommon but they are seldom worth worrying about and usually disappear fairly soon.

Within a few hours of birth, the pediatrician makes a thorough examination of the baby. This general examination, the tests which are usually carried out and the various reflexes that a normal baby will display, are explained and illustrated, enabling parents to understand why the tests are done.

Premature babies are those who are born after a shorter than normal period of time in the uterus; small-for-dates babies are those who have grown slowly during their time in the uterus whether they are born early or at the normal time. Although most premature and small-for-dates babies will turn out to be healthy individuals, these two types of baby are subject to greater risks and will require special care and attention. Premature babies also differ physically at birth from babies born at the normal time (mature babies) – for example in respect of their skin color, the development of their feet and ears and their characteristic sleeping posture.

These differences and the nature of the special care units in which premature and small-for-dates babies may be cared for are explained in detail. Some mature babies also need to be cared for in the intensive care unit, and this section of the chapter should help the parents of such a baby to understand in advance what to expect. Postmature babies are now very rare, but a brief section on the particular problems associated with such babies is included.

Only a few people have twins, let alone three or four babies, but a chapter on the newborn baby would be incomplete without talking about this rewarding experience. Multiple pregnancies are a challenge during gestation because of the increased risks compared to a singleton (one fetus) pregnancy. They are also a challenge after delivery, because their management requires organization, stamina and ingenuity. But ask the parents and the answer is always the same: "These babies are wonderful!"

The effects of labor

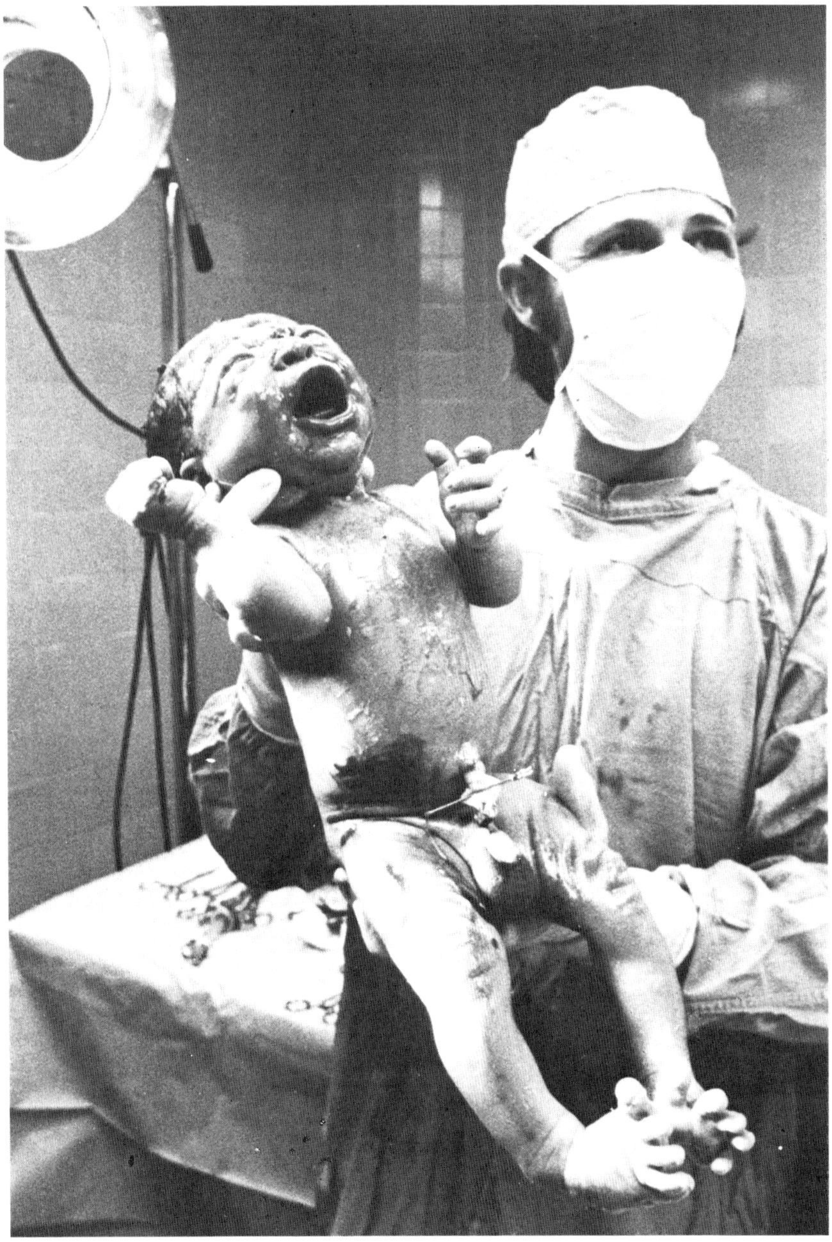

The culmination of the whole pregnancy is often the moment when the mother hears the first cry of her newborn baby.

What controls the length of pregnancy is not yet understood, but it does seem that the baby plays an important part in starting labor – probably by producing hormones.

Although the mother exerts a great deal of energy in the second stage of labor, literally pushing the baby out, the baby is not usually upset by the process of labor itself. During the contractions of the uterus the baby and the placenta are squeezed and this temporarily reduces the blood flow to the placenta. The effect of this is equivalent to holding your breath for a few moments. Provided the placenta is working well and the uterus relaxes fully between contractions, the baby has plenty of time to receive oxygen between contractions.

Sometimes, if the placenta is not working perfectly – perhaps as a result of high blood pressure of the mother during pregnancy – the flow of oxygen to the baby may be interrupted for longer periods. The same thing happens if the contractions are abnormally forceful or prolonged: this may cause "fetal distress", i.e. the fetus is not getting enough oxygen.

Fetal distress will show itself by a slowing of the baby's heart rate, which is constantly checked during labor. The lack of oxygen is potentially very serious but fortunately, once it has been discovered, it can be dealt with quite easily by expediting the delivery with forceps or vacuum extraction or, occasionally, by performing a cesarean section.

During the birth the shape of the baby's head is changed by the process of molding. There are five bones which form the upper part of the baby's skull, and these are joined together by tough membranes. (Later in life these bones will fuse together.) As the head is pushed into the birth passage, the skull bones move slightly, allowing the head to adopt a more narrow and elongated shape. At this time, the brain is temporarily flexible enough to accommodate this change.

The appearance of molding is made more striking by the caput succedaneum. This is a soft swelling which develops over the foremost part of the head as it is squeezed through the birth passage. The pattern of molding is rather different if the baby is born by the breech, for example, where the head passes through the birth canal last, and comparatively quickly (*see* p. 74). Babies born by cesarean section do not have this molding.

Molding and caput only appear if the birth is fairly slow. The gradual molding over a period of time makes the delivery of the head much easier. If the delivery is very rapid, the head does not have time to mold properly. Molding and caput disappear after a few days.

Although the baby is not usually affected by the process of labor, he has to make profound and rapid adaptations at birth. Throughout pregnancy he has been in darkness, hearing the whooshing noises of his mother's blood and comfortably supported in warm fluid. He has kicked his legs and moved his chest as if breathing, has drunk some fluid and passed urine, and he may even have sucked his thumb, but his existence has been essentially passive and has depended entirely on his mother who supplied all his needs by way of the placenta. Very soon after birth, he must breathe for himself and then start to feed. He must begin to cope with all his bodily functions, and he must also start to make sense of all the new sensations of noise, light, movement and cold which rush at him from the moment of birth.

The baby's first cry is the climax of the whole pregnancy and many mothers forget their discomfort the moment they hear it. Now nothing else matters. However, while the mother is thrilled the baby is making his first great effort as an independent individual, because the first breaths are extremely hard work. Before birth the lungs, mouth, nose and air passages are full of fluid. As the head is delivered, the fluid drains out of the mouth and

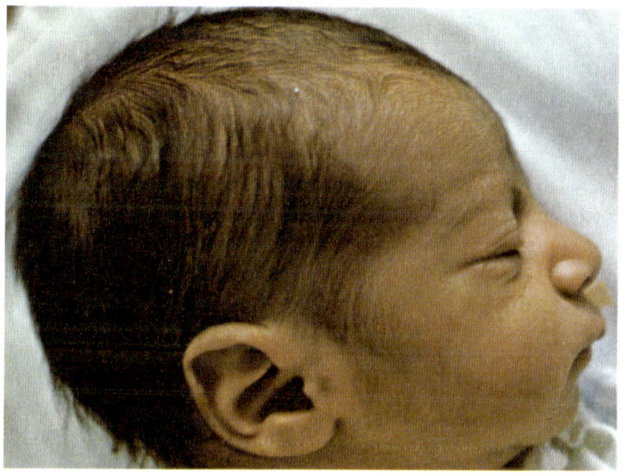

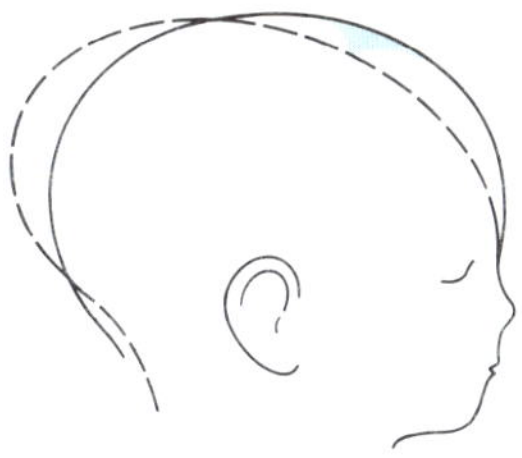

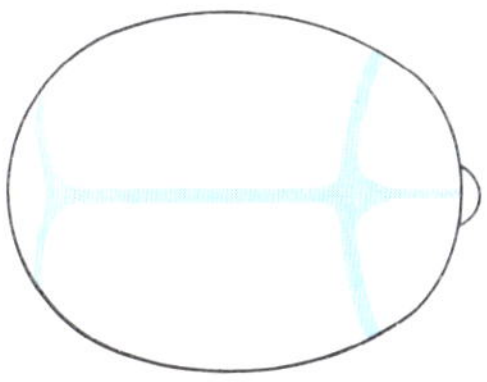

The baby's head changes shape during birth. The photograph (above) shows one example of molding, illustrated by the broken line (right). The blue triangle represents the fontanelle – the soft spot between the skull bones. Molding is made possible by the structure of the five skull bones (below right) which move slightly as the head is squeezed.

nose, and then the chest is squeezed as it is born, forcing some fluid from the lungs. Nevertheless the lungs still contain fluid and it requires a much greater effort to draw air into lungs that contain no air than to draw more air into lungs which already contain some. After a few mighty gasps have partly expanded the lungs, breathing becomes easier. The remaining fluid is removed by small vessels in the lungs, and over the next few days full expansion of the lungs is achieved.

Not all babies cry at birth. Some just begin to breathe quietly. The cry possibly expresses real distress; when one thinks how suddenly he or she is born – naked and wet – into a cold, bright and noisy world, it is easy to see why he is so upset. A lot of this distress may, however, be caused by a feeling of suffocation which is probably present at birth. It is difficult to avoid this as it probably makes the baby take his first breath. It is nevertheless reasonable to make birth as gentle as possible by minimizing light and noise in the delivery room and by keeping the baby warm.

Most babies are able to breathe at birth despite the amniotic fluid which is still in their mouth. They soon swallow this anyway. It is, however, usual practice to clear the mouth gently with a bulb syringe as soon as the baby is born so that he has an absolutely clear airway. Occasionally, a baby does not breathe within a few moments of birth and if this happens he may soon become short of oxygen. This is treated by blowing air with added oxygen into the lungs, either through a mask or by means of a small tube which is passed through the mouth into the trachea (windpipe). Once this is done the baby usually starts breathing quite quickly and there should be no further problem.

With the first few breaths there are also changes in the circulation of blood. Before the birth the baby received oxygen through the placenta, which acted as his "lungs". His real lungs were not yet used for breathing, and so most of the blood bypassed the lungs. At birth this must change. After the baby is born the uterus contracts. The placenta becomes detached and ceases to function and is passed out of the vagina. The arteries in the umbilical cord constrict and close, stopping the blood flow to the placenta. At the same time some of the blood in the blood vessels of the placenta passes into the baby's circulation. This "placental transfusion" takes a few moments, and it is usual to delay tying and cutting the umbilical cord to allow it time to occur – although it is not essential to do this.

With the placenta's job finished, and the lungs now responsible for breathing, the blood flow to the placenta through the umbilical cord stops and the blood flow to the lungs increases. The change involves a switch from the single blood circuit (heart to body and placenta and then back to heart) of the fetus, to the more efficient double circuit of the child (heart to lungs and then back to the heart before being pumped around the body). The change is brought about by the removal of the placenta and the closure of the ductus arteriosus shortly after birth (*see* diagram).

The cardiovascular changes are not the only major adjustments the newborn baby is making. He must adjust to the environmental temperature. If he is wet he will lose heat rapidly through evaporation. This is why the obstetrician dries him off before placing him on his mother's abdomen. His body surface to volume is large compared to an adult's so that he will lose body heat faster and therefore he must be kept warm. The bassinet into which he is placed usually has a radiant warmer positioned above it with a thermostat connected to an electrode placed on the baby's skin.

Once the baby is born he is cut off from his automatic source of energy, transplacental transfer of nourishment. Until he receives his first meal he will rely upon his stores of liver glycogen for nourishment. If he is premature or a small-for-dates baby he will probably have a decreased amount of glycogen stores in the liver and require special care.

Some babies actively cry at birth, others lie quietly. Generally, the baby starts to move all of his extremities shortly after birth. The doctor observes this movement as he makes a cursory neurological check-up. Frequently, the hands and feet are slightly blue: the most common reason for a nine rather than a 10 Apgar score. After the baby takes several breaths the hands and feet start to turn pink.

FETAL CIRCULATION BEFORE AND AFTER BIRTH

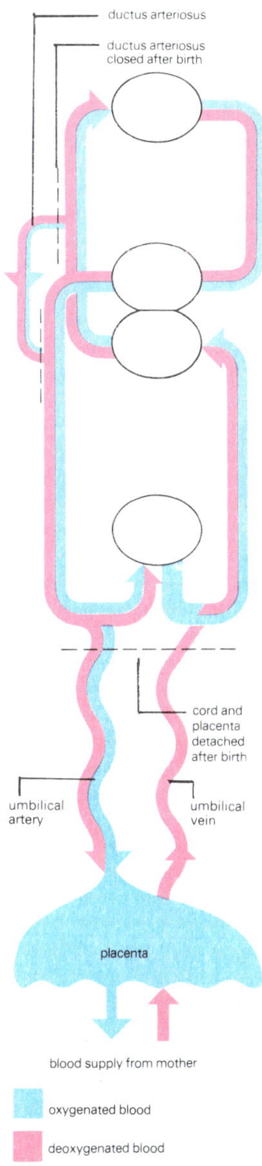

At birth, with the removal of the placenta and the closure of the ductus arteriosus, the circulation of the blood changes from a single circuit (heart to body and placenta and then back to the heart) to a double circuit (heart to lungs and then back to the heart before being pumped around the body).

The baby's appearance

To begin with the baby is asleep much of the time. Gradually he spends more time awake, but for the first week or so he may only wake up for brief periods – mainly at feeding times. A baby tends to sleep curled up in a position similar to that adopted in the uterus. If his position was unusual then it may remain so a few days. For example, some babies born by breech delivery (*see* p. 106) will have been in the uterus with their legs out straight and their feet up by their chins. They will continue to lie in this awkward position for several days after the birth.

It is sometimes said that a newborn baby cannot see or focus properly until he is about six weeks old. This is because at that time babies begin to look intently at their mothers and to smile freely when talked to. However, before this, even in the first few days of life, his or her attention can be engaged for short periods, and he will look at his mother's face. There is actually no doubt that he can see at this early age, though only objects about 10 in (25 cm) from his eyes are clearly in focus. You will notice that this is about the distance you hold the baby from your face when he or she is in your arms. It is particularly nice for the baby if you align your face with his so that he can see your face clearly.

In the first days of life some babies show enlargement of the breasts. This is the result of the hormone changes which stimulate the mother's breasts, and may affect male as well as female babies. It may even be possible to express a drop of milk, but the baby's breasts should be left alone as any handling might cause an infection. The breasts gradually flatten during the first few weeks.

The mother's hormones sometimes also stimulate the lining of a female baby's uterus and, after birth when the hormones are no longer reaching the baby, this uterine lining is shed as a small "period". This is quite normal but will not happen again until puberty.

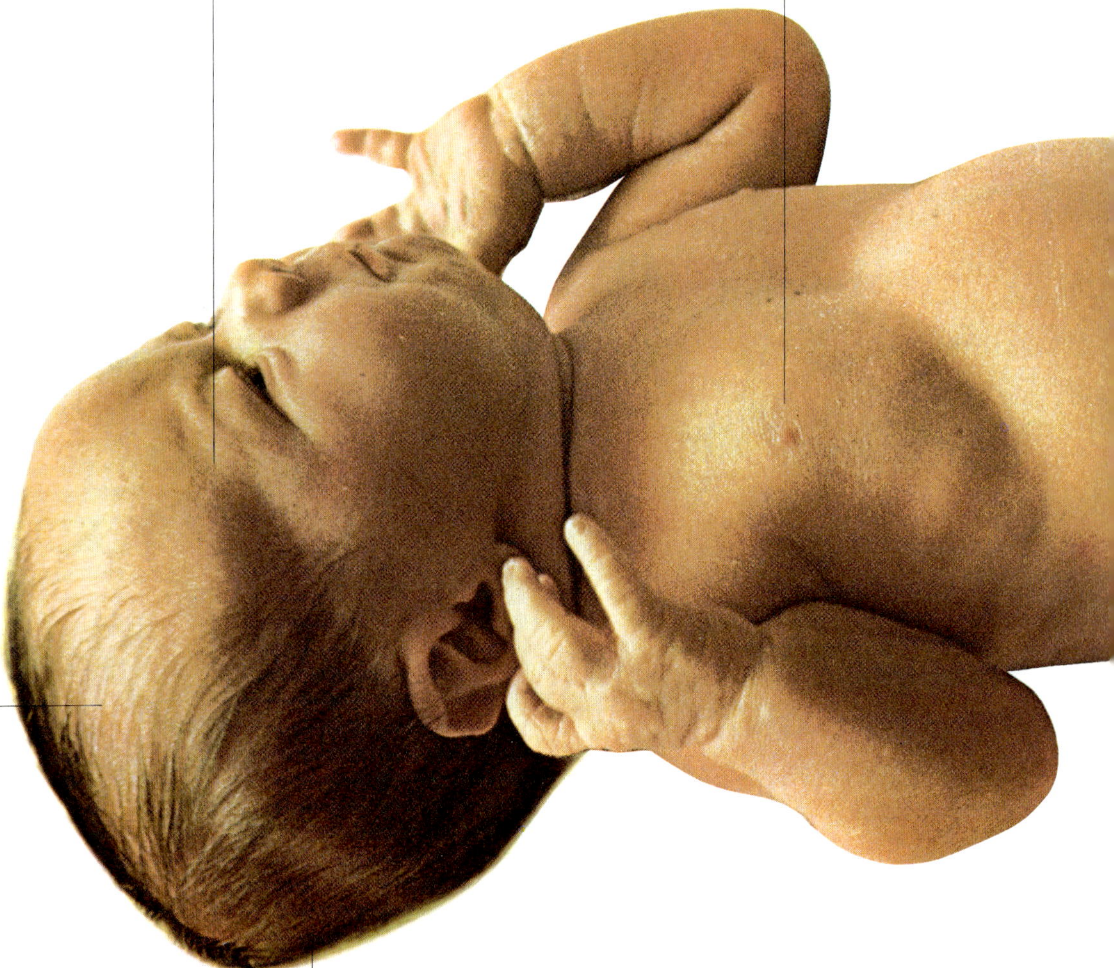

By the time of birth the baby's brain is more than one third of its full adult size whereas the body is little more than one twentieth. Thus the head appears large in relation to the body. On top of the head, at the point where the rounded corners of the skull bones just fail to meet, there is a gap known as the fontanelle, or soft spot. This area is in fact covered by a tough membrane and the baby is not at all vulnerable there. As the bones grow, the fontanelle gets smaller and it closes at around one and a half years of age – although the exact time at which this happens varies considerably.

Many babies are born with quite a mop of hair, which is usually dark even though it may later turn fair. The hair is in a resting phase and new hair does not begin to grow until the latter part of the first year. By this time much of the original hair will have fallen out. Many babies develop a completely bald patch at the point where they rub their heads on the mattress. Once the hair grows again this patch will be covered.

Soon after the birth the umbilical cord is cut quite short and securely clamped. Initially the cord is translucent and jelly-like but it soon begins to dry and after a few days it will fall off. This is quite painless. The area should be kept dry and clean. To avoid infections, the cord should be handled as little as possible. When the cord separates there may be a little bleeding, but so long as this is no more than a few spots, it is unimportant.

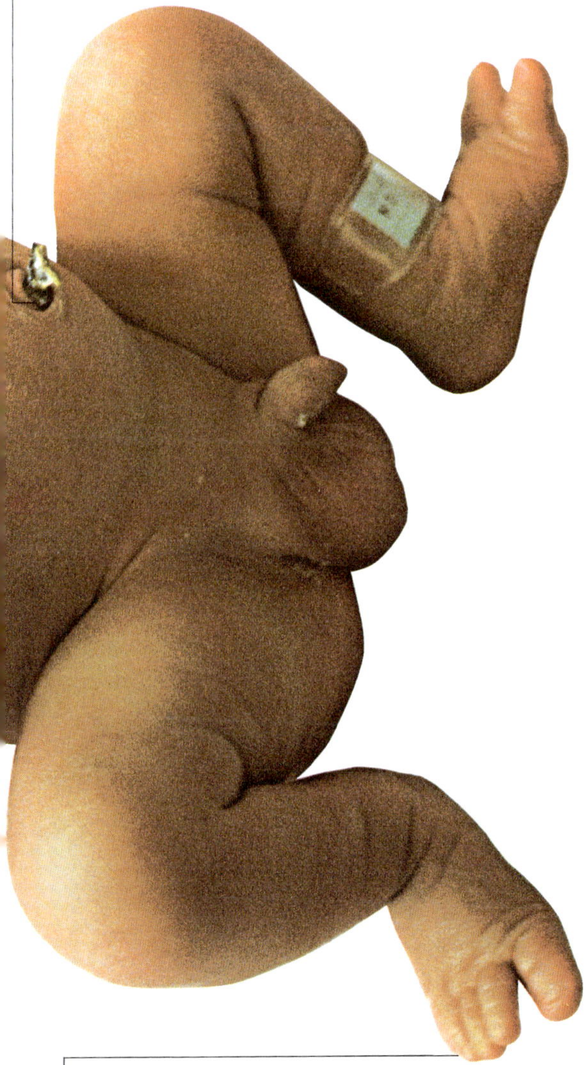

The finger- and toenails are fully formed at birth, and are a constant source of wonder to the baby's admirers. Sometimes the nails are quite long and it is then a good idea to trim them with very fine scissors to prevent the baby scratching his face. If the cut nails are still sharp, as they often are, a pair of mittens will solve the problem.

A newborn baby's skin is less smooth and clean than many parents expect. At birth the skin is usually covered with vernix caseosa **(a)** (*see* p. 50 – a greasy white substance. It is usually best to allow it to come off on its own accord over the first few days. Sometimes, however, vernix becomes rather dry and hard in the creases of the neck and under the arms and may irritate the skin; it can then be gently washed off with soap and water.

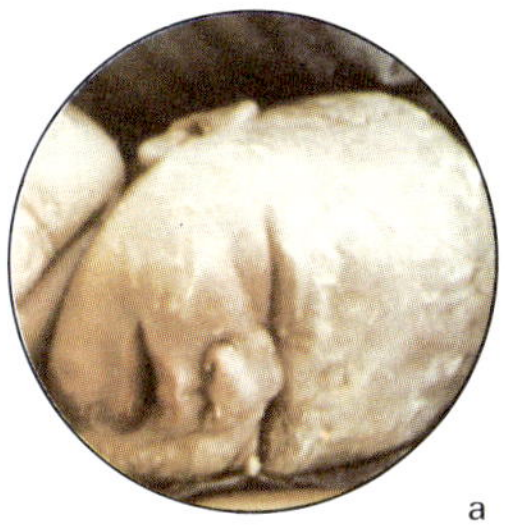

a

Following a forceps delivery there may be marks, usually on the cheeks, left by the blades of the forceps. These disappear in a few days. The pressures of birth may be sufficient to cause rupture of minute blood vessels in the baby's skin. This causes small purple spots – usually on the face. As they fade, jaundice may result (*see* p. 166), but this is rarely a cause for concern. Rupture of a blood vessel in the white of the eyes is also common, and may make the eye rather frighteningly red, but these marks are also harmless and disappear after a couple of weeks.

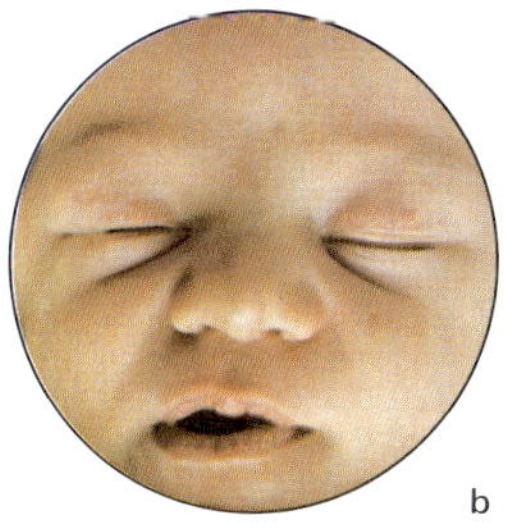

b

Stork bites **(b)**, or nevus simplex, (nevus means birthmark) are common. The mark is so called because the small reddish patch just above the bridge of the nose (which may also spread on to the upper eyelids) and a similar mark at the back of the neck are supposedly caused by the bill of the stork which brings the baby. The mark at the front soon fades and although the mark on the neck may persist it will in time be covered by hair.

Another fairly common birthmark is the strawberry nevus. This is not actually present at birth, but appears after a few days. It is a dusky red raised patch that really does look like a strawberry. It gradually fades and by about three years of age will have disappeared altogether without any treatment.

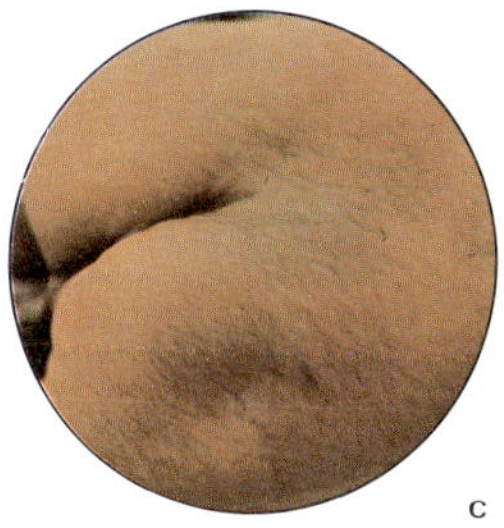

c

The mongolian blue spot **(c)** is a dark mark, usually on the lower back, and may look like a bruise. This mark has nothing to do with Down's Syndrome (mongolism), is quite harmless, and becomes less obvious in time. Such marks are more common in darker skinned babies – nearly all Asian and black babies have them.

Many newborn babies have a dramatic but harmless rash known as urticaria neonatorum or toxic erythema **(d)**. This consists of red blotches with slightly raised yellow centers. The spots come and go with amazing speed, and a baby who was covered in blotches may have barely a trace left half an hour later.

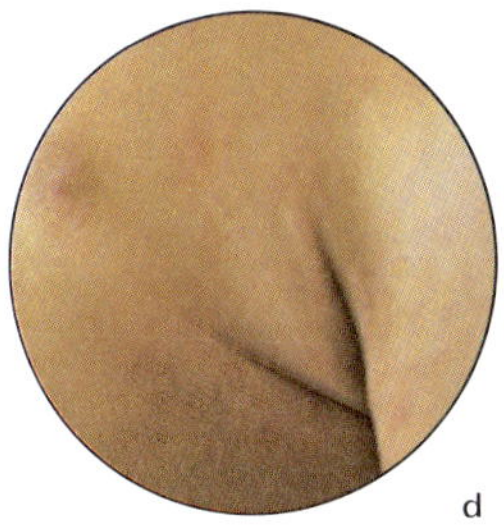

d

Milia (milk spots) **(e)** are tiny pearly white spots about the size of a pinhead which occur mainly over the nose. These actually look quite attractive, rather like a few freckles on an older child. They gradually disappear.

You may now have gained the impression that your baby's skin will be an unrecognizable patchwork of birthmarks, rashes and scratches. It will not be anything like as bad as that. However, for the first few weeks a baby's skin is often quite spotty. Later the skin will be clearer but still more delicate than an adult's.

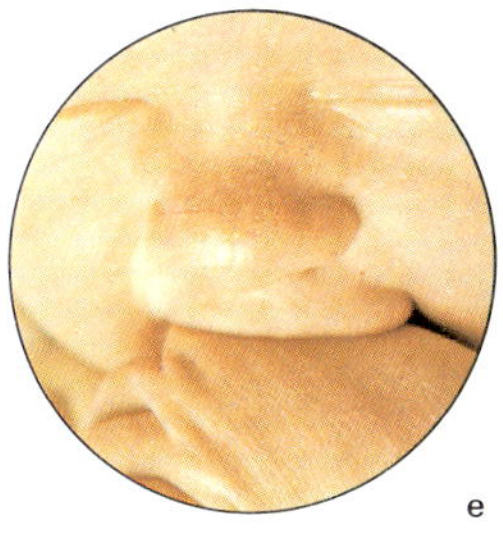

e

Examining the newborn

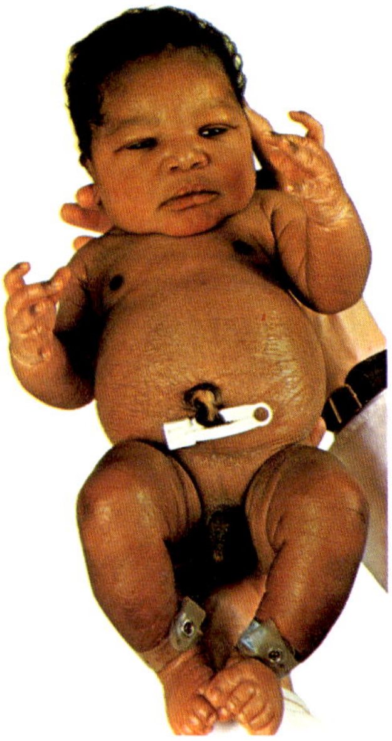

The medical examination of a newborn baby is most important in order that any abnormality may be diagnosed and treated as soon as possible.

Within a few days of birth, your doctor makes a full examination of the baby. You should try to see the examination, if at all possible, as this is also a good opportunity to ask advice and raise questions. It is not unusual for mothers to have dreadful fears about their babies, and a brief explanation might set your mind at rest and allay any such fears.

The doctor often begins the examination by undressing the baby himself. Simply by doing this he can learn much about the physical state and alertness of the baby. The way the baby stirs as he or she is disturbed, the way he moves, the way he cries or simply wakes up and quietly allows himself to be examined – all these things will tell the doctor a great deal.

Next comes a detailed inspection of the baby, looking at all the external features, such as the skin, hands and feet, and the eyes. The heart is checked by listening with a stethoscope. Many babies have a heart murmur, but these are usually quite innocent and do not mean that the heart is abnormal. The pulses are felt, in particular the femoral pulses in the groin. If these are absent, it suggests a blockage in the main arteries from the heart.

Various organs can be felt through the baby's soft abdominal wall and these organs will also be examined.

Checking the baby's hips to make sure that the joints are secure usually makes the baby cry, and is therefore best left until the end of the examination. It is important that this slightly unpleasant test should be done, because the treatment of dislocated hips is much more successful if it is started as soon as possible after the birth.

The doctor will want to know the baby's weight and how he or she is eating. Babies normally lose a little weight during the first few days, and this may amount to as much as ten per cent of their birthweight. After about five to seven days they begin to gain weight again, and normal weight gain is a sign of a healthy baby.

The PKU Test

On the third day of life and during the first newborn exam at two weeks, a sample of blood will be taken by making a small prick in the heel. This is for the Guthrie (or other similar) test, which is concerned with phenylketonuria, a rare disorder in which the body is unable to metabolize (i.e. use) phenylalanine. If this substance (which is present in most foods) is not metabolized it will accumulate in the body, harm the developing brain and cause mental retardation. This damage can be prevented by giving the child a special diet which contains very little phenylalanine.

The Guthrie test is a simple screening test which has been devised to divide babies up into those with a negative result, who definitely do not have phenylketonuria, and a small number with positive results who might possibly have the disorder. The latter group is then tested in more detail to determine which babies are in fact affected by this disease.

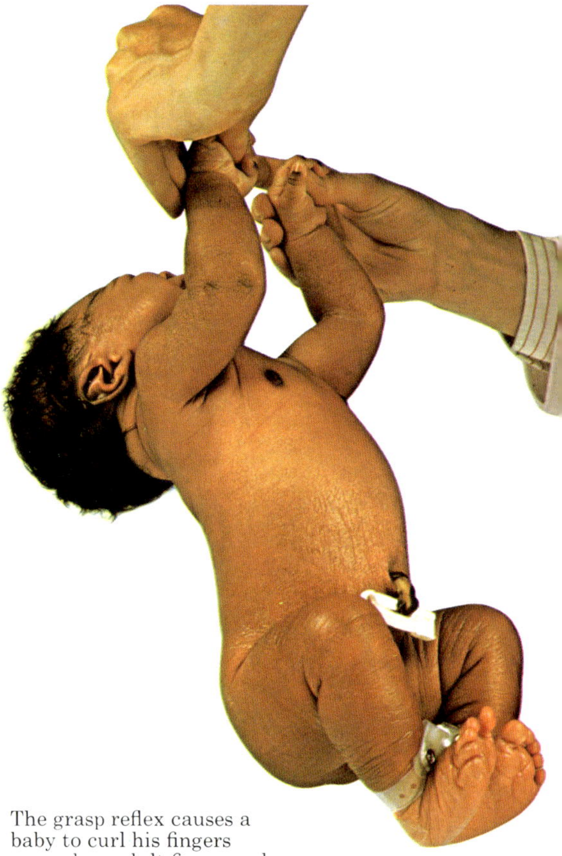

The grasp reflex causes a baby to curl his fingers around an adult finger and to grip it tightly. If his grasp is tight enough, he can actually be lifted up by the grasp of two hands (above).

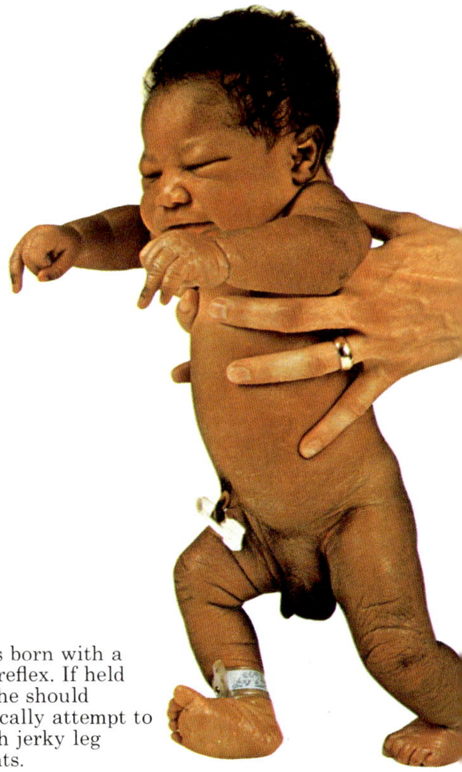

A baby is born with a walking reflex. If held upright, he should automatically attempt to walk with jerky leg movements.

It is naturally upsetting for parents to find that their child has phenylketonuria, but with early diagnosis and a proper diet the child will be able to grow up normally. The Guthrie test can also be used for other metabolic diseases which could cause mental handicap if not diagnosed early in life.

As well as the Guthrie test, a check for thyroid deficiency (done on the sample of blood taken for the Guthrie test) and a test on the meconium (the first stool passed by the baby) for cystic fibrosis are sometimes done. Treatments are available for both these conditions once they have been detected.

Reflexes

A newborn baby shows a number of reflexes. They are not all routinely tested in the medical examination, but they make a fascinating study, and one can see how the complex, coordinated voluntary movements of later childhood develop from some of these instinctive "primitive reflexes".

The rooting reflex is a good example. If the baby's cheek is gently touched, his head automatically turns to that side and his lips move in an effort to get his mouth around whatever touched him. When his mother's breast touches his cheek this reflex makes sure that he gets the nipple into his mouth. As he grows and gains greater control of his movements he will be capable of much more elaborate maneuvers, but until that time the rooting reflex reaction will suffice.

The grasp reflex is shown by gently touching the baby's palm. His fingers will curl around and grip firmly. Pulling against the grip strengthens it, and the grip is often so strong that he or she can be lifted right up by the grasp of both hands.

There is another similar, though much less dramatic, grasp reflex in the feet. The grasp reflex probably has more to do with the need to hold on to mother than with grasping objects. Indeed, it is not until the baby has begun to acquire voluntary control over his grasp that he is able to open his hand so that he might be able to grab hold of any object which catches his attention.

Although a baby cannot walk until he or she is about a year old, he has a walking reflex at birth. If held upright with his feet in contact with a firm surface, he will make rather jerky, high-stepping movements. A similar reflex is evoked if, held in the same way, his shin is brought into contact with an edge – of a table, for example. He will step up to place his foot on the table, as if mounting a step.

The Moro reflex occurs when the baby is startled. It is usually tested by holding the baby's head about an inch from the pillow and then suddenly letting it drop back, though some babies respond to milder stimuli such as a sudden movement or noise. The baby reacts by flinging out his arms and spreading his hands wide. The hands then begin to clasp and the arms are brought back a little as if clutching. This reflex is rather frightening for babies when it happens, and therefore the doctor only elicits it very gently.

The reflexes just described, and others, are useful for testing whether the baby's nervous system is functioning properly. For example, the walking reflex tests the ability to move the legs and the Moro reflex tests the arms. As the baby develops, and learns to coordinate his movements, these and other primitive reflexes will disappear gradually.

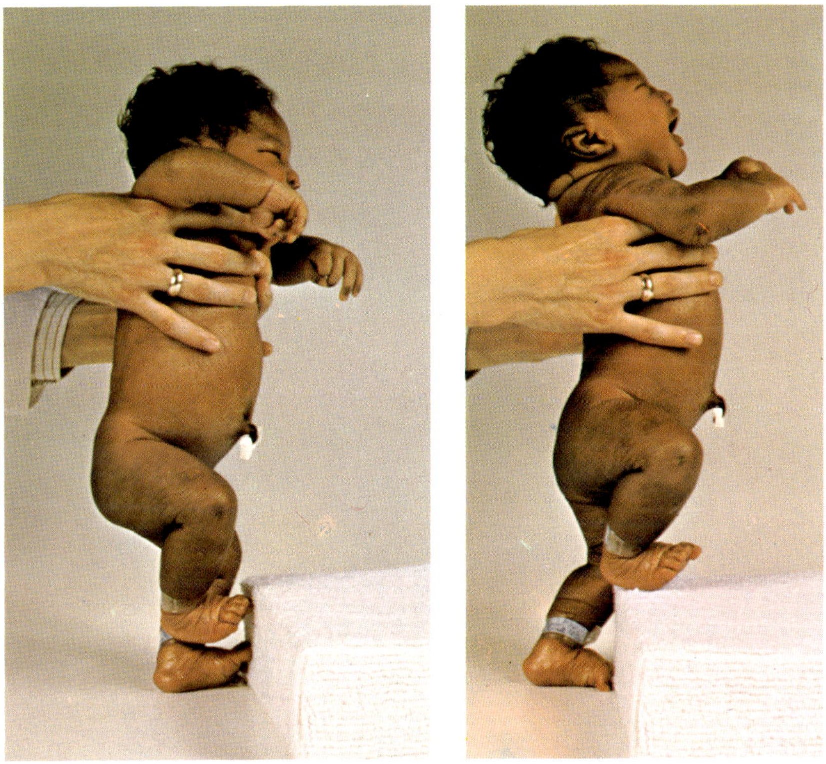

If a baby's shin makes contact with the side of a step, his walking reflex will cause him to step up and place his foot on top of the step.

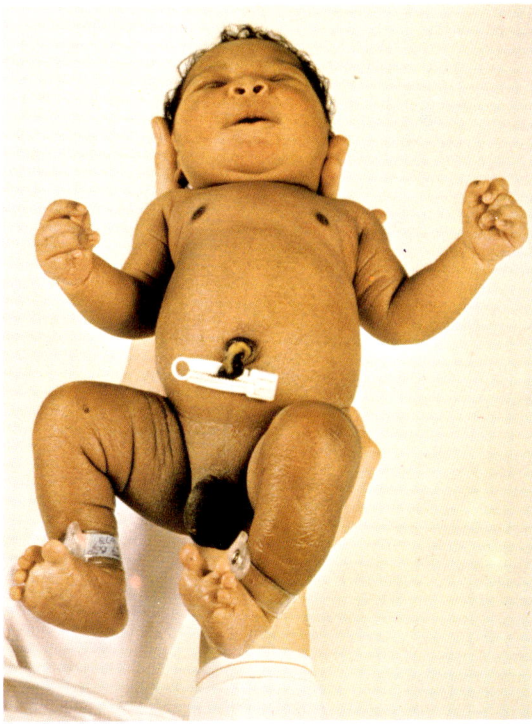

The Moro reflex takes place when the baby is startled. The baby flings out his arms and spreads his hands out wide. He then begins to close his hands and to bring his arms back a little.

Premature and small-for-dates babies

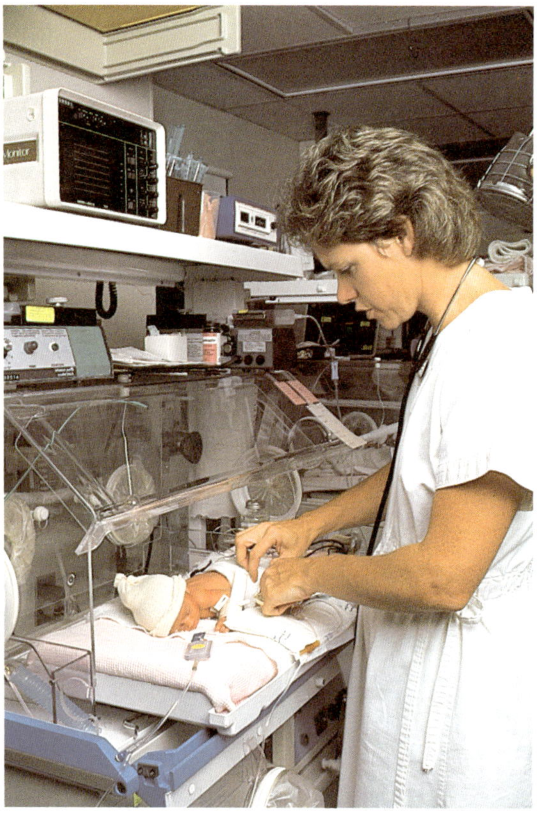

A baby who is born before term, if he is very premature and has a low birthweight, should be given close medical attention in a special care unit.

Roughly seven per cent of babies are born after pregnancies of less than 37 weeks. They are usually called premature. Whether they are likely to have serious problems depends on just how early they were born. Babies born after 34 weeks of pregnancy will normally do well, whereas those born before 24–25 weeks rarely survive. Fortunately the former are more common than the latter and the chances of survival for even very premature babies are improving all the time.

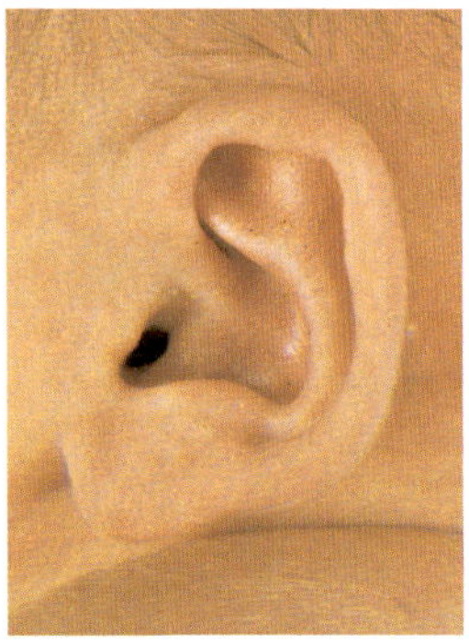

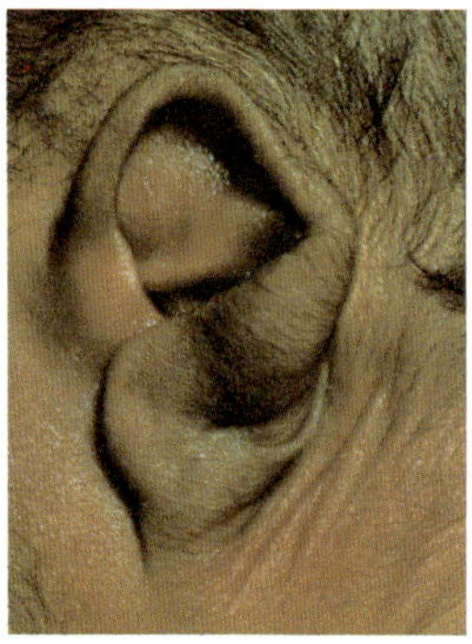

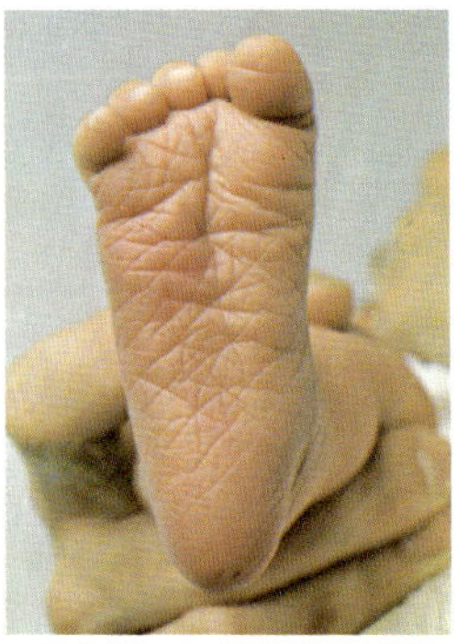

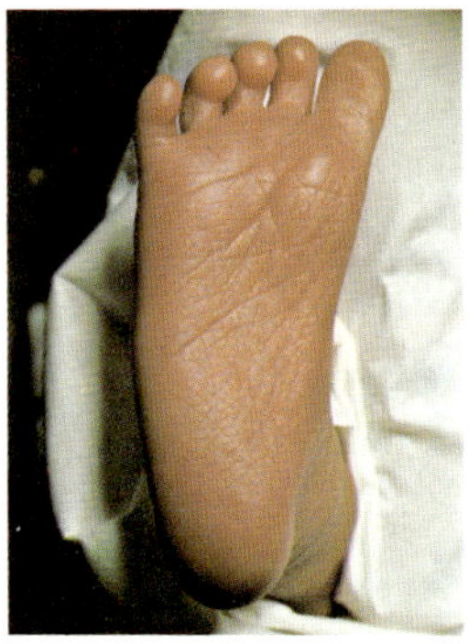

A premature baby's ears are softer and more pliable (above) than a full-term baby's ears (above left). When the lobe is pushed forward it will remain in position.

The soles of a full-term baby's feet have developed lines and creases (far left) whereas a premature baby's soles are much smoother (left).

A premature baby is small and skinny as he or she has missed the last part of pregnancy when extra layers of fat would have been built up. The baby's skin is thin and (since the blood vessels show through more as a result) usually pinky red. Being small and delicate, he may be bruised during birth but the bruises soon fade. As the muscles are underdeveloped, he tends to be floppy and weak and to lie sprawled out rather than curled up in the position typical of a full-term baby. He also often has more difficulty in breathing.

The hands and feet of a full-term baby have begun to develop creases and lines along the skin folds. The premature baby has smoother palms and soles; a slight swelling which occurs during the first few days makes them look still smoother. The ears are soft and may be rather flat, lacking the complex folds which are typical of the full-term baby's ears. Premature babies are often quite hairy, keeping much of the downy hair (lanugo) which the fetus has in the uterus and which normally disappears in the latter weeks of pregnancy. A doctor looking at these and other features should be able to estimate roughly how premature a baby is.

The more premature babies need careful attention, which is best given in an intensive care unit. Most large hospitals have one, and usually babies weighing less than 5 lb (2.2 kg) or those born more than five or six weeks early may go into the unit.

Because he or she has less insulating fat, a premature baby is particularly vulnerable to cold and will need to be cared for in an environment which is only a few degrees below body temperature. Very small babies are kept naked or lightly clothed in an incubator where they can be easily observed in the nursery and where the temperature can be readily adjusted.

Babies born before about 35 weeks of pregnancy do not usually suck well enough to feed from either the breast or a bottle; they need nasogastric tube feeding. The tube is not uncomfortable and as they grow and suck strongly they begin to feed normally.

Premature babies are prone to a number of complications; one of the most common being difficulty with breathing as a result of immature lungs (respiratory distress syndrome). The baby may need oxygen or, if seriously ill, an artificial ventilator to help him breathe. Sometimes the baby is so severely affected that he dies, but in milder cases the breathing gradually improves and recovery is complete.

Jaundice is another common complication in premature babies. Their livers are not yet able to get rid of the yellow substance, bilirubin, and the most obvious symptom is the yellowing of the skin.

It is disappointing for you if your baby has to go to an intensive care unit. However, you should be able to visit the baby at almost any time, and to help look after him, perhaps by feeding or changing him.

As soon as your baby is feeding well and attains a good weight he will be allowed home. How long this will take varies but it will be when he or she weighs about 5 lb (2.2 kg). You can make a rough guess by allowing two weeks before the baby regains his birth weight and then another week for each 3 oz (85 g).

Parents are naturally anxious to know if their baby is likely to grow up normally if born early. A small number of babies who are born very early or who develop serious complications will die and a few may survive with serious handicaps. But the great majority turn out fine. After the initial period, the physical health of most premature babies is good – though they may have more infections, especially coughs and colds, during the first year of life. Prematurity itself does not seem to have any effect on subsequent mental development. In the first few months, remember to subtract the number of weeks that the baby was born early before calculating the age of development. By two to two and a half years the development of the premature baby and the full-term baby are no longer distinguishable.

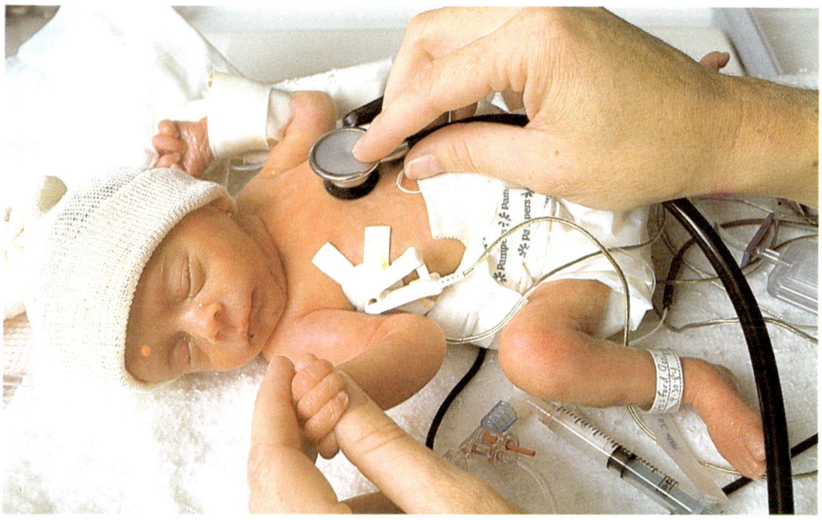

All the bodily functions of a premature baby are constantly monitored and tested so that any complications that may arise can be dealt with immediately.

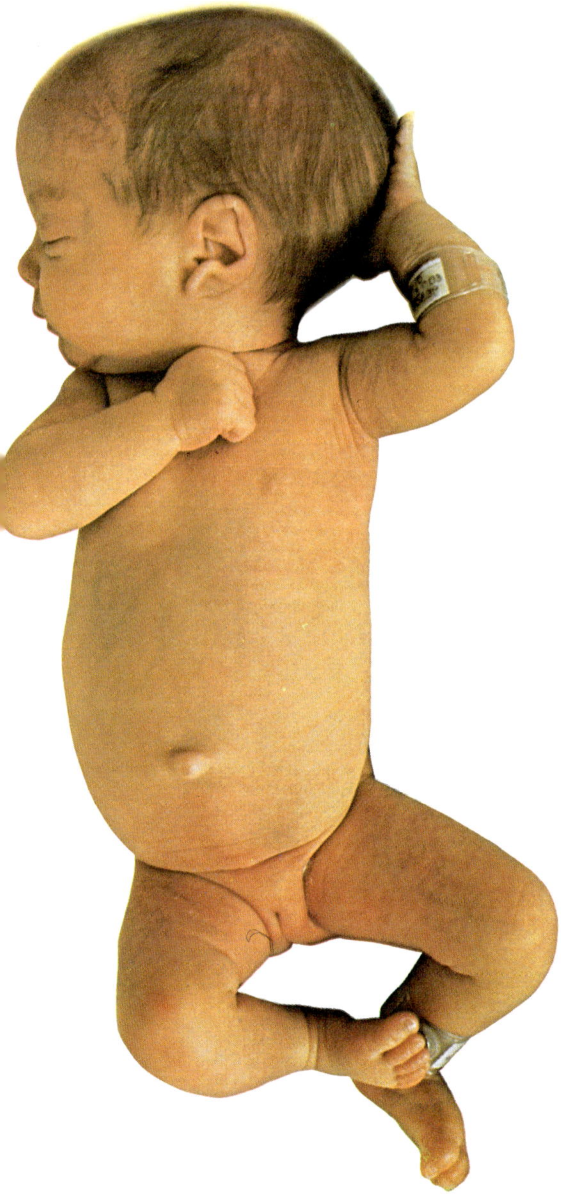

A premature baby is small, thin, and rather pink, because his skin is thin and his blood vessels are therefore very visible. He will tend to lie stretched out rather than in the curled-up position which is characteristic of full-term babies.

Small-for-dates babies

Premature babies are small because they have not stayed long enough in the uterus. Other babies are small because they have grown too slowly. These are called small-for-dates since they are smaller than would be expected for the duration of the pregnancy. They have grown slowly either because of some inherent tendency or, much more commonly, because they did not get enough food via the placenta. Slow growth of the fetus can usually be detected during pregnancy (*see* chapter 3), and it is generally agreed that if pregnancy is well advanced it is better to deliver the baby early so that he can be fed, rather than letting him remain undernourished inside the uterus.

A small-for-dates baby resembles a premature baby in size, but there the resemblance ends. He is skinny, but his loose flesh makes him look as if he had recently lost weight. His skin is thicker and paler. His head will be large in proportion.

These babies have fewer problems than premature babies. Serious breathing difficulties are rare, but small-for-dates babies are more prone to develop a lack of glucose in the blood. Feeding within an hour or two of birth will help. The doctor will check the level of glucose in the baby's blood for the first 48 hours after the birth. If a low level is found, it can be corrected by extra milk, formula, or by intravenous glucose. The long-term outlook for small-for-dates babies is good. It has been suggested that their development may be a little slower than that of babies of normal birthweight but this is not certain.

Postdatism and postmaturity

Most normal pregnancies last an average of 280 days. A term pregnancy is one which is completed between 38 and 42 weeks of gestation. Postdatism implies a pregnancy that goes beyond 294 days or two weeks or more beyond the estimated date of delivery, whereas postmaturity is the result of the fetus remaining in utero after the placenta is no longer functioning with normal efficiency. Postdatism occurs in approximately 10 per cent of pregnancies, but actual postmaturity in only about 4 per cent.

The syndrome of postmaturity consists of a fetus which begins to lose weight, has decreased subcutaneous fat, long fingernails, and wrinkled skin which sloughs off. The amniotic fluid volume is decreased and the placenta may have an increased amount of fibrous content.

Postmaturity is a serious condition. Some fetuses may die in utero prior to labor, whereas others can die during labor. Besides the risk of fetal death, there are other problems. The fetus is more susceptible to distress in labor and the newborn to metabolic problems.

The clinical problem of postmaturity is relatively easy to solve; simply deliver the baby. The dilemma arises in trying to determine whether the pregnancy is truly postdates, or whether the dates are simply incorrect.

Dating the pregnancy

In recent years, because diagnostic ultrasound can be used to confirm gestational dates whenever there is doubt, the accuracy of estimating gestational age has improved considerably. In the past, many of the patients believed to have postmaturity merely had incorrect dates. Today, by carefully noting the date of the last normal menstrual period, the size of the uterus on the first exam, the time when quickening (initial feeling of fetal movement) occurs, and by obtaining ultrasound measurements, very accurate dating of pregnancy can be achieved. In the first trimester, the crown-rump-length may be measured by diagnostic ultrasound, giving an accuracy of three or four days for gestational dates. During the second trimester, the biparietal (head) diameter and the femur (thigh) lengths may be measured, providing an accuracy of ± 1 week.

When a mother visits her doctor at approximately 41 to 42 weeks of gestation, the question of whether she will go beyond 42 weeks is usually raised. As she approaches the 42nd week, fetal surveillance is initiated. If the cervix is favorable at 42 weeks, labor may be induced. If the cervix is not, then biweekly non-stress tests or contraction stress tests with ultrasound scanning are done. With such a program it is extremely unlikely that there would be a fetal death. Plans are made to evaluate the pregnancy for signs of postmaturity, should she not deliver spontaneously in the next few days. The doctor schedules several tests which will tell whether the fetus is safe remaining in utero. If the tests are unfavorable, then the baby is usually delivered, and if the tests are favorable, the fetus is allowed to remain in utero. Estriol determination is one of the commonly used tests. It is measured either in the serum, or by a 24 hour urine collection. The serum specimen is faster because the 24 hour urine requires one day to collect and is therefore a day late in reporting.

Biophysical tests, such as the non-stress test or the contraction stress test with an ultrasound estimation of amniotic fluid volume, are the best way to follow fetal well-being. With a non-stress test, the fetus is observed with an external electronic fetal monitor. The desired favorable finding is an acceleration of the fetal heart rate by 15 beats per minute for 15 second duration, caused by fetal movement. If this is non-reactive (unfavorable), it may be only because the fetus is sleeping; therefore, commonly it will be repeated after a meal, when the fetus may be more awake and active. If it is still non-reactive, then a contraction stress test may be done. This may be performed either by stimulating the nipples by rubbing, which releases oxytocin from the mother's pituitary and causes uterine contractions, or by the administration of oxytocin by a intravenous drip. In either case, the oxytocin causes the uterus to contract and the desired result is slowing of the heart rates (decelerations) caused by uterine contractions. Generally, three contractions in ten minutes are required to have a valid test. Additionally, an ultrasound scan of the pregnant uterus is performed to observe the volume of amniotic fluid and any placental changes. If the amniotic fluid volume seems adequate or normal, this is a favorable sign. If it is considerably decreased, this is an indication of postmaturity. Finally, if the placenta contains many calcium deposits and echo-free areas, this indicates that the placenta may no longer be functioning efficiently and it is best to deliver the fetus.

Risks and effects

During the delivery of a postmature baby, there is an increased risk of fetal distress. Accordingly, it is imperative that electronic fetal monitoring be employed in order to identify any potential fetal hypoxia (oxygen deprivation), which would be indicated by late decelerations on electronic fetal monitoring. If the fetus is not tolerating labor well then delivery by immediate cesarean birth is the preferred course of action.

Numerous studies have been done on postmature babies to determine the long-term effects of postmaturity. Field and co-workers reported lower developmental scores at four months of age. Usually, by eight months, there is developmental "catch-up", but the mental scores are slightly lower. It is important to remember that many babies have postdatism, but far fewer have postmaturity. Today, unfavorable effects due to postmaturity are much less likely because of sensitive monitoring techniques. With any indication of fetal deterioration, a delivery may be accomplished to prevent serious complications.

Twins

Multiple gestations are relatively common in human pregnancies. Twin gestations occur in 1 out of 80 pregnancies. Triplets are much less common, occurring in 1 out of every 6400 pregnancies; and the odds for having quadruplets are a remote 1 out of 51,200. Blacks have a 20 to 25 per cent greater chance of producing twins, a 70 to 75 per cent greater chance of triplets and four times greater chance of quadruplets.

Twins can originate from either one or two eggs. Identical twins (monozygotic) are the result of fertilization of a single ovum by a single sperm. The fertilized ovum splits into identical halves which give rise to twins sharing the exact same genetic makeup. Therefore, identical twins are always of the same sex and can be expected to have the same hair color, eye color and blood type. Identical twins result from a temporary delay in development of the ovum prior to implantation and are relatively rare.

Fraternal twins (dizygotic) are the result of the fertilization of two different ova by two sperm. The ova are released from separate follicles that mature at the same time; these follicles may be in one or both ovaries. Fraternal twins may be of the same or opposite sexes and can differ in characteristics as much as single gestation brothers and sisters do.

Signs and Symptoms

Because the twin pregnancy has two fetuses and commonly two placentas, there will be increased levels of hormones and the uterus will be larger. Therefore, it is logical to expect the symptoms of pregnancy to be exaggerated: often, urinary frequency, nausea and vomiting are increased; there is more rapid weight gain; the abdominal distention may be increased compared to a singleton pregnancy (i.e. only one fetus).

In the past, as many as 30 per cent of twins were diagnosed as late at the time of delivery. Today, with realtime ultrasound scanning most twins are diagnosed early in pregnancy so that the clinician can assign the correct expected date of delivery. Usually the uterus grows more rapidly with multiple gestations. On the initial examination, for instance at eight weeks since the last normal menstrual period, it is possible that the uterine size may be equivalent to 10 or 12 weeks gestational size. This is very suggestive of multiple gestation. The diagnosis can be made by performing an ultrasound scan. At this stage two gestational sacs can be identified.

Complications

From the obstetrical standpoint, there are numerous challenges. The incidence of preeclampsia, prematurity, and malpresentation are increased. The overdistention of the uterus can lead to dysfunctional (sluggish and inefficient) labor and the possibility of a postpartum hemorrhage. Premature labor is a major risk in multiple pregnancy. The average gestational period for twins is about 20–21 days shorter than for singleton pregnancies. The physician will probably check the cervix at regular intervals to detect shortening or dilation. The value of routine admission to the hospital for bed rest at 28 to 34 weeks of pregnancy for reducing premature labor is not established; however, with any complication or a suggestion of prematurity or preeclampsia, admission to the hospital is necessary.

There are numerous variations in the way twins grow in the uterus. The part closest to the cervix is called the presenting part. The first baby to deliver is termed Twin A and the second baby is Twin B. In 45 per cent of twin pregnancies, both babies have their heads (vertex) down. In 38 per cent, one baby has its head down and the other the breech down. In 9 per cent of pregnancies, both babies have the breeches presenting. In the remaining 8 per cent, there is a combination of head first and transverse or breech first and both babies lying in a transverse position.

As might be expected, carrying two fetuses takes its toll on the mother. The incidence of anemia, chance of developing preeclampsia, polyhydramnios (excess amniotic fluid) and postpartum hemorrhage are all increased, but the mother's health is rarely in true jeopardy. Maternal mortality is only very slightly increased over that of a mother having a single baby. The perinatal mortality rate, however, is 3 to 4 times higher for twins. The major reason for this is prematurity. The mean gestational age at birth for twins is 35 weeks.

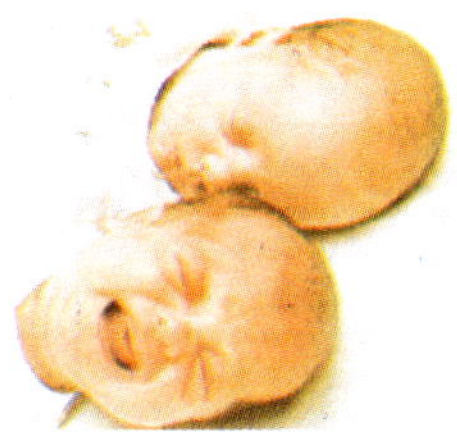

A multiple pregnancy is usually detected early, and the exact number can then be established by an ultrasound scan.

Delivery

Women having twins should deliver in perinatal centers when possible. If both twins present as vertex (head down), vaginal delivery will probably be chosen. If the twins have abnormal presentations the obstetrician may judge that cesarean section is the safest route for delivery. Additionally, extreme prematurity may influence the choice for cesarean section.

If a vaginal delivery is planned, electronic fetal monitoring of both fetuses should be done. Twin A may have internal monitoring with a scalp electrode. Twin B may have external monitoring. After the delivery of Twin A the cord is clamped and marked Twin A. The fetal heart rate of Twin B is carefully monitored. The best results occur if Twin B is delivered from 5 to 15 minutes after Twin A.

A neonatologist should be present at the delivery to take care of any of the potential problems that occur with twins, e.g. hypoxia, congenital malformations or anemia from a twin to twin transfusion.

The placenta(s) is then deliverd and inspected. Visual inspection may reveal if the twins are identical, e.g. one placenta with membranes between twins consisting only of two layers of amnion. Following the delivery of the placenta, the top of the uterus is palpated and massaged through the mother's abdominal wall to prevent excessive bleeding from the over-distended uterus.

Feeding the newborn baby

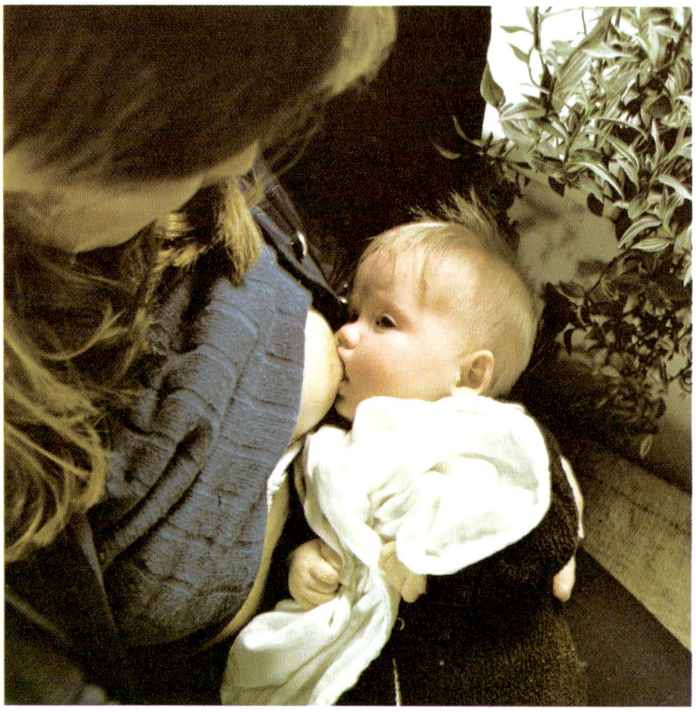

CHAPTER 10

How you will want to feed your baby may be influenced by your childhood. If you come from a large family, for example, you may have watched your own mother or an elder sister breast-feed, and you will have grown up unconsciously expecting to do the same when the time comes. Or nowadays you may have friends who are happily breast-feeding. If you have not had these experiences, or been exposed to the idea of breast-feeding as natural and enjoyable for both mother and baby, the whole idea of breast-feeding may seem primitive or distasteful.

The opinions of close relatives are also likely to influence an expectant mother in her view of breast-feeding. Her husband's attitude is of course crucial, and he will probably have been conditioned by his upbringing. To a lesser extent, the influence of mother and mother-in-law may be important. They can give a mother tremendous support when she wishes to breast-feed, so much so that success may depend heavily on their attitudes and general supportiveness.

It is useful to know something of the history of artificial feeding before making up your mind. Bottle feeding began to spread in developed countries at the beginning of this century, and became more and more common, reaching a peak in the 1960s. The decline of breast-feeding went hand in hand with the increase of hospital births; the separation of baby from mother, regimentation and hospital routines such as four-hourly feedings all made it difficult if not impossible. It was not until the majority of women were bottle feeding that the disadvantages of "formula milks" for the baby's health became apparent, and this has led to recent changes in the attitude of doctors, who are beginning to realize the incalculable advantages of

Cross references

See also	Chapter
Feeding in the first year	13
The newborn baby at home	11
Hormones	2
The puerperium	8

The birth cycle ends not with delivery, but with weaning; breast-feeding is an extension of the nourishment given by the mother's body to the baby in the uterus.

breast milk. So a mother who wants to breast-feed may receive more encouragement from them now than she would have a few years ago.

Another blow to the prestige of bottle feeding was the revelation that many third world babies were dying because their mothers had been persuaded to use artificial feeding. In the Western world it is comparatively safe; sterilization of bottles is easier, people are more likely to use it correctly, and infections can be treated with antibiotics. So a baby can thrive on bottle feeding if the necessary care is taken. But it is misleading to present the two kinds of feeding as equal alternatives, with practical considerations dictating the choice. Breast milk is perfectly designed for the baby's needs; for instance, the fat content changes to meet the demands of his growing brain, and the antibodies it contains are a valuable protection. Formulas, however "improved", are still based on cow's milk, and the needs of calves are quite different from those of human babies.

It is unfortunate that many nurses and doctors who attend young mothers in the hospital have not yet had the experience necessary to give informed advice, which is essential for a newly-delivered mother who has never breast-fed before. Although it is a natural process, it is not enough to learn about it from books; help and advice are needed to get the baby "on" in the right position. Breast-feeding is a skill which mother and baby both learn. But as experience in supporting breast-feeding grows, this should lead to fewer women changing to bottle feeding because of "failure" in breast-feeding. Some mothers, who do not want to breast-feed because of previous feeding problems, may decide to give it another try; they may well be delighted that they did.

Breast-feeding is a splendid process of adaptation between mother and child – an extension of the ways in which the mother's body has nourished the baby in the uterus. The birth cycle ends not with the birth, but with the weaning of the baby; and seeing the baby thrive on her breast milk alone can give the mother a sense of achievement almost as great as giving birth. For most women, breast-feeding is uniquely pleasurable – many live in a state of pleasant anticipation of the next feeding. Although women may fear feeling tied down, they are amazed how flexible the pattern of feeding becomes; and there is another advantage: fat stores built up in pregnancy are used up during lactation, so most women can eat what they want while they are breast-feeding and not put on any excess weight.

In some areas, there are special classes for breast-feeding mothers. There are groups of mothers who are willing to help with the problems that can face a newly breast-feeding mother; if you do not know of such a group locally, contact the La Leche League.

A few mothers should not breast-feed – those, for instance, who have a history of certain rare illnesses, or who need to take one of the few drugs which can affect the baby when passed into the milk, or those who really do not want to breast-feed.

You may choose to bottle feed your baby so that you can go back to work. But you could still start by breast-feeding, so that the baby gets many of the advantages in the early days of life. When you go back to work it may be possible to find a relation, a babysitter, or a day care center near your place of work, so you can breast-feed in the middle of the day. Or you can use a handy small breast pump and express a supply of milk for the following day.

Breast-feeding: facts and fallacies

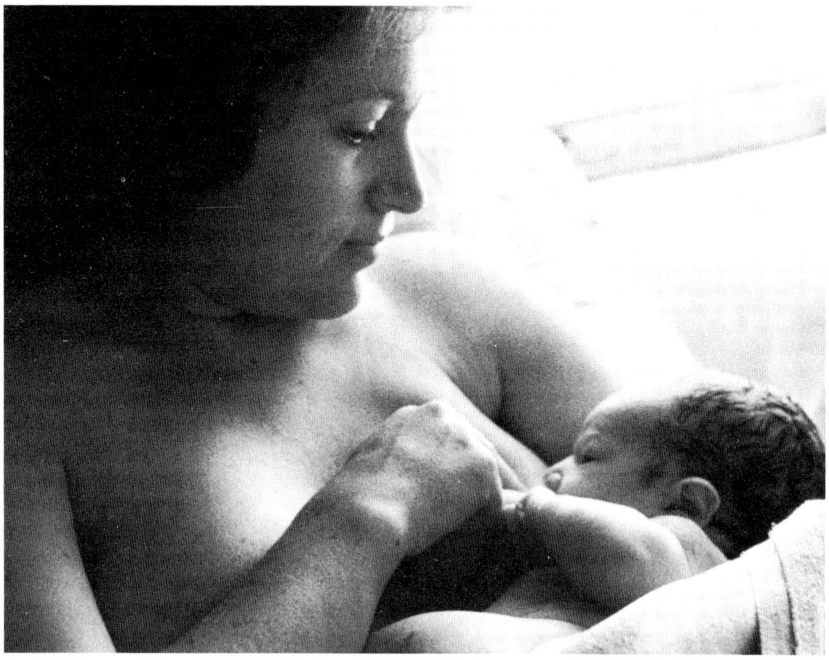

It is important, during feedings, to be comfortable and able to relax completely. Breast-feeding will soon become a pleasure you and your baby can both enjoy.

For mothers who wish to breast-feed their babies, it is helpful to know what happens in the breasts immediately after the birth.

After the birth

During the course of pregnancy, the breasts grow larger as a result of hormonal changes in the body (*see* p. 30). When the baby is born, the breasts contain colostrum – a protein-rich substance which is usually creamy yellow in color and quite thick. Colostrum contains all the food the baby will need until the milk itself "comes in". It also contains important antibodies and acts to help your newborn infant have a first bowel movement.

Within a day or two hormones trigger further changes in the breasts so that they start to produce milk. There is a dramatic increase in the blood supply to the breasts, which lasts about 24 to 48 hours. During this time the breasts swell and become very tender and uncomfortable. This is usually more marked with a first baby. Do not be alarmed; this is perfectly normal and they will soon settle down. By the time the baby is about two weeks old you will find that your breasts will be soft all or most of the time.

While your breasts are adjusting, the milk-colostrum balance in them is changing all the time. By about four weeks, the milk usually ceases to be creamy yellow and gradually becomes whiter until it closely resembles skim milk. In small amounts it might even seem transparent. As the baby grows older, the milk becomes almost colorless, although it still gives the baby all the nourishment he needs. It is important to remember that these color changes are natural; the milk itself actually alters to meet the changing needs of the growing baby.

The baby should be put to the breast as soon as possible, taking colostrum in the first few days and then the milk as it is first produced in the breasts. The baby's needs are small just after birth, but he still gets great pleasure from sucking at the breast. There should be no need for the baby to be given water and glucose, although this is a practice which is followed in some hospitals.

It is worth noting that it is quite possible to breast-feed a baby who has been given bottle feedings in the first few days, but it is better for mother and baby to start from the beginning together. There are a number of reasons why a baby may not be able to breast-feed at first: the baby may be in a special care unit, or have an illness such as severe jaundice; so he may be unable to suck, or the mother herself may be ill. In all these cases the baby is separated from the mother and it is necessary for the nurses to feed the baby his mother's milk in a bottle or by tube. She expresses her milk with a breast pump (*see* below) which also helps to establish lactation.

If you are worried about whether you will have enough milk for the baby later, it is worth knowing that as a result of the baby being put to the breast women have lactated even when several months or years have passed since they were pregnant or nursed a child. In some developing countries, where the large extended family is the rule rather than the exception, it is not at all unusual for post-menopausal grandmothers to share the breast-feeding routine with their daughters.

Many people believe that if the baby has had to be fed by bottle for a period, you cannot get him on to the breast. Certainly, there can be a problem getting the baby adjusted to your nipple, once he has gotten used to that of the bottle. It is important to tease the baby with the nipple so that he is able to get a large mouthful and respond to the new stimulus. You should have a bottle ready to give him if he becomes very hungry or upset, then try again at the next feeding. Eventually, in most cases, the baby will take the breast; and once breast-feeding has started, the process of getting the baby on to the breast becomes easier and easier.

Common fallacies

Many of the ideas that are quoted about breast-feeding are ill founded. In particular, there are several fallacies about breast-feeding that we can dispel now.

One of the common fallacies is that small breasts may not produce enough milk. In fact, they are at least as bountiful as large ones. If you are healthy, there is no reason why your breasts cannot produce milk, whatever their size or shape. The mother's supply of milk responds to the amount the baby takes and adapts to his needs.

When starting to breast-feed, women are often encouraged to feed the baby for a few minutes only on each breast and to increase the length of feedings very gradually. The reason given for this is that the nipples need time to harden or they will become sore. This idea is based on a misunderstanding about the reasons for sore nipples. Sucking will not damage your nipples if the baby is in the right position. In fact, restricting the length of feedings can hamper the development of an easy feeding relationship between mother and baby, distress the baby and lead to engorgement of the breasts.

It is sometimes thought that the concept of feeding "on demand" applies simply to when you feed, though in fact it applies also to the length of the feeding. It used to be thought that feeding a baby "on demand" in this way led to greedy and uncontrollable behavior by encouraging his "insatiable" appetite. But in the first few months, babies do gradually take more food at fewer meal times and sleep through most of the night, and they seem to have been programmed to do this since birth. They seem to know when they have had enough; it is possible that this is because of the changing quality of the milk during the feeding. The fat content is higher at the end of each breast. If mothers can accept that this is how it happens, they will be able to relax and enjoy breast-feeding.

Another erroneous idea connected with the timing of feedings is that hunger is the most common cause of crying. Curiously it is much more common for a baby to cry after a feeding than before, surely a sign that babies do not cry simply because they are hungry. In the young baby this crying seems to stem from some inexplicable discomfort that occurs after a good feeding; what makes this confusing for an inexperienced mother is that the baby may open his mouth frantically and shove his fist in, or seem to be searching desperately for the nipple. A mother will soon learn to differentiate this behavior from the way the baby behaves when he is genuinely hungry before a feeding.

Mothers may imagine that the length of the feeding time gets longer as the baby grows older – this can be worrying with a new baby who takes a long time to feed. In actual fact, the feeding time will become shorter and shorter as both mother and baby gain experience and become expert at the procedure. For a first-time mother, the time from when her newborn baby wakes for a feeding to the time when he is settled down again after it, may be up to an hour; but by as early as the second week of breast-feeding this time may be down to as little as half an hour.

It is also said that the breasts should be emptied at each feeding and that if the baby does not empty them the mother should express the milk. This is not true either. Since the milk supply adapts to demand, emptying the breasts merely causes more milk to come in. Comfort for the mother and baby lies in the natural rhythm of the baby's needs.

Many people imagine that the baby sucks the nipple, but this is not true. In fact he squeezes the milk from the breast by pressing with his hard palate and tongue on the ducts that lie behind the areola. The milk flows into the baby's mouth in response to the pressure, while the baby uses suction to stay in position. This suction, the lack of pain and the pattern of the baby's sucking are unmistakable once you have experienced them.

The baby uses different sucking patterns for bottle feeding and breast-feeding. A baby taking cow's milk will suck rhythmically for long continuous periods; a baby taking human milk will suck for short periods, with pauses in between. With breast-feeding, the baby must use his jaws, tongue and palate and breathe during this motion. With bottle feeding, the baby's tongue must only stop the continuous flow of milk. It is a suck, swallow, breathe motion. Too often the bottle-feeding pattern is taken as the norm and breast-feeding mothers are advised to rouse the baby if he pauses and to keep him feeding continuously. This is almost always unnecessary; but if the baby at the breast does need encouragement, a gentle nudge or bounce should be sufficient.

Many mothers are led to believe that the breast may suffocate the baby. This is impossible as the channel between the top lip and the nose provides a space for air. If this continues to worry you, however, you can gently draw back the top of the breast with your free hand as the baby drinks, but be careful not to compress the breast in such a way that the baby loses his grip.

Another fallacy is that breast-feeding can only continue until the baby cuts his teeth. In fact, as the mouth is wide open in the correct sucking action, the teeth do not meet during normal sucking, though the baby may sometimes take a playful nip!

Breast-feeding requires that the mother rests, eats well and gets enough liquid to drink. Mothers may worry, however, that the food they eat will affect the baby. No food will harm the baby but certain foods may give the baby loose bowel movements – for instance, onions, red wine or chocolate – if they are eaten to excess. Many mothers are told that they must drink a certain number of glasses of water a day while they are breast-feeding. This is unnecessary, and there is some evidence that too much fluid can suppress the production of milk. Breast-feeding does make one more thirsty than usual but your own thirst is the best guide to how much fluid you should drink. You will often find that you are thirsty as the baby begins to feed, so it is worth having a glass of some liquid (such as milk or water) handy to drink at this time.

Lastly, there is talk of breast-feeding making women tired or of the milk drying up once the mother starts to get up and around. Neither of these is true, but in the period after the birth the mother will be tired anyway and must have enough rest and eat well. Fatigue and tension are the worst enemies of breast-feeding, so mothers should try to rest whenever they feel tired. Relaxation techniques learned in pregnancy (*see* chapter 2) can help here. Breast-feeding is very relaxing and a superb opportunity to enjoy your baby.

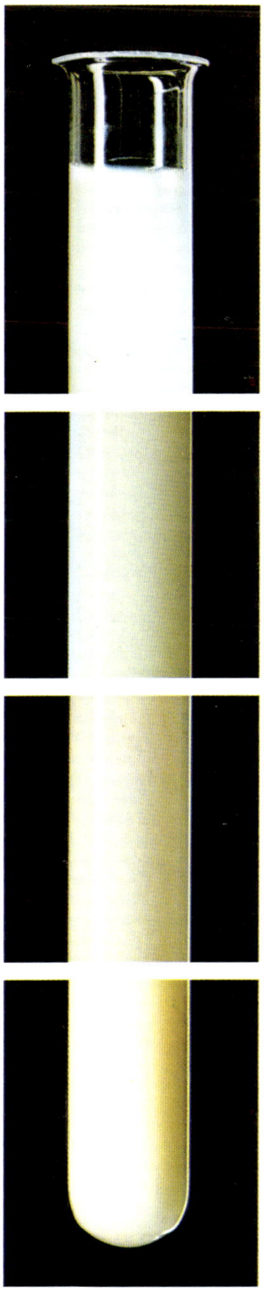

The appearance of breast milk changes considerably as time goes on. Compared with cow's milk (top), colostrum (bottom) appears very thick and creamy. Breast milk at six months (second from top) looks almost transparent and much thinner than a sample of early breast milk below it. At each stage, the milk is perfectly suited to the baby's nutritional needs.

How to breast-feed

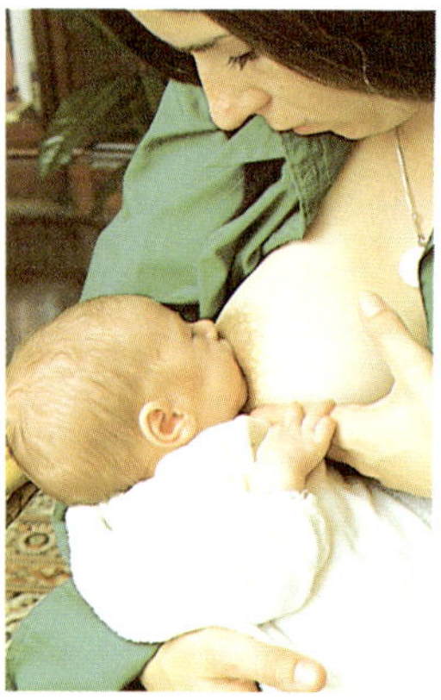

Feeding times should provide not only nourishment but an opportunity for play and discovery as the relationship between mother and baby develops.

At the beginning of a feeding make sure that you and the baby are both relaxed and comfortable. The first few feedings may take place in bed; and if it is difficult to sit upright because of a sore perineum, it is possible to feed lying down. This position is also excellent after a cesarean section. Once mobile, try to find a chair with a firm back and which is low enough for you to rest your feet flat on the floor, and cradle the baby in your arms. Failing this, sit on the edge of the bed with your feet on a chair. You may find that it helps to place the baby on a pillow at first so that you don't have to support his whole weight. Once you have learned to breast-feed you can discard the pillow.

Once you are both settled comfortably, move the baby toward you holding his head in one hand or in the crook of your arm. Hold the baby so that his mouth is in line with the nipple. Then move the baby toward you holding him so that his head is tipped back slightly and his bottom lip is nearest to the nipple and below it. Lean forward slightly while putting the baby to the breast.

The baby opens his mouth when his lips touch the nipple, so tease him with the nipple until his mouth is wide open before putting him on the breast. Aim his bottom lip at the bottom of the areola and his top lip will be in the right position to take the breast. Remember that the baby is mobile, so put the baby to the breast rather than the breast to the baby. If the nipple hurts, this may be a sign that the baby is not in the right position, because the nipple should be so far back in the mouth that there is no friction on it.

One of the first signs that things are going well is that after a few sucks, which initiate the let-down reflex, the baby falls into the typical rhythm of breast-feeding. This consists of long, deep sucks interspersed with rests during which he remains attached to the breast. His body is relaxed, but when sucking his ears wriggle, his scalp moves, and his cheeks remain full. (If the baby's cheeks are drawn in this means that there is not a good vacuum between his mouth and the breast.)

After the first short period on the breast the baby will often want to come off and rest. This is because the "let down" reflex of the milk is often too much at the beginning of the feeding. The baby swallows air to keep up and may need to burp at this stage.

If babies are burped at this stage it is often not necessary to burp them after the feeding, as the flow of milk steadies after the initial rush. Sit the baby up on your lap and rub his back so that he burps and brings up the air. The baby will then want to go back to the breast. He will stop of his own accord and then he may or may not want the second breast. This is a good time to change a diaper. As many babies have a bowel movement while on the first breast, and fall asleep on the second one, this timing has many advantages. Just remember to wash your hands carefully after you change the diaper.

One breast – frequently the left with the right-handed woman – is often easier to feed with at the beginning because the mother finds it easier to guide the baby with her right hand. Indeed, women who suffer from sore nipples often find that it is the right side (if they are right-handed) that is sore. This seems to confirm the notion that sore nipples are caused not by long feedings but by the way the baby takes the breast. If you are right-handed and find it difficult to feed the baby on the right breast with your left hand there is a simple solution. Instead of turning the baby around you can move the baby across in front of you with his feet under your right arm and still use your right hand to guide him. If you are comfortable and relaxed the baby will not be restless. Left-handed women will often find that the right breast is easier.

If you want to detach the baby while he is feeding, slip a finger between his mouth and the nipple to break the vacuum.

When to feed your baby

When to feed your baby and how much to give him is something only you and your baby can decide! You will be happiest if you feed him whenever you know he is hungry. You can judge this by the amount of time since his last feeding and how he ate then. It is often possible to feed a baby before he cries; babies are often awake and looking hungry before they start to cry. This is a good reason for not changing the diaper before the feeding, but giving the first breast without delay. If for some reason you have been delayed and baby gets very hungry, he may become upset. When this does happen, comfort him before you feed him. Once he is calmer he will find it much easier to eat, and you yourself will be more relaxed.

It is best if you start to breast-feed your baby from the first day so that he becomes used to the breast before the milk comes in. It is also likely that feeding in this early period helps to prevent engorgement. When the breast becomes engorged it is overfull and fluid swells the tissues beneath the areola making it difficult for the baby to suck. If this happens, gently compress the tissue underneath the areola with your finger and thumb. This pushes away the extra fluid in the tissues.

It is important to remember that each baby has a variable pattern and that this will change from day to day until a regular pattern emerges, usually after about two weeks. Thereafter the pattern will change more slowly and you will find that the number of feedings will begin to drop gradually.

Most babies are fed six to eight times in 24 hours at first. The gaps between feedings average two-and-a-half to four hours; some will be closer together than others, with a gap as short as two hours. The pattern of feeding might be a feeding before breakfast; during the morning; early afternoon; early evening; mother's bedtime; and one in the middle of the night. The first long gap between feedings to emerge in a large proportion of babies is often

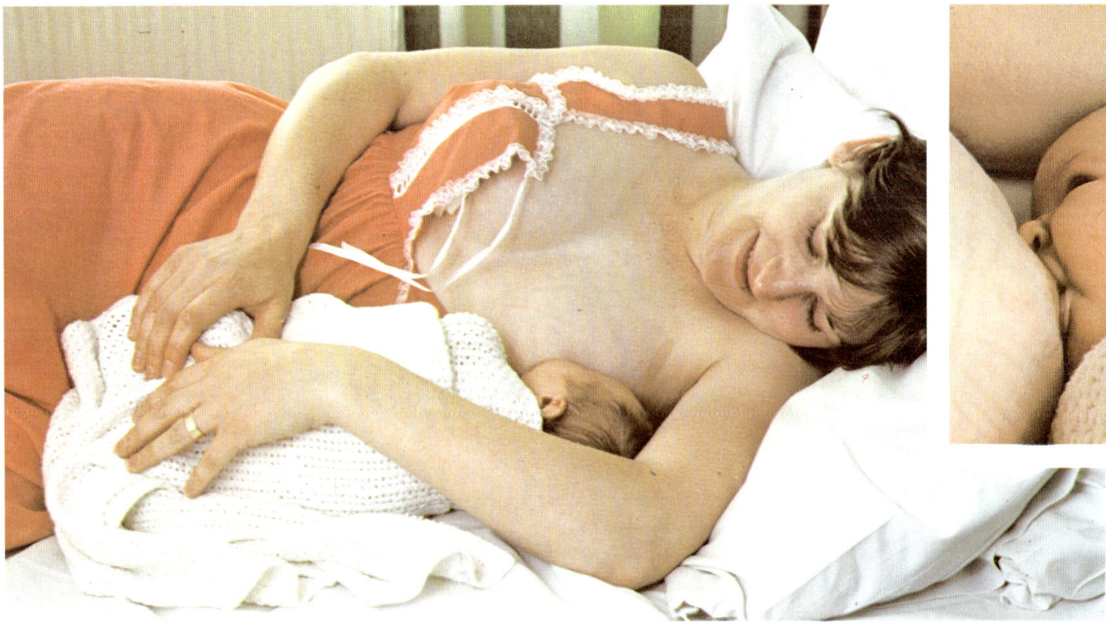

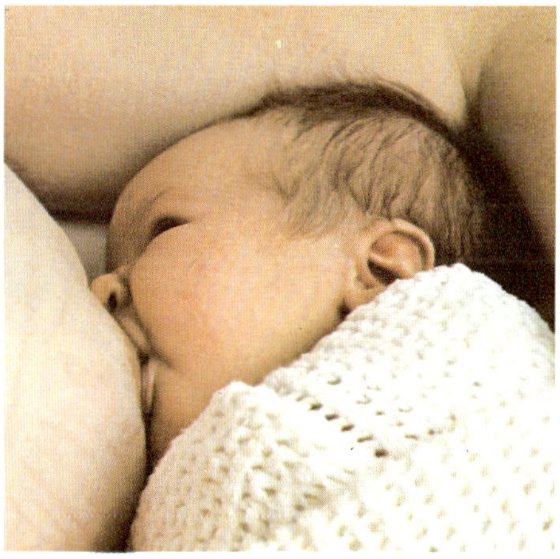

A good grip by the baby on the breast ensures that the sucking action is well rewarded! He should not suck on the nipple but on the areola.

If her stitches are sore, the new mother may be more comfortable feeding her baby lying down, well supported by pillows.

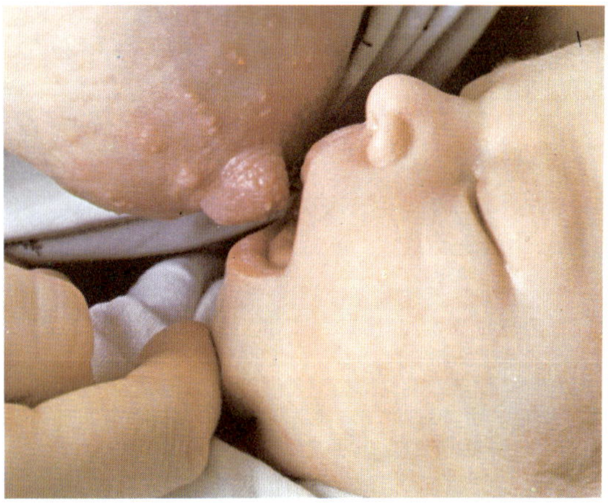

The sucking reflex is very strong in a newborn baby. If you gently stroke his cheek, he will turn toward the breast, lips pursed, ready to take the nipple into his mouth.

after the early evening feeding. This means the baby will wake for his next feeding in the middle of the night. The advantage of this pattern is that mothers can get some sleep either side of the feeding, instead of having to give both a late night feeding and an early morning feeding. This middle-of-the-night feeding tends to get later and later and eventually merges with the morning feeding.

Another pattern is the classical one where the first long gap is after the late evening feeding. If you try to persuade your baby to fall into this pattern by waking him to feed at 10 or 11, when he would have slept through till 2 or 3, you may find he still wakes to be fed in the middle of the night.

As at least one of the feedings in the early months will be at night, it is most important that you should get some sleep during the day.

Feeding may create problems during the day. New babies are easy to carry with you, especially if you use a sling or a front pack.

If you can take the baby with you, it is easy to feed in public discreetly. There is no reason why breast and nipples should show. If you wear a loose fitting garment that opens easily down the front, the baby can be slipped inside it. You may also find it helps to carry a shawl to throw over one shoulder, covering the baby and your breasts.

Care of the breasts

Breast-feeding is a natural process and the breasts adapt to it. The sebaceous glands in the areola produce a natural oil which serves to protect the breasts during breast-feeding. If however, you have particularly sensitive skin, it may help to rub a little cream into the breasts in the days after the birth while you and your baby are learning to breast-feed. It is also important not to use any soap while washing the nipples as this can remove the natural oils and make them more likely to become chafed. The breasts should be air-dried carefully after feedings for the same reason.

It is important to wear a bra which is comfortable and easy to undo for breast-feeding. Suitable bras designed especially for breast-feeding are widely available.

Contraception

Breast-feeding usually delays the resumption of the menses, but should not be relied upon for contraception. It is uncertain what effect any oral contraceptive has on the milk. Although the supply may not diminish, research has suggested that the quality may change. Since there are numerous barrier contraception options as well as the I.U.D., it is more prudent not to take a chance that steroid contraception might have some unfavorable effect on your baby. Most doctors won't prescribe the Pill during breast-feeding.

Drugs

Many substances, including drugs, pass to the baby in the milk. Few drugs should definitely not be taken while breast-feeding, but knowledge on this subject is still far from complete. If you need to take medication tell your doctor that you are breast-feeding. It is also better to avoid smoking while breast-feeding.

Expressing milk
There may be occasions when the mother needs to go out and cannot take the child with her. In these cases it is possible for the mother to express the milk by hand or with the help of a breast pump and to leave it in a bottle for someone else to feed to the baby. It is necessary to express a bit at previous feedings to accumulate enough for the baby to take at the missed feeding. Breast milk can be kept for up to 24 hours in a refrigerator, or for up to six months in a separate door freezer compartment.

It is possible to express by hand but some women find this laborious, and even unpleasant. It also has the disadvantage that it is difficult to trap the milk into a bottle. Expressing with the help of an electric or hand pump is easier. There are various designs of small hand pumps and electric pumps, which can be found in supermarkets and pharmacies.

Inverted nipples
If your nipples are flat, or inverted, they can be teased out by gently pulling with the finger and thumb or with the help of breast-care shields. This is best done during pregnancy, however, so that by the time the baby arrives the nipples are ready for breast-feeding.

Special care units
If your baby needs to be cared for in a special care unit immediately after birth it is still possible to give him breast milk by using a breast pump (*see* below). The milk can then be fed to the baby in a bottle, and when he is well, he can go to the breast. The advantage of this is that lactation will have been established.

Teething
There is no need to stop breast-feeding once the baby starts to teethe, provided that he is taking the breast correctly (*see* p. 140). At times, the baby may take a playful nip, but this rarely causes concern.

The problems

There is no doubt that breast-feeding can be simple, fun and give the mother and baby a great deal of pleasure and enjoyment. Yet it would be wrong to gloss over the fact that there can be problems. If you do have difficulties, seek advice.

Colic or irritable crying
We do not understand what causes babies to have bouts of discomfort. It is not uncommon for a baby to have a restless period between some of his feedings. In manageable cases the baby can be comforted by being held and talked to; it is amazing how often it happens in the evening, when there are other people to share in the comforting.

If the baby seems to suffer severe discomfort a doctor may be able to prescribe an antispasmodic or other medication.

Cracked and sore nipples
Cracked and sore nipples usually occur when a baby is not taking the breast correctly. Start with short, frequent feedings. If you develop sore nipples, consult your doctor and keep trying. In nearly all cases, once you have found the best position for the baby, the nipple will heal. Remember that the baby should not grasp the nipple while breast-feeding. Instead the gums, hard palate and tongue should press on the areola and the nipple should be well back in the baby's mouth.

Sore nipples may develop if the breasts become overfull. This sometimes occurs in the early days of feeding before the mother's breasts have adjusted to the baby's requirements. If this happens you may find that it helps to express some of the milk by hand. Standing in a hot shower can also help to relieve the soreness.

Dripping
About 10 per cent of women may drip milk from the other breast when the baby feeds from the first side. The milk can be absorbed by a bra padded with tissues or a nursing pad or a standard 4 × 4 sterile gauze pad.

A woman may also leak when a feeding is "due" or in response to her baby's (or even

EXPRESSING MILK

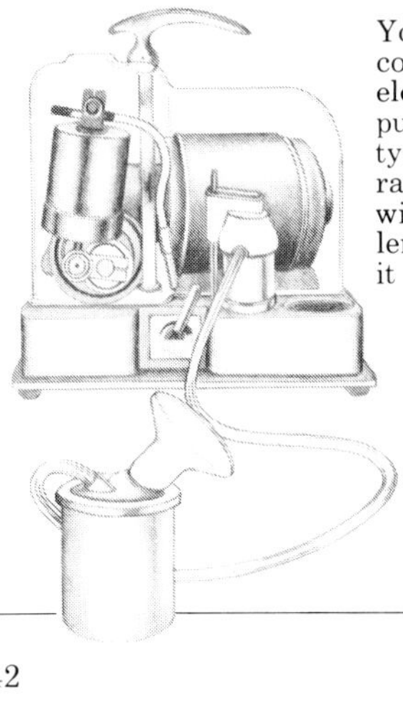

You may find it convenient to use an electric pump. As the pulling action of this type of pump can be rather strong, you may wish to limit the length of time you use it on each breast.

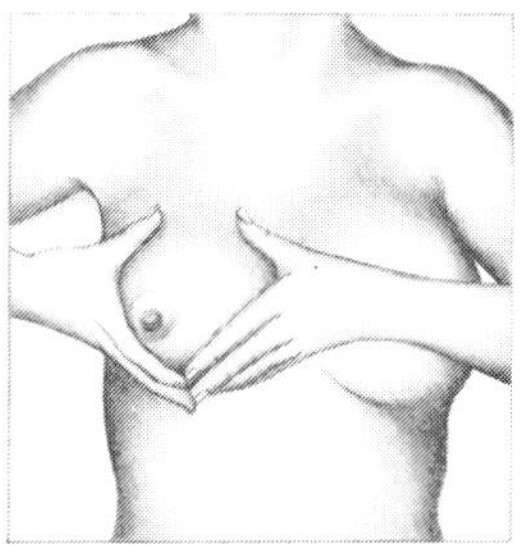

To express milk manually, gently massage to start the milk moving down the ducts. Work evenly around the breast, stroking repeatedly downward toward the areola.

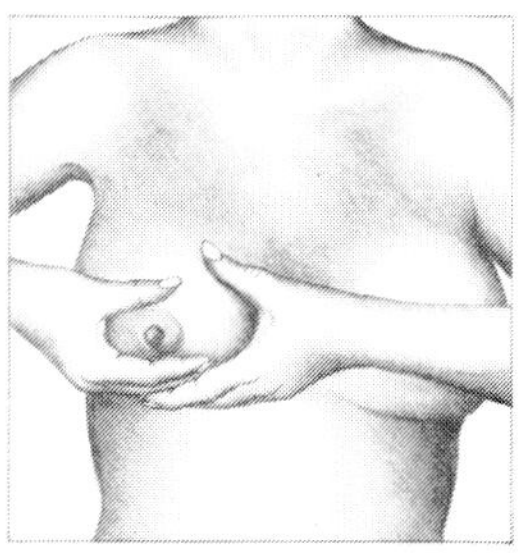

Starting about halfway up the breast, run your thumb firmly down. As it reaches the edge of the areola, press in and up and the milk will squirt from the nipple.

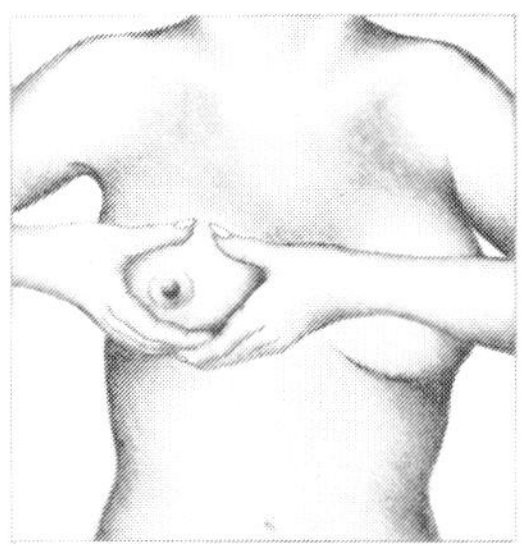

Do not squeeze the nipple, as this will close the ducts, or continue expressing until you think the breast is empty. Stop when the milk starts coming in drips rather than jets.

some other baby's) cry. This reaction tends to happen much more frequently during early lactation; with experience and the establishment of a routine, it eventually settles down.

Engorgement
The breasts can become engorged when the milk supply and the feeding pattern of the baby are out of phase during the first week after birth when the milk first comes in and the blood supply to the breasts increases. Engorgement means that the breast itself is too full for the baby to be able to take milk. It may also mean that the breast behind the areola is swollen, with fluid in the tissues.

It is possible to press the fluid away from behind the areola by squeezing it gently between the forefinger and thumb. Occasionally it is necessary to express milk by hand or with the help of a breast pump (*see* below). If your breasts are also painful you may find that it helps to take hot baths, which will encourage the milk to flow, or to use cold compresses or ice packs, which will soothe the pain.

Gas
Your baby will certainly swallow some air along with his or her milk. When the stomach becomes uncomfortable, he will "burp" to relieve the pressure. Give your baby the opportunity to bring up air after a feeding by holding him upright against your shoulder and rubbing or patting his back gently. This will encourage the lighter air to rise above the level of the milk in the stomach and escape, possibly bringing a little milk with it. Do not, however, feel you must sit there doggedly until the magic sound is heard. If your baby is uncomfortable, put him to sleep lying on his abdomen; he will burp later if he needs to.

Insufficient lactation
Insufficient lactation is thought to occur quite frequently because it is the reason so commonly given for giving up breast-feeding. An apparent shortage of milk seems to be an acceptable explanation for the baby's normal disturbed behavior after some meals – whereas this is frequently a sign of being well fed. Once doubts have crept in it isn't long before supplementary bottle feedings are given and then the supply will definitely begin to diminish. There are two situations when the baby may actually not be getting enough milk and both may ultimately lead to an inadequate supply. Firstly, the baby may not have a good grip so the milking action is not good and the baby receives only a small amount of milk for each sucking action. Secondly, the duration and frequency of feeding times might have been restricted and this can lead to a diminished supply. The solution is to make sure that the baby is well "on" and is allowed to suck as frequently and for as long as he or she requires. If the baby has actually lost weight and is sleepy, it might be necessary for a day or two to wake him regularly for feedings. Frequent feedings on both breasts is recommended.

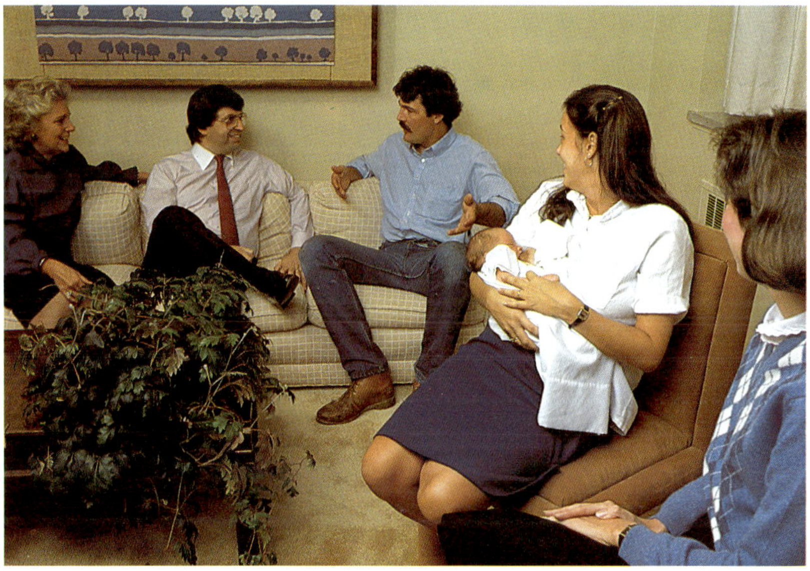

Some people fear that breast-feeding in public will be a problem, but there is no need for the breast and nipple to show. It is worth persevering, as it greatly increases the mother's ability to get out and about.

Mastitis
Mastitis (*see* pp. 120–3), is a painful red area on one of the breasts. This is initially caused by a blockage in one of the milk ducts and milk leaking into the tissues. This area then may become infected and cause inflammation of the breast tissue and on rare occasions an abscess. If either of your breasts become inflamed in this way, apply heat to the area and contact your doctor immediately. Early treatment can prevent mastitis from progressing to an abscess and the condition usually clears in a few days. One of the first signs of mastitis is aching and shivering like the onset of flu. If you develop mastitis, your doctor will usually prescribe some antibiotics. You may continue breast-feeding even on the breast which is affected by the inflammation.

Weaning
Some mothers may be anxious about how long they should breast-feed. The process of introducing the baby to solid food and the changing pattern of feeding is described in chapter 13. Ideally the mother will breast-feed until her baby can be fed entirely by cup and spoon, probably at about eight to ten months. But the baby's own reactions are the best guides. Some babies give up the breast suddenly. Others will continue to take one or more feedings a day until they are one or even two years old. Breast-feeding can happily continue even when it is no longer nutritionally necessary.

Weight gain
It is almost impossible for a breast-fed baby to be overfed. It is, however, possible that he or she will not gain weight fast enough. Do not worry unnecessarily about your baby's weight, your doctor will advise you about how much your baby should gain. It is possible that your doctor or pediatrician may recommend waking the baby for more frequent feedings to boost the weight gain.

Bottle feeding

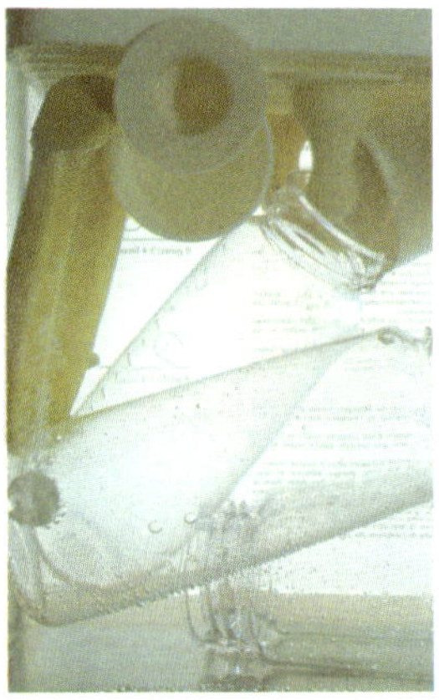

Not every mother wants to breast-feed her baby. Some cannot do so for a variety of reasons, e.g. wanting to return to work, or having to take medication, or some simply prefer bottle feeding. Bottle feeding is quite satisfactory if the right precautions are taken, and most babies will thrive on it.

There is a wide variety of specially prepared formulas for babies, but almost all are based on cow's milk. Milk, whether human or from a cow, is 90 per cent water, and it is in the remaining 10 per cent that the differences in food substances lie. Cow's milk may be modified to bring it closer to human milk.

If you are bottle feeding, then your baby will be started on this method with a commercial formula. In the United States, such a formula is available to everybody regardless of the family's financial means. Most families can buy the formula at a local store. But, if their means are limited, they can obtain such a formula through the WIC program. Commercial formula comes premixed in a bottle ready to feed or as a powder to be added to sterile water, or as concentrated formula to be diluted with water. The nipple-bottle premixed formula unit is the most convenient and the most expensive. The powdered formula requires more preparation but is less expensive.

Breast milk comes "ready mixed". There is no way of succumbing to any temptation of "adding one for the pot," or putting in that "spoonful of sugar" because "he likes it sweet". The pharmaceutical manufacturers have carefully prepared artificial feeding formula to simulate human milk. It is important to mix formula according to the manufacturer's instructions, always to use the scoop provided, and never to add sugar unless specifically told to do so by your doctor.

Breast milk is sterile, and breast-fed babies have added protection through their mothers' antibodies which a bottle-fed baby cannot receive. It is therefore important to develop a routine for the sterilization of bottles and nipples. Remember that scrupulously clean hands are most important. It is wise to use paper towels, if possible, for drying them, as a less than clean hand towel will undo all your good work.

One advantage of bottle feeding is that the mother need not always be available to give it in person. This is of course true, but it is not necessarily a good thing. If nature's way is to make sure that this particular mother-baby couple (the "nursing couple") is together at regular intervals, day in, day out for the first few weeks then truly successful bottle feeding may also depend on just this regularity and closeness. Obviously, there are bound to be exceptions, and one of these will be the night when the mother is desperately tired and the father gives the night feeding. For most of the time, however, it is probably better if the nursing couple remains the same, and the time the mother spends cuddling and talking to her baby is most important. However, some fathers like to join in this relationship by assuming one of the feedings each day.

It is the inevitability of close physical contact during breast-feeding which constitutes one of the major differences between breast- and bottle feeding. But, if the mother is careful to provide cuddling and eye-to-eye contact with her baby, there should be no less mother-infant bonding with bottle-feeding. It is all a matter of attitude. This is a time for physical contact and love. Bottle feeding, however, is the father's only chance to take part in the feeding process.

In summary, follow the instructions for preparing a feeding and for sterilizing equipment meticulously. Then bear in mind what your baby could miss in terms of contact with his mother – make sure you do not let this happen, and he will thrive.

Sterilizing

The only way to be sure of absolute safety for your baby is to follow the sterilizing instructions for your feeding equipment. They may sound laborious at first, but will soon become second nature.

Sterilization of feeding utensils can be stopped at about nine months or as soon as the baby starts to crawl; boiling milk and water can also be dispensed with at this time. Feeding bottles should always be sterilized, however. More information is given in chapter 13.

Cleaning equipment Whatever method you are using to sterilize your equipment, whether by the boiling method or by the dishwasher method; routine cleaning after a feeding is a must. Traces of milk left on bottles or nipples can breed germs and hamper proper sterilization which may endanger your baby's health.

Rinse the bottle and nipple in cold water before removing the nipple, and start by scrubbing the outside of the nipple in order to rid it completely of any mucus. Take off the nipple, turn it inside out, and scrub the inside. Rinse off the nipple. The nipples should be boiled for two or three minutes and then stored in a sterile jar.

Rinse the inside of the bottle with cold water, as you would with an ordinary milk bottle, as hot water makes the milk stick. Wash the bottle in warm water with a detergent, and brush well with a bottle brush, then rinse in clear water. This brush also has to be kept very clean. Then you may sterilize the bottles by boiling or by running through the dishwasher.

The boiling method If you have glass bottles and wish to use the boiling method of sterilization, clean the bottles and put the equipment in a pan of cold water that covers it completely. Put on a lid; bring to a boil; and keep boiling for at least five minutes. Leave to cool in the pan with the lid on until it is needed. Equipment should be boiled after each feeding. It can be safely left in the pan for up to 12 hours, after draining the water; but after that needs boiling again. Boil nipples separately for two to three minutes only.

The dishwasher method In the United States most modern dishwashers reach temperatures that are adequate to cleanse and sterilize the bottles and feeding utensils. The nipples should be boiled separately for two to three minutes because the dishwasher cycle could cause them to crack. Clean the items before placing them in the dishwasher. Place them well away from the heating element and stack the bottles securely in the racks so they will not flip over during washing.

Equipment

Bottles: Buy a dozen 8-ounce bottles. You will only need six to eight a day. But over the months you are going to misplace or break a few bottles. You can purchase two or three 4-ounce bottles for water or juice feedings, but you can use the 8-ounce bottles just as well and then you will have only one size to contend with. Pyrex bottles have the advantage of not breaking if they are heated or cooled too quickly. Although they cost slightly more, the problem of cracking due to rapid temperature changes is real, so they are good value. Plastic bottles have the advantage of not breaking when they are dropped.
Nipples: Buy at least a dozen. You will probably prefer the kind with one or more holes on the top. If the nipples contain silicon they will tolerate boiling better and last longer.
Sterilizing container: This can be a roasting pan or a pot designed specifically for sterilizing baby's bottles. It must have a lid and be big enough to accommodate a rack that holds eight bottles.

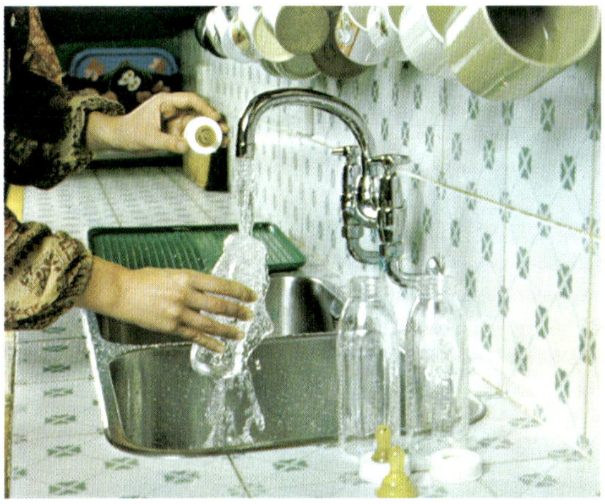

1. Routine cleansing of feeding equipment is most important. Rinse the inside of the bottle with cold water, as hot water makes the milk stick.

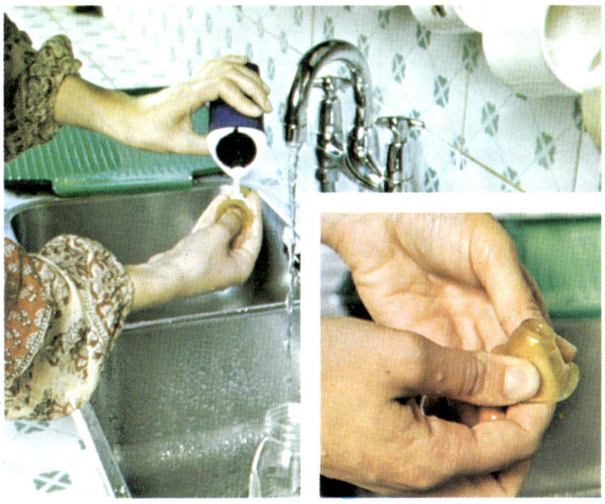

2. After scrubbing the outside of the nipple while it is still on the bottle, remove the nipple, turn it inside out, and scrub the inside as well. This removes any mucus. Rinse off with warm water.

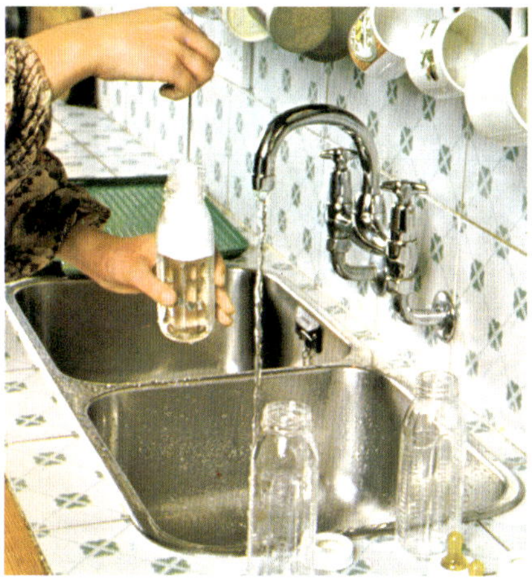

3. Wash the bottle in warm water with a detergent, and brush well with a bottle brush, then rinse in clear water. You must make sure that this brush is also kept scrupulously clean, either by boiling or by using a detergent solution.

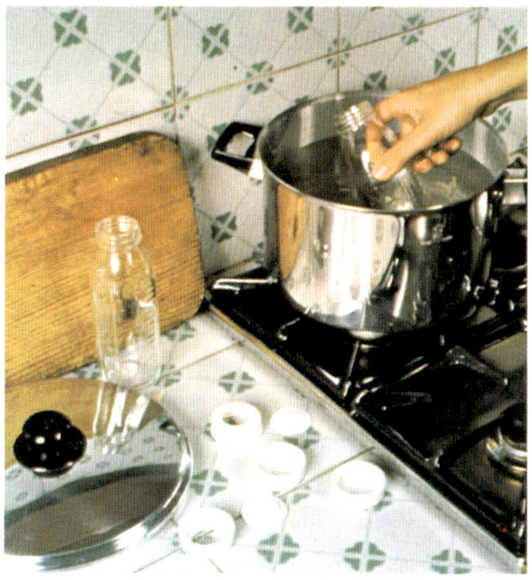

4. To sterilize by boiling, put the equipment in a pan of cold water that covers it completely. Put on a lid; bring to a boil and keep boiling for at least five minutes. Leave to cool in the pan with the lid on.

Preparing a feeding

The bottle-nipple formula unit

The easy pre-packaged formula is available at a local supermarket. This comes in a bottle-nipple formula unit which is as hassle-free as breast-feeding. There is no need to mix the formula, to sterilize or refrigerate. This formula unit can be bought in handy 6-pack quantities or in larger cases. These ready-to-use bottle-nipple formula units come in 4-ounce, 6-ounce and 8-ounce disposable bottles.

The extraordinary convenience of these formula units has made this type of bottle feeding very popular. If this is so convenient, why don't all bottle-feeding mothers use these units? The answer is obvious: the cost is considerably more. But, to many parents, it is well worth the expense to have a convenient and hassle-free method of bottle-feeding.

Commercially prepared formula

Prepared formulas can also be purchased in your local pharmacy. They make the routine of preparing a baby's formula simple and, generally, foolproof. They require mixing, sterilizing bottles and refrigeration for storage once the formula is prepared.

The prepared formula comes in ready-to-use content reduced and sugar (lactose) added to make them more like human milk. Vitamins A, C and D and minerals have been added. Your doctor may request that you purchase prepared formula with added iron.

The prepared formula come in ready-to-use 32-ounce cans which is poured directly into the bottles without the addition of water. Prepared formula also comes in concentrated form in a 13-ounce can which must be diluted with water. Finally, there is a concentrated prepared formula that comes in powdered form, requiring the addition of sterile water.

Mixing a formula requires precise measuring and meticulous adherence to sterile technique. Whether you use concentrated prepared liquid or powder formula, careful measuring is essential. Follow the instructions precisely. The bottles may be sterilized in advance and the formula prepared by the addition of sterilized water. Or the formula may be mixed with tap water and added to the bottle. Then, the bottles containing formula are sterilized. This is called terminal sterilization. Whatever method you use, remember that if you allow the formula to be contaminated with even a small number of bacteria, these bacteria will multiply and can cause severe illness.

If a mother has enough bottles she may save herself a lot of time by preparing several feedings at once, cooling them quickly and keeping them in the refrigerator. When it is nearly time for the baby's feeding, she can warm it up, either by standing the bottle in hot water, or by using one of the commercial sterilizers. A feeding should always be heated (or cooled) quickly because germs thrive in

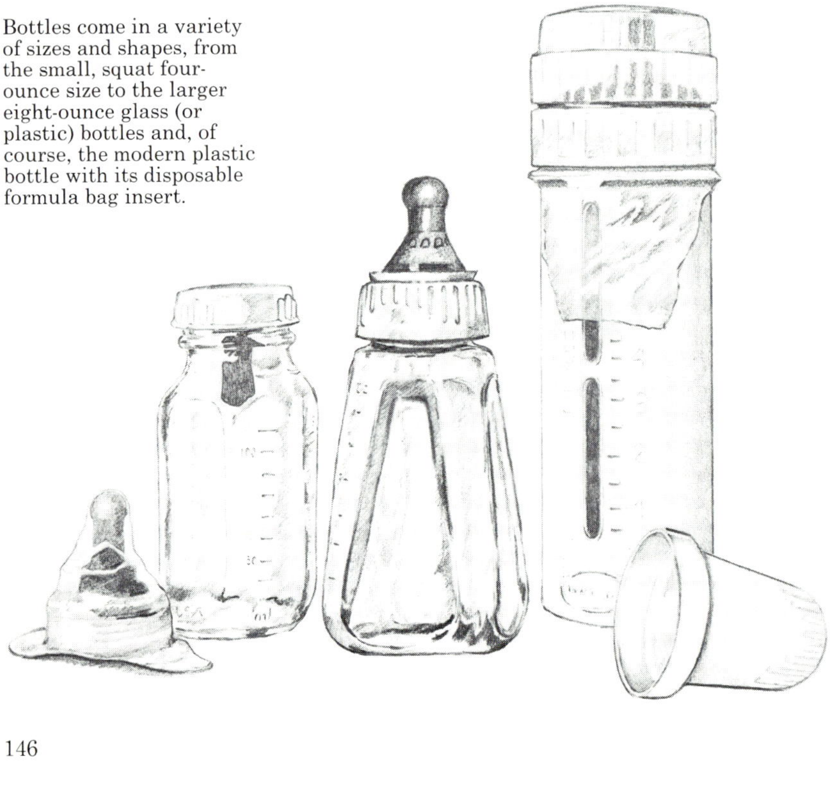

Bottles come in a variety of sizes and shapes, from the small, squat four-ounce size to the larger eight-ounce glass (or plastic) bottles and, of course, the modern plastic bottle with its disposable formula bag insert.

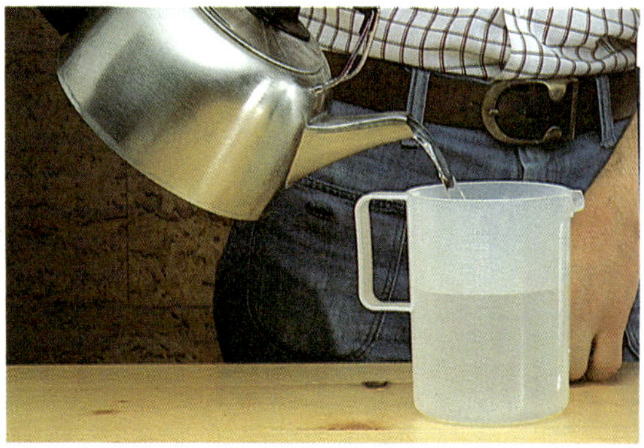

1

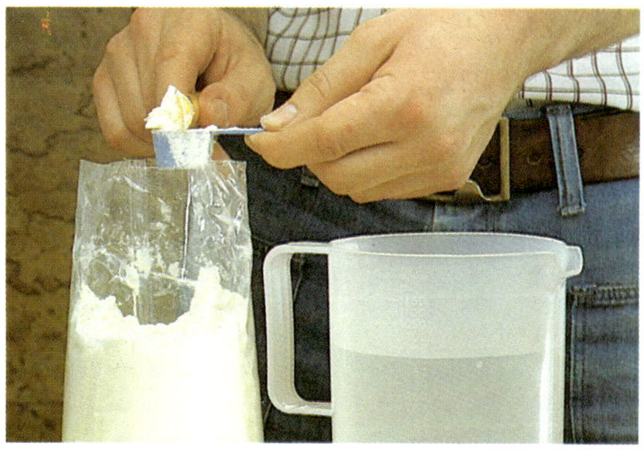

2

1. Sterilize the water by boiling before measuring as some will evaporate. Let it cool to hand-heat. Take measuring cup, mixing spoon and knife from sterilizer. Pour water into cup, checking the quantity carefully.

2. Use only the scoop provided for the milk powder and level off each measure with a sterile knife. Do not be tempted to "heap" the measure in the belief that it is more nourishing for the baby. Over-concentrated feeds lead to overweight babies, and can be dangerous.

slow temperature changes. The useful bottle insulators on the market are to make sure that the bottle remains cool while traveling, or as an alternative to a refrigerator, and not, as some people suppose, as an alternative to a thermos for hot liquids.

If the feedings are going to be kept in the refrigerator, prepare them as usual, and put on the bottle cap with the nipple inverted. Remember to hold the nipple by the outside rim only, or it will no longer be sterile.

Cool the feeding as quickly as possible and put the bottle in the refrigerator.

Breast milk always comes at the right temperature, but when you are getting a bottle feeding ready, you may have to cool it, or warm it up if it comes out of the refrigerator. It is important always to test the temperature against the back of your hand or inside of your wrist and, if in doubt, give the baby too cool rather than too warm a feeding.

Even when a bottle is being warmed from very cold, it is still important to test the temperature on the back of the hand, or wrist, as the milk can easily get too hot.

The breast-fed baby often comes to his or her mother to find that the breast is already dripping with milk because her "let down" reflex has been set off by his cry, or by the realization that the feeding is due. To be fair, the bottle-fed baby should not have to struggle for his feeding either, so it is important to make sure that the milk really does drip when the bottle is held vertically, and without being shaken, although, of course, the drip does stop after a few seconds. Try counting the drips and, if they are just too fast to count, the hole in the nipple is about the right size. If the milk comes out in slow drips, the hole in the nipple is either blocked or too small. The same is true if the baby takes longer than 20 minutes to feed, unless he is one of those sleepy babies who has to be cajoled all the time.

Modern nipples do not often block, but the hole may be too small. To enlarge the hole, stick the blunt end of a needle into a cork (so you have a firm hold and will not burn your fingers). Heat the point to a white heat and place it into the hole in the nipple for a short time – be sure not to enlarge it too much.

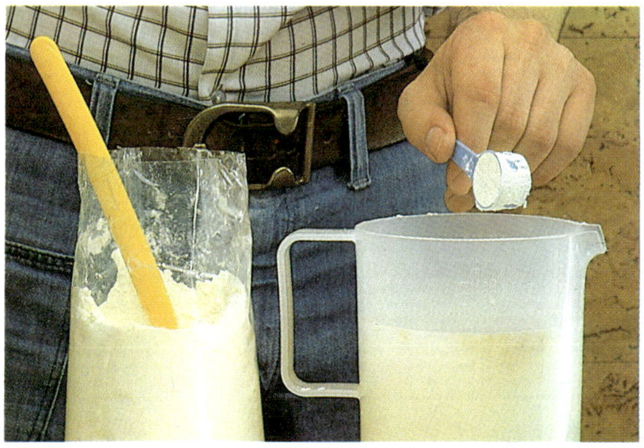

3

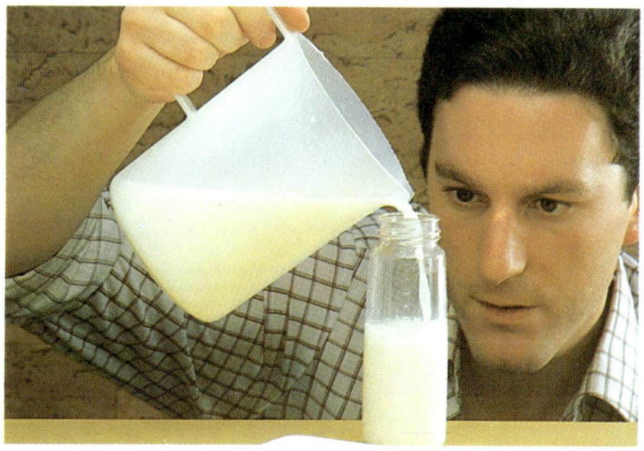

5

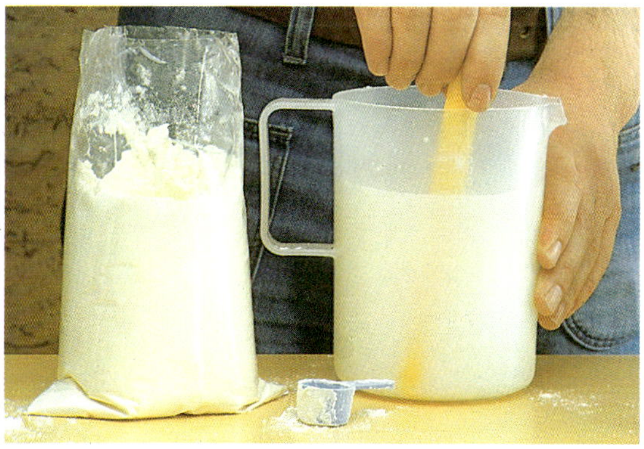

4

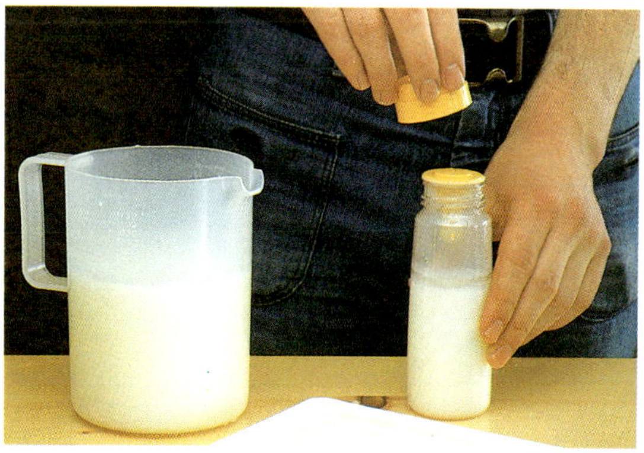

6

3. Add the required number of measures to the water. Do not add "one for the pot" as this will make the feeding too strong. If the formula you are using needs added sugar, measure this very carefully.

4. Stir the mixture very thoroughly with a sterile spoon. Some formulas are more easily mixed than others. You should keep stirring until the mixture is completely free of lumps as these will block the nipple, and interfere with the flow of the milk.

5. Remove the bottle from the sterilizing solution and drain. Do not rinse. Pour the required amount of milk into the bottle. It is a good idea to put in a couple of ounces more than you think the baby will need as his appetite will vary a little from feeding to feeding.

6. Screw the nipple upside down on the bottle. Cover with their sterile caps. If you wish to make up several bottles at once, store either a covered container or the filled bottles in a refrigerator. Never leave feedings standing at room temperature.

How to bottle feed

If the hole in the nipple is too small, you can easily enlarge it. Push eye of needle into a cork, so it can be held easily. Heat the point of the needle until it is white-hot then insert it into the hole in the nipple. Milk should come out at several drops per second.

A lot of research has been done recently on the first few minutes and hours of life. When mothers and babies are left alone at this time (hopefully with the father too), a gentle dialogue may take place, with the baby wide-eyed and awake, looking at his or her mother, and the mother caressing and looking at her child. This eye contact is very important. The baby at the breast lies with his gaze at exactly the right distance from his mother's face for him to see her, for his still immature ability to focus means that he can only do so at this distance. So, in the bustling confusion around him, the one point of contact is his mother's face, at which he gazes with such rapt attention.

The traditional way to bottle feed a baby is by cradling his head in the crook of one arm and holding the bottle with the other. If you remember to hold the bottle up and to lean slightly forward so that you and the baby look directly at each other, you will establish excellent communication. This achieves the same body and eye contact as breast-feeding. An alternative way to bottle feed is the "*en face*" position. Sit on a bed, sofa or chair, comfortably propped up, and with knees bent. Lay your baby with head against your knees and his feet up against your abdomen. Then support his head with one hand, using the other to hold the bottle. If you feed him in this position, he can look at you, and you can look at him, talk to him and get to know him. But what this position gains in eye-to-eye contact it loses in cuddling and baby contact.

Some babies seem to need their mother's whole attention while feeding, and will go on a hunger strike if they have to compete with the television or radio. Mothers, too, will soon find that they can enjoy their babies more when they concentrate in this way. Occasionally, in a moment of stress, a mother may leave the bottle propped up against the side of the crib or a cushion. But the practice could lead to the baby choking so it is potentially dangerous, as well as depriving the baby of a few precious moments with his mother who is, after all, the center of his universe.

Most mothers use wide necked bottles which stand upright, and are made either of glass or plastic. When the baby is taking a feeding, it is important to check that the bottle neck contains milk and not air, as the baby who swallows a lot of air, either for that reason or because he is taking the feeding too fast, is often sick with the large amount of gas he has to bring up.

A baby usually indicates when he has had enough, and the sensible mother will not worry too much about how much he has taken. The exact intake cannot be measured in breast-feeding, when there are only subjective "feelings" to go on, but the bottle feeding mother cannot fail to see how much, or how little, the baby has left. The maxim of $2\frac{1}{2}$ oz/lb body weight (175 ml per kg body weight) per day is a useful guide, though it is only a guide. The amount taken may vary from feeding to feeding.

It is worth giving the baby enough milk at any one feeding so that he leaves just a little in the bottle when he has had enough. The baby who appears to demand feeding every two hours, or more frequently, is either not getting enough, or is thirsty or upset.

When to feed

Bottle feeding makes possible the strict scheduling of feedings in a way that breast-feeding cannot. In the past, the conventional pattern of feeding at 6am, 10am, 2pm, 6pm and 10pm was undoubtedly adhered to far too rigidly; feeding "on demand" was supposed to lead to spoiled and demanding children, whereas feeding "on schedule" disciplined the baby right from the start into a socially acceptable pattern. Such concepts as "discipline" and "spoiling", however, are virtually meaningless when applied to the newborn baby: probably much of the success claimed from feeding "on schedule" from the very beginning was a result simply of the baby's maturing digestive system. After a few weeks, once the baby has become accustomed to the pattern of hunger/feeding/satisfaction, he will probably only demand food every three to four hours as it takes this long to digest a full feeding. In the early days however it is best to treat the bottle-fed baby as if he were breast-feeding. Leaving him to cry until it is "time" for his feeding will leave you both in such a state that he won't be able to calm down for the feeding, will swallow an ounce or so and then be screaming for more in another hour. Until a pattern emerges, a certain amount of flexibility will be easier on everyone's nerves.

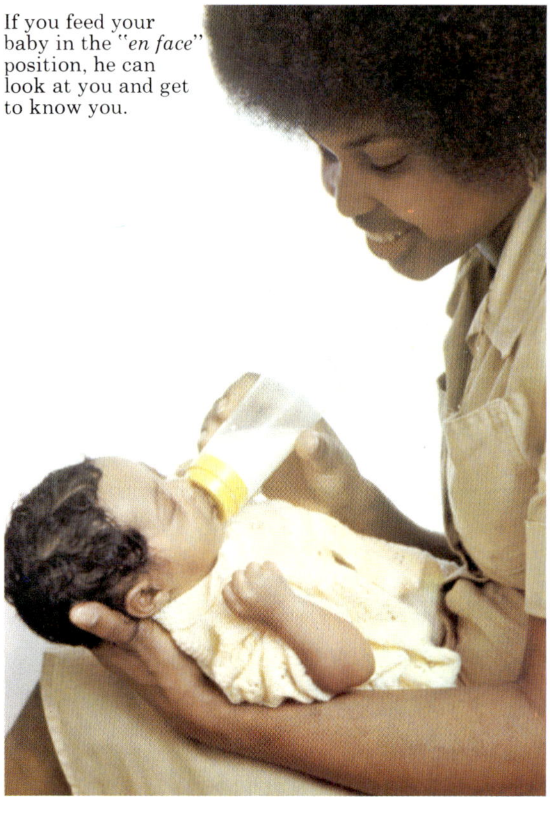

If you feed your baby in the "*en face*" position, he can look at you and get to know you.

The problems of bottle feeding

Stools

A mother who has breast-fed a previous baby may be concerned at the appearance of the stools in her bottle-fed baby. The breast-fed baby's stool has a particular color, consistency and a unique, aromatic smell (*see* p. 160). The bottle-fed baby's stool is often pale green, fairly formed, crumbly, and smells quite different. He is likely to pass a little each day, unlike the breast-fed baby who may produce nothing for several days, then have a large stool. The bottle-fed baby's stool may be hard and look difficult to pass, although this may not be the case. If the weather is warm, and the stools are hard, it will do no harm to give the baby a little extra fluid, in the form of cooled boiled water, either on its own or in a diluted fruit juice drink.

Travel

Although it is true that bottle feeding while traveling does not entail the embarrassment sometimes caused by breast-feeding, it may involve more in the way of preparation and special equipment. The amount of luggage required seems out of all proportion to the size of the individual needing it! It is worth planning carefully before you set out in order to keep the amount of "clutter" to a minimum while making sure that no vital piece of equipment is left behind. This may reduce the spontaneity of excursions, but it will also reduce the degree of "wear and tear" on the parents', and the baby's, nerves. Don't stay at home simply because it all seems too much bother. Keep a comprehensive checklist of items you will need to have with you. You can refer to this list both quickly and easily, and after your first trip, preparation will become second nature.

The safest, and simplest method, if there are going to be several feedings during a trip, is to buy premixed ready-to-use formula like Enfamil or Similac from a local store. These come in handy six-packs and are extremely convenient for traveling. No additional equipment is needed. There is no need to warm up your baby's milk while traveling and *never* try to keep it warm for any length of time as any germs will multiply rapidly. It is better to give your baby a cold feeding. This will do the baby no harm and you can be reassured that he is getting a full meal.

When traveling abroad, particularly in countries with a warmer climate and perhaps a water supply of questionable safety, hygiene is the most important point to remember. Sterilizing of equipment (*see* p. 145) is of course essential at all times. Bear in mind also that the bacteria in less temperate climates, while not necessarily more virulent than those of your own environment, are certainly less familiar and possibly less easily dealt with by the body's own defense systems.

Weight gain

Some mothers fear that their babies will get fat on the bottle. This is not necessarily the case, but does sometimes happen. In the past, mothers were not so strongly urged to follow the formula manufacturers' instructions, but rather to follow their instincts and the baby's individual demands. This led to a generous attitude toward a spoonful of extra sugar "for energy", and sometimes even more. A dangerous situation could arise, particularly in hot weather, or if the baby had a fever. The feeding became too strong, and the baby's kidneys had difficulty in excreting all the salt. The baby also put on too much weight. The popular practice of adding cereal to the late-night bottle, in the hope that the baby will sleep longer, should also be avoided as this can cause a great weight gain.

Nowadays, mothers are advised to follow manufacturers' instructions; to use the correct scoops, to level them off, and never to press the dried milk down in order to add more. They are advised against adding sugar. The baby should be offered a feeding which holds just that much more than he or she will take, and then be left to demand his next feeding after a reasonable time. If he cries within an hour of a good feeding, he may have gas, or have a pin sticking into him, or just be lonely. He is unlikely to be hungry. Mothers who resist the temptation to respond to every cry with another bottle will make sure that their baby is not overfed and, as a direct consequence, overweight.

Sometimes a baby may get thirsty, particularly in hot weather, or if he has diarrhea or a fever. He may thus accept a bottle-feeding although what he really wants is plain water. It is advisable to keep boiled water in the refrigerator in a sterilized bottle at all times so that, if the baby is crying and it is not yet time for his feeding, you can give him some cool, boiled water, which may, in fact, be all he wants for the time being.

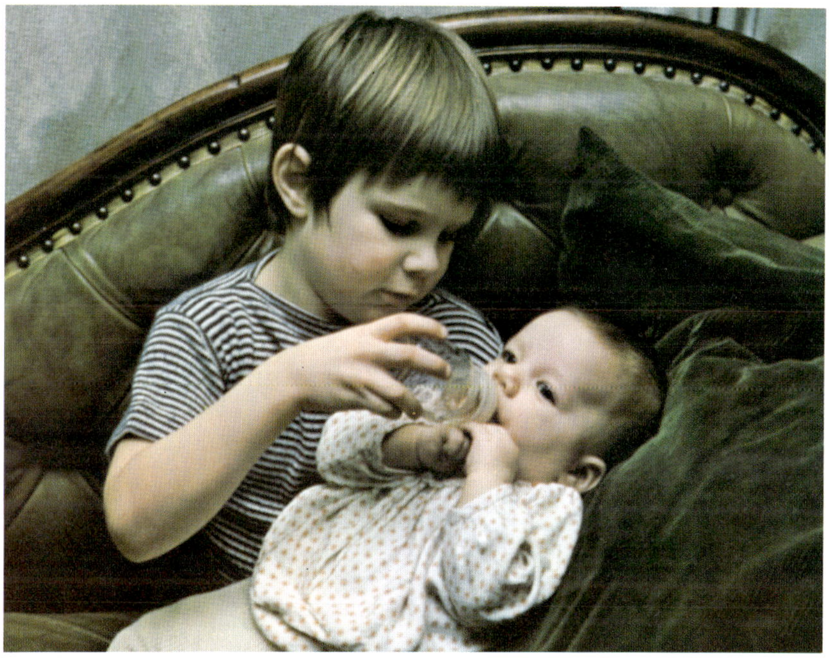

Overweight can be a problem with bottle-fed babies, if every cry is interpreted as hunger. He could easily be thirsty and would welcome a drink of cooled boiled water or diluted fruit juice. Other members of the family can help with these refreshments.

The new baby at home

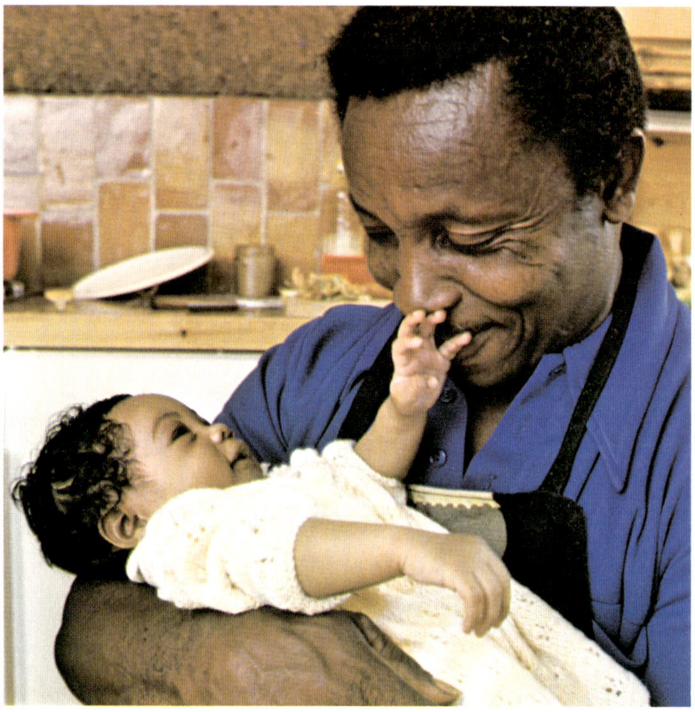

CHAPTER 11

Organizing the routine

Fathering

Bathing the baby

Elimination

Changing diapers

Every new mother looks forward to the day when she takes her baby home from the hospital. She cannot wait to have her baby all to herself at last. Once home, however, many women feel less sure of themselves and confidence begins to slip away. Friends and relations offer conflicting advice and, ultimately, a mother must make up her own mind about what is best for her baby – but how does she know? She is, after all, still tired after the hard work of labor. Sitting down may feel uncomfortable and if she is breast-feeding, her breasts may appear to have a life of their own.

A baby often seems to cry more once at home, and when he or she cries the mother feels sure there must be something wrong. He must be sick to keep crying like that. When it stops, it is even worse – he must be dead! Common sense says this is nonsense: of course he is all right, he has just gone to sleep. But the mother must make sure, so she creeps over to have a look at him. Usually this is enough to reassure her. Occasionally she is still concerned by his color – babies are often very pale in sleep – and she may have to touch him lightly to make sure he is still alive.

Any new mother who feels this way should take comfort from the fact that she is not alone, but one of countless new mothers – probably the majority – who have such worries. Nor is it solely the experience of a mother with her firstborn; it may happen again with subsequent children. The birth of a baby brings a woman face-to-face with the knowledge of birth and death. She may find even in her joy that there are moments of uncertainty and emptiness.

Added to this, the new mother is still physically, as well as mentally, very involved with her baby. If she is breast-feeding, the rush of milk (the surging and

Cross references

See also	Chapter
Breast- and bottle feeding	10
The child and the family	15
Common problems in newborn babies	12
The newborn baby	9

Playing with the new baby not only gives both parents much enjoyment, but is also one of the best ways of developing his social awareness and physical skills.

tingling of the milk coming toward the nipples) occurs when her baby cries – and sometimes when someone else's baby cries. She is preoccupied with thoughts and experiences of the baby which was until so recently a part of her own body. Dr. Winnicott, the child psychiatrist, called this experience "primary maternal preoccupation". It does not last forever: within four to six weeks she will find that the intensity of this feeling wanes. Then other people can share the absorbing responsibility for the baby which, at first, seems to be hers alone.

Once these early few weeks have passed, the mother will come back into life as a person in her own right, but for the time being she may concentrate on nothing which does not concern her child. She may be unable to read, or make small talk, and offers from kind friends to babysit while she and her husband "go out and enjoy themselves" seem irrelevant. Her sexual life may well be at a low ebb, and this is where the current trend of involving the father in pregnancy, as well as in labor and after the birth, is so valuable. It helps him understand that at a time when he is longing to have his wife to himself and wants to make love to her, he must wait a little longer if he is to arouse her response.

Such are the emotional factors that dominate the first few weeks. The chief practical factor is that, at first, the baby is the center of life and all else is secondary. Don't try to entertain in the first few weeks at home; it will be too exhausting. If there are other children in the family, then the most helpful friends are those who take them out for a special treat, although parents too should make a point of setting aside a special time to be with them.

The most important part of the day is that spent feeding the baby. A full discussion of breast-feeding and bottle feeding appears in chapter 10. Here we are mainly concerned with the impact of feeding on the mother's day. In the past mothers were told to feed their babies from the start at regular four-hourly intervals. But babies are not machines and a more flexible approach can better combine the needs of mother and baby. If the baby is fed according to his own rhythms from his birth, it should soon be possible to sense what this rhythm is and plan around it. Later, knowing that it takes between three and four hours for the baby's stomach to empty completely, the mother can try to console him in other ways if she finds he cries less than two hours from the end of a good feeding. She can try changing his diaper, altering his position, propping him up a little so he can see, or providing him with another person with whom to play, and only if these strategies prove ineffective feed him again. This is not necessarily true for a very small-for-dates baby, or one born prematurely, who may need feeding more often.

A baby who cries a lot, who will not settle and who demands feeding often, but is obviously thriving, can be very tiring. In this case it is wise to plan the chores of the day around the beginning of his sleep, so there is someone available to nurse him, or rock him, or take him out in a carriage when his next crying session starts. But even such a baby as this will finally fit into a routine.

Everyday, indeed almost every hour, with her baby will bring a mother moments of joy and wonder, but also moments of great anxiety. Looking back later, mothers are often surprised at the things which gave them the greatest concern, because these are the happenings which are repeated day after day.

Organizing the routine

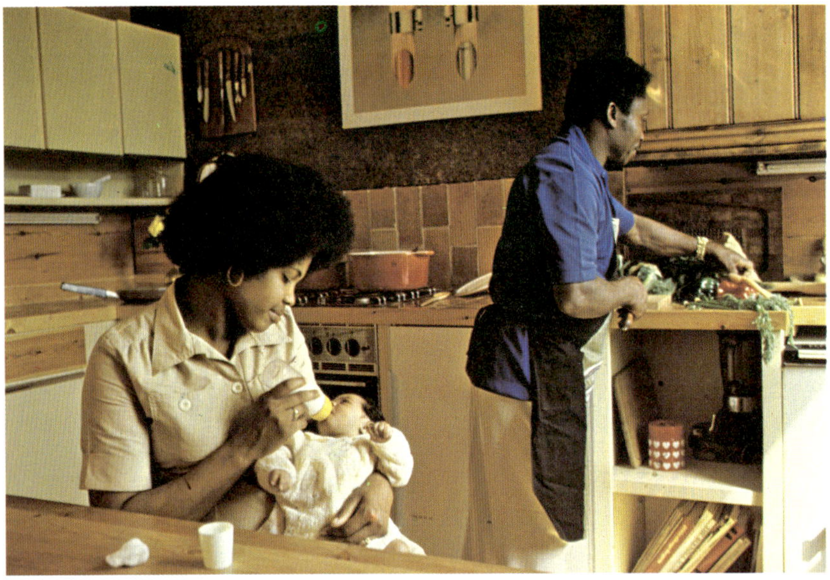

The baby's father can be a great help, especially when the baby needs feeding just as a meal is being prepared.

A young baby is very helpless and needs a great deal of attention. For the time being the household must revolve around his waking, sleeping and feeding times but, after the first few weeks, the baby will gradually fit into the family pattern of living. Soon he will be just as important as, but not more important than, other members of the household, although, because of his age and helplessness, he will still need more than his share of attention. How do you begin to get him into the family routine?

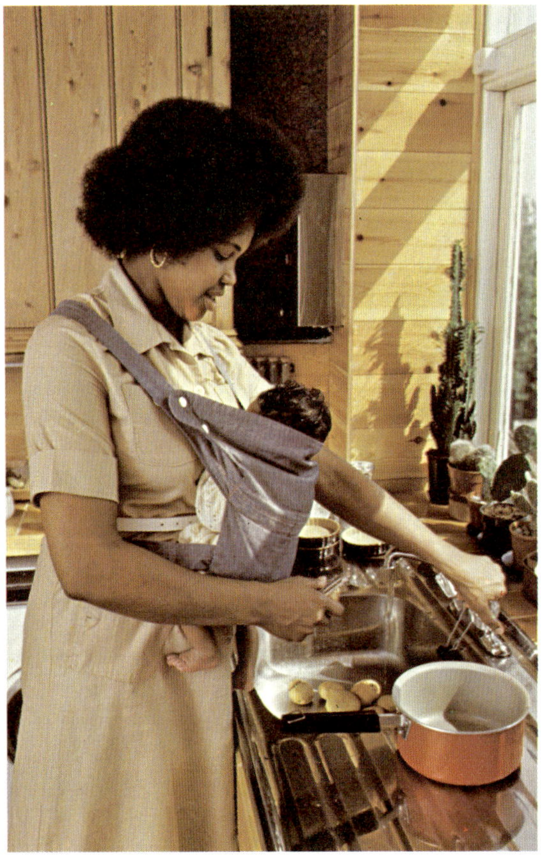

A baby carrier allows the mother to carry her baby but leaves her hands free. The baby is lulled by the mother's movements and the close contact with her body. For a very young baby the carrier should be worn at the front, with a head support.

The baby's feedings are the events which take up most of the time. Breast-feeding and bottle feeding, described in detail in chapter 10, have different rhythms. Whichever method you use, once the baby is thriving and contented, it is worth trying gently to work the feedings into a pattern. When you begin to do this will depend on you and the baby. Start by trying to fix the time of just one feeding a day. Look at your day and decide where is the one point when you would like the baby always to have a feeding at the same time. For instance, you may choose 9 am as a suitable time.

If the baby wakes then for a feeding, that is fine. If at 9 am he is still fast asleep, pick him up and wake him gently; bathe his face and bottom; then give him as much milk as he will take before settling him back for sleep.

If he wakes at 8 am the problem is more difficult. It is worth trying to make him last out another hour if possible and this may involve the help of someone else to amuse and pacify him. A carrier in which you can carry the baby while you work can be a great blessing at such a time; the pleasure of being close up against you may do short-term wonders for his pangs of hunger. A bath too may help to distract him. Should all these delaying tactics fail, however, it is better to feed him and abandon the routine for that day, rather than struggle to maintain it at all costs.

Gradually most babies will begin to conform to a pattern and you can set out to fix the time of another feeding. Some babies do not fit into a pattern; you have to be patient if this is the case with your baby.

It is not just a baby's lack of routine which causes problems in a family. Nights are worrying when there is a new baby in the house. Mothers who say they have never lost a night's sleep are either very forgetful, or they have unusual children.

Once they have passed the first week of life babies do not usually sleep through the night until they are about a month old. This is where the breast-feeding mother is in a very strong position for she can give her baby instant satisfaction which will often send him back to sleep immediately.

If the baby is bottle-fed, the father may be able to take charge some nights to enable the mother to sleep, but if he is working during the day this can be very demanding on him, except perhaps on the weekends.

Mothers get very tired when they are having disturbed nights and it is worth fitting in a regular rest during the day at some time when the baby is asleep. This is not always possible if there are other children in the family.

A new mother should take all the shortcuts she can where cooking and housework are concerned; anything that can make the daily domestic routine easier should be adopted. Eat sensibly (*see* chapter 8) but make maximum use of frozen and canned foods. If you have a deep freeze, now is the time to use up the meals prepared when you had more leisure. Dust will come off just as easily after a month as after a week and by that time you and your baby will be settling into a more regular routine. If you can afford it, employ a cleaning lady or hire a cleaning service on a time schedule that fits in with your needs.

Your partner can help by relieving you of much of the shopping and some of the cooking, leaving you free to concentrate on the baby. If he can take part of his vacation or if he gets a paternity leave which he can take during his child's early weeks, his presence can be of great practical, as well as emotional, support to you. And a great joy to the new father.

Any offers of assistance from relations and friends should be eagerly accepted. The most helpful person is often an understanding mother or a family friend who has had her children recently enough to remember what it was like, and who is prepared to deal with the day-to-day details which you don't want to bother with. When the first six weeks or so are over, mother and baby can emerge as a happy partnership, prepared to share one another with the rest of the world.

All but very tiny babies are, by the time they are under their mother's care, spending at least a third of the 24 hours awake, and so have more opportunity to cry. Why, you may ask, do babies cry? A baby cannot fend for himself, so discomfort evokes a cry for help. Soon he will learn to manipulate his environment but, for the moment, crying demands a response from his mother. Crying is sometimes blamed on loneliness, boredom or "exercising the lungs" but these are adult concepts.

There are three cries which a mother will come to recognize. The ordinary cry is sometimes called the "hunger" cry. The cry is followed immediately by a deep breath and then a pause, giving it a characteristic short, staccato rhythm. The second type of cry may follow the ordinary cry if this is ignored. Mothers may call it a "temper" cry, superimposing, as do most people, adult attitudes where none are possible. The rhythm is similar to the ordinary cry but the noise is more intense. The pain or distress cry starts suddenly and continues, often interspersed with bouts of breath holding so that the rhythm is different from the other two cries.

The ordinary, or hunger cry mothers usually find very irritating and respond by doing something to stop it. But there is no need to rush to the baby right away. Sometimes the cry becomes less, then stops and the baby goes back to sleep. Alternatively, it may be possible to console him by propping him up so he can see his mother, by changing his diaper, altering his position or giving him to someone else to play with. But if after a little while the crying does not stop, a wise mother will feed him. This will probably satisfy the baby, and the mother is richly rewarded by her ability to give comfort. She has also increased the time spent in physical contact between the two of them which is so important to them both.

The "temper" cry that can follow if the "hunger" cry is ignored may be harder to comfort, and the baby may need a lot of cuddling and reassurance.

The pain cry cannot be ignored; here there is no waiting to see if it stops. Unlike the other two cries, this one makes the mother, and everyone else, very anxious. It is particularly worrying if the baby also holds his or her breath and goes slightly blue – even though everyone knows he will breathe again. Colic, open diaper pins, overheating, sudden loud noises or unexpected movements may be responsible for the baby's distress and eventually he will respond to warm, close reassurance. If the crying persists beyond half an hour and the baby will not be comforted it is wise to contact your doctor for advice.

For a mother on her own, a crying baby can be a source of worry. Sharing the responsibility with her own mother, or with a friend, will help her to keep a sense of proportion. A new mother may worry about her own tiredness: how will she ever hear the cry of her baby when she is in a deep, much needed sleep? The answer lies in an awareness which all human beings have when there is something important happening. If you know you have to catch an early train, and worry that the alarm clock will not wake you, often you wake just before the alarm sounds. In the same way, the tired mother will sleep through the doorbell and the fire engine, but almost before the tiny cry (and the later softly whispered "Mommy") she becomes fully conscious.

Sleep

Babies, at about the time they come home, can spend as much as two-thirds of each 24 hours in sleep. At first short, random periods of sleep are interspersed with shorter periods of wakefulness. Gradually the baby comes to stay awake for longer periods and sleeps at regular times in the day and night. At the same time, parents will almost unconsciously introduce into the baby's pattern some of their family routine. They will respond to daytime crying by attention and feeding; nighttime crying may be briefly ignored, or at least received less enthusiastically.

For all humans there are two kinds of sleep. One is a deep sleep; the other a lighter sleep known as rapid eye movement (REM) sleep. These two types of sleep are by no means fully understood and both can be affected greatly by different drugs. We dream during REM sleep.

Babies in utero have a lot of REM sleep. Within the first month of life, they have more deep sleep and as time goes on the amount of REM sleep diminishes still further. The significance of this changing pattern of sleep in babies is not yet known.

For practical purposes babies are described as having five stages of consciousness, ranging from deep sleep to thrashing and crying. Halfway along this spectrum, there is a point where the baby is alert, peaceful and wide-eyed. It is in this state that the baby's response to his mother, and also to other people, is greatest. Talking to him; playing with him;

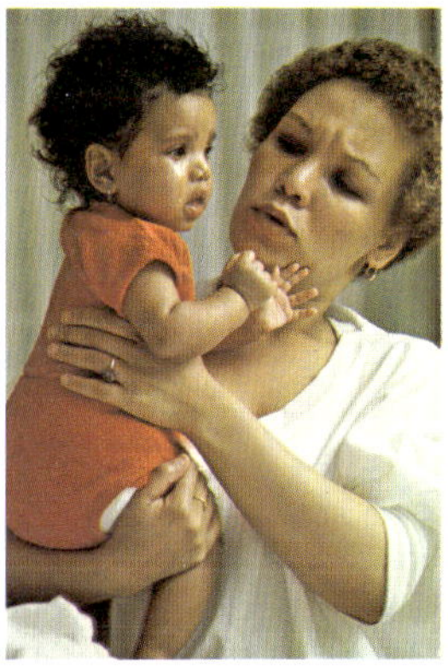

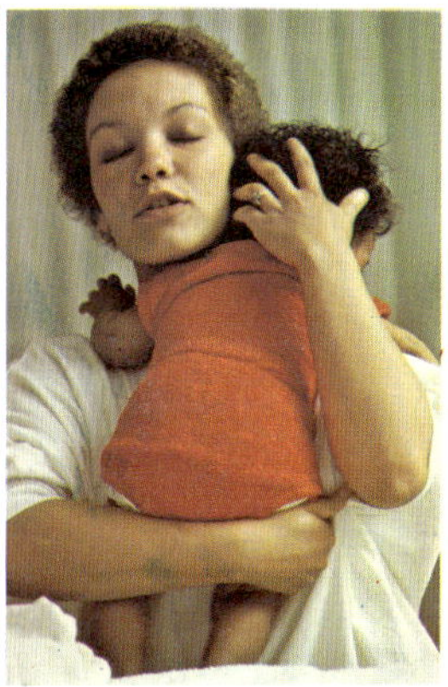

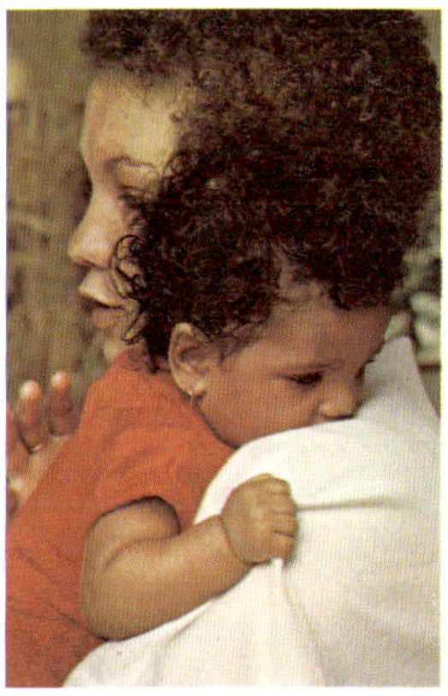

A mother comforts her crying baby. Sometimes a bit of love and attention is all he wants. Parents soon learn to distinguish between the cries of hunger and real distress.

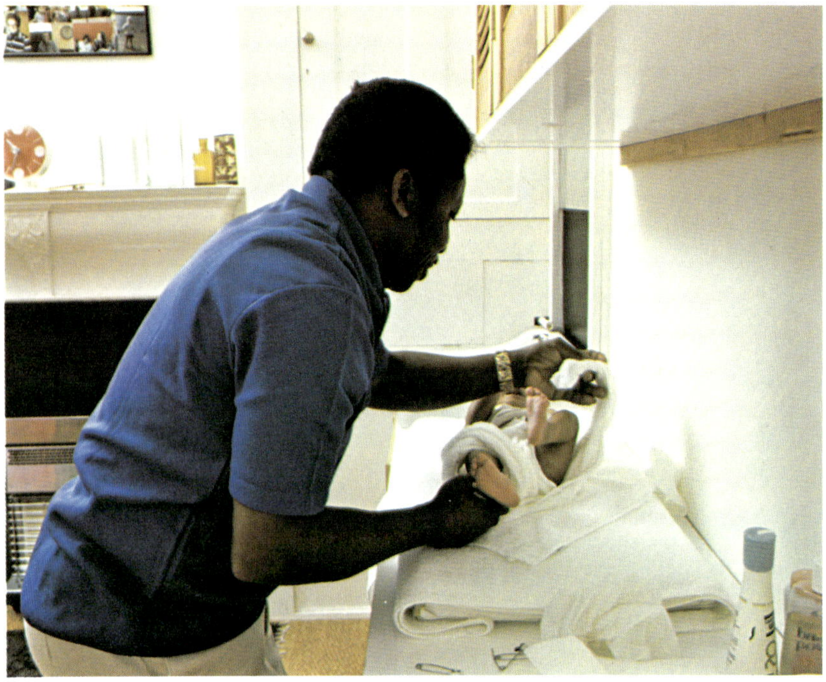

Once diaper-changing is fitted into the daily routine it becomes a quick and simple operation.

making tongue movements which he will watch and try to copy; repeating the sounds he makes and pausing for his reply – are all means by which he learns about his environment.

All babies are individuals and will therefore need different amounts of sleep and wakefulness. Nothing will disturb them in their deep sleep, and they are easily alerted in light sleep. Do not encourage silence in your home during the day "in case the baby wakes". On the contrary, he needs to hear the television, the foot on the stairs, the noise of laughter, both as a natural background and later as a reassurance. Although at first the baby does not distinguish between day and night, he comes to expect silence at night, and this too will help establish a diurnal rhythm.

Temperature control

Overheating can occur in a temperate climate as some babies may be overdressed. Usually babies fret and fuss when they get too hot, however, they tend to suffer in silence if they are very cold. In this case the skin may become pinkish, giving a false appearance of good health. As babies cannot shiver and the surface area they present to the world is so great relative to their size, over-cooling, or hypothermia, develops quite rapidly without even a protest.

Ideally the room temperature should be constant at around 65–70°F (20°C). In this case, the baby may be lightly dressed, with a single blanket, and he will maintain a body temperature of approximately 98°F (37°C). A small baby (less than 5 lb or 2300 gm) is particularly at risk from cold; a bigger one is not nearly so vulnerable. By six months all babies should be able to stand lower temperatures.

Good insulation including draft excluders under doors, molding along baseboards and lined curtains all help to maintain a constant room temperature. You can fit the crib with padded bumpers, which also act as draft excluders.

In the early weeks an infant seat, or Snugli, is best for keeping a baby cozy. Lightweight clothes and a warm crib in a warm room are ideal but not always possible. To test if the baby's temperature is correct lift up his or her clothes and put a hand on his tummy. If he is cold, his tummy will feel cold; if he is too hot, it will feel slightly sticky.

Baby clothes

Two of the most important things to remember when you start on the exciting business of collecting your first layette are that babies remain tiny for a surprisingly short time; and that what you buy should depend very much on your way of life.

This first point means that it is worthwhile spending some time and effort (and money) on larger garments. Kind friends and relations who want to knit or sew for you will be just as happy to make something for a six-month-old baby as they would be for a much younger one. If you try to put a 12-month size undershirt onto a newborn baby, however, he will quickly be swamped, so some small things are necessary. If your house is very warm, a sweater may not be essential at all in the beginning. A checklist for your first layette is found in the margin of the page opposite.

Choose clothes that are easy to put on. Snap-on undershirts and things that button or tie are best. They do not need to be made of pure wool and, in fact, it is often better if they are of cotton. Wool can irritate your baby's skin.

Sweaters or a sleeping bag are useful if the room gets cold or you are taking your baby out. Again, simple styles that are easy to put on, with front openings, or with one or two buttons, are better than those with ribbons which get hard with washing, or with lacy patterns which trap tiny fingers.

Stretch suits are a boon, and make the baby so much more compact and easy to carry. Some of the small sizes have attached "mittens", and these can be helpful in preventing the baby from scratching his face and making it sore. It is essential to have a suit which is too large rather than too small.

Mittens and bootees are all fairly unnecessary and can be left to kind aunts to provide. If the baby is very small, a hat may, however, be useful, as tiny babies lose heat easily from their heads. This is particularly important if the baby is taken outside in the winter.

Dresses or overalls can be left for a while as the baby is not going to need these right away. He is going to need nightgowns, and these are best with easy back or front closings, preferably coming off without going over the baby's head. Make sure that they are easy to wash and dry, and again cotton is better than wool. Nylon or Dacron are very practical, although it is wise to use cotton garments next to the skin.

Diapers are basically of two kinds – cloth and disposable. There are obvious differences in cost and work involved but most mothers use both at different times; perhaps cloth at nighttime for absorbency and disposable during the day. In many communities commercial diaper services provide the most economical option for families.

Plastic pants are important at times – no matter what many doctors may say! Some babies do get rashes easily, so the time spent in plastic pants for them must be strictly limited. A short time each day without a diaper on at all is good for all babies, especially those with a tender skin. Plastic pants should be rather baggy so the air can get in. They should be discarded as soon as the leg hole edges begin to harden. Almost all disposable diapers have a built-in plastic cover, which is also disposable. These are very useful. Do not turn this plastic lining in so that it comes in direct contact with the baby's skin.

Equipment

The larger items you need to buy depend very much upon your way of life. If you travel by car all babies and infants should be in a properly installed car safety seat. Holding a child in your lap can be very dangerous. If you are using a carbed in a car, you must use a special restraint which prevents the carbed from being thrown to the floor with a sudden movement.

If you choose to buy a carriage, remember you may need to use it for shopping; if you buy one with a special basket for this, you will find that heavy shopping will actually make the carriage more stable.

Most well-made carriages are fitted with good quality mattresses and harnesses. If not, buy these when you buy the carriage. It is always a good idea to start using the harness before you think it is really necessary. If you have a springtime baby, you may need a sun shade as well.

Never be tempted to put a very young baby into a stroller. He needs to be able to sit up securely on his own, without overbalancing, before he is safe in one of these.

Cribs

You may not need a crib right away as a small baby bed or bassinet will do instead. Some cribs have a dual life as cribs and then junior bed; others have two levels for the mattress – a higher one to make handling a little baby easier, and a lower one to make it difficult for him to climb out when he gets more adventurous. There is yet another type which incorporates useful storage space. Mattresses need to be firm and waterproof and are usually bought with the crib. Babies do not need pillows; they can be harmful at first. It is possible to get foam-padded, easy-to-clean "bumpers", which can not only be fitted inside the crib but also do a double duty as draft excluders. Finally, make sure the catch of the crib side is child-proof.

Chairs

Babies love to look around from a very early age, and are particularly interested in what their mothers are doing, so a molded plastic infant seat, which can be picked up with the baby in it and carried from room to room, can be a great help. This will be especially valuable if it is used later as a high chair with its own table or a high chair which can be brought to the family table.

If the seat does not have a really secure safety harness provided, you must buy one, and it must always be used. Even with a harness, never leave a baby alone while the seat is fixed in the high position, nor if the seat is standing on a table for feeding, as it is very easy for a baby to upset the balance and knock the seat over.

Other practical items

A changing mat is most useful and so is a box, which may be made for the purpose or adapted from a wicker basket, in which all the baby's things, from pins to bibs, can be kept. You may wish to buy an all-in-one changing table, complete with mat and storage areas for clothing and all bathtime needs. Two plastic buckets – one with a lid for soiled diapers – are almost indispensable.

There are excellent baby carriers on the market. The ones for the back are ideal for a young child who can sit securely on his own. There are front carriers that a mother can use for a new baby, with a good support for his head. These may look uncomfortable, but they do provide warmth and a cozy nest for the baby, and his mother can get on with her work moderately unhindered.

SUGGESTIONS FOR THE LAYETTE

- 3 undershirts – 6-month size
- 3 nightgowns, back- or front-opening
- 2 or 3 stretch suits
- 2 dozen cloth prefolded diapers
- Safety diaper pins
- Supply of disposable diapers, if preferred – newborn size
- 3 waterproof pads
- 3 pairs plastic pants
- Hat
- 2 or 3 sweaters
- 4 lightweight receiving blankets to use as shawls or blankets
- 3 bibs

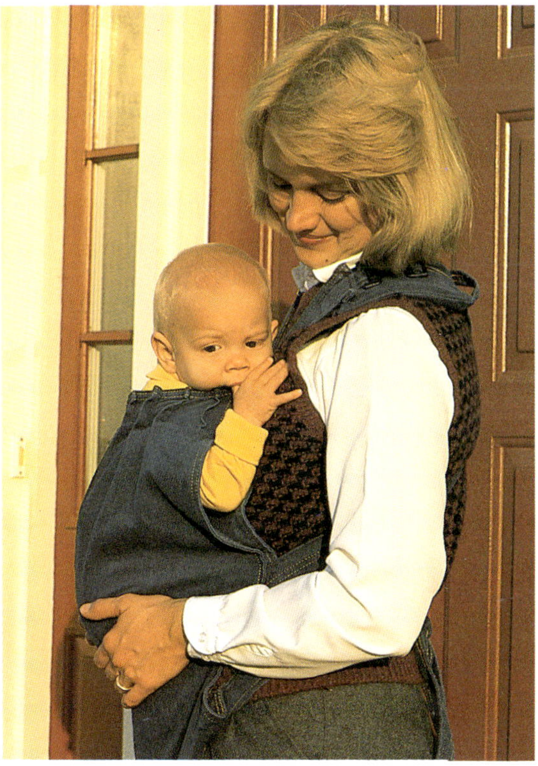

This Snugli is an ideal way to carry your baby. You have almost complete freedom of movement, yet you are as close to your baby as you possibly can be. And your baby is comfortable and secure.

Fathering

Every new parent greets the arrival of their baby with exhilaration and apprehension, yet most books and magazine articles still only deal with the mother's role in parenting – relegating the father to the periphery. However, judging by the current trend, the periphery is not where many fathers want to be!

For having taken an interested and supportive role in their partner's pregnancy and the birth experience, they don't want their involvement to end there. Indeed many new fathers envisage a rather more equal and flexible arrangement – one which allows them to share in the pleasures and the responsibilities of parenthood.

Unfortunately, the majority of new fathers have no role model on which to base their participation – their own fathers and their fathers before them having been distant figures, whose sole functions were to dole out punishment to the children and act as economic providers for the family. No wonder, then, that today's new fathers are confused about what fathering could – or should – entail.

Establishing a relationship

The first few weeks after the birth of the baby are the most exciting and disruptive time for both parents. Nothing could have possibly prepared them for this immense undertaking – the care of their baby, who has suddenly become the center of their lives. During this period lending mutual support and assistance is not just desirable but necessary: for the parents, who will need the time together to become skilled in the practicalities of babycare and to work out the sharing arrangements, and for the baby, who will need to be settled into some routine.

Moreover, it is during this crucial period that the bonding relationship is established: never again will fathers be able to devote their undivided attention to the baby, getting to know him or her on such intimate and all-embracing terms and finding out what being a father is really all about. For this reason it is recommended that fathers should try to make sure that they can take a week or two off work, using this period as vacation time. Perhaps a more enlightened age will see the concept of paternity leave becoming a reality.

During this period the bulk of time and energy will be devoted to the caretaking of the baby whose demands will appear never-ending. Traditionally such childcare activities were considered to be "woman's work," but fathers who wish to become fully involved should accustom themselves to taking on the role – and not view it as a threat to their masculinity! What should be appreciated here is that few, if any, first-time parents are "naturals" in the spheres of feeding, diaper changing and bathing the baby, and a great deal of time, patience and trial and error will be necessary to perfect these skills.

Moreover, both partners should recognize that each is as capable as the other (and likewise may have a similar fear and distaste) of grasping the essentials of childcare; in any event practice does make perfect, and if both partners do the necessary often enough they will eventually do it well.

For these reasons it is important that parents learn together the routine care of the baby if sharing is to become a fact of life and not a concept to which only lip-service is paid. Mothers, no matter how anxious and impatient, must make a conscious effort to stand back and allow their partners to play an active role in babycare. This way a rhythm can be developed between them for carrying out the routine duties – thus avoiding the twin problems of mothers quickly becoming adept while fathers stand on the sidelines feeling helpless and isolated, or of mothers saying, with some dissatisfaction, "He can do it but he has to be asked."

A changing partnership

The partnering involvement with babycare will also provide another added bonus to the parents' relationship to each other. During the early weeks of parenthood the dynamics of the partnership will change dramatically because of the addition of a third person. The transition to the new roles of "mother" and "father" is never a simple one and women, especially, will need all the consideration and support they can get from their partners. Working out a flexible arrangement will do much to alleviate the anxiety, exhaustion and sense of dislocation that many new mothers feel and this will do much to further the teamwork effort and deepen their own relaitionship. At the same time it will provide the baby with two fully participating and nurturing individuals, each of whom can contribute, in their different ways, to the baby's ultimate development.

Coming to grips with the practicalities of babycare is imperative for both parents during this period. True, the initial burden will be divided between the partners, but once the father returns to work, perhaps with the mother following at some later period, the bulk of parenting will fall on the mother's shoulders, together with all the domestic duties. From the start some arrangement should be worked out whereby a mutual support system can be maintained so that while one partner does the cleaning, cooking, laundry and so on, the other can spend time caring for and playing with the baby. Some fathers may balk at taking on a domestic role in addition to their career, but unless some sharing arrangement of domestic duties can be arrived at and/or help brought in, then the burden will fall unfairly and entirely on the mother, who will feel that the all-consuming mothering/housewife role has made her lose sight of the independent existence she had before the baby's birth.

Again, working out an arrangement to both partners' satisfaction will have additional benefits. Fathers who, because of heavy work commitments, have less time to spend with the baby, may be able to cope with the domestic

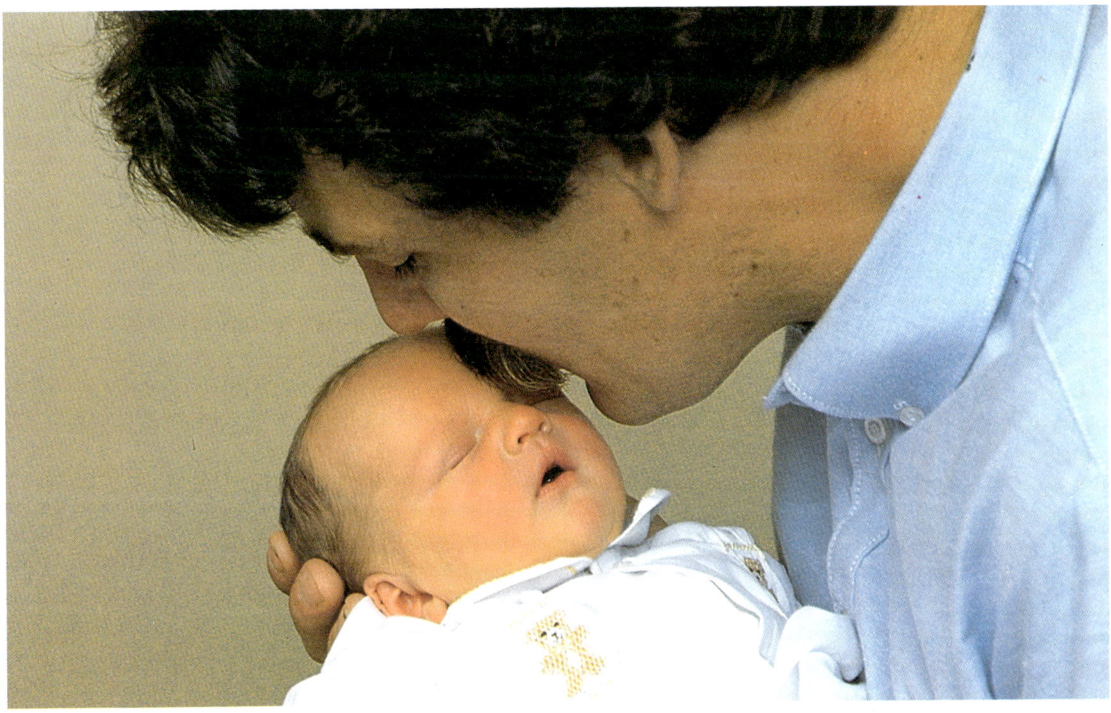

The very basis of parenting must surely be the tenderness and love you feel for the tiny new human being that is your child. And what greater joy can there be than the freedom and ability to express those feelings.

duties during the week and then, on the weekend, take over the babycare completely, giving his partner a welcome rest and a chance to be herself. During these concentrated days of fathering an even closer attachment can develop between father and baby. Indeed many experts have said that it isn't the amount of time a father spends with his baby that counts, rather that it is the quality of the time that is all important. Very rapidly a great intimacy will spring up between fathers and babies – even more so, as studies have shown, once the baby gets a bit older and develops a personality in his or her own right. Fathers who make it their business to participate actively in the care, nurturing and development will make the baby more "real" to themselves in terms of a person they have helped to create and for whom they feel great love and affection. Simultaneously, fathers will gain incalculable pleasure from the all too rapid and truly wondrous transformation of this helpless, demanding creature into a little person in his or her own right, complete with a character and personality.

Fatherhood – a growth opportunity

What's to be remembered – all through the horror of sleepless nights and soiled diapers – is that fathering is a unique experience, and that each man, given his own personality, his maturity and the worldly experience he can bring to the role, and the time he has available from his work commitments, has something very individual to contribute. The impact fathers have on their baby's life will very often be decided in those first few weeks and months when the baby's needs are so great and the emotional pull so strong. By opting out of this vital period a distance may be set up that may never be closed to either the father's or the child's satisfaction.

Further, sincere interest and involvement with the baby will, in addition to lightening the practical burden of babycare for the mother, help to cement further the relationship between partners. Fathers, like mothers, will be entirely changed by the parenting experience, and both will recognize that neither will ever be the same person again. Fathers who take an active part in parenting will become much more attuned to their partner's ever-widening array of thoughts and feelings through this experience that they share so deeply and fully with each other. Because of this they will never forget that in addition to their roles as parents that they are lovers and friends to each other. For if fathers allow their partners to create a very private world between themselves and the baby they will be foregoing the one great common interest that they have together – the child.

Fathering, when it is considered in these terms, is therefore a rather different experience than it was for men in previous generations, with the role reflecting the more equal and flexible partnership between themselves and women. Shared parenting is – or can be – viable in practical, emotional and, indeed, financial terms, as apart from the common interest that partners have, both can retain a certain measure of freedom and independence, which can only serve to make them both happier as people.

Finally, by this alteration of roles from the traditional to the modern approach, which provides more satisfaction, a strong family bond can be created, which, for the majority of couples, was one of the more important reasons for having the baby in the first place!

Bathing the baby

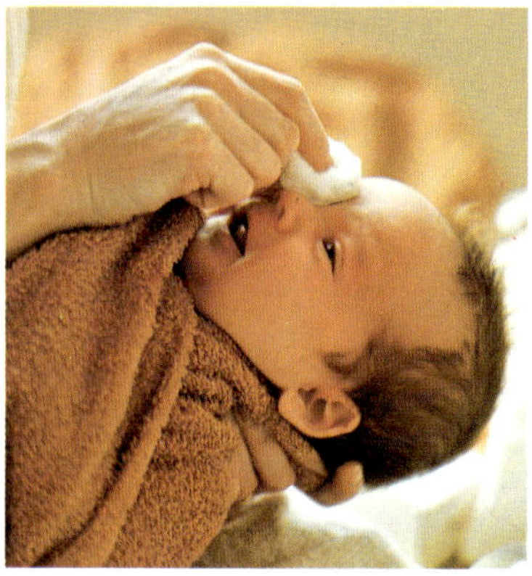

To avoid infection, wipe each eye from the nose outward, using a separate piece of absorbent cotton, wrung out in warm boiled water. Wash the face with another piece of damp absorbent cotton.

Wash the head first (right), keeping the baby wrapped in a towel. If you use soap or baby shampoo, rinse the hair with clean water from the bath.

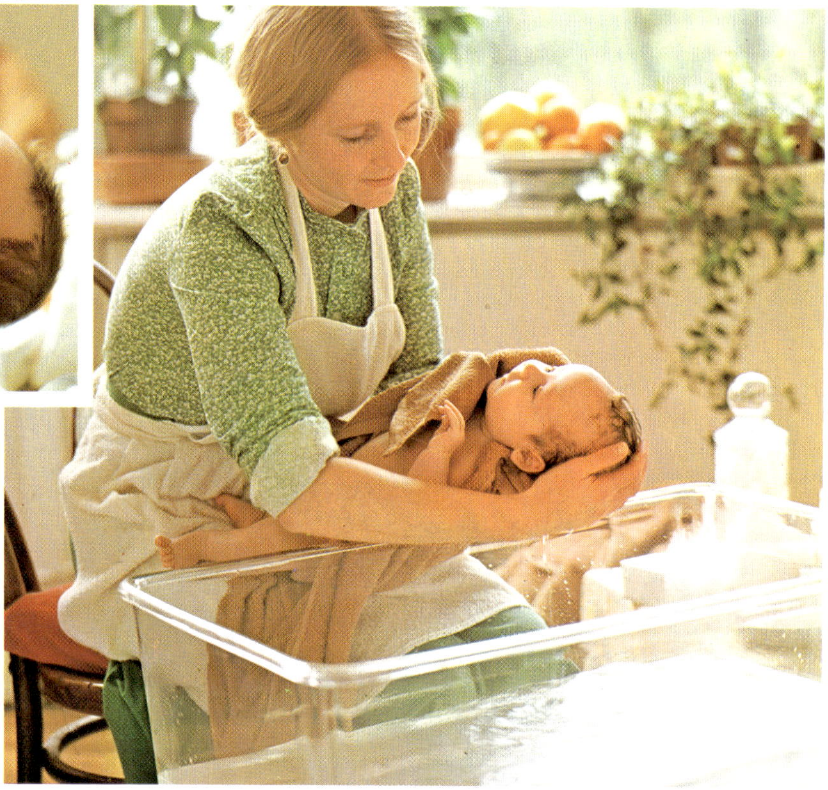

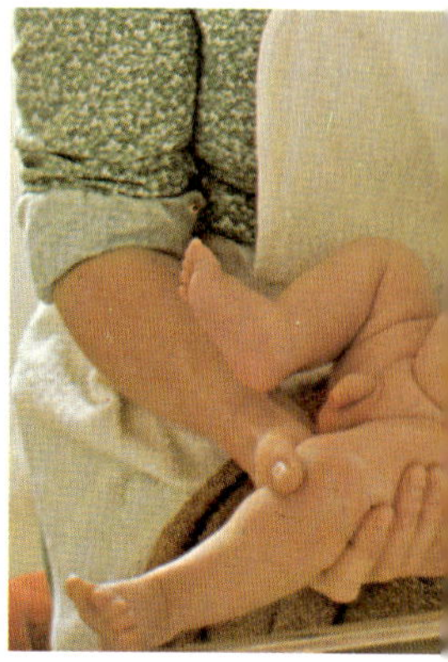

When lifting the baby into the bath (above), cradle the neck in your left arm, with your left hand holding the baby's left arm against his chest. The right hand supports both the baby's legs. Support his back and head in the water (right) and be sure to talk to him as you soap and rinse him.

For bathing the baby you will need:
- a comfortable chair
- large soft towel
- pail for diapers
- disposal bag for soiled items and clothing
- clean clothes
- small bowl of lukewarm water
- soap
- cream
- powder (if you use it)
- absorbent cotton
- sponge
- diaper and safety pins
- plastic pants

The first thing to remember about bathing a baby is that it is not necessary. If at first the idea worries you, give him a partial bath and wait until you feel confident about "proper" bathing.

The next important point is to make sure you have all the necessary equipment on hand before you pick up the baby (*see* checklist in the margin of this page).

All the descriptions given here are for a right-handed person. If you are left-handed, read left for right and vice versa.

Partial bath. This is done by sitting the baby, dressed, on your knee, his head resting on your left arm. Take absorbent cotton, wrung out in cool water, and wipe it gently over his face. If his eyes are all sticky use two more pieces of absorbent cotton, moistened in the same way – one for each eye – and wipe gently away from the nose. This avoids the possibilty of any cross-infection. Never use soap on your baby's face.

If the baby has any dried secretions in his nose, wipe them away with absorbent cotton, gently pressing below the nostril to dislodge them. There is no need to dig into a baby's nostrils, for even absorbent cotton, which seems soft to an adult, can scratch the delicate membranes inside the nose. When you have finished, pat the child's face dry with a soft towel. (By the time the baby is about six to eight weeks old, you can use a soft sponge for washing his face.) Now take off his lower clothes and diaper.

Then place a towel under your baby's buttocks and, holding up his feet with your left hand, wash his bottom with the other. Use soapy absorbent cotton. Sponge off the soap, pat dry and rub powder carefully into the creases. Many mothers like to give a partial bath, and to do all diaper changing, on a special mat. Others prefer to sit down and use their laps.

Towel bath. One way to bathe a baby without actually immersing him is to give him a towel bath. Undress the baby and lay him on a towel, on your lap or on a changing mat. Wash his face as described earlier. Then wash his body, especially in the armpit creases and arm and neck folds. Wash his bottom, paying particular attention to the groin creases and the one between the buttocks. Lightly sponge his legs and arms and pat him dry by cuddling him in the towel.

If you find the umbilicus at all red or draining dab it with a cotton swab soaked in warm water. If this does not clear it up, you should see your doctor.

Bathing. The temperature of the bathroom should be around 75–80°F (24–27°C) and the water 95–97°F (35–36°C). It is wise to put cold water into the bath first, both to avoid putting the baby in water which is too hot and because the tub itself may retain the heat of the hot water, so the baby could possibly burn himself on it.

Test the temperature of the bath water with a thermometer or, more conveniently, with your own elbow. If you can't decide whether your elbow feels hot or cold the temperature is correct.

Undress your baby, wrap him in a towel and wash his face. Then unwrap him and cradle him in your arms with his head – the heaviest

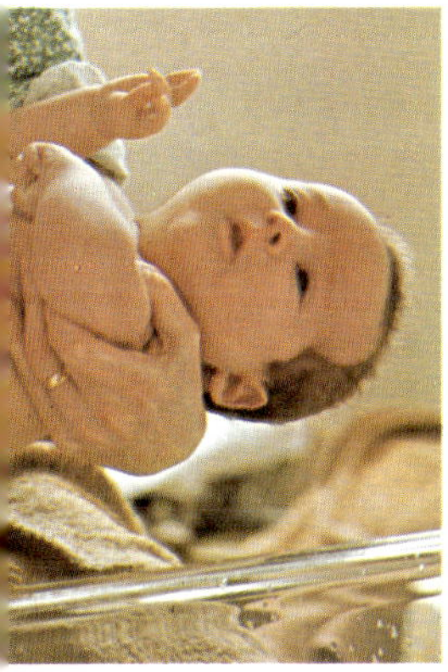

Choose a baby bath to suit your needs, but if you buy one which supports the baby's back, still keep hold of him in the bath.

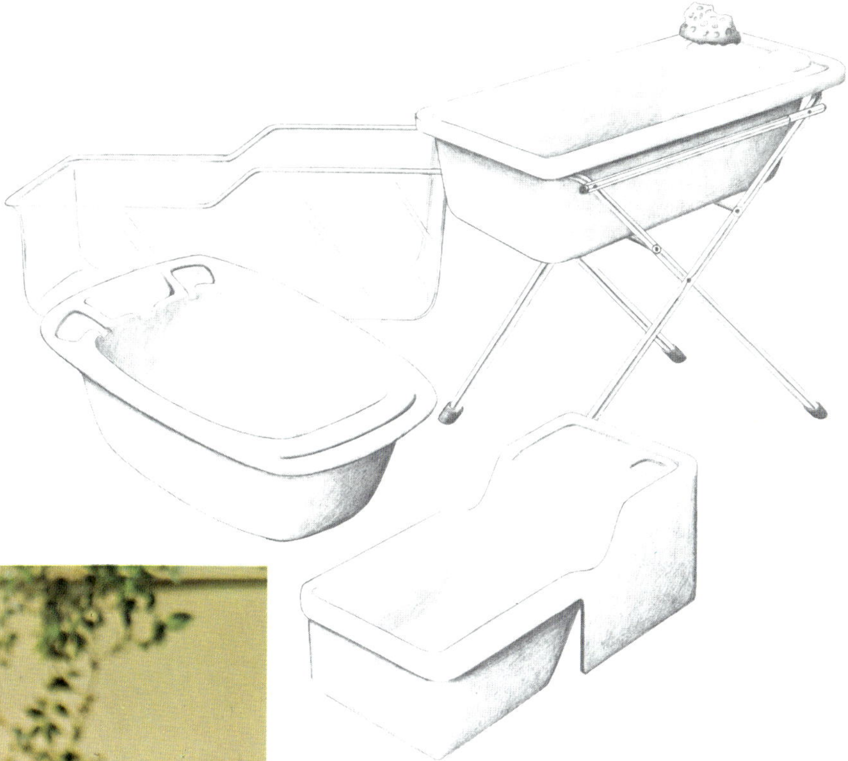

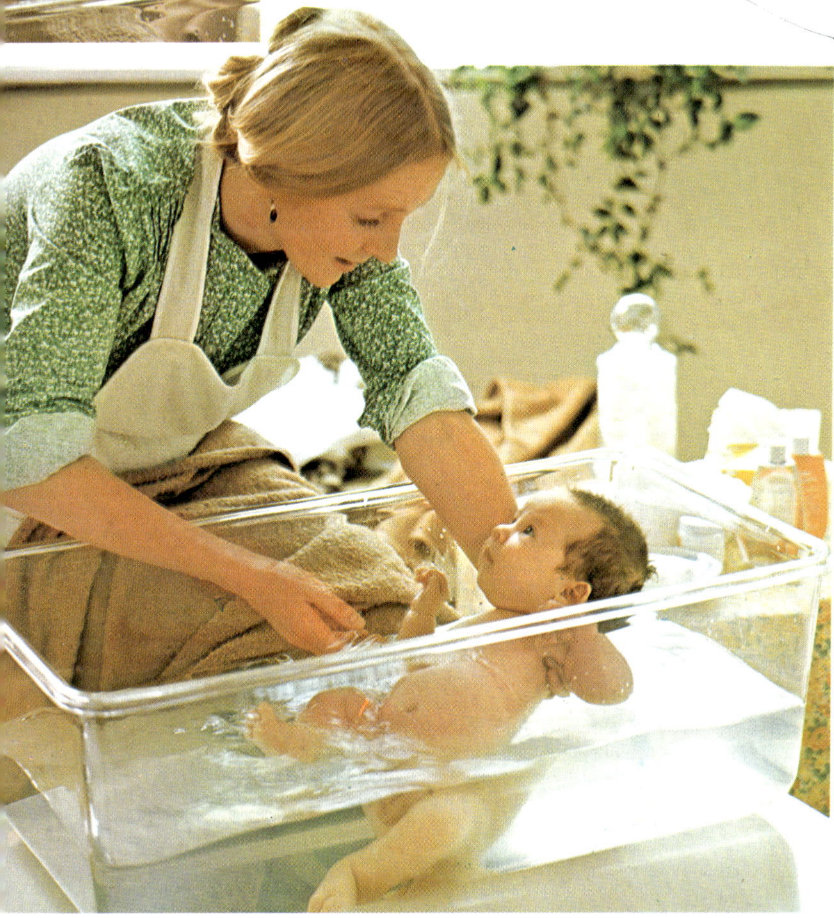

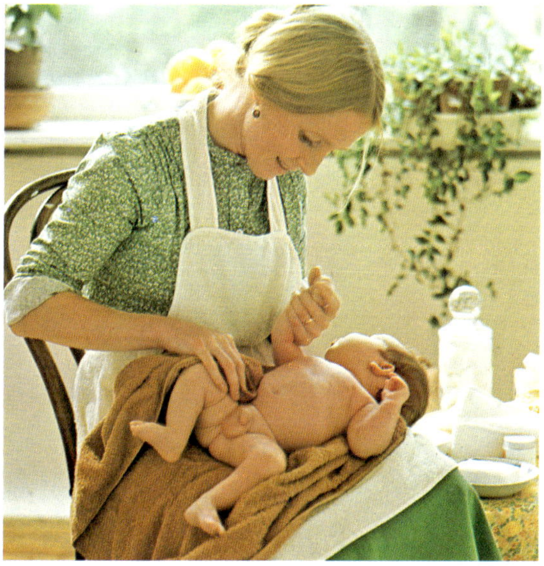

part of him – supported by your left arm. Hold his left arm firmly against his chest with your left hand, support his legs and bottom with your right hand and lift him toward the water.

With your right hand splash him gently on his tummy and his toes, so he gets used to the water. Then gently lower him into the water. Soap him, splash him, rinse him, and talk to him all the time. Even at this age it is worth talking about what you are doing as well as telling him what a lovely baby he is.

Mothers usually like to wash their babies' hair every time they bathe them because it looks pretty standing up. This can be done either before or after bathing the baby. Remember that soap is not essential for washing the hair and scalp.

When you have finished giving your baby a bath, lift him onto your lap and cuddle him dry in the towel. Make sure you dry in all the creases. Never use cream and powder together as they tend to mix, forming hard irritant lumps. Little girls sometimes accumulate white dried talcum powder in the folds of the vulva and this material needs to be gotten out very gently.

Most babies love bathtime and soon begin to splash and kick. Once they get to this stage it is worth thinking about using an adult bath, or putting the baby bath into it. It is important, however, to consider your own back muscles. A happy solution is to give the baby to his father while he is having a bath, or to an older brother or sister. This way the baby will feel safe and secure in their arms, he will have plenty of opportunity to kick and splash, and washing is made all that much easier. Bathtime should be fun for all.

If you are drying the baby on your lap (above) always lay him across your knees, not along the line of your thighs. If you prefer to use a firm surface, such as a baby mat, always make sure that the baby cannot roll off. Wrap the baby in a soft towel and dry him by patting, rather than by rubbing vigorously which may break the skin.

Elimination

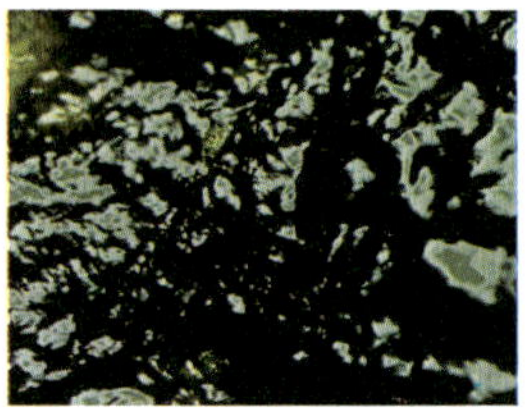

The meconium stool of the newborn baby.

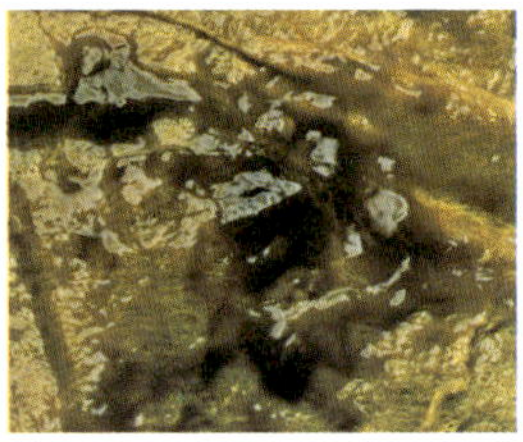

There is still some meconium left in the stool of this breast-fed baby.

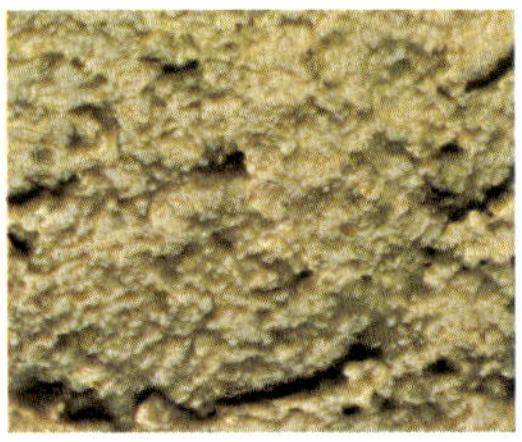

This bottle-fed baby's stool also still contains some meconium.

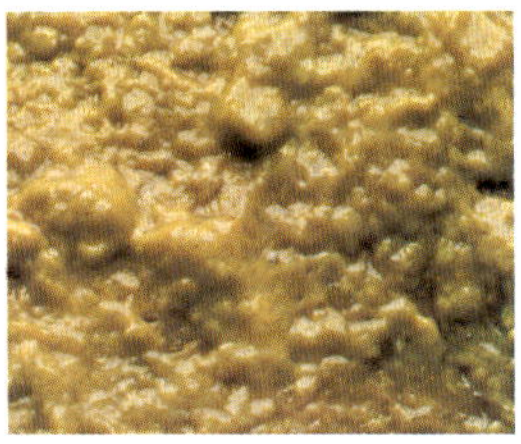

A normal breast-fed baby's stool.

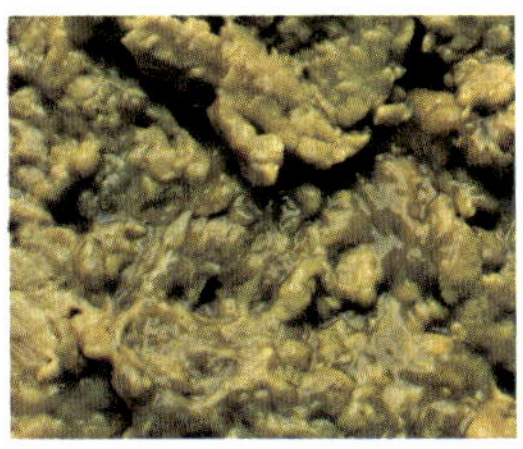

A normal bottle-fed baby's stool.

A fetus has urine in its bladder from very early on and is known to urinate into the amniotic fluid, although most of its waste products are removed via the placenta (*see* pp. 32, 46).

Babies usually pass urine at some time around the moment of birth. Thereafter the amount they pass depends on how much they drink. For the first three or four days they may pass it only three or four times a day; by the seventh day the frequency has doubled; and by about the tenth day a baby will be wetting at least a dozen times a day.

A baby often wets as the diaper is removed and, as far as little boys are concerned, this is an opportunity to see whether the urine comes out in a good stream or "dribbles". Constant dribbling needs medical attention as it suggests there may be a blockage of some sort in the outlet system.

With birth, a baby's kidneys have to take on a great deal more work than they did in the uterus. This they do with nature's (almost) customary efficiency. "Almost" because, although the baby's kidneys can cope with normal conditions, for a few months they will be too immature to respond immediately to stress situations. This is why it is important to be sure that babies receive only milk which is suited to their special needs.

The color of the urine varies slightly depending on how concentrated it is. The urine passed in the morning may be slightly darker than that passed during the rest of the day. If the urine looks concentrated all the time, it may mean that the baby needs more fluid.

In the early days, when the baby may have some physiological (naturally occurring) jaundice (*see* p. 166), the urine may look slightly brown due to the presence of bile salts.

Stools are more variable in color and texture. The meconium stool of the newborn – sticky, dark olive green – will be a thing of the past by the time mother and baby are home from the hospital.

During the early days at home the baby will probably pass two or three stools a day, often in response to a feeding (whether the baby is breast-fed or bottle-fed). If this happens, it is wise to carry on the feeding and not interrupt it for changing the baby.

If the baby is breast-fed the stools will have a characteristic aromatic smell and may look like soft scrambled egg. After a few weeks their appearance changes and the stools generally become pale yellow and of a pasty consistency. Occasionally, without warning, and with no significance, the baby produces a loose green stool with curds and mucus. This is quite normal.

Breast-fed babies, after a few weeks, may have a day or several days without passing a stool. Suddenly they will fill a diaper – perhaps two in rapid succession – and again lapse into inactivity for a few days. This is completely normal. Some babies, particularly in the first week, may pass a watery stool many times a day, at almost every feeding.

Bottle-fed babies have rather different-looking stools from those who are breast-fed. They may be harder, more gray-yellow in color and of the consistency of clay, or they can be green in color. Really hard, pellet-like stools, whether the baby is breast- or bottle-fed, may suggest a lack of water or possibly underfeeding.

Hard stools themselves are unimportant except that they occasionally cause slight bleeding from the anus.

Mothers often think their babies are constipated because they seem to have problems passing a stool. Remember that a baby in the early days of life works neurologically in one piece, so that if his head drops back slightly and unexpectedly he will respond by throwing out his arms and even his legs. In the same way his whole body will respond to discomfort in his rectum. He will go red in the face, grunt, and even push with his eyebrows. To everyone's surprise, the stool that labors out is quite soft and normal. As the months go by he will gradually learn to use muscle groups selectively, and to use a lot of effort only for a really hard stool.

Gastroenteritis

The main characteristic of a stool which could mean an infection is that it is so watery that even the cloth diaper is soaked through and appears greenish on the outside. The stools are more frequent than normal and may be dark green with mucus. If your baby has this kind of diarrhea, or is vomiting with diarrhea, take him to the doctor, as babies lose fluid very quickly and this can be dangerous.

Diapers

Some people are concerned that a bulky diaper between the baby's thighs causes discomfort, but this is really not important so long as the baby can move his or her legs and spends some time each day diaper-free (*see* p. 161). The main purpose of a diaper is to absorb liquid and so far no material has been invented which will do this without bulk.

Mothers also worry about diaper rash. This is almost unavoidable at some time during infancy, but there are points worth remembering. A sensitive skin reacts whatever you do. Find a cream which suits your baby, preferably a very soft one which you can rub lightly into your hands and then onto the baby. It is worth doing this at every diaper change.

Even though the baby's urine is harmless, it is possible for germs to develop in the wet diaper which produce an ammonia substance from the urine. For this reason it is best to change the baby when you know he is wet, although it is quite harmless to wait to change him until he wakes up, should you notice a wet diaper when he is asleep.

Quite often, mothers will use two cloth diapers when putting the baby to sleep for the night. Plastic pants can be used as you feel necessary, but not all the time. Wash plastic pants frequently and discard them once they get hard. Do not use too small a size on your baby or the legholes will rub, possibly causing skin irritations but certainly making the baby uncomfortable.

Set aside some time during the day when the baby can kick on a towel, blanket or quilt on the floor without a diaper. All babies enjoy this. If there are many drafts, lay him in his crib instead, but protect the mattress against the inevitable puddle. The more sensitive a skin your baby has, the more important is this diaper-free time.

There are many different types of diapers and plastic pants. Some are useful only for young babies, others can be adapted to all ages. The basic choice is really between cloth diapers and the disposable type. Each has advantages and disadvantages and many mothers use both at some time.

The problem with using a cloth diaper on a young baby is to avoid enveloping him completely. But if there is a lot of material to spare there will be a lot of it to soak up the wet. Modern prefolded cloth diapers simplify things and are easy to use.

Initially, cloth diapers are expensive but they can be used for years and for more than one child. Disposable diapers are very good for traveling and for going out – and for mothers with no washing machine or limited drying facilities. The outside plastic layer protects and yet allows free air to flow. The cost of disposable diapers is more than compensated for by the sheer fact of their convenience and the work they save. They are available in sizes to fit growing babies.

Washing diapers and clothes

Have a pail filled with a mild antiseptic solution for keeping wet diapers in until it is convenient to wash them. It is advisable to remove most of the dirt from a soiled diaper as soon as possible to avoid staining. Remove any solid matter and then rinse well in cold water. This can be accomplished by holding on tightly to the diaper then placing it in the toilet and flushing. Then put the diaper in a solution of soap and detergent and rub over the stained part. Rinse and then put it in the antiseptic solution.

When washing diapers use detergent and very hot water and make sure you rinse thoroughly. The object of washing is to get rid of the ammonia from the urine and all bacteria in the cloth diapers. If you have an efficient washing machine there is no need to boil diapers, and the machine should be capable of giving them a proper rinse. Some people like to use a fabric softener to improve the color and feel of diapers, but this may cause a mild skin rash.

If possible diapers should be dried on a line in the open air. The action of fresh air and sunshine is not completely understood, but it certainly seems to improve the color and feel of diapers. Sunlight may also help kill any remaining bacteria. Tumble drying is also useful for shortening the time of drying and for making diapers softer.

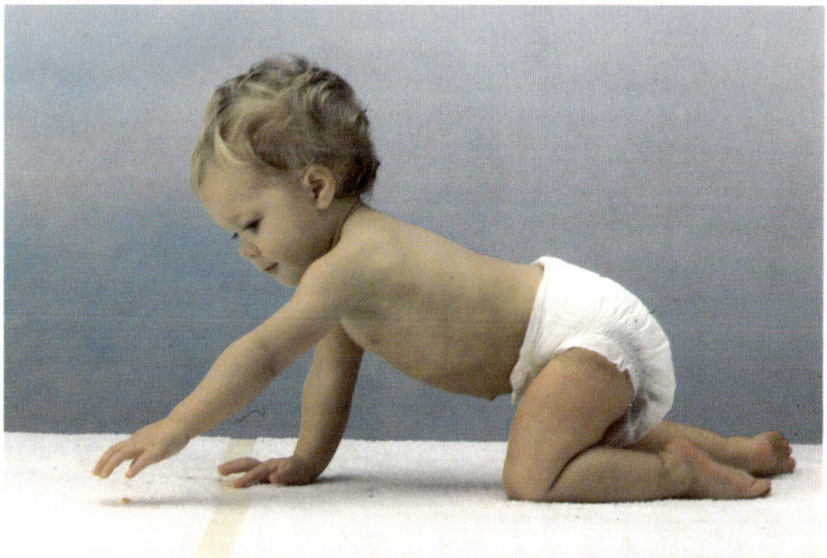

Disposable diapers have a plastic outer layer that protects the baby's clothing, yet allows air to circulate freely. Elasticated legs give further protection from seepage. Although more costly than cloth diapers, disposable ones are invaluable when traveling with your baby and are very convenient for mothers with limited washing facilities.

The rules are much the same for other baby clothes. Use a good detergent sparingly and rinse well. Do not change laundry products frequently. Find one product that works (cleans well and causes no skin irritation) and stay with it. Woolen clothes need hand washing and drying first of all inside a towel. Clothes made from man-made fibers are practical but can be too warm and irritate a baby's skin.

A word of caution about laundry detergents and soaps. A new baby has tender and sensitive skin. There are many washing soaps that are not caustic, clean well and cause no skin irritation. Use of a mild, low suds soap or detergent is fine. Should the baby develop a rash remember the name of the washing preparation you are using. Tell this to your pediatrician when you call him.

The baby's sheets and blankets should be given the same meticulous care during laundering as is given diapers and clothing. Use a good but mild soap or detergent and be certain to rinse these bulky items very thoroughly. Your baby's face and other areas of exposed skin will be in direct contact with bed sheets. It is very important that they are not soiled from old spit-up food or urine.

Blankets and bedpads need frequent laundering especially during the time when the baby is very young. An infant will soak several spots in his bed during the period of rest and sleep between feedings. These spots may dry before you look in on your child or the child awakens and cries for you. Change the baby's bed often. Wash soiled blankets and pads thoroughly and rinse twice as bedding is thick and tends to retain soap. Many mothers find the use of a sleeping bag very convenient especially as the baby grows older. These bags are cozy, warm and cannot be kicked off leaving the baby uncovered. Sleeping bags are generally made of soft blanket material. Therefore, the same careful and frequent laundering given to the baby's other bedding should be given to them.

Changing diapers

FOR CHANGING A DIAPER YOU WILL NEED:

bucket for dirty diaper and clothes
absorbent cotton
baby ointment
clean cloth diaper, **or** disposable lined diaper, if used
clean plastic pants
clean stretch suit or other clothes

Diapering used to be one of the great skills of parenthood. It consisted of experimenting with several different methods of folding the very large cloth to find which one was best suited to your baby's size and particular shape. The cloth was folded to create a multi-layered pad for absorbency. The folding method was up to you.

With the advent of the prefolded washable diaper, all that has changed. The diaper itself has been folded into layers and stitched closed at the top and bottom. It has two lines of stitching which run the length of the diaper to prevent the cloth layers inside from shifting. The result is a neat, soft, thick rectangular pad, easy to use and comfortable for your baby. Prefolded diapers come in varying sizes from newborn to toddler.

To use the prefolded diaper: lay it flat on the changing mat and fold both ends toward the middle, lengthwise. Make a thicker part for extra absorbancy by folding one end down, inside the diaper. This should be at the back for a girl, at the front for a boy. Place the baby on the diaper, overlap the corners at both sides and, when you have made sure the fit is snug but not tight, pin with diaper safety pins.

Changing diapers may be at first a clumsy, awkward process but in no time you will become very proficient. Indeed, there will be sufficient opportunities to practice this new skill! There are many different techniques and all are acceptable if the end result is a snug fitting, comfortable diaper safely secured on the baby.

Use the techniques shown in these pictures as a guide but also invent tricks of your own so that the process becomes easy for your baby. A few changes in folding and some adjustments in ways to secure the diapers may be required before this routine is accomplished with ease. Remember always to wash your hands after changing a diaper, just as you do after using the toilet yourself.

Bonding

The changing of diapers should be an opportunity for much more than just a quick, perfunctory clean-up. This is an opportunity to interact, to communicate with the baby. It is a good time for a warm, loving social exchange. So, talk to the baby, smile at him and show him how special you think he is. This is an excellent opportunity for finger play and discovery games. (Remember to keep a spare diaper handy because little boys when they are uncovered have a proclivity to sprinkle – with good aim!) As an experienced parent do not take the job of caring for your baby so seriously that you forget to enjoy it.

Today both parents share in much of the care of the new baby. It is very rewarding to care for an infant who is by nature a warm, loving creature initially so dependent on you and so very responsive to your efforts. Actually, the routine of diaper changing provides an excellent time for the parents to become involved with their baby.

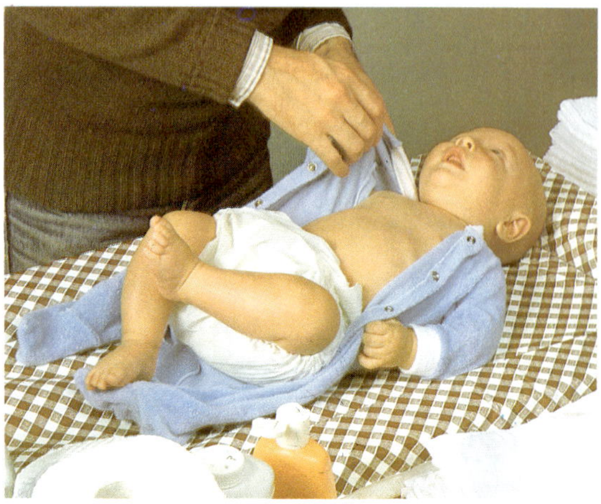

1 First, remove the old diaper and plastic pants.

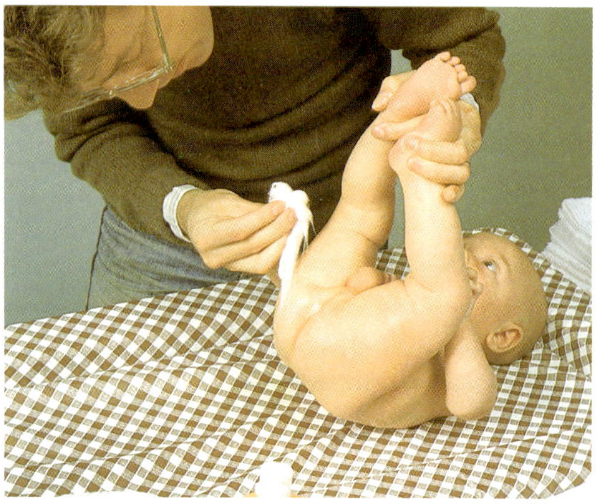

2 Lift up the baby's bottom, holding both ankles in one hand, with a finger between the ankle bones to prevent them from rubbing together.

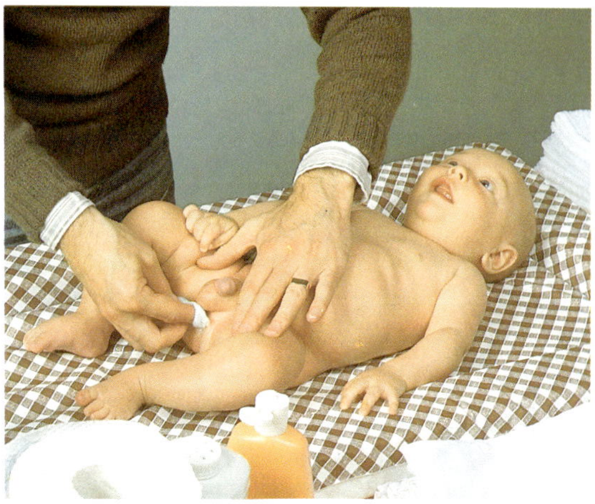

3 Wipe the baby's bottom with absorbent cotton and baby oil. Then lower the baby onto the mat and clean the genital area in the same way.

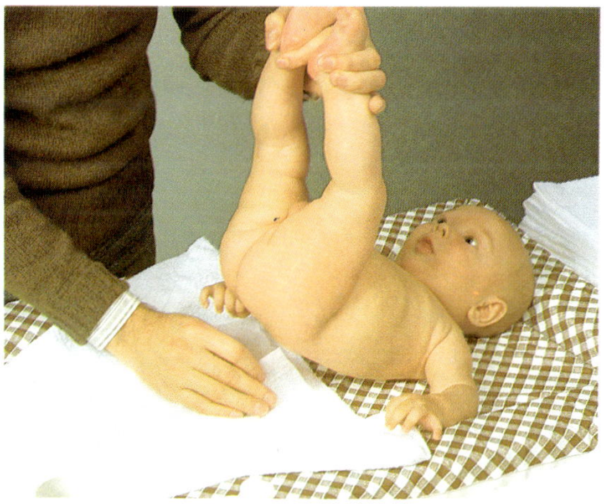

4 Lower the baby's bottom onto the diaper.

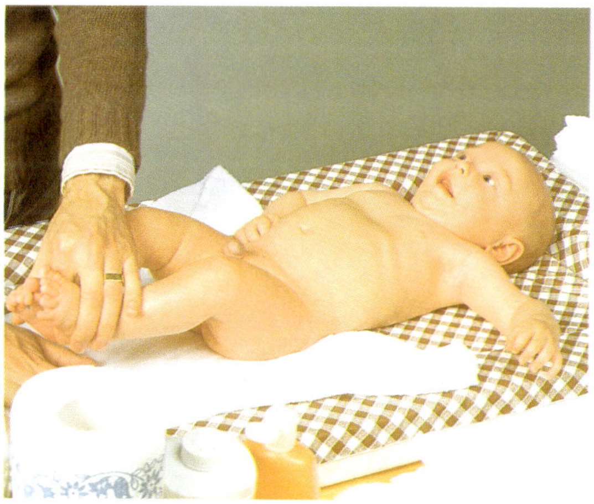

5 Position the baby in the centre of the diaper.

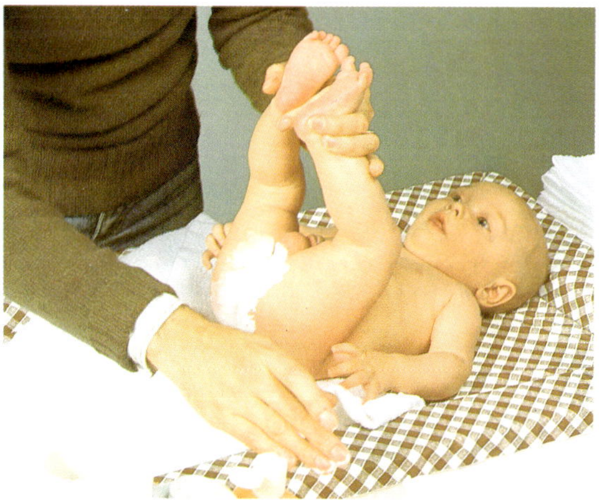

6 Apply baby powder liberally to the baby's bottom.

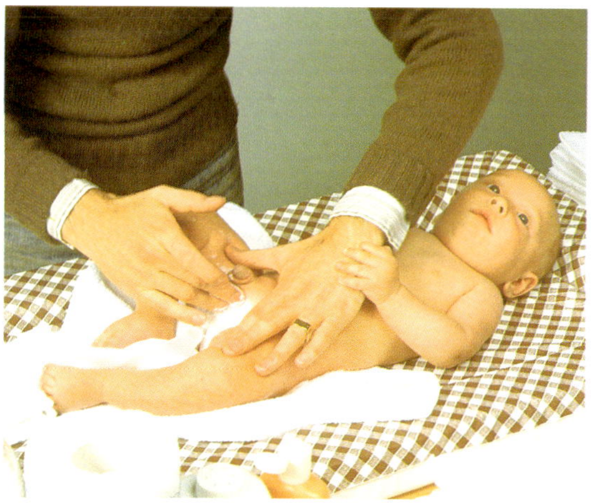

7 If irritated, apply baby ointment to the genital area.

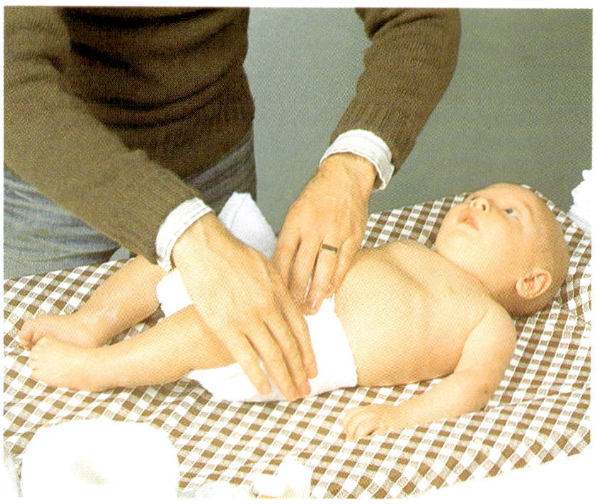

8 Bring the central portion of the diaper up between the baby's legs and overlap the corners at both sides. Make sure that the diaper fits snugly and is not too tight.

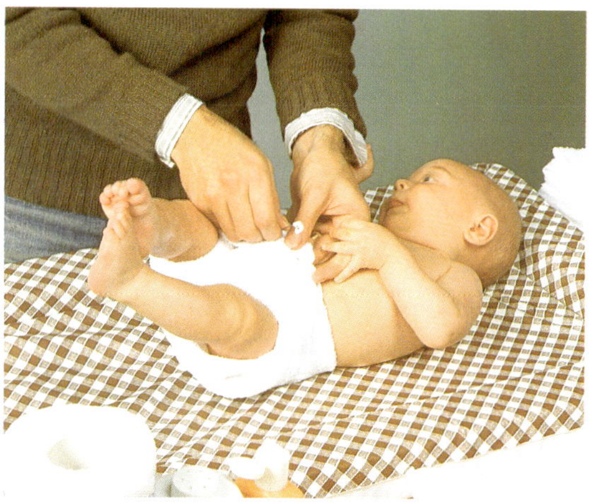

9 Pin, catching all layers of the diaper with a plastic-headed diaper pin. Keep your hand between the pin and the baby's skin.

Chapter 12 Common problems in the newborn

This discussion of problems which commonly occur during a baby's first few weeks of life is not intended as a substitute for seeking expert medical advice. It would be impracticable to suggest that every problem should be taken to a doctor. Friends and relatives can still be a great help but you should consider carefully before following their advice. If in doubt consult your doctor.

Most of the symptoms mentioned here can indicate one of several conditions and they can also occur in perfectly healthy babies. It requires experience to decide whether a symptom is harmless, and the purpose of this list is simply to give enough information to enable parents to decide whether they need to get in touch with their doctor. Some of the conditions covered here occur in babies throughout their early years, but the causes of illness in young babies and their reactions to them are often sufficiently different to require quite special advice. This separate checklist has therefore been drawn up to supplement the longer guide to your baby's health which is given at the end of the book.

ABNORMAL STOOLS *see* Diarrhea; Constipation

ANEMIA
Often characterized by pallor and lassitude, anemia is caused by a fall in hemoglobin concentration – the substance that carries oxygen in the blood. Premature babies and babies who have been ill are especially prone to anemia. Mild cases are harmless and cure themselves. If lack of iron or of a particular vitamin is the cause, then medicine can be given to effect the cure. Occasionally, severe anemia may require a blood transfusion – a simple and safe procedure.

ASYMMETRY of the head *see* Head asymmetry
BILIRUBIN *see* Jaundice

BLEEDING
Female babies sometimes have vaginal bleeding like a period for a few days after birth. Slight bleeding may also occur when the umbilical cord separates, staining the diaper. Loss of more than a few drops of blood should be taken seriously as a tiny baby cannot afford to lose much blood. Severe bleeding from any site in the first few days of life due to a vitamin deficiency is now rare. It can be corrected by giving vitamin K prescribed by the doctor.

BOILS *see* Spots
CANDIDA ALBICANS *see* Monilia

CEPHALHEMATOMA
Bruising of the baby's skull during delivery sometimes causes a little blood to be trapped between one of the skull bones and the membrane which lies over it. As the blood is broken down, fluid accumulates and a soft swelling appears a few days after birth. Some babies may have two swellings. The swelling is quite harmless and usually disappears within a few weeks, though it may persist two or three months.

CIRCUMCISION
Circumcision is done to improve hygiene. It involves cutting the foreskin off a baby's penis. In most instances it is done the day before the baby is discharged from the hospital; in others, it may be done in the delivery room. The procedure causes very little pain, so anesthesia is unnecessary. Over 90 percent of male babies have this procedure in the United States. If a Jewish couple plans to have a ritual circumcision this is done on the eighth day of life. There are those who maintain circumcision is not necessary. If a male decides, in later life, he wants to be circumcised this operation will cause increased morbidity.

COLIC *see* Crying

CONGENITAL DISORDER
This is any disorder which is present at birth – often a physical malformation of some kind. Early detection and treatment are important, and this is the reason for the detailed routine examination of all newborn babies.

CONJUNCTIVITIS
During the first few days of life many babies have a slight yellow discharge from the eyes which dries as loose crusts on the eyelids and inner corners of the eyes. This is harmless and the crusts can be cleaned off with cotton and warm water.

A similar, but more profuse discharge usually indicates conjunctivitis. The eyelids may also be swollen and red. Such an infection could damage the eye, but antibiotic drops or ointment will normally cure it. Intensive treatment is sometimes necessary, involving injections of antibiotics and very frequent eye drops, but even in severe cases the eye is very rarely damaged if adequate treatment is given.

The ducts which drain tears from the eyes into the nose are not always fully formed at birth. If they are blocked, tears tend to spill out of the eyes all the time and the baby may be prone to mild attacks of conjunctivitis. Antibiotic ointment may therefore be prescribed to prevent this. The ducts can be opened by gentle probing by a surgeon using a general anesthetic, but this is delayed for some months since spontaneous opening often occurs.

CONSTIPATION

A perfectly healthy breast-fed baby may move his bowels only once a week. A baby is therefore said to be constipated only if the stools are abnormally hard and difficult to pass as well as being infrequent. Passing a hard stool may be painful and sometimes causes a crack in the lining of the anal canal which bleeds a little.

There are many possible causes of constipation, though often no definite cause will be found. Underfeeding or loss of food by vomiting may be responsible. A rare but important cause is Hirschsprung's disease, a partial obstruction of the lower bowel. The importance of recognizing this is that laxative treatment will not help and, in fact, may even be harmful.

It is important to check if there is an underlying cause of constipation which requires special treatment. If no such cause exists and constipation continues, various simple remedies can be tried. Give the baby plenty to drink, such as boiled water or diluted fruit juice, which usually softens and loosens the stools.

COUGHING

A baby may cough a little during or after a feeding but persistent coughing at other times is not normal; it may indicate that the baby has a chest infection.

CRADLE CAP

Cradle cap is the name given to the slightly greasy scales or crusts which sometimes collect on the baby's scalp. It is quite harmless and disappears of its own accord during the first few months. Picking, scratching, washing or brushing the scalp usually has no effect. Washing the scalp with a shampoo recommended by your doctor can help keep it at bay, and persistent crusts can be removed by applying baby oil overnight and combing gently.

CRYING

All babies cry at times. This may be simply because they want company, are hungry or are uncomfortable in a dirty diaper, in which case attending to these basic needs will settle the baby. Parents should not be rigid about only feeding their baby when the feeding is "due". Picking up a crying baby to comfort him is not "spoiling" but simply supplying a basic need. If the crying seems to indicate that the baby wants to be picked up often, then carrying him in a baby sling may be the answer.

Occasionally the baby cries excessively and this will cause anxiety. However, even when a baby suddenly starts to cry far more than usual, a physical illness is seldom the cause. It may be that a vicious circle has been set up in the following way. The baby is uncomfortable and therefore fails to take a full feeding. He goes to sleep but wakes up soon because he is still hungry. Not having slept enough, he again does not take a proper feeding. After crying for his feeding, he may gulp his milk greedily along with a lot of air. Before he has finished his stomach feels full and so he does not want any more. He may belch up a lot of air and at the same time vomit. When he eventually goes to sleep again he is still underfed and once more wakes up too soon feeling hungry and crying.

The mother is naturally upset, and this makes it more difficult for her to comfort the baby. Add to this the fatigue that the mother feels during the first few weeks, and it is not difficult to see why the problem can be so hard to cope with.

One of the most helpful things in this situation is for all parties to have a good sleep and regain their composure. Of course the reassurance that there is nothing wrong with the baby, and that the whole problem will soon pass, is a great help. If the baby is crying excessively and the feeding routine is very irregular, it may help to try and establish a regular regimen. If the baby is being bottle-fed, the father or another relative or friend may be able to lend a hand so that the mother can catch up on her rest. If the baby is breast-fed nobody else can take over, but an occasional bottle feeding can give the mother a much needed break.

Babies who cry a lot are often said to have colic – a pain experienced when the intestine is distended, or contracting forcefully. It is often said that three-month colic (the problem tends to ease after three months) or evening colic are responsible. The supply of breast milk is rather less in the evenings and this may be why babies cry more then. There is, in fact, little evidence of abnormality in the intestines of babies who cry frequently.

Crying babies are sometimes said to have "gas". There is no doubt that babies swallow air when they feed and that passing gas sometimes makes a baby more comfortable. It is, however, unlikely that gas will make a baby cry for days on end. It is more a case of the crying causing the baby to swallow excess air in the first place.

DIAPER RASH

As a baby's bottom is almost always wrapped up in a diaper which is soaked in urine part of the time, it is no wonder that the skin gets irritated.

Often the urine itself, and its ammonia content in particular, is responsible for a rash called *ammoniacal dermatitis*. The soap used to wash the diapers may not have been rinsed out properly and may irritate the skin. *Candida albicans* (monilia) may infect the area and a skin condition called **seborrheic dermatitis** often begins there.

It is important to change diapers regularly in order to avoid rashes. Several creams to protect the baby's skin are available. Fresh air is helpful if the baby has a rash and it is worthwhile to leave the baby without a diaper for a time. Plastic pants should be avoided if a rash is present.

DIARRHEA

This is the frequent passage of abnormally fluid stools. Since a baby's stools can often be quite soft and frequent, you need not be concerned unless they are very different from usual and much more frequent. If the baby is not taking fluids, or if the diarrhea is combined with vomiting, there is a danger of dehydration and you should see the doctor immediately.

Diarrhea is not usually due to overfeeding or to the type of milk. However, if a mother who is breast-feeding takes even a mild laxative this may be passed to the baby in the milk and cause mild diarrhea.

The most important cause of diarrhea in babies and young children is infection. The infection may be within the intestines (gastroenteritis) or elsewhere, in the ear for example.

The treatment for the diarrhea itself is to give the baby only clear fluids to drink. Stopping the milk can stop the diarrhea and the fluid replaces that which has been lost. Once the diarrhea has ceased, milk feedings can be gradually started again.

It is best to seek advice if you think your baby's diarrhea is severe enough to need treatment. It is unwise to give homemade mixtures or family remedies, as giving the wrong substances could be harmful. Kaopectate, paregoric and other remedies used by adults should not be used; some such preparations might be extremely dangerous.

DIMPLE, SACRAL *see* Sacral dimple
EVENING COLIC *see* Crying
EXCHANGE TRANSFUSION *see* Jaundice
EYE DISCHARGE *see* Conjunctivitis

FEVER

Fever is one of the most common signs of illness in children. If there is any doubt about the cause of a baby's fever, and especially if he or she seems otherwise sick, you should call your doctor. Perfectly healthy small babies may, however, develop a high temperature simply because they are wearing too many clothes. (Too little clothing may cause a baby's temperature to fall below normal, and this is more dangerous than overheating.) As a rough guide: a baby will need about double the thickness of clothing that an adult would want to be comfortable.

FLUORIDE

It has been shown that fluoride helps children to develop teeth which are more resistant to decay. Fluoride is beneficial while teeth are developing (the permanent teeth actually start to develop before birth), so, if supplements are to be given, this should start soon after birth.

FOOT DEFORMITY *see* Talipes
GAS *see* Crying
GASTROENTERITIS *see* Diarrhea

HEAD ASYMMETRY

It is quite common for a young baby's head to become asymmetrical because the skull bones are quite pliable and the side that usually rests on the mattress may become flattened. In time, the baby is able to move his head more freely and the tendency for continued pressure at one point is less. At the same time the head is growing and the skull bones are becoming firmer and less susceptible to the effects of pressure. Thus the asymmetry gradually disappears. This may take several years, and may never be quite complete – very few adults have absolutely symmetrical heads – but long before that the child's hair will hide the asymmetry.

HERNIA, Inguinal and Umbilical

A hernia occurs when part of an organ protrudes from its normal position through a gap in the layer of muscle which covers it. In a hernia in the groin (an **inguinal hernia**) the intestine can become blocked and its blood supply cut off (strangulated). This can be very painful.

A hernia at the umbilicus, or navel, is quite common and much less serious. It may not be apparent during the first week or so but may eventually reach quite a size – protruding more than an inch. For unknown reasons these hernias are particularly common in black children. They may sometimes cause a baby a little discomfort but, since they usually disappear during the first year or two and since complications do not develop, there is no need for an operation. If such a hernia does persist (and this is very rare), it can be repaired at a later date.

HIPS, dislocation of

Some babies are born with abnormally lax hip joints. Usually these are not actually dislocated but the hip slips easily in and out of joint. This is what the doctor is looking for when he tests the newborn's hips (*see* p. 130). If the hips are not properly in joint at birth, they are likely to become more unstable as the baby grows and a permanently dislocated hip could result.

Treatment aims to hold the hips firmly in joint so they can develop normally. The earlier treatment is started, the easier and more successful it will be. Keeping the legs well apart by putting on two diapers may be adequate, or splints can be used to do the same thing more effectively. If the condition fails to respond to this treatment, a physician may advise an operation at a later date.

HYDROCELE

A hydrocele is an accumulation of fluid around the testes, which causes a swelling of a baby boy's scrotum. This may look similar to an **inguinal hernia** but the distinction is important since a hydrocele is quite harmless. No treatment is required and most hydroceles disappear during the first year of life. If one does persist it can be removed by an operation at a later date.

INGUINAL HERNIA *see* Hernia
INTESTINAL OBSTRUCTION *see* Vomiting

JAUNDICE

As a result of the continuous breakdown of aging red blood cells, a yellow pigment (bilirubin) is produced in the body and is removed by the liver. Before birth the bilirubin produced by the fetus is removed across the placenta and excreted by the mother's liver. After birth, the baby's own liver must excrete the bilirubin, but it takes a few days for this to begin. During this time the pigment accumulates, which gives the baby's skin a yellowish tinge known as jaundice. Nearly all babies become at least slightly jaundiced in the days immediately after birth.

There are several situations in which jaundice may be prolonged or more pronounced. The premature baby's liver, being less mature, takes longer to begin excreting bilirubin; infection may reduce the liver's efficiency; and, very occasionally, a substance in breast milk has a similar effect.

The production of a greater than usual amount of bilirubin can also exacerbate jaundice. This may be caused by bruising, when the blood under the skin (that is what bruising is) is broken down to bilirubin. Similarly, antibodies from an Rh-negative mother destroy the red blood cells of an Rh-positive baby, producing extra bilirubin (*see* p. 221).

Severe jaundice in the newborn period can impair hearing and cause brain damage. Fortunately treatment is available which can prevent these consequences. Light changes bilrubin into a similar but apparently harmless chemical, and if the baby is under lights (phototherapy), bilirubin is cleared from the body more rapidly. If this is not successful, exchange transfusion can be performed. By repeatedly removing a small volume of blood and replacing it with fresh blood the baby's blood is gradually changed. This process replaces the red cells as well as removing the bilirubin itself. This is important in Rh-disease because it is the breakdown of these cells which causes the jaundice.

JITTERINESS

This is the term used to describe a baby who is easily startled, perhaps irritable, and whose movements are very jerky. Such babies are also likely to be difficult to feed as they find it difficult to control their sucking movements.

Jitteriness can be the result of a difficult or rapid delivery or of a lack of glucose or calcium in the blood, though in many cases no cause can be found. The condition can be quite distressing for the baby and mother, but it appears to be harmless and disappears in time.

LASSITUDE *see* Sleepiness

MONILIA

This is an infection caused by the fungus *Candida albicans*. It takes the form of white patches, looking rather like curds of milk, which are firmly attached to the tongue and the inside of the cheeks. *Candida albicans* can also cause a diaper rash.

Often the baby is not upset by monilia, though sometimes the mouth appears to be sore and he is reluctant to eat. Treatment with an antifungal medicine is simple and clears the infection quite quickly.

NAVEL *see* Umbilicus

OVERFEEDING

Provided the supply of milk is adequate (and it usually is), a breast-fed baby will take just as much as he needs and will not get really fat. The same applies to a bottle-fed baby, but there are ways in which the latter can be persuaded to overeat. Although when a baby has had enough he tends to show this by sucking less strongly, stopping altogether or in some other way expressing his lack of interest, he can nonetheless sometimes be coaxed into taking more. This is a mistake.

Some babies are naturally restless; if the mother thinks he is hungry every time he stirs she may tend to overfeed him. Making the formula too rich is another cause of overfeeding. The overstrength formula leaves the baby thirsty. He cries, and so is given another feeding, still too strong, and the cycle continues. Care should be taken every time a formula is mixed and the temptation to make the feeding a little stronger in order to help "build up" the baby must be resisted. A bottle-fed baby – or any baby in particularly hot weather – should be offered plain water or dilute fruit juice once or twice a day; if the baby is only thirsty, he will happily drink this. Introducing solid food too soon (i.e. before about four months) can also cause excessive weight gain (*see* chapter 13).

PALLOR *see* Anemia
PHOTOTHERAPY *see* Jaundice
PYLORIC STENOSIS *see* Vomiting
REGURGITATION *see* Vomiting

RESPIRATORY DISTRESS

The "respiratory distress syndrome" is a condition which affects premature babies. Mature babies are almost never affected. It is caused by lack of a chemical called surfactant which helps to keep the lungs expanded. Without it, breathing is physically more difficult and less efficient. Oxygen treatment is often required and in more severe cases the baby may need a ventilator to help him breathe. The condition can be fatal, but in most cases it will get better in time as the lungs begin to produce surfactant.

RH-DISEASE *see* Jaundice

SACRAL DIMPLE

Many babies have a dimple over the base of the spine, visible in the upper part of the cleft between the buttocks. This is generally harmless and, as the baby grows older, the dimple will disappear. Some dimples, usually rather higher up, are much deeper and extend right down to the spinal cord. These can be the cause of meningitis and so need to be repaired surgically.

SEBORRHEIC DERMATITIS *see* Diaper rash

SLEEPINESS
The newborn baby usually spends most of his day asleep. As he grows older he will stay awake for longer periods. Some normal babies are very sleepy and falling asleep in the middle of a feeding is quite common. Sleepiness in the first few days of life can also be caused by certain drugs taken by the mother during labor. A moderate degree of jaundice (*see* p. 166) will also make the baby more sleepy than usual, but as the jaundice clears, so the baby will become more alert. Undue sleepiness, however, especially if the baby had not previously been so sleepy, may indicate that the baby is sick. If there is any doubt advice should be sought.

SNEEZING
This is the normal way for a baby to clear his nose and does not indicate that he is sick. Dried crusts of mucus in the nose may cause discomfort to the baby and can be gently removed with damp absorbent cotton, but do not poke the baby's nose as this only causes further discomfort.

SPOTS or BOILS
Babies do not often develop boils but they sometimes have more superficial septic spots. These appear like little white or yellow blisters and are usually found in the skin folds of the neck and under the arms. They are mostly harmless but, as they can lead to a more serious infection or infect other babies, it is usual to treat them if there are more than two or three spots. Washing the skin with a dilute antiseptic may be sufficient but antibiotics are sometimes required. Consult your doctor.

SQUINT
If each eye looks in a slightly different direction rather than being exactly parallel, the baby has a squint. Squints are common in the first few weeks of life. Most are due to a slight imbalance between the six muscles which move each eye, and are no cause for concern. As the baby's vision develops he is able to control his eye movements more accurately and the squint should disappear. If the baby has a very marked squint or if it persists beyond three months, he should be seen by a doctor.

STICKY EYES *see* Conjunctivitis

SUCKING BLISTERS
Sucking may cause some thickening of the baby's lips, known as "sucking pads". These look a little like blisters, though they are not. They are harmless and disappear in time.

TALIPES
A child's foot is naturally held at about right angles to the shin, but a newborn baby's foot often points downward and inward. However, the foot can normally be pushed to at least the right angle position. When it cannot, the deformity is known as talipes.

Sometimes the baby's foot lies at a narrower than normal angle to the shin and cannot be pushed to the right-angle position. This can quite easily be corrected by gently manipulating it downward at fairly frequent intervals – at every feeding, for example. Sufficient pressure should be used to cause slight discomfort to the baby but not pain. The range of movement of the foot soon increases and the deformity does not recur.

Less commonly, the foot is turned down and inward. This is a more severe deformity which needs expert treatment. Possibly the doctor will strap the foot and the sooner this treatment begins (within a few hours of birth is not too soon), the better the result will be. So long as adequate treatment is given, the baby should eventually have normal feet.

TEAR DUCT OBSTRUCTION *see* Conjunctivitis
TEMPERATURE *see* Fever
THREE-MONTH COLIC *see* Crying
UMBILICAL HERNIA *see* Hernia

UMBILICUS
The stump of the umbilical cord usually dries cleanly and after a few days it separates, leaving a very small raw area at its point of attachment, which quickly heals. Sometimes, due to the presence of bacteria, the umbilicus is "sticky" and there is a slight discharge. Healing usually takes place naturally but the bacteria can cause a more serious infection. The area must be kept clean and dry. If infected, see doctor.

Most babies have navels that retract after the umbilical cord drops off. Actually, there is little that can be done to affect whether your baby has an "inner" or an "outer" navel. The odds are overwhelmingly in favor of the navel retracting.

In some babies, the umbilical ring, the opening through which the umbilical vessels passed, is enlarged. If the enlargement is pronounced a small portion of the baby's intestine can protrude through it when the baby cries (umbilical hernia). This is a rare problem and if the protrusion is small (pea-size), it is of no consequence. It usually closes in a few months. If the protrusion is larger, it may be cosmetically displeasing, but should not cause the baby any harm.

VITAMINS
Since a normal varied diet contains all the vitamins necessary for health, taking extra vitamins is usually unnecessary and can even be harmful. There are, however, some conditions in which vitamin supplements are required and, while a baby is taking only milk he can suffer from lack of vitamins.

Breast milk does not contain an abundance of vitamins, but, provided the mother is well-nourished and the baby well-fed, he should be healthy. Nonetheless, there is no harm in giving a breast-fed baby small supplementary doses of vitamins as a precaution. Artificial milks have added vitamins and supplements are therefore unnecessary unless the baby is premature. Premature babies are prone to deficiencies during the first few months of life and extra vitamins A, C and D are usually given.

VOMITING
During the first few days of life, milk can quite easily flow back from the stomach to the mouth and trickle out. This regurgitation often happens soon after a feeding. Regurgitation usually stops after a few days but in some babies it will continue for much longer. It is a harmless condition although it can cause considerable inconvenience.

Practically every baby vomits at some time or other, yet vomiting can be an important sign of illness. As a general rule, if the vomiting is frequent or severe enough to prevent the baby gaining weight or if the baby is sick in any other way, then medical advice should be sought. Vomiting should not be blamed on the type of milk. It may be caused by infection (not necessarily of the intestine, i.e. gastroenteritis), or by intestinal obstruction. The latter is sometimes present from birth because of congenital malformation of the intestine.

One form of obstruction, pyloric stenosis, develops only after a few days or weeks. It is more common in boys. The pylorus, a muscle which controls the passage of food from the stomach into the intestines, becomes overdeveloped and almost completely blocks the outlet from the stomach. The only way the stomach can be emptied is by the milk being vomited back. This usually happens soon after a feeding and the milk tends to shoot out with some force. The diagnosis can be confirmed by the doctor feeling the pyloric muscle, and a minor operation is usually required to cure the condition.

WEIGHT LOSS
Babies normally lose a little weight during the first few days of life – between five per cent and ten per cent of the birthweight. By the seventh day, the baby should have begun to gain weight. Greater weight loss or a longer delay before weight gain commences may mean that the baby is not getting enough food or it may mean the baby is sick (*see* chapter 14). Obviously, should a baby suddenly start losing weight after previously gaining normally, medical advice should be sought. A reduction in the milk supply, if the mother is breast-feeding, sometimes coincides with an appetite spurt in young babies, and efforts may have to be made to stimulate the supply.

Mothers have an excellent intuition about babies who are losing weight. Most mothers do not have a baby scale in their home but this is not necessary as weighing the baby is a regular part of the checkup at the doctor's office.

Feeding in the first year

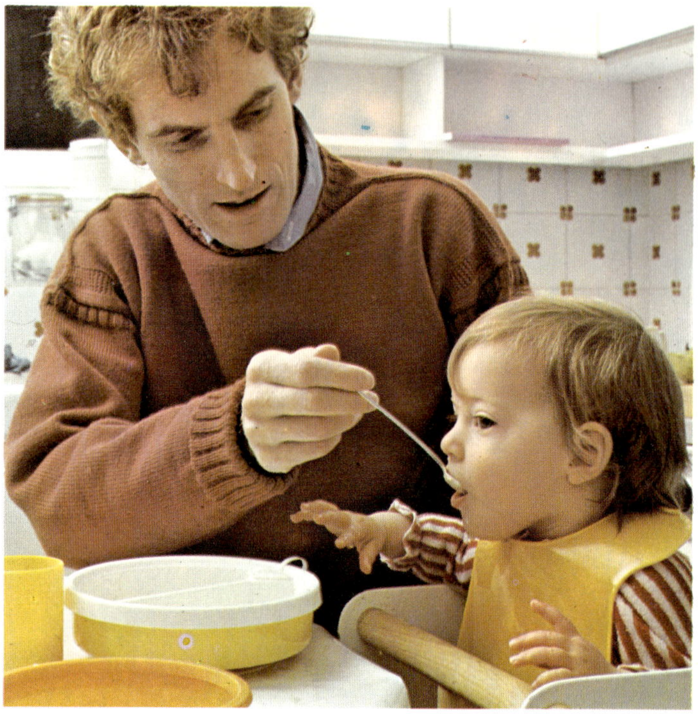

CHAPTER 13

One of the first changes a mother will make in feeding her baby is the addition of some solid food. The first step in this process is usually the adding of cereals to an infant's milk-based diet and is generally followed by the gradual introduction of other foods, such as fruits and vegetables.

When and how the change is accomplished has been the subject of much controversy. In the 1920s, after concerted efforts to improve child nutrition, a type of enriched cereal was devised that became the basis of baby food in the Western world. By this time, the long-standing custom of weaning babies after a year was gradually giving way to weaning at the age of six months. In the 1940s this became earlier still, so that in some places meat was offered at fourteen days, vegetables at ten and cereals at two days.

There were probably two main reasons for the trend toward the early introduction of solids: first, the belief that the baby would be more content, and second, an obsession with adequate, and in some cases rapid, weight gain. Inexperienced mothers were, and indeed still are, sometimes influenced by the advertising of baby food companies, advice from other mothers with fat babies and from nurses, who suggested solid foods as a "cure for crying".

Recently it has become increasingly clear that it is best not to begin mixed feeding at a very early age. There are several areas in which problems may arise. First, the younger the baby, the more likely it is that his enzyme systems and immunological (or defense) mechanisms, are immature, causing problems in the short term in digesting certain foods. There is also a suggestion that in the long term some chronic allergic illnesses may be caused by eating certain foods at an early age.

Cross references

See also	Chapter
Child health	12,16
Food values	2
Physical development	14

The introduction of solid or semisolid food, usually in the form of cereals added to the milk – is the first change in a baby's diet.

The second problem area is connected with the salt, or sodium, intake of the baby. The early introduction of solids, particularly the type of tasty foods that may be used as the first course of an infant's meal, generally increases sodium intake. Sodium is not stored by the body; any excess is passed out in the urine. As an infant's kidneys are not able to pass very concentrated urine, this means that excessively large volumes of urine have to be passed to excrete excess sodium. If this happens the baby loses water it needs and can become dehydrated. Severe dehydration may create a high sodium level in the baby's blood; and this high sodium level can, in turn, be dangerous to the brain.

The dehydration becomes even more serious if a baby is losing water, or fluid, in other ways – such as vomiting and diarrhea, or by excessive sweating in hot weather or during a feverish illness. The situation is frequently worsened because the baby, being short of water, becomes thirsty and cries. A mother will often assume that he is hungry and not thirsty, and she may therefore give him food, which may itself be salted, and this creates the establishment of a vicious circle.

The third problem is obesity. The introduction of cereals, rusks and mixed feeding too early, and the addition of too much sugar to these foods, can mean that the baby takes in more calories than he needs. The extra food is then stored in the form of fat. It is now known that 80 per cent of fat children will carry their obesity into adult life, although it has not been proven that all fat babies become fat children. There are, however, more immediate dangers for fat babies. They are more likely to suffer from acute respiratory, or chest, infections; extra weight often makes it difficult for them to move around; and, if they become dehydrated, this is difficult to detect as fatty tissue contains little water and the skin and subcutaneous tissue therefore show little change. For this reason a dangerous situation may go unrecognized. It is far easier to see your baby has a sensible diet.

Fourth, it is known that approximately one in 1,800 people suffers from celiac disease – a sensitivity to the protein of wheat, called gluten. If a child is sensitive to gluten, the early introduction of cereals containing wheat may well cause the child to develop celiac disease earlier in life than would otherwise occur. Although the diagnosis of this condition has improved, a child may nevertheless fail to thrive for a considerable time before the parents suspect that something is wrong.

The early introduction of solids caused a lot of concern in the mid-1970s. Introduction of cereals and other solid foods to the diet of babies before they have reached about four months of age should be strongly discouraged.

Practices in infant feeding are the result of a number of different factors, but whatever the external influences, it must be remembered that there are no average babies nor average parents; all are individuals, with varying needs. Parental – especially maternal – satisfaction is very important, and often underrated. Parents usually know better than anyone else what should be introduced into their baby's diet. If they use common sense and consult their pediatrician when a serious concern arises, they should have no major problems. In this way, they will know not only what new foods to introduce, but also what schedule of adding foods is best for their baby.

Changing patterns

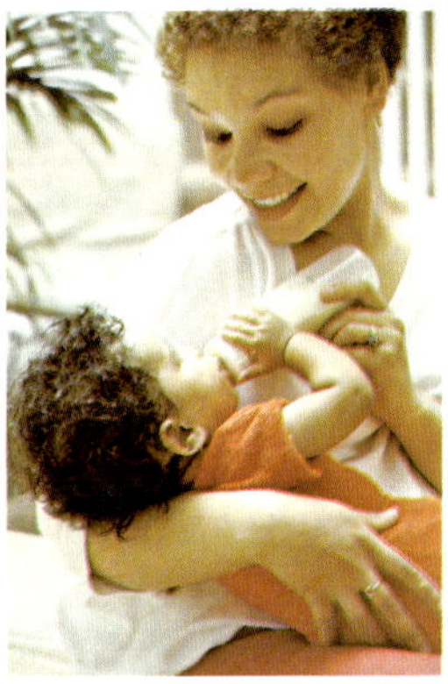

A baby does not need cereals or solids before the age of four months.

In eating, as in other things, a baby learns new skills and has new experiences during the first year. In fact, parents will see more dietary changes in this period than at any time in the future. The baby's diet gradually progresses from milk feedings to the addition of small amounts of solids, which become larger both in quantity and variety, before being completely integrated into the normal meals of the rest of the family. With new feeding skills it is important to give a free rein to individuality, remembering that all babies develop at their own pace; the natural rate of development should neither be hurried nor compared with that of other children.

At all stages, your attitude is very important; eating should always be regarded as an enjoyable event for both baby and parents. There is no need for mealtime to become a battle or a race against time. On the contrary, babies need to take their time to become accustomed to the new foods that they are given; touching food, playing with it and then rolling it around the mouth before swallowing are all part of this process.

If a baby refuses or spits out a food with a new taste or texture, this may have nothing to do with the flavor and the feel of the food; it may be simply that it is different and the child does not know what to do with it. Be patient and try again slowly. If it becomes obvious that the baby doesn't like it, stop and try again the next day. Never force your baby to eat a particular type of food.

Always try to keep calm, and if in doubt use your common sense. For example, if a baby is sick, upset or having teething difficulties, introducing new foods or making changes in routine will only add to the problems, not solve them. Making more than one change at a time may only confuse a baby and could result in you achieving nothing. Patience will therefore reap more rewards in the end.

Whether home-cooked or commercially prepared baby foods are used, the final aim is the same – to accustom the child to new tastes and textures and to ensure that he or she will grow up to like and eat a wide variety of foods.

Early changes (four to six months)

As described above, it is unwise and unnecessary to begin mixed feeding before the baby is four months old, but it should be begun at or before six months, as his own supplies of iron begin to run out about then.

The first taste of solid food will be a completely new experience for the baby and, quite naturally, he or she will take a few days to become accustomed to it and to taking food from a spoon.

Only a very small amount of food, of a smooth, semi-fluid consistency, is needed to start with, and you will still give a breast- or bottle feeding as well. Broth, strained baby foods and cereals are all suitable. Cereal should always be mixed with expressed breast milk, or milk from the baby's bottle, and fed with a spoon. It should never be added to the milk already in the bottle. If the baby will not take foods from a spoon, then he or she is not ready for solids.

Commercial baby foods are a good idea at this stage, when only small amounts are required. They are easily prepared, economical and the right consistency for a baby. Instant powdered foods are particularly economical.

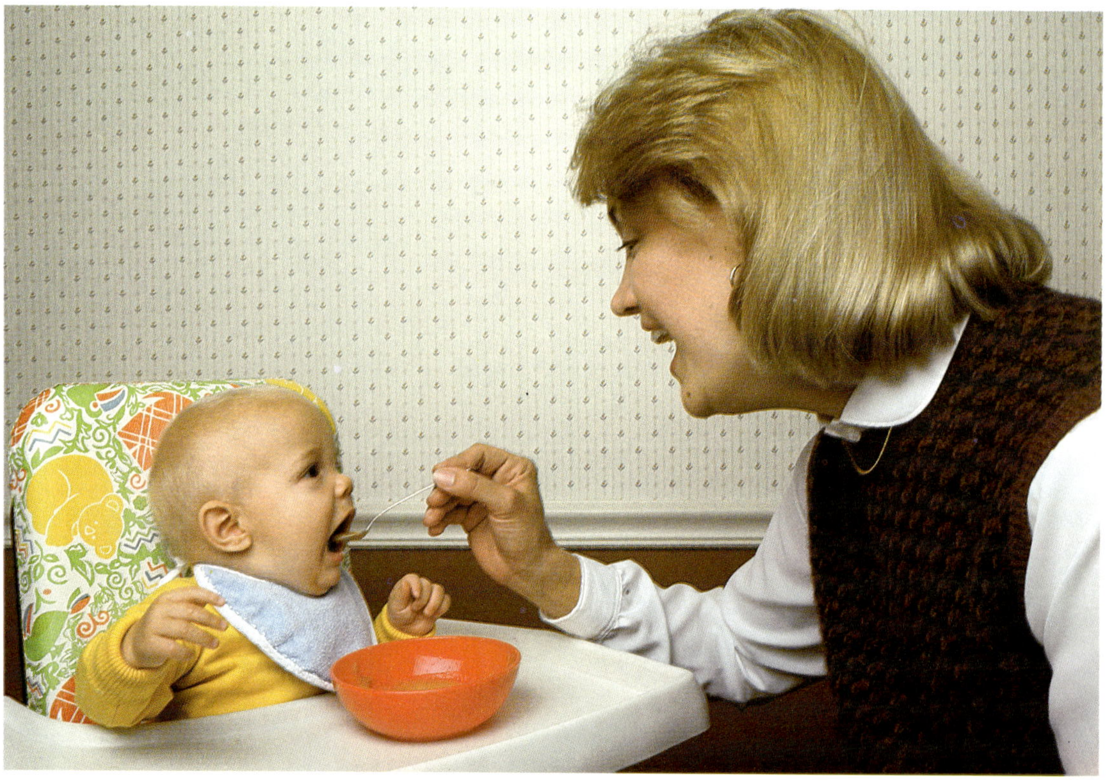

You may like to accustom your baby to eat with a spoon before teething begins at six or seven months, though this is not really necessary.

Remember, however, that opened jars should be stored in the refrigerator.

Sugar should not be added to foods, as this encourages a sweet tooth, which might lead to obesity and dental decay. Try to encourage an interest in various flavors, but do not add salt to the baby's food or use excessively salty foods. Many mothers taste food before feeding it to their babies and often try to season or sweeten it to their own taste. This is potentially dangerous (*see* p. 173).

As nutritional requirements are covered initially by milk alone, there is no need to worry if the baby takes only very little additional food. After a few weeks, however, more solids will be required, and the amounts given should be increased gradually and new food introduced. Eventually, the quantity of milk given can be decreased, but it is still essential that the baby be given enough fluid as water or fruit juice.

The amount of food a baby wants can vary enormously from day to day. Mothers should not be worried if the baby leaves most of his food one day because he is not hungry. He should not be made to eat it.

Changes from six to nine months

As the baby gradually becomes more independent and more active there are an increasing number of changes in his diet.

Babies may try to feed themselves any time from the age of six months and their efforts should be encouraged. Needless to say, this can be very messy: the floor, baby and mother all need some kind of protective covering.

Usually, babies start to chew when they are about six to seven months old, although teeth may not appear for several months. As definite chewing motions become regular, chopped foods of a familiar flavor can gradually be substituted for the more smooth-textured.

It is been suggested that there are critical periods when children are developmentally ready to learn certain skills, for example – chewing and coping with lumpier foods. Failure to introduce suitable foods at this time may mean that a critical, or sensitive, learning period has been missed, and may even result in lazy eating habits in later life.

With the baby's increasing independence comes an increasing awareness and interest in food. He will watch his mother preparing his food, perhaps chuckling with glee that it is yet another mealtime. As the purées give way to ground meats and liver, fish, mashed fruit and vegetables, whole eggs, grated cheese and bread and butter, special care should be taken to make the meals look attractive.

Interesting colors and shapes as well as textures are important characteristics of food at this time. White fish in a white sauce with mashed potatoes and cauliflower, followed by vanilla pudding, looks as pale and uninteresting a meal to a baby as it does to an adult. Colorful vegetables and colorful and unbreakable dishes can make all the difference to a baby's reaction – and desire to eat.

As the baby progresses to larger quantities of ground and mashed foods, home cooking becomes worthwhile – and cheaper than commercially prepared foods. During this stage the child can enjoy more items from the family menu, but perhaps not fried or spicy foods, onions or baked beans, as he may have difficulty in digesting them.

An adequate fluid intake is essential. If the baby cries between feedings, always consider that he or she may be thirsty rather than hungry and try a little natural fruit juice diluted with water or simply cool water. Remember that he cannot help himself to an extra drink like an adult. Natural fruit juice is better than many of the vitamin C-enriched syrupy fruit drinks, as these can harm the developing teeth because of their high sugar content. If a pacifier is used, never fill it with sweetened juice or syrup, as this encourages tooth decay.

When teeth begin to show, the baby can be offered plenty of hard foods, such as raw apple or carrot, instead of a teething ring. Never give small pieces of food, however, as the baby may choke on them.

Drinking from a cup is another skill that is acquired during this period. Many mothers like to let the baby practice with a cup in the bath tub. As the baby becomes more proficient with a cup it is possible to think of stopping breast- or bottle feeding altogether. Drinking from a cup is a major step forward in the social development of a child. He will be able to participate more in family meals. He may be more willing to attempt other new foods.

Later changes (nine to twelve months)

By this time a child is even more independent. He or she will be crawling and climbing, and may well be on the way to standing and walking unsupported. He should be able to feed himself reasonably well and drink from a cup on his own. All these efforts should be applauded and encouraged.

By this stage a baby's diet often contains a large variety of foods and gradually comes more into line with family meals, both in timing and food content.

Breast- and bottle feedings can cease when the baby is quite happy drinking from a cup, but milk is still a very important part of his diet. Many babies enjoy breast-feeding well into the second year; there is certainly no need to stop breast-feeding if both mother and baby enjoy it.

Some mothers continue to use approved infant formulas until the first birthday, but there is little or no advantage in giving such milk, which is meticulously modified to resemble breast milk, when mixed feeding is well established. If commercial milk is used, vitamin supplements may be indicated. Consult your physician about this.

The amount of milk needed varies from one child to another, and diminishes as more solids are included in the diet. At one year the baby will need about 1 pint (500 ml) a day.

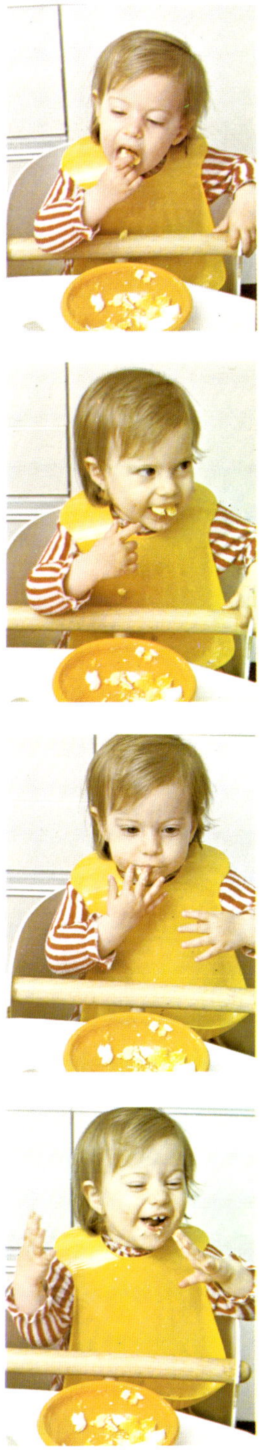

The baby should have time to enjoy his food and to become accustomed to its texture and feel as well as its taste. Let your baby play with his food and enjoy his mealtimes as much as possible.

Techniques and tools

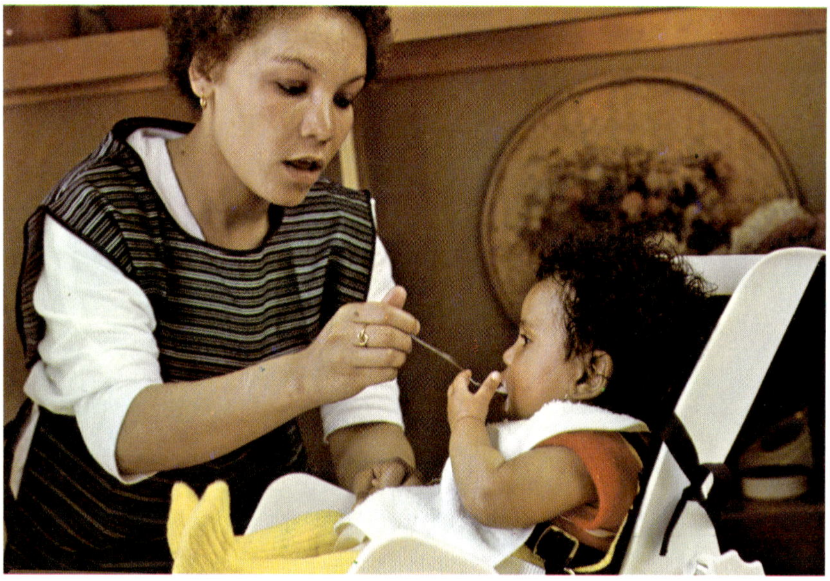

During mealtimes, protect your own clothes with an apron, and your baby's clothes with a bib.

Each step in introducing your baby to new foods will be easier if you make use of a set of simple aids – whether these are plastic spoons, bibs or waterproof floor covering – and make sure that you have them on hand for each feeding.

How to introduce solids

If you decide to use commercially prepared baby foods make sure you follow the manufacturer's instructions about opening and storage. Collect together all the utensils you will need before picking up the baby: a small spoon and cup or bowl and a pan containing some water. Take great care when opening jars to use a lever; insert it under the edge of the lid and turn as if unlocking a door; never attempt to open it by ramming a pointed instrument up under the cap and levering outward, as this can break the rim of the jar and shatter tiny pieces of glass into the baby food.

At first the baby takes only very small quantities of food. After he becomes accustomed to this new adventure he will take progressively more.

If you use a jar, only part of it will be used at one time. Open the container and spoon the right amount into the cup or bowl; cover the jar and store it in the refrigerator, and discard after use the following day. Place the cup or bowl in the pan of water and warm through. After finishing one variety of strained food, introduce another.

Protect your clothes by wearing an apron. It is unnecessary to buy one specially, many mothers find their husband's old shirts or pajama tops ideal cover-ups. They must, of course, be clean and soft to touch.

The baby's clothes are best protected by a waterproof bib with sleeves and a pocket the full width of the bottom to catch any spilled or dropped food. Flimsy plastic-covered bibs should not be used as these can easily adhere to the baby's mouth and are difficult for him to remove himself. Never leave any plastic bib on a child when you put him back in his carriage or crib thus avoiding any danger of suffocation.

Before starting, always make sure that your baby is comfortable and, preferably, in a dry diaper. It is probably better for the baby to begin by feeding him sitting on your lap, although some babies are able to sit in a high chair or baby chair by the time solids are introduced. If you use either always use a secure harness.

Sit the baby in a slightly more upright position than for breast- or bottle feeding, with his or her head against your shoulder and your left arm cuddled around him if you are right-handed. (If you are left-handed have your right arm supporting him.)

Have a table by your chair on which the bowl or cup can be safely placed, out of the baby's reach. Some people prefer to hold the cup or bowl in their supporting arm's hand, but you will probably find that you need this hand to keep the baby's arms under control and out of his mouth.

Start with a very small amount of food on the tip of a teaspoon and place it in the middle of the child's tongue about halfway back. The positioning is important; if it is placed too far forward the baby will almost certainly spit it out, and if it is placed too far back, he may choke slightly.

Do not force the food off the spoon but allow the baby time to suck it off. Your first attempt is likely to be ejected anyway. This is quite normal, as it takes the baby a little time to get used to this new method of feeding and the new taste of the food.

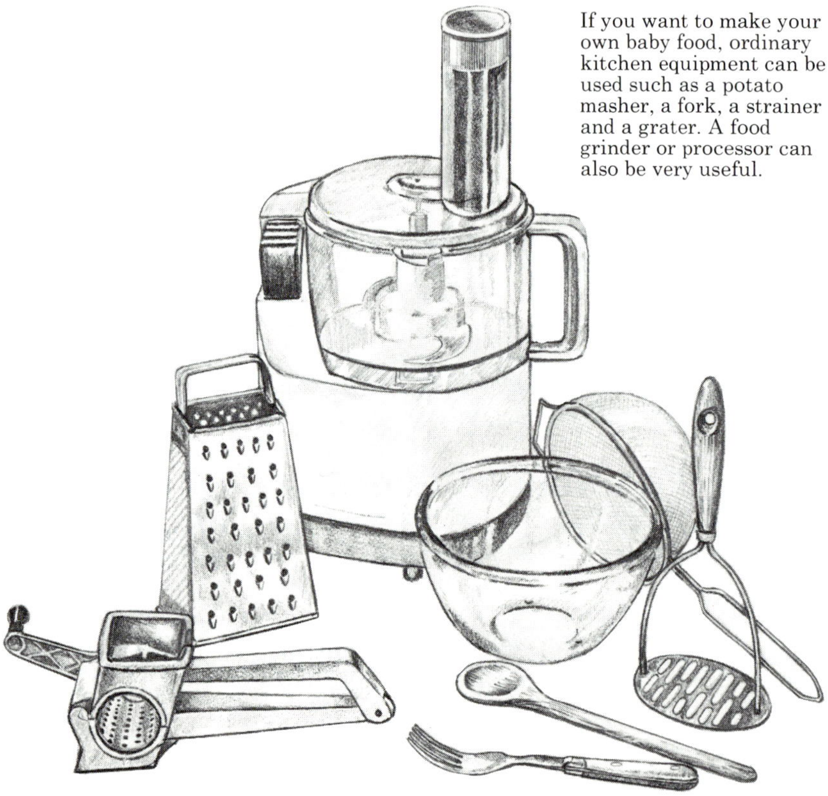

If you want to make your own baby food, ordinary kitchen equipment can be used such as a potato masher, a fork, a strainer and a grater. A food grinder or processor can also be very useful.

Your attitude is important. Try to be relaxed; if you are anxious the baby will soon become aware of your tension. Never try to encourage a baby to eat by the unhygienic practice of first taking a spoonful yourself and then offering the same spoon to the child; this can be a source of infection.

Making your own baby food
If you want to make your own strained or puréed foods, you can use a blender. But for the small quantity required you may well find that the blender blades are above the food.

Very high standards of hygiene are essential, both for yourself and your equipment. Only really fresh food should be used and it is important not to add any salt or a lot of sugar. Do not season food to suit yourself; a baby has much blander tastes than an adult.

As the child gets older, the family's food can be finely ground, chopped or mashed. No special equipment is required.

Freezing
Even when the baby is having chopped or mashed food from the family meal, quantities will still be relatively small. If you have a freezer you will find it saves time to prepare and cook double quantities or even more and freeze the excess. You can freeze it in an ice cube tray and take out the number of cubes that are needed.

When freezing food for a small baby, it is even more essential than usual to follow the instructions given by the freezer manufacturer. It is vital also to make sure that only sterilized utensils are used.

Individual plastic containers are suitable for freezing food and can be sterilized in the same way as baby bottles. Plastic freezer bags and freezer foil are also suitable, but should be used only once, as they are virtually impossible to clean adequately.

Warm food is an ideal breeding place for bacteria, so after cooking, food should be chilled rapidly and then frozen quickly. Similarly, food should always be reheated straight from the freezer, not thawed out first. To do this, put the frozen food into a bowl or pan of boiling water.

Other useful items
When about six months old, the baby will want to feed himself, so make sure that both his and your clothes are well protected. As he gets older and more proficient, a washable, strong plastic bib with "catch pocket" should suffice.

Put the baby in his high chair and make certain that he is securely harnessed. At all mealtimes, it might be better to let him concentrate on the job at hand and not have his attention diverted by such distractions as television or pets. If the floor within range of the baby is not washable, cover it. Old newspapers, or a plastic tablecloth, make a splendid "carpet".

Give the baby his own spoon. It should have a straight handle with a shallow bowl and rounded, not sharp, sides; a plastic spoon is ideal. Continue to keep a spoon for you to feed him, as his spoon is likely to be used as a toy until he starts to copy you.

A baby dish with straight sides makes it easier for the baby to push food onto his spoon. "Pushers" were once fashionable, but these are unnecessary and would be used for only a short time, soon being superseded by a fork. It is a good idea to use a bowl with a suction cap attached to its base to anchor it firmly to the tray of the high chair. This avoids the problem of the baby having to "chase" his bowl around the tray.

Drinking cups
There are various types of cups available, and much disagreement as to which is best. But there are general guidelines to bear in mind.

A cup needs to be unbreakable, as it is likely to be dropped when the baby has finished drinking, and thick enough for him to be unable to bite through it. Many parents like the non-spill baby cups. These have a cap to prevent spilling. The cap has a mouthpiece through which the baby may suck or allow fluid to flow when he drinks. These non-spill cups are convenient and should be considered a transition from the bottle to the regular cup which the child must eventually master.

A more conventional type of cup should be wide enough not to bump the baby's nose, but small enough for him to see over the top – for example, a plastic juice cup. The two-handled variety of cup is very practical: one handle for mother to hold onto – for greater security – and one for the baby.

A plastic bib with a "catch pocket" will protect the baby's clothes from spills.

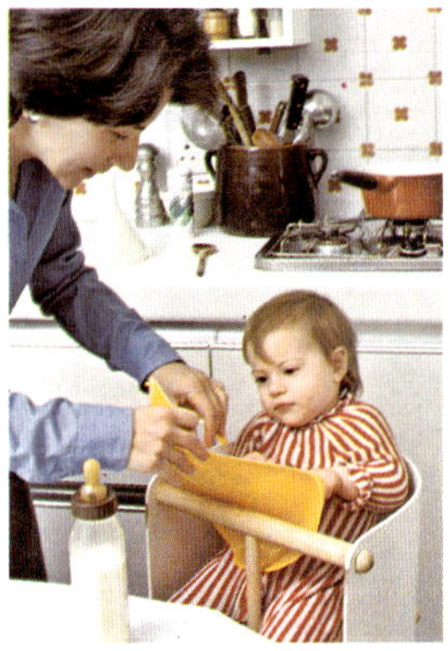

Special plastic feeding equipment is useful for feeding your baby. It is easy to clean and does not break easily. Forks and spoons should be rounded with no sharp edges. Dishes with straight sides make it easier for the baby to push food onto his spoon. Non-spill baby cups are particularly useful for a young baby, though he must eventually get used to a conventional cup.

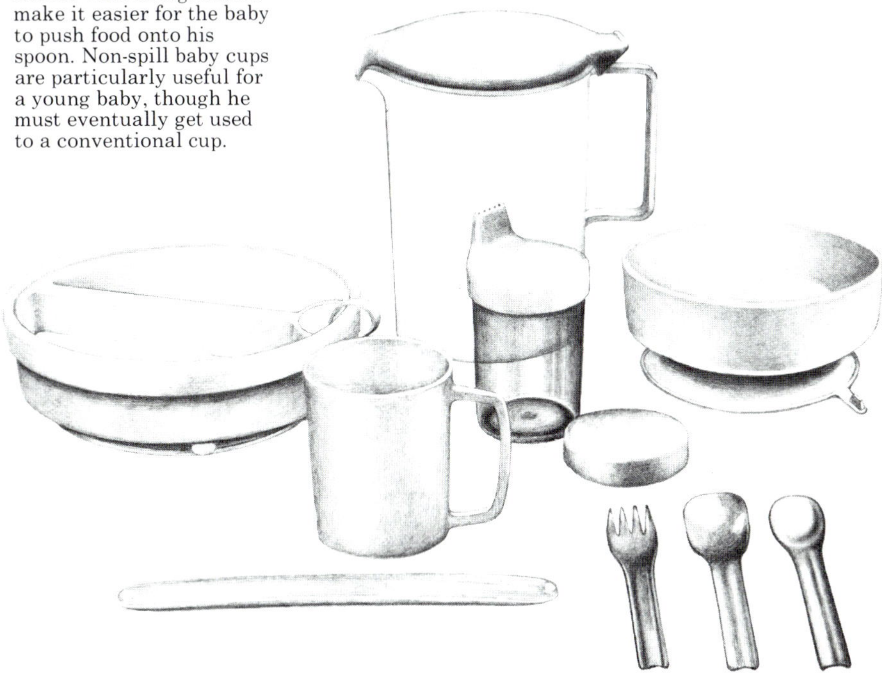

Landmarks

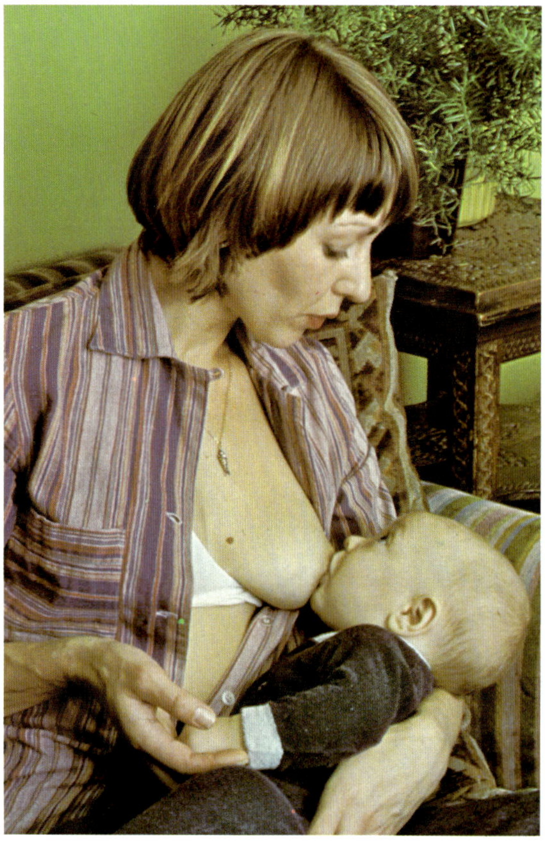

Breast-feeding can generally be continued as long as it suits both mother and baby to do so.

There are two types of changes connected with feeding which occur during the first year, one affecting the other. First, the changing patterns or landmarks of development (*see* chapter 14), and second, the changes of the daily routine, which depend on the landmarks. No two children, not even twins, acquire the same skills at exactly the same time. All timings are therefore only a guide to parents, who soon come to know what is right for their child.

Obviously it is easier to manage if there is some sort of routine, but it must be flexible. As long as the baby is well and contented, and most of the chores eventually get done, it certainly does not matter if days are organized chaos. Any time spent playing with and cuddling your baby is always well spent.

There are four major landmarks in the first year: (1) starting semisolids when about four to six months old; (2) learning to chew and cope with lumps and small pieces of food at any time from about six to seven months; (3) the baby learning to feed him or herself, at around the same age; (4) from about nine months old, becoming gradually integrated into family mealtimes, both in terms of what is eaten and when. As these changes are made, the baby progresses from five milk feedings a day (before starting solids) to three meals a day and two or three cups of milk daily by one year. As the amount of solid food increases, the amount of milk decreases and some feedings are therefore dropped.

The chart on the opposite page is a rough guide to changes in daily routine.

Introducing solids

It is probably easier to introduce solids at the middle of the day feeding, offering a small amount before the baby's breast- or bottle feeding, while he is still hungry. On the other hand there is no reason why you should not start at the morning feeding if the baby appears hungry then. Some parents start with the evening feeding, hoping that extra food at that time might help the baby to sleep through the night. This may not be such a good idea as he may be rather tired by then, and evenings are a busy time in most households. Whatever time is chosen, be ready to give a breast- or bottle feeding immediately after the solids, as the baby will not want to be kept waiting.

Increasing quantities

About a week after you introduce solids, the baby will be taking about four teaspoonfuls before his breast- or bottle feeding. You can then try adding solids to another feeding, probably the morning one. A breakfast variety of strained baby food, cereal mixed with breast milk or milk taken from the bottle feeding, or a little egg yolk are suitable. After another week, you can introduce either strained baby food – vegetable or fruit purées – or cereal to the remaining daytime feeding. During this time, the quantities of solids given at all feedings will be increasing slowly.

The time for dropping the late evening or early morning feeding, or both, varies a lot, but it is unlikely to occur before mixed feeding has been established three times a day. If you find that you have to wake your baby for his late evening feeding, try dropping it and see if he or she sleeps through the night.

Alternatively, the baby may wake in the evening and sleep through until breakfast time, in which case, try dropping the early morning feeding. Again, you can always return to giving it if necessary. If bottle feeding, remember, when you drop feedings, not to decrease the baby's daily supply of milk; offer the same amount of milk by dividing it between the remaining feedings.

Altering times

When the baby is about five months old, he will probably sleep longer in the morning, and his first feeding will be later in the day. (If he wakes earlier, he can be given fruit juice and cool water to tide him over.) The middle of the day feeding can then be given at about lunchtime, making suppertime around 4 to 4:30 pm. A bedtime feeding ends the day.

When to stop breast- or bottle feeding

Breast feedings or feedings of sophisticated modified formulas are usually stopped when certain landmarks have been reached. Mixed feeding should be firmly established with substantial amounts being taken at each of the three main meals. The baby should be quite happy drinking from a cup and the night and early morning feedings discontinued. These landmarks are all likely to be reached between

months 0 1 2 3 4	5 6	7 8 9	10 11 12
Milk only	Introduce semisolids Accustom baby to eating from a spoon	Baby begins to feed himself Baby begins to chew Introduce lumpier, ground foods	Baby feeds himself and drinks from a cup Integrate baby's feeding into family meals

Less than 4 months	At about 4 months	From 5 months	At about 8 months	By 1 year
5 milk feedings breast- or bottle Approximate times: (6 am–10 am–2 pm–6 pm–10 pm)	5 milk feedings breast- or bottle (6 am–10 am–2 pm–6 pm–10 pm 1) small amount of solids once daily (2 pm) 2) small amounts of solids twice daily (2 pm *and* 10 am or 6 pm) 3) Increased amount of solids three times daily (10 am–2 pm –6 pm)	4 milk feedings breast- or bottle (8 am–12 pm–4:30 pm–6:30 pm) Solid three times daily (8 am–12 pm–4:30 pm)	3 milk drinks (8 am–4:30 pm –bedtime) Solids three times daily (8 am–12 pm, including 2 courses–4:30 pm)	2–3 milk drinks (8 am–bedtime –possibly also in the evening) 3 Meals (breakfast–midday–evening)

Chart showing the four stages of the change to solid foods. The mealtimes given are to be taken only as a rough guide.

six and nine months. It is then quite safe to change to ordinary cow's milk, providing vitamin supplements are given (*see* p. 171). At first milk, and water, should be boiled and then cooled before they are given to the baby.

Breast- or bottle feedings are discontinued when the baby becomes uninterested in them. Breast-feeding can be continued as long as both mother and baby remain happy and content to do so. Sometimes mothers breast-feed for a year or more. If breast-feeding stops before a baby is drinking easily from a cup then bottle feeding will be necessary.

Unless advised by your doctor, it is unnecessary to take drugs to stop breast milk production: breasts might feel a little tight at the time a feeding would have been due, but this feeling subsides after a few days and the milk "dries up" naturally.

When to stop sterilizing and boiling

Feeding utensils which can harbor germs should be sterilized. This can generally be accomplished by your electric dishwasher. The time to stop this precaution ranges from 6–9 months depending on the development of the child. Once the child is active and mobile it seems rather pointless to continue sterilizing feeding utensils, as at this stage the baby is coming into contact with numerous non-sterile objects and, naturally, putting them into his mouth.

Although sterilizing can be stopped, high standards of hygiene and cleanliness are still essential. As long as you have a safe supply of water and pasteurized milk, boiling water and milk can be dispensed with when you stop sterilizing utensils. If you have any doubts about the safety of supplies, then continue to boil water and milk until the baby is over a year old – and consult your doctor.

By the age of one year, the baby will be having breakfast, lunch and suppertime meals with the family, and some milk with breakfast, at bedtime and possibly in the afternoon.

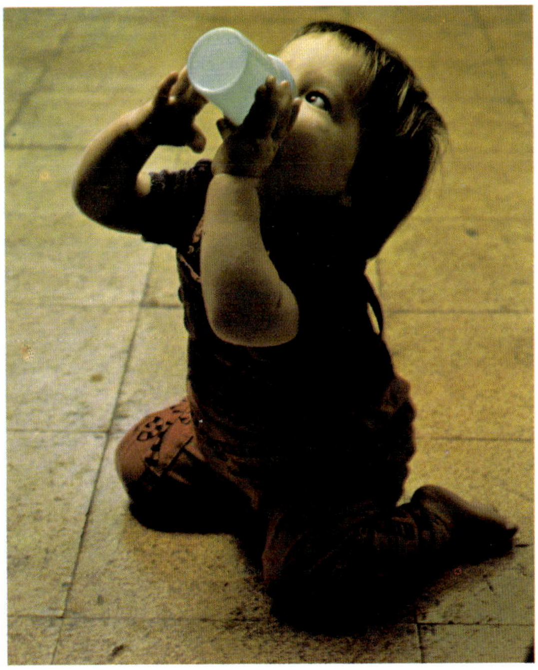

A baby should learn to drink from a cup at about six to seven months.

Menus for the baby

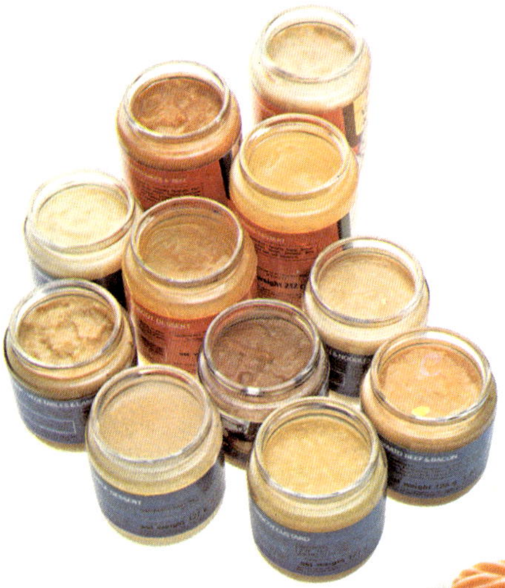

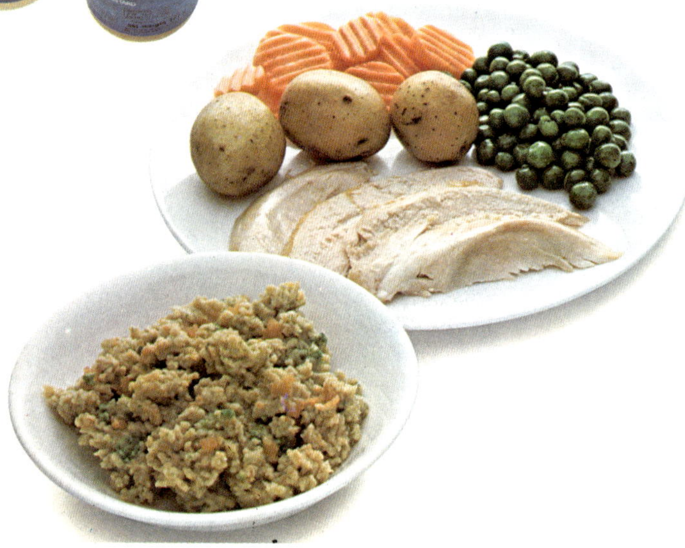

As your baby gets older and becomes accustomed to solid foods, it is important to introduce a variety of different foods into his diet, whether they are homemade or commercially prepared baby foods. By about 8 months you can start giving him a mashed-up portion of your own adult meal.

SUITABLE MENUS FOR EARLY AND LATER MIXED FEEDING		
	From about five months	**From about eight months**
Early morning	Breast- or bottle feeding (the baby will soon be ready to drop this feeding)	
Breakfast	Baby cereal (with egg yolk or applesauce) *or* baby-food breakfast *or* strained fruit Breast- or bottle feeding (when early morning feeding has been discontinued)	Certain adult cereals, Boiled, poached or scrambled egg Fingers of toast Cup of milk
Lunch	Strained meat and vegetable dinner *or* home-cooked puréed meat Strained fruit *or* egg custard *or* fruit dessert Breast- or bottle feeding	Home-cooked, chopped ground meat with potato and vegetable Yogurt Cup of diluted fruit juice
Supper	Mashed banana *or* Jello Breast- or bottle feeding	Tasty sandwiches Fruit and custard *or* pudding Bottle feeding or cup of milk
Bedtime or late evening	Breast- or bottle feeding (if this feeding has not been dropped)	Breast- or bottle feeding

Breakfasts

Breakfast time can begin to fall in line with that of the rest of the family when the baby is about five months old. If he has cereal, which is economical and easy to prepare, it can be made more interesting by adding a little applesauce, or strained fruit. Cereals are easy to mix with milk which is already familiar. High protein or fortified cereals are often not best for the baby as too much supplementation can cause problems. Egg yolk can also be added. It is a source of iron and encourages acceptance of new flavors (*see* p. 174). Egg white should not be given to a baby until he or she is at least six months old, as some young babies are sensitive to the albumen in egg white.

Strained fruit alone makes a welcome change for a baby, and is, of course, a natural way to prevent constipation.

From about eight months certain adult cereals can be introduced, without the addition of sugar. By this time the baby will probably have some teeth coming through and will appreciate something hard to chew on: try giving him a piece of toast cut into fingers, for example.

Lunch

Midday seldom presents problems, as there is a wide choice of suitable foods. Commercial strained foods are useful to start with, and the baby will take increasing amounts until he is eating a whole jar by six months.

Ground meat or baked fish, well-mashed vegetables and a little potato with gravy are the next stage, although special care must be taken to remove any fish bones.

Desserts of fruit, custard, milk puddings and yogurt add more variety and can be regularly added after about six months.

Suppertime

The time when most mothers find they run short of ideas is suppertime. When the baby is still quite young the commercial baby food may well be the best choice for supper. For a busy mother there is nothing more soul-destroying or frustrating than spending a great deal of time preparing special or elaborate foods for her baby only to have them refused or regurgitated by an "ungrateful" baby who isn't hungry.

Jello, mashed banana and strained fruit are simple to prepare and can always be used if a mother feels twinges of guilt about using too many commercial foods.

When the baby is over six months old, little simple sandwiches, cut into finger-sized pieces are excellent for training him to feed himself. Use fillings such as chopped meat, peanut butter, jelly and cream cheese.

As the baby gets older, sweet foods, including cake, cookies without nuts, and chocolate may be given *in moderation*, but only after a meal. As sugar causes tooth decay, it is not wise to encourage a liking for any type of sweet foods.

Eating problems

All normal infants go through phases in which they may go on a hunger strike, refusing food altogether; slow eaters, taking an abnormally long time to eat; or just fussy eaters, refusing many foods they previously accepted happily and eating only a very limited number of foods. Although these problems commonly occur during the second, rather than the first, year of life, they can start any time after the baby is seven to nine months old. This type of problem should not, however, be confused with a refusal of either a new food or a new texture, or the fact that some days a baby is simply less hungry than others.

A desire for certain foods or refusal of food is normal. Usually the child involved is perfectly well, within the normal height and weight ranges, and the fad appears to do no harm even when his dietary history becomes bizarre enough to alarm even the most phlegmatic expert. Parents, naturally, become concerned and often go to desperate lengths to tempt or bribe the child to eat. Bullying and even battering have been known to become the weapons of some frustrated parents.

The problems of food refusal are usually short-lived if they are virtually ignored by the parents and treated in a calm, matter-of-fact way. But, if parental anxiety persists, so may the hunger strike, slow eating and special desires, which then act as attention-seeking mechanisms. In addition, if the mother is upset then the baby may become upset.

Your parental attitude from the outset is the key factor; once a baby has gained the upper hand, it becomes very difficult for the parents. If mealtimes become a battlefield, allow a reasonable time for the child to eat if he wants to, then just remove any uneaten food without a fuss. Do *not* replace it with a food you know the child will eat. The rules are quite simple – just keep calm and never substitute, because any self-respecting baby soon realizes that, in order to get his favorite food, all he will have to do is to refuse what is first offered. Similarly, if a first course is picked at or refused, remove it and then give only the usual sized helping of dessert. Never compensate for the uneaten food or you will find yourself with a baby who eats only desserts.

During any problem phase, it is helpful to the mother to keep meals as simple as possible. Parents may feel that as most adults have one or two minor dislikes where food is concerned, it is reasonable to allow their baby to have genuine dislikes. This is fair enough, but it is worth remembering, even in this situation, that it is still unnecessary to provide a whole string of alternatives.

Coping with these feeding problems can be very difficult for a busy mother, but try and be rational and convince yourself that you are establishing your child's eating pattern for a long time, possibly for life. The knowledge that babies do not starve themselves to death can be very reassuring. If, however, your baby is not well or obviously losing weight, then be sure to consult your doctor.

Vacation and travel

Traveling with a baby, whether on a long trip or just a short trip, need not be a problem. Plans can be made in advance for what is required on the trip and, once away from home, it helps to keep as close as possible to the baby's normal feeding and daily routine. This will mean that the child is more likely to adjust without any problems. In many respects car travel is simplest; you can stop when you want to and carry all necessary equipment.

If you are undertaking a long trip, whether by road, rail, or air, make sure that you have an adequate supply of suitable (non-carbonated) drinks on hand. Always carry plenty of water or diluted fruit juice in feeding bottles, as babies get hot and dehydrated when traveling. Small cans of fruit juice and cartons of milk that do not require refrigeration are helpful.

It is common to see infants traveling with their mothers by airplane today. Most airlines, given prior notice, will also provide a sleeping facility or portable crib, baby food and milk for a long trip, even though the baby is officially traveling on a parent's lap. On short flights, cabin staff are usually very busy, so take your own baby food and prepared or commercial formula. Babies (and toddlers) may get slight ear discomfort on take-off and landing. Do not discourage a baby from crying, at such times, as this helps to "pop" his ears. A drink sucked from a bottle may also help.

Whichever form of travel you take, try to make your journey at off-peak, less busy times and always be prepared for unscheduled delays by having extra food available for the baby. When traveling a baby will usually accept food from a jar without it being warmed, so long as it is not too cold.

Once you are at your destination, remember that the warmer the climate the more fastidious you have to be with hygiene. Be very careful when sterilizing and cleaning bottles and feeding equipment. Handy portable sterilizers are widely available. If you travel to a place where the water is of questionable purity buy bottled water. Use it for drinking, cooking, brushing teeth and making ice cubes. Use premixed formula or buy only pasteurized milk. Take your usual baby foods unless you are sure you will be able to buy them.

If you are feeding your baby with home-cooked foods, always prepare his food yourself rather than risk someone else's lower standards of hygiene, or use commercial baby food for the duration of the trip. Jars are particularly convenient as you can serve the food straight from them, but do not keep opened jars unless they are put straight into the refrigerator.

Accommodations with a kitchen may be less restrictive as you will not have to fit in with other people. Many hotels, however, are very helpful to parents with babies and may even provide special foods for babies. However, in most instances you may have to bring your own baby food supplies from home.

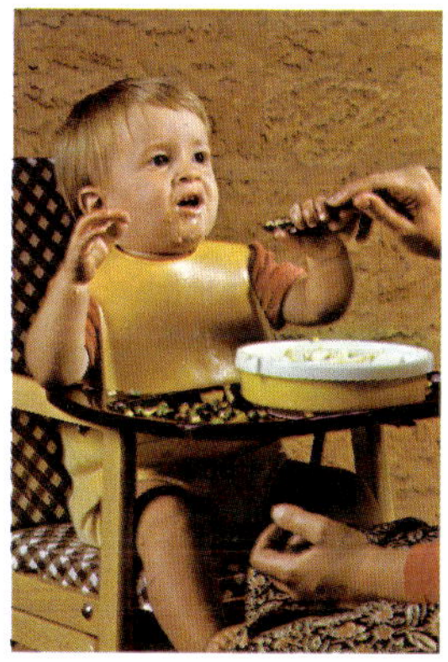

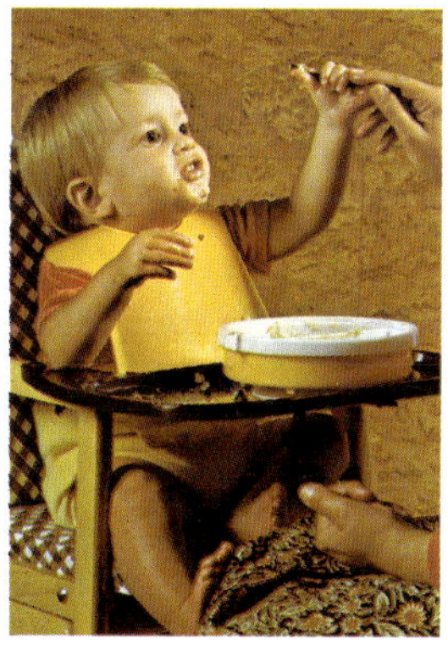

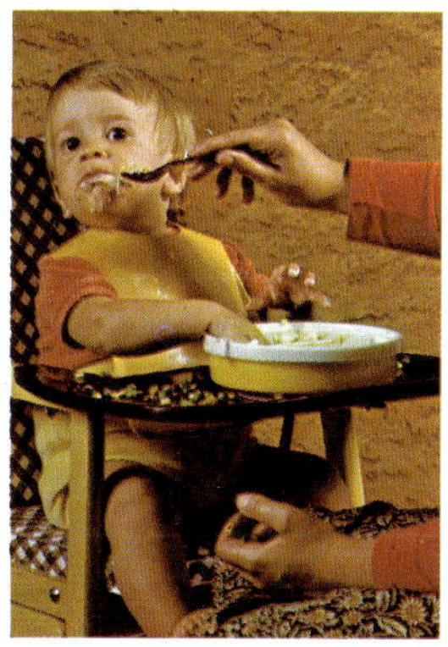

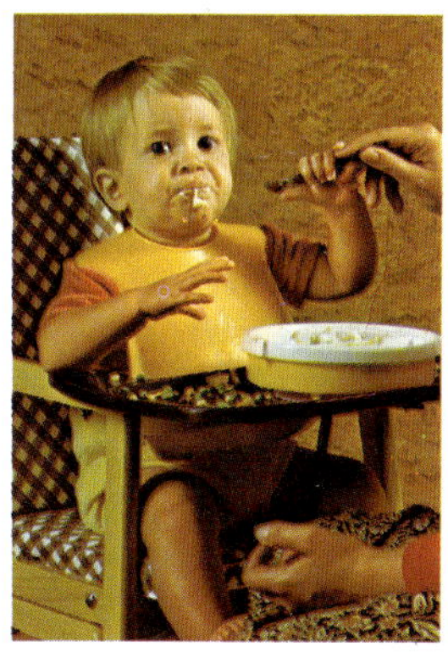

Most babies go through phases of food refusal. It is better not to offer him his favorite food instead, but wait until he is hungry and try again.

Development in the first year

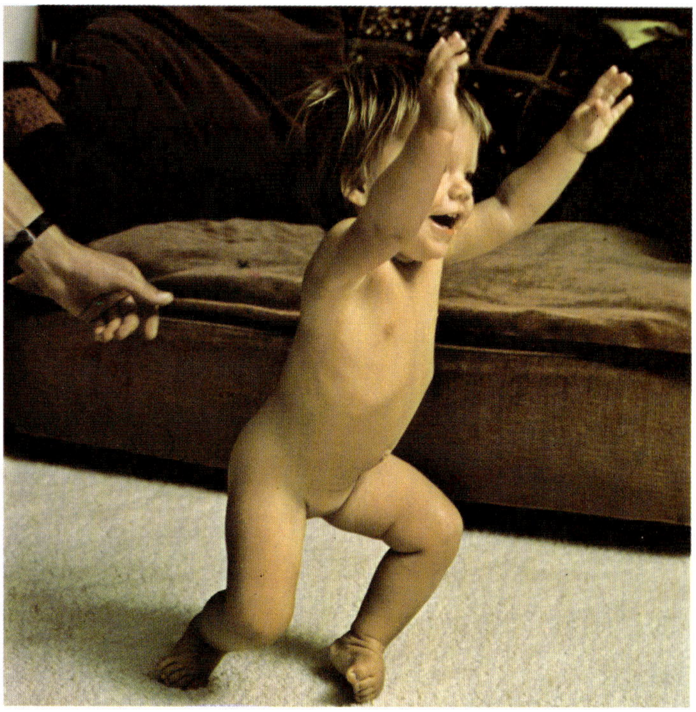

CHAPTER 14

Growth

Learning to control the body

Use of the hands

Vision

Hearing and speech

One of the most exciting things for parents is to watch the growth of their child's abilities. In the first year a baby learns something new nearly every week. These landmarks in development are soon forgotten unless you keep a diary and write down each event as it happens. If you include photographs you will end up with a fascinating record of these vital early months.

The rate of a child's development depends both on inherited characteristics and on having the appropriate opportunities to learn and practice new skills. On the one hand, the rate at which the nervous system matures is an inherited characteristic and there is, for example, no point in expecting a child to walk before the nerves supplying his or her legs have matured. On the other hand, it is not enough for a child to possess the inborn abilities necessary to be a great mathematician if the child is never given suitable opportunities to learn about numbers.

Parents are often worried that their child is slow to learn a particular skill, but it is actually quite common to be advanced in one skill, such as walking, and slow in another, such as talking. Provided he is average in most other abilities, there is no need for anxiety because progress seems to be slow in one area. Einstein was apparently five years old before he spoke and was still not fluent at nine!

If your baby does seem to be developing slowly, however, take him to the doctor for a check-up since there is sometimes a physical explanation. For instance, delayed speaking may be due to a hearing difficulty which can be treated. It is worth remembering that babies born prematurely will seem slow unless you allow for the number of weeks they were born early. Illness causes a temporary slowing down

Cross references

See also	Chapter
Child health	12, 17
Feeding in the first year	13

The baby's first unsupported steps are a memorable landmark. This 11-month-old baby cannot walk yet but is enjoying her first attempt.

of development, though the baby will usually catch up rapidly as soon as he recovers.

A new baby begins life with very little control over his actions and with many reflexes (*see* pp. 130–1). Some of these reflexes remain throughout life – we all blink if a fly buzzes close to our eye or quickly pull our hand away if it is touched by a hot plate or a sharp needle. We keep these reflexes because they are useful. Most of the protective reflexes, however, are soon replaced by controlled action and some play an important role in helping the baby to learn new skills. For example, a new baby will turn toward something which touches his cheek and open his mouth. This "rooting" reflex helps him to find the nipple when the breast touches his cheek and it also teaches him to recognize his mother's smell.

Another reflex (the asymmetric tonic neck reflex) helps babies learn to use their eyes to coordinate the movements of their hands. You may notice that if a baby lies on his back and faces in one direction, say to the right, then his right arm and leg will be stretched out while his left arm and leg will be bent close to the body. When a baby looks to the right and sees a toy beside him, his right arm is already stretched out toward the toy and this helps him to touch it and eventually to pick it up.

During the first year a baby loses most of these automatic reflexes and learns to move his body voluntarily, so he can reach out for the toys he wants, move around on his own and communicate with others. Development takes place from the head downward; babies always learn to control their heads first, then their bodies and finally end up with the use of their legs. It seems that the shortest nerves, which supply parts of the body close to the brain, mature first and that the longest nerves, which supply the legs and the feet, mature last – because they have the greatest distance to travel from the brain. This sequence of development is also the most logical since it is obviously important that a baby should learn to see and understand his environment before he is able to move around in it.

The first muscles which a baby is able to control are those of his eyes and face. Shortly after birth the infant will look at his mother's face for a couple of seconds and in a few weeks will start to smile and make cooing noises. Gradually he will discover how to overcome the effects of gravity and to maintain an upright position. He will learn to hold his head up steadily, to sit up with a straight back, to use his arms to prop himself up or to grasp a toy, and – finally – to stand up and walk.

The different aspects of development are closely related. For instance, once a baby is able to hold his head up steadily, he can start to use both eyes together. This helps him to judge distances more accurately and makes it easier to coordinate hand movements. A steady head also helps him to sense more clearly where sounds are coming from so that he can turn and see what is making the noise. In this way the baby begins to associate sounds with certain people and actions. Soon he will become very excited when he sees a feeding being prepared.

Each aspect of development will be treated separately, although the way in which progress is made in one area depends on advances in another. The different sections show the stages through which a baby passes during his first year and create a picture of how the child learns to control the faculties of the body: hands, eyes, hearing and speech.

Growth

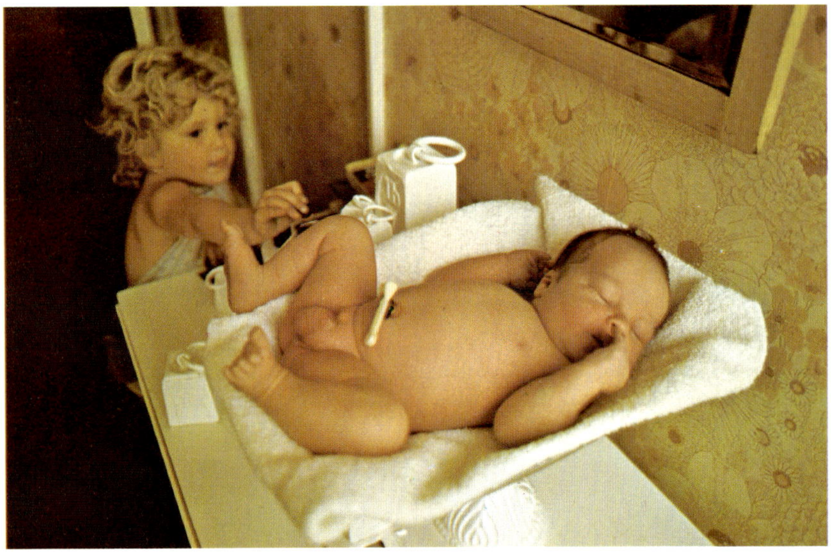

If you wish to chart your baby's growth yourself, you will find it invaluable to have an accurate scale at home.

Parents are often surprised at how much babies of the same age vary in size. Provided that a baby is both healthy and well fed, his growth will be determined by characteristics inherited from both mother and father. In general, tall parents will have tall children and short parents will have short children, though it takes about two years before the inherited growth patterns are clearly seen.

The normal range of growth is so wide that doctors always use growth charts to decide whether an individual baby is growing satisfactorily. These charts have been derived from measuring hundreds of babies at different ages. The curves on the charts are called centile lines. If you look at the girls' weight chart for example, the 50th centile line gives the average weight of girls at each age; one half will be heavier than the point on the 50th centile and one half will be lighter. In the same way, 10 girls in every 100 would be lighter than the 10th centile at each age, and three girls in every hundred would be heavier than the 97th centile. Usually you will find that your own baby follows one of the curves marked.

Weighing and measuring your baby

You must weigh and measure your baby accurately if you would like to use the growth charts. Babies should always be weighed naked, since wet diapers can be surprisingly heavy. Make sure that the scales are carefully balanced first, or, if they are ones with a spring balance (like bathroom scales) check that the dial is on "0" before beginning. Balance scales are usually the most accurate. Weighing once a week is quite enough – unless your doctor advises otherwise. Ideally, you should weigh your baby at the same time of day (because the child's weight will depend on whether he has just been fed or has just soiled his diaper). This may not always prove possible in practice.

The baby's length is difficult to measure because babies prefer to lie curled up; so two people are needed. Your pediatrician may use a special measuring table. This is a long thin table with a fixed headboard at one end and a movable footboard at the other end. The baby lies on his back on the table. A nurse holds his head, so that it touches the headboard. The doctor, or another nurse, straightens the baby's legs so that they lie stretched out flat on the table and then brings the movable footboard up against his heels. The length is read off from a gauge attached to the footboard.

At home, you can get a rough idea of your baby's length by laying him on a table next to the wall. The wall serves as the headboard and a hardback book can be used as the footboard. Simply measure the distance between the two with a tape measure.

In the office the doctor will also measure the circumference of the baby's head. This is done by putting a tape measure around the forehead just above the eyebrows and then passing it around the widest part at the back of the head.

Using the growth charts

All babies have their weight, length and head circumference measured at birth. In some hospitals the figures are written on a label which is stuck onto the baby's bassinet. If you do not know your baby's measurements, and would like to, ask your doctor.

You can begin by plotting these birth measurements on the growth charts. Read the instructions below the chart carefully and make sure you use the appropriate one; since boys are slightly bigger than girls, there are separate charts for each. You can then see how your baby compares with other babies. You may find the child has an average length (50th centile) and is light (25th centile). This pattern, or its reverse, is quite normal. Babies, like adults, are seldom perfectly proportioned. Our shape usually follows a family pattern.

Babies born several weeks prematurely may seem very small if their birth measurements are plotted in the normal way. Measuring such a baby again on the date you *expected* him to be born, and plotting these as his birth measurements, will give you a better idea of how big he is in relation to other babies. If the premature baby experiences medical complications, growth may be slower until he recovers.

When several measurements have been plotted on the growth charts, you will begin to see how your baby is growing. During the first week of life most babies lose weight. They catch up quite quickly once they start to drink more milk. Thereafter growth is very rapid. The steepness of the curves at the beginning of the growth charts indicates just how rapid. After a few weeks, most babies have growth curves that run parallel to the centile curves, although head circumference, weight and length may be on different centiles.

Some babies grow faster than expected during the first couple of months, and their growth curve will therefore move up from one centile to another on the charts. This is quite normal so long as weight, length and head size are increasing equally rapidly. Babies who

GROWTH CHART I: WEIGHT (Girls)

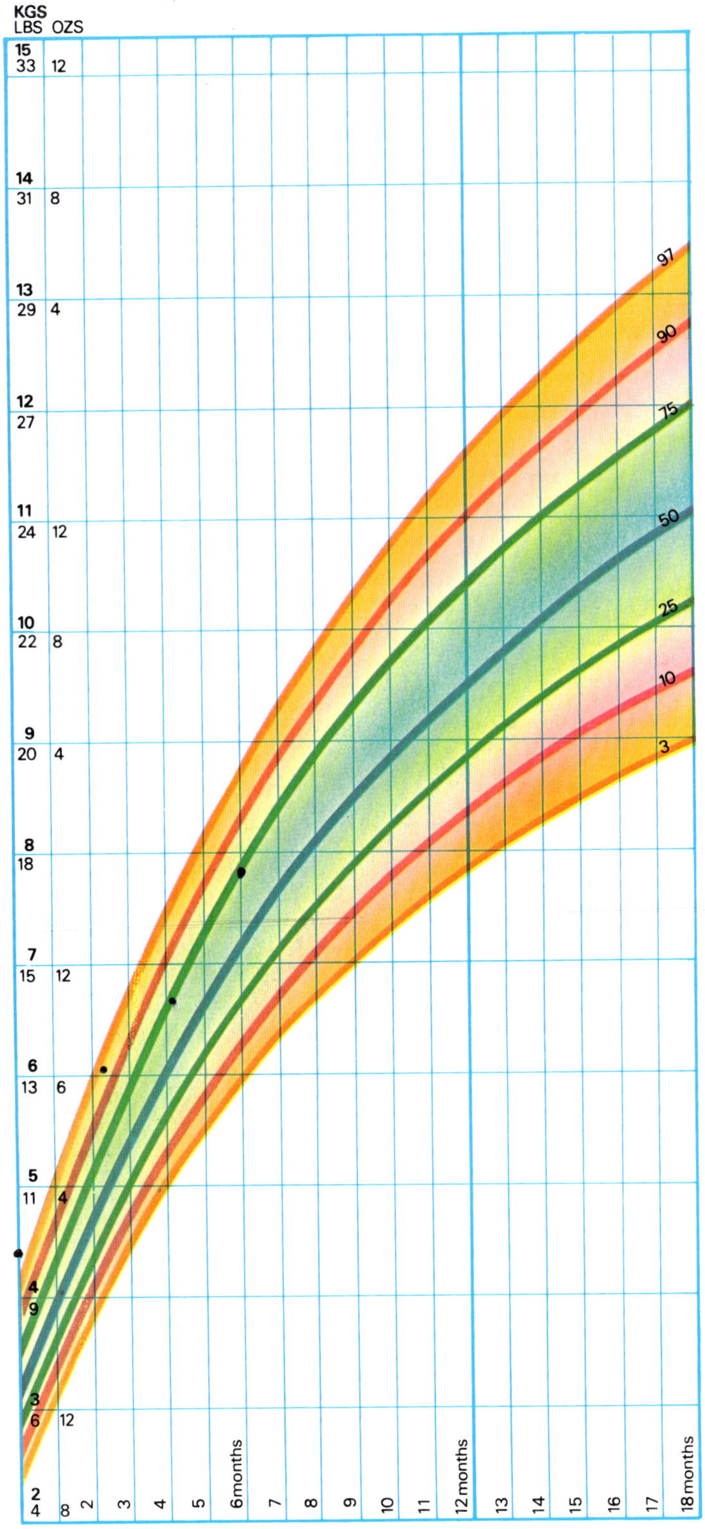

GROWTH CHART I: WEIGHT (Boys)

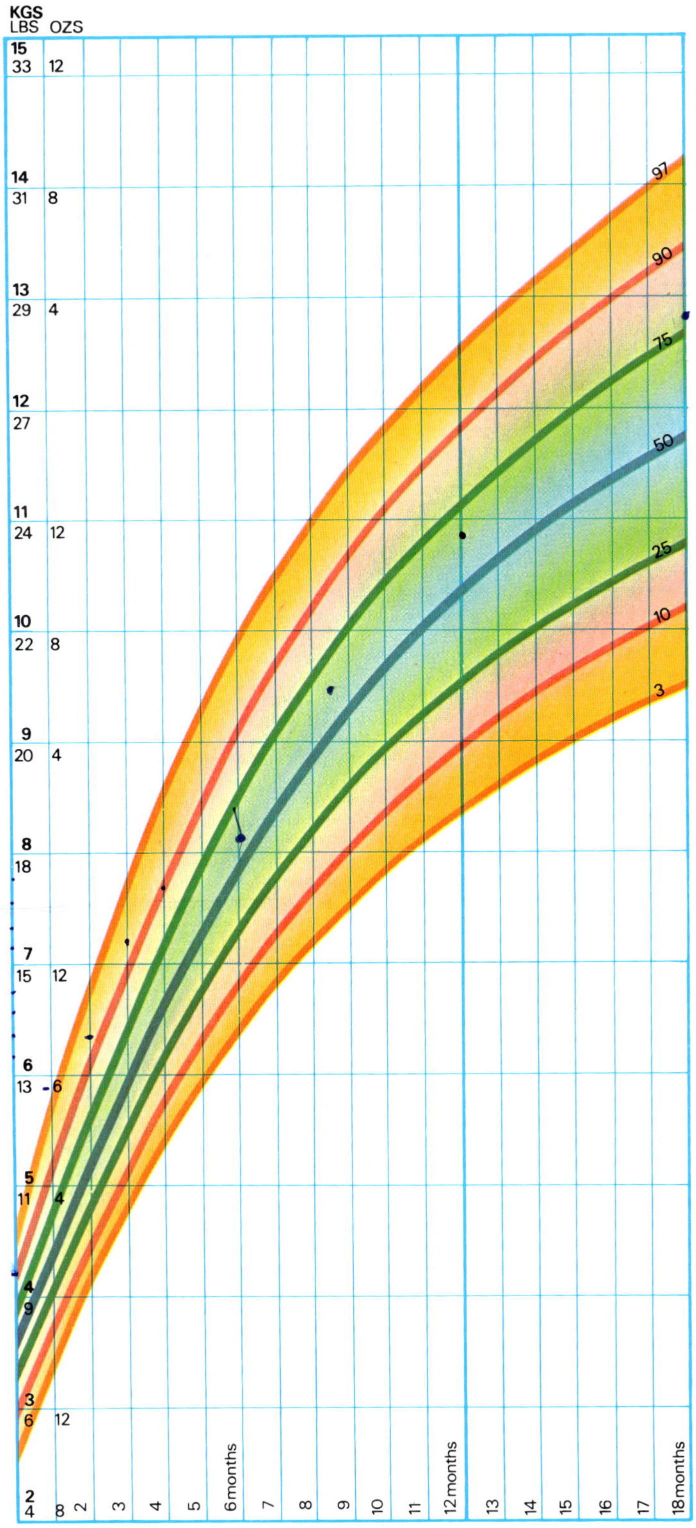

grew slowly at the end of the pregnancy and who were therefore lighter than expected at birth often grow very fast in this way until they reach their normal growth curve.

Slow growth
Parents often worry because their baby seems much smaller than that of their friends. You

YOUR BABY'S WEIGHT
To plot your baby's weight, first choose the appropriate chart – the left-hand one for a girl – then find her age at the bottom and her weight at the side. Follow the two lines until they cross and mark this point on the chart. If you do this once a month and join up the points you will get her growth curve for weight.

The curves on the chart are called centiles. They indicate how many babies, out of 100 normal babies the same age, are likely to be lighter than the weight shown. Taking the 97th centile on the girls' chart as an example, at the age of 17 months 97 girl babies out of 100 are likely to be lighter than about 29 lbs (13 kg), and three heavier.

GROWTH CHART II: LENGTH (Girls)

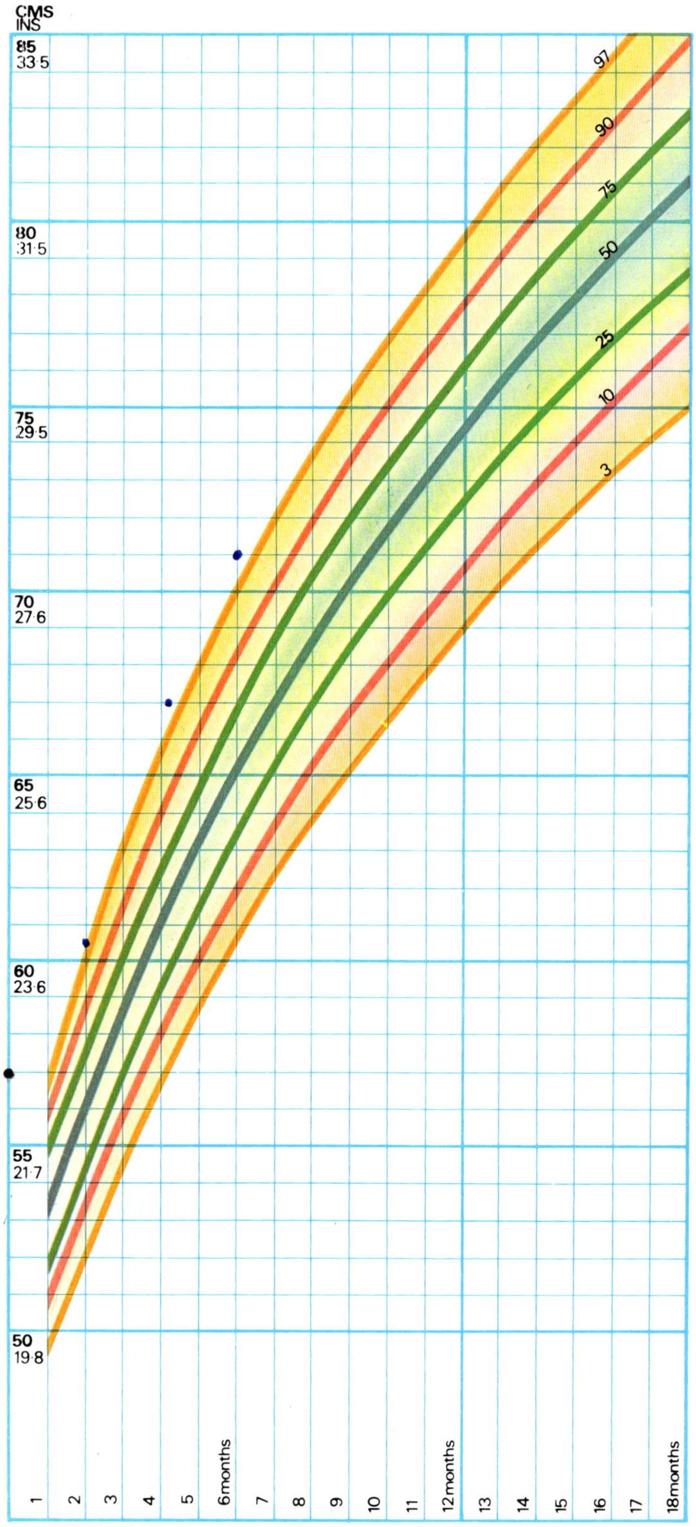

GROWTH CHART II: LENGTH (Boys)

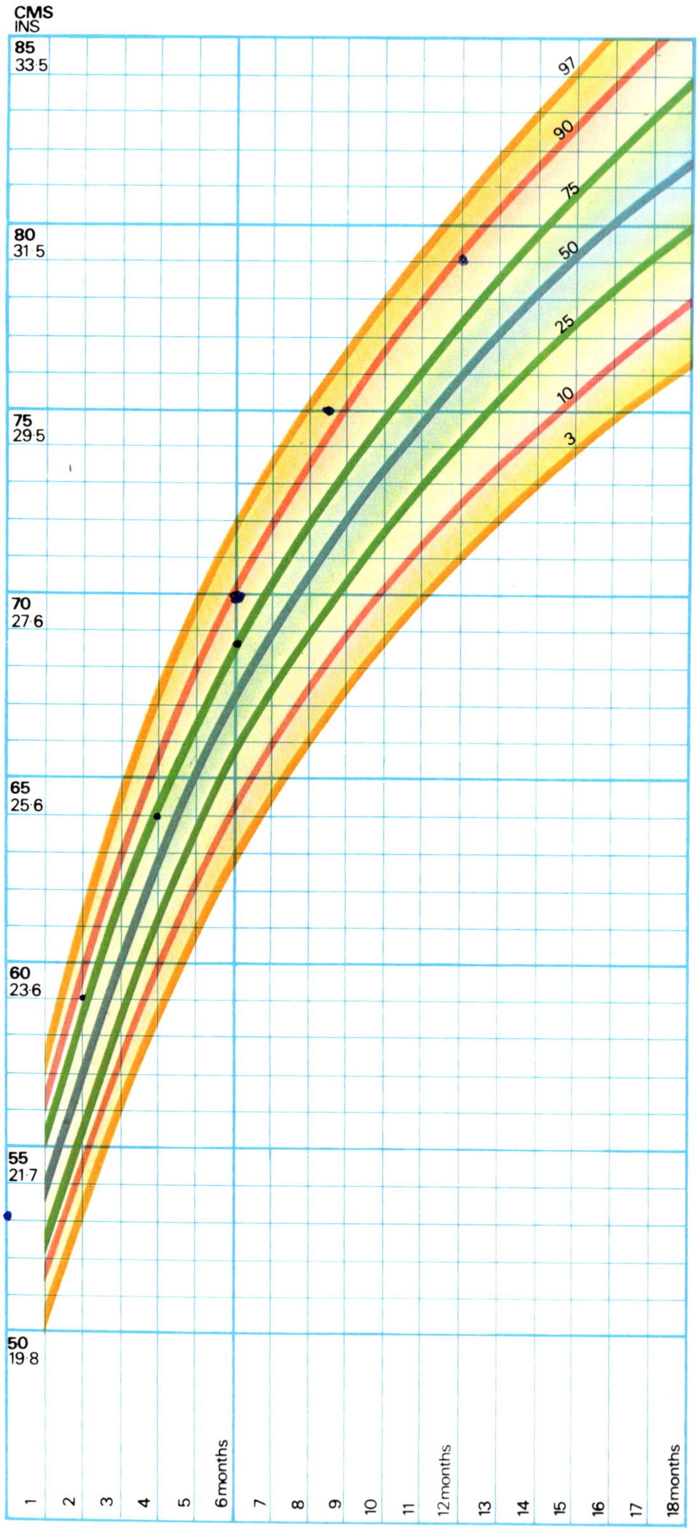

YOUR BABY'S LENGTH

To plot your baby's length, the procedure is the same as for the weight chart on the previous page. Choose the appropriate chart – the right-hand one for a boy – then find his age at the bottom and his length at the side. Mark the point where the two lines cross. Do this periodically and join up the points to make a curve.

These weight and length charts are based on hundreds of measurements taken from average children. Most babies follow a growth curve like the ones shown, although some healthy babies have growth curves outside the 3rd and 97th centiles. If you are worried about your baby's progress it is best to check with your doctor.

can easily tell if your baby is growing too slowly. Instead of the baby's growth curve running parallel to the centiles on the charts it will start to cross them in a downward direction. Slow growth is usually associated with obvious ill health and most parents would consult a doctor. The baby's weight reacts quite quickly to illness. Even minor illnesses like colds or diarrhea and vomiting can cause the baby to lose weight. The smaller a baby is, the less weight he can afford to lose. Doctors usually admit babies to the hospital if they lose more than five per cent of their weight – that would mean 17 oz (500 gm) for a 22 lb (10 kg) baby, but only 5 oz (150 gm) for a 6 lb 8 oz (3 kg) baby. The baby will, however, usually catch up rapidly as soon as he becomes well again. More prolonged ill health affects the baby's length as well as his weight. But length will also catch up once the baby has recovered.

Occasionally babies grow slowly but do not appear to be sick. This may happen if they lack some of the hormones necessary for growth, or if they have an allergy to the proteins in cow's milk or wheat cereals which interferes with the absorption of food from the intestinal tract. Slow growth may be the only visible symptom of these conditions.

Obesity

Babies are naturally round and chubby at birth and remain so until their second year. The layer of fat beneath the skin helps to keep the baby warm and is an important source of energy. But excess fat, or obesity, is undesirable since some fat babies grow up into fat adults and these people have a much greater risk of developing heart disease and dying early. Apart from judging by looking, you can tell how fat a baby is by picking up a fold of skin between your finger and thumb; if the baby is too fat, the skin fold will feel thick.

When a baby is gaining weight very quickly, he is in danger of becoming too fat. You will be able to see if this is happening by comparing the growth charts. The weight curve will start to cross the centiles in an upward direction, whereas the length curve will hardly change. If this happens you should check your baby's diet. Most babies can be adequately fed on milk alone for the first four months. When solids are introduced, avoid giving too much rice, cereal or high calorie baby foods. Avoid baby desserts and other selections that include sugar or starch.

Growth of the head

A baby's head grows very rapidly during the first 12 to 18 months – reflecting the increase in size of the brain. The heads of premature or small-for-dates babies often grow so quickly that it is difficult to decide whether growth is normal or excessive and for this reason doctors always watch their development closely. The skull bones do not start to fuse until most of the rapid brain growth is over. You will be able to feel the "soft spot" or fontanelle between the bones (*see* p. 131) getting gradually smaller. Remember that it is quite safe to touch or wash the fontanelle since the brain is protected by a tough membrane. When the baby is quiet, the fontanelle can sometimes be seen pulsating but this is no cause for alarm.

Teeth

Most babies cut their first tooth between six and ten months of age. The accompanying diagram shows the order in which the teeth usually appear. It seems that bigger babies cut their teeth early and that twins, triplets and premature babies are later than average. Most children have cut all 20 of their "milk teeth" by the time they are three years old.

It is very important to look after these primary teeth carefully since they stimulate the growth of the jaws and thus give the adult teeth room to come through. If one of the primary teeth is lost, the adult teeth may be overcrowded and more difficult to keep clean. Good dental hygiene should therefore start early. Avoid giving your baby too many sweet foods or drinks. A drink of water after each feeding will help wash away food particles from around the teeth. Some babies enjoy playing with a soft toothbrush which can be tied onto the side of the crib. Once they get used to the toothbrush they often become eager to start cleaning their own teeth.

Fluoride helps to prevent dental decay. Ask your doctor if it has been added to the drinking water supply in your area. If not, he may suggest giving fluoride drops in water or the baby's vitamins, daily, from two weeks after birth. Sometimes a baby will have cut a tooth before birth. This may be very troublesome and cause ulcers on the tongue when the baby sucks. It is therefore best to remove it. There is no danger of overcrowding later since any tooth present at birth is usually additional and not part of the normal primary dentition.

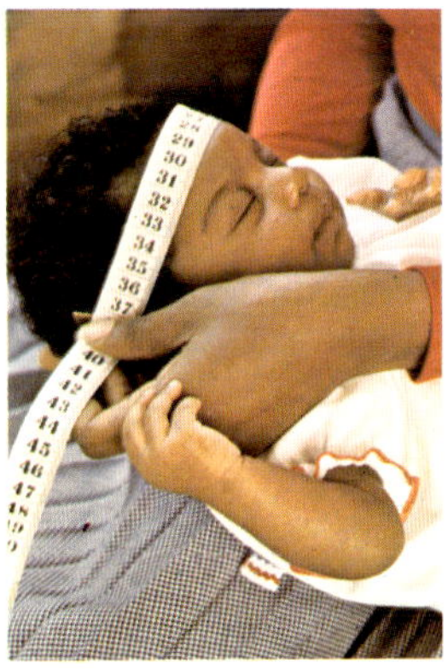

All babies have their head circumference measured at birth. The doctor may measure it as the baby grows older, and head circumference can be plotted on a growth chart similar to the length and weight charts.

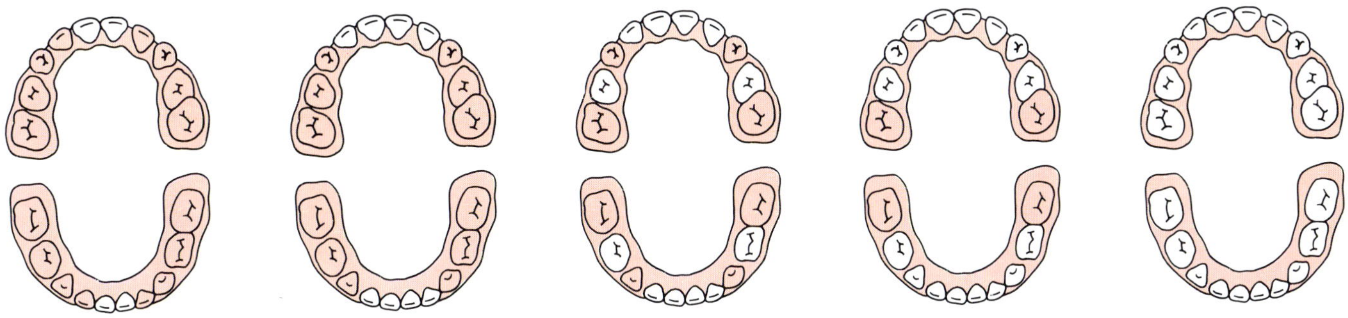

The central incisors appear at about 6 to 8 months.

The lateral incisors appear at about 9 to 11 months.

The first molars are cut at about 14 to 17 months.

The canines (eye teeth) follow at about 18 to 20 months.

The second molars appear at about 24 to 26 months.

Learning to control the body

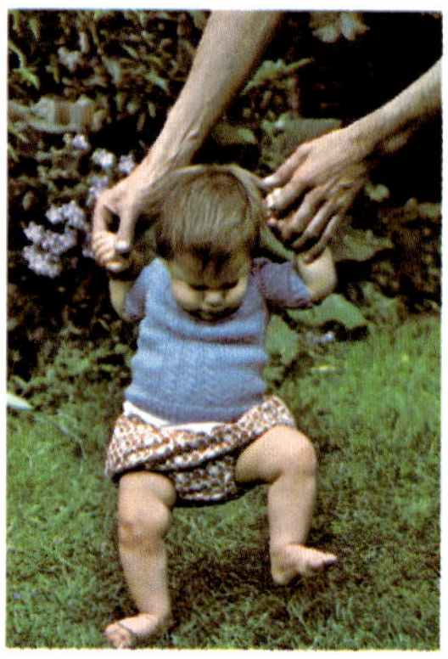

This baby can already stand if her hands are held, and is beginning to take steps. She keeps her feet wide apart for balance and watches their movements.

In the first few weeks of life, babies lie curled up, with their arms and legs close to the body. When a newborn baby lies on his front, he is just able to lift his head up from the bed and turn it to one side; this prevents him from burying his nose in the mattress and suffocating himself. Babies should always be put to sleep on very firm mattresses without a pillow. For safety, the crib mattress should fit tightly and the slats should be no more than $2\frac{1}{4}$ inches apart. If the crib (or playpen) sides are mesh, they should never be left down in the first eight months.

Six weeks to six months

By the time your baby is six weeks old, he will be able to turn his head to the side so he can follow your face as you feed and change him. When lying on his stomach, he will lift his head just off the bed and hold it there for a few moments. He will also start to take an interest in his surroundings and will watch intently anything that moves near him. If you sit him up, his head will still be very wobbly and, if not supported, his chin will fall forward onto his chest. As you pick him up, cradle his head firmly in your hand or against your arm.

After three months a baby can hold his head up steadily and, if you hold his hand firmly and pull him up into a sitting position, his head will come up easily with very little lag. From now on you will find your baby eager to sit up and see more of his surroundings and he may cry with frustration if not allowed to do so. On the other hand, he can be kept amused for a long time so long as he can see his mother moving around. When your baby lies on his abdomen, he now stretches his legs out behind him and can lift his head and shoulders off the bed by using his forearms to prop himself up.

Between three and six months, most babies try to sit up on their own, but usually only succeed in lifting their head from the pillow. If you hold your baby's hands, he will pull himself to a sitting position, keeping his back quite straight, and may balance there briefly. Lying on his front, he can now lift his chest clear of the bed. If he pushes with a hand and foot on the same side, he may accidentally roll from his stomach onto his back. Rolling from the back onto the stomach is more difficult, but, once this has been learned, he will soon find that rolling over and over is a useful way of moving around. This happens quite suddenly; parents may leave their baby in what has always been a safe place – like the center of a double bed – and discover a few moments later that he has rolled off onto the floor.

By the time they are six months old, most babies are struggling to move around. They usually lie on their stomachs and attempt to pull themselves forward or to push backwards using their hands. Moving in this way, only using the hands, is called creeping. Sometimes the baby only manages to pivot around on one spot. Six-month-old babies also enjoy being held upright and bounced up and down on their feet. Their leg muscles get stronger by relaxing and contracting. This is good practice for coordination and learning to stand.

Six to twelve months

Most babies soon discover how to sit up on their own and how to balance in a sitting position. Initially a baby sits with his legs wide apart as this gives him a firm triangular base and leaves his hands free to play with toys. He will topple over if pushed but after a while learns to put out a hand to prop himself up. At first he can only stop himself from falling

From the age of six weeks, a baby who is lying on her stomach will learn to lift her head just off the bed (right). As she grows older, so she will be able to prop herself up with her arms (far right).

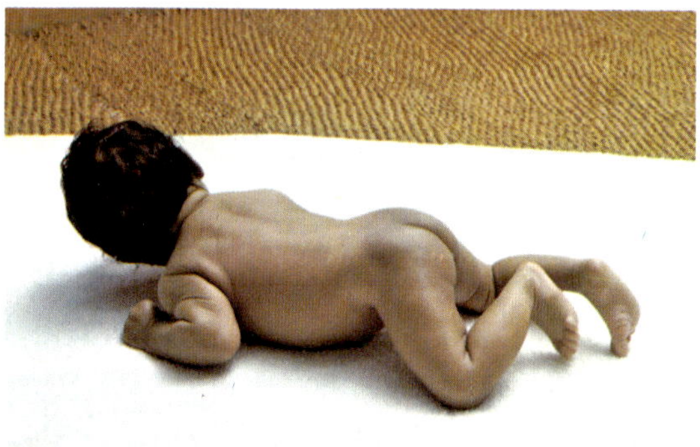

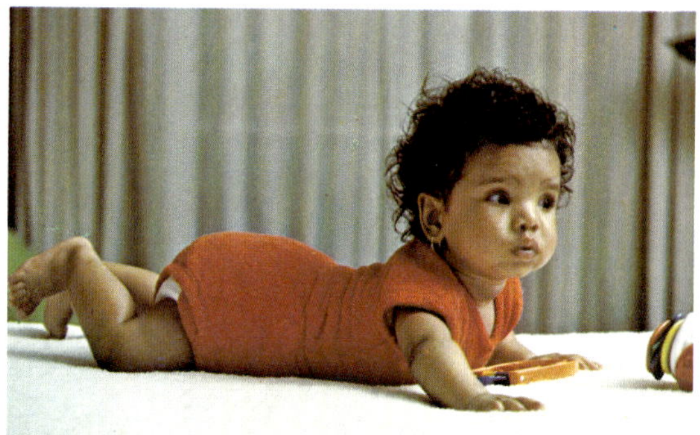

Given a firm hand hold, a baby will learn to pull herself up into a sitting position (right). Babies also discover that they can roll over from their front onto their back (far right).

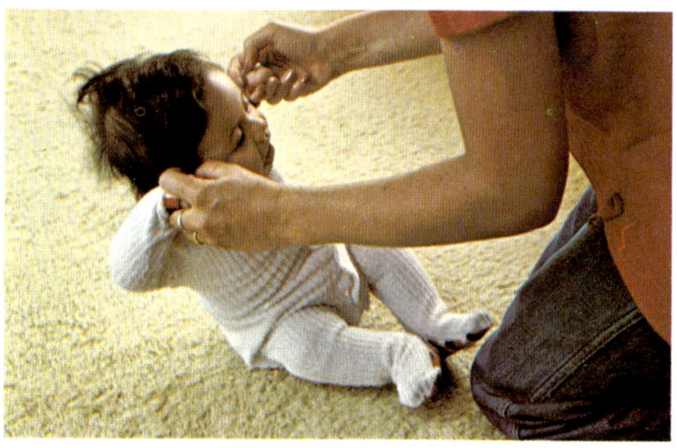

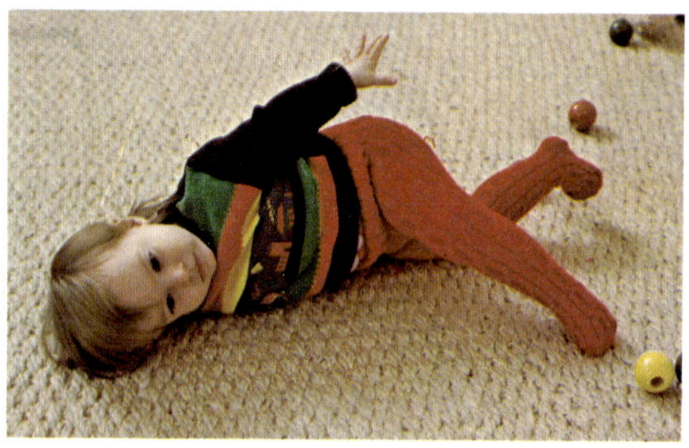

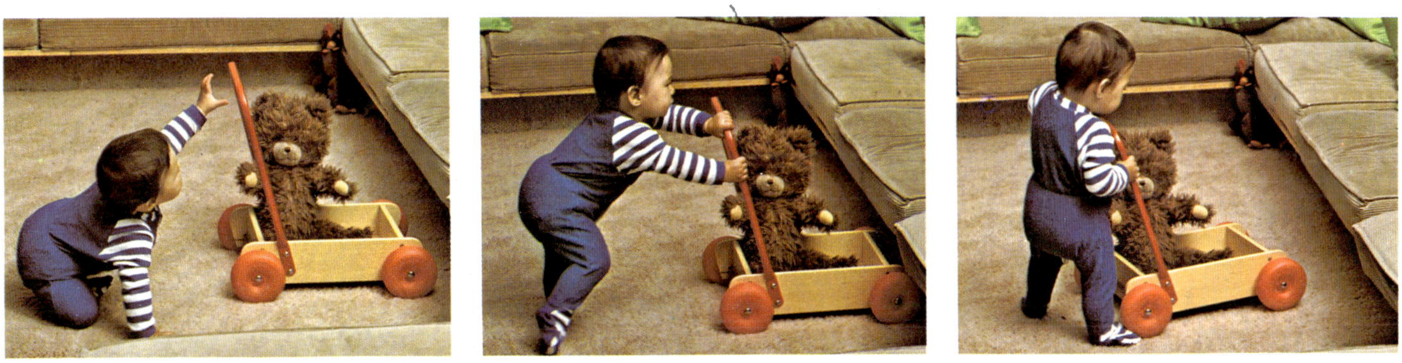

A baby will soon realize the advantages of standing on his own two feet and walking. His interest in toys will gradually help develop this ability.

forward, then sideways and finally he learns to put a hand out behind him to stop himself from falling backwards.

The way in which babies move around before they have learned to walk varies a lot. Your baby may use his arms and legs to creep around on his abdomen, crawl with his body off the ground, roll over and over, shuffle along on his bottom, or try to pull himself to a standing position and walk around holding on to the furniture. Some children seem to skip the preparatory stages and just stand up and walk.

The majority of babies, in fact, learn to creep on their abdomen first, then crawl, then pull themselves to standing and cruise around, and finally walk alone. The first steps usually look very awkward; the feet are kept wide apart and the arms are held out for balance. The baby has to watch his feet very carefully and will fall over if he is distracted and looks up. This often happens when a mother encourages her baby to walk to her; he looks up at her face and promptly falls into her outstretched arms.

The time it takes babies to learn to walk varies and may depend on which method they first used to move around. Both those who creep and crawl and those who just stand up and walk usually learn to stand by 13 months and to walk alone by 15 months. Some babies, however, go on creeping on their stomachs for a long time and are over one year old before they begin to crawl. Others seem to prefer to lie on their backs and tend to cry if left lying on their stomachs. Some of these babies move around by rolling over and over, and do not learn to crawl until they are over one year old. Others prefer the sitting position and shuffle along on their bottoms, never learning to crawl at all. They may continue to move around in this way until they are 16 months old. Most "creepers", "rollers" and "bottom shufflers" are slower than average in learning to stand up and walk, although most are walking soon after their second birthday.

A baby learns by discovering that there are definite advantages and disadvantages to the different methods of moving around. Imagine your baby trying to reach a toy on the other side of the room. If he rolls over and over, he will keep losing sight of the toy. If he creeps on his stomach he can see where he is going, and crawling is even better because he can travel faster. With each of these methods, he has to use his hands to move and will therefore find it difficult to carry a toy with him. Bottom shuffling leaves the baby's hands free and this may explain why some babies continue to move in this way for so long before walking. Walking is clearly the ideal method; it is quick, vision is uninterrupted, both hands are free and the baby soon realizes that it is socially acceptable since parents show how pleased they are and praise him when he learns to walk.

Patterns of learning to walk seem to be repeated in members of the same family. If your baby has one of the less usual patterns of development, you may find out that some of your relatives had a similar pattern. Most grandparents can remember whether their sons and daughters learned to walk early or late and whether, for example, they shuffled around on their bottoms for a long time.

By the end of the first year, most babies have achieved quite good control of their bodies: they have learned to overcome gravity in standing upright and have gained some independence by discovering how to move on their own. This allows them to use their senses of vision, hearing and touch much more fully, and thus increases all their opportunities for learning other new skills.

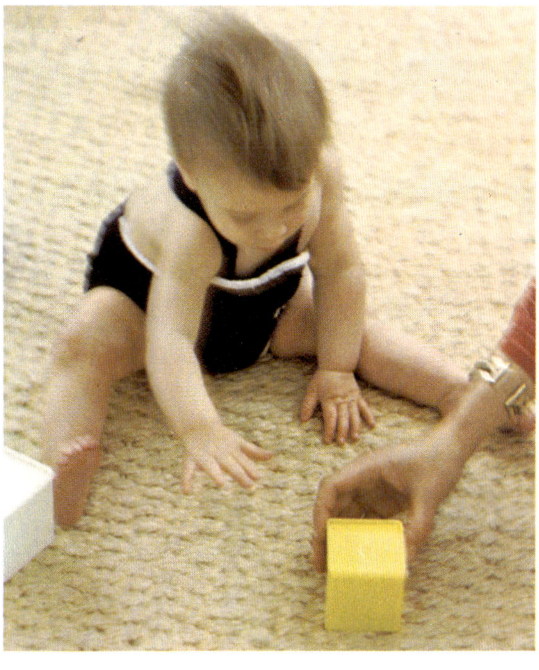

A toy placed in a baby's line of vision but just out of his reach will encourage him to move forward of his own accord. This baby is sitting up well with legs wide apart and one hand on the floor to help him balance.

Use of the hands

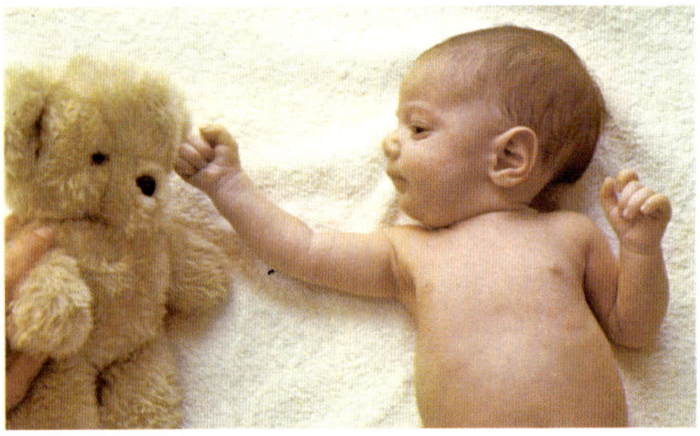

The asymmetric tonic reflex causes a baby to stretch one arm in the direction in which he is facing and so accidentally to touch the toy he is looking at (left).

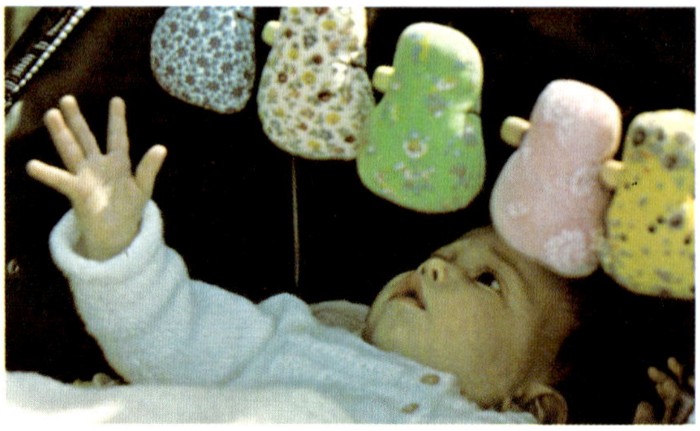

Colored toys, or mobiles, hung over a baby's crib, will help to coordinate vision and movement (right).

At a certain point in human evolutionary development, men and women learned to balance upright and move around on their hind legs. Once they could do this their hands were free and they were able to perfect manipulative skills which were more sophisticated than those of any other creatures. First of all humans learned to bring the thumb across the palm to meet the other fingers. This made it possible to pick up objects of varying sizes. They also learned to use their fingers independently of each other. Typing and playing the piano are good examples of this skill. If you watch a baby's development during the first year, you can see changes taking place which are similar to these stages in the evolutionary process.

From birth to six months

A newborn baby shows a strong grasp reflex if you touch the palm of his or her hand with your finger (*see* pp. 130–1). Whereas the baby will readily grasp a finger or a thin pencil, it is difficult to persuade him to grasp a larger object as he will not allow his hand to be opened wide.

By three months, a baby's hand will open more freely because the grasp reflex is disappearing. At this time, however, the baby is not yet able to grasp objects voluntarily. If you put a rattle in his hand, he will hold it for a few moments and then drop it accidentally. Having just learned to control his head movements, he may fix his eyes on a brightly colored toy, obviously fascinated; but though he looks as if he would like to pick it up, he does not yet seem to understand that he could reach out his hand and grasp it.

The asymmetric tonic reflex is an important aid to learning at this stage. When a baby lies on his back and stretches his arm out in the direction he is facing, he may accidentally touch the toy he is looking at. This helps him to realize that he could reach out for it deliberately. Once he can hold his head steady he will also start to use both eyes to judge distances more accurately when he reaches out for a toy.

Watch your baby when he first tries to pick up a toy: he will make wide waving movements with his arm, vaguely in the direction of the toy, and will probably knock it over or out of reach. As he learns to control his arm muscles and to use his eyes to coordinate movement, he discovers that he can reach straight out and touch the toy he wants. It is a good idea to hang colored toys or a mobile across your baby's crib, just within reach – he will enjoy trying to grab them.

Six months

A six-month-old baby should be able to see the toy he wants, reach out accurately with either hand and pick it up. His grasp will still be rather clumsy, however, and he will press the toy into the palm of his hand, using all his fingers. Only objects which fit into the palm of the hand can be picked up; larger objects will just be knocked over and very small ones will be pushed away.

From four months onward, a baby develops a tendency to grab everything in sight and to put it in her mouth. Her feet are no exception.

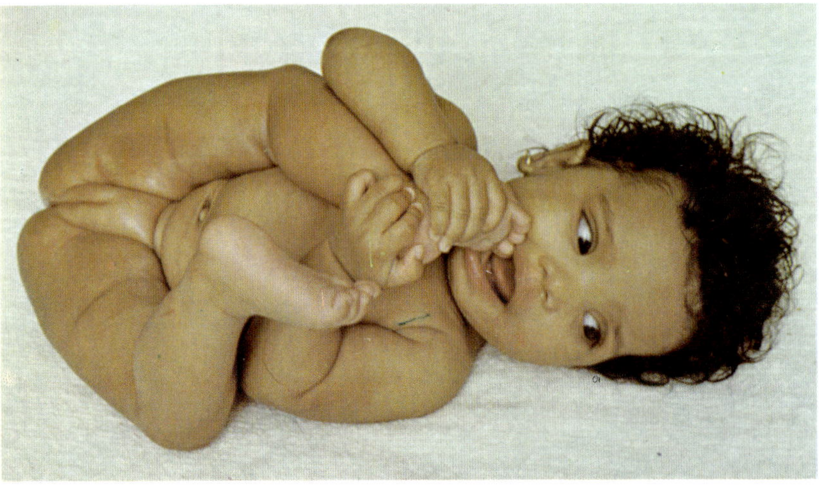

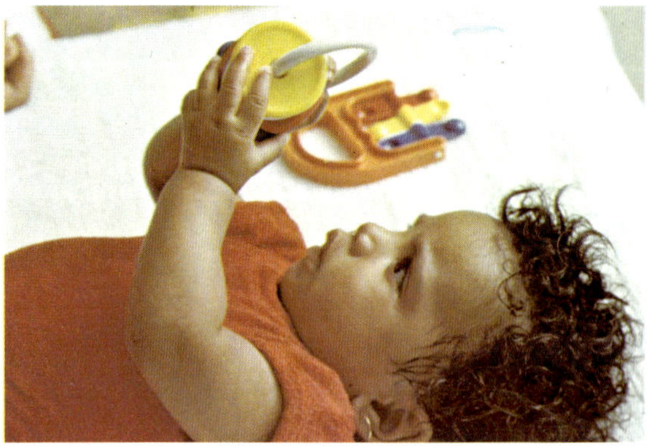

From the age of four months, a baby is able to grasp an object with both hands and to bring it in front of her face (above). She will probably look at it briefly before putting it into her mouth.

From four months onward, the asymmetric tonic reflex starts to disappear so that a baby is able to bring both hands together in front of his face. You may notice that your baby plays for a long time just watching his hands as he waves them in front of his face. When he reaches out to grasp a toy he will bring it in front of his face and may look at it momentarily before putting it into his mouth for a more thorough exploration of its size and shape. He may well grab hold of his toes and put them into his mouth too!

In between six and nine months of age, a baby's hand movements become more skillful. The thumb increases in size and the baby discovers how to pick up small objects by pressing them between the fleshy part at the base of his thumb and his fingers. This is a primitive pincer grasp. He also learns how to transfer toys from one hand to the other.

Nine months

As a baby gradually becomes better at manipulating toys with his hands, he cuts down on putting everything in his mouth and increases looking carefully at his toys and manipulating them with his fingers. If you give the baby a small hand bell, he or she will poke the clanger as if curious about how the ringing sound is made.

Babies also enjoy playing with small blocks at this age – those with sides about 1 in (2.5 cm) long are good because they are easy to pick up. At first a baby is only able to play with one block at a time. He then learns to move it from hand to hand and he will examine it carefully. If a second block is offered he may ignore it or drop the first block in order to pick it up.

As his awareness increases, so he will be able to pick up two blocks, one in each hand. Initially the baby has to concentrate hard in order to hold two blocks at once and he or she may drop one or both of them if distracted. After a while he will start to compare the two blocks and may bang them together.

Dropping toys is still accidental at this stage. But see whether your baby has begun to peer around the side of a table to search for the toys he has dropped on the floor. At about this time, most babies come to realize that even though a toy has disappeared from view it has not gone forever.

Twelve months

By the time a baby is one year of age, he should be able to use all the fingers separately and will often point at a small cookie with the forefinger, and then pick it up delicately between the tip of the forefinger and thumb. This is the mature pincer grasp.

At this time the baby is also learning to release objects from his hand and may play a game of giving toys to his mother. At first he will put a toy in her outstretched hand, then take it away without letting go. Later he learns to let go of the toy. As soon as he can let go easily when he chooses, you will find that your baby starts throwing all the toys onto the floor, and then shouting until someone comes to pick them up. Luckily this tiresome game is short-lived. Larger plastic containers that can be emptied, filled with blocks, large beads or wooden or plastic shapes can provide hours of enjoyment.

In a few weeks the baby will start to play more constructively with toys. Then you can show your baby how to make a tower of two blocks and encourage him to copy it. Building a tower demonstrates all the manipulative skills the baby has learned in the first year. Good control in reaching out with his arm, accurate judgment of distances, and fine control of the fingers enable him to pick up the block with a pincer grasp and to release it in the right place and at the right moment. Coordinating these movements he learns to balance one block on top of another.

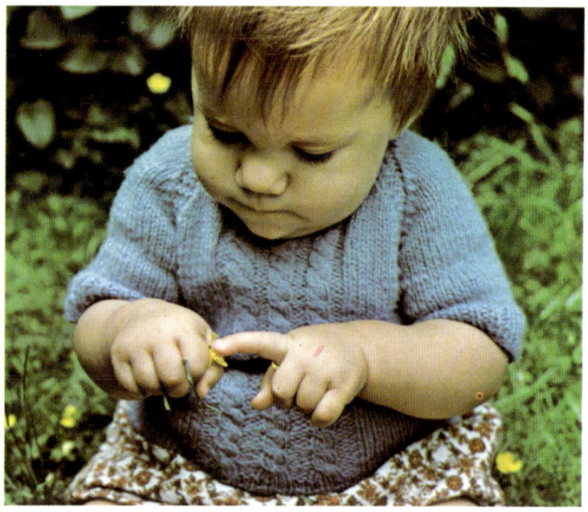

From six months, a baby's grasp gradually matures. This baby shows that she can already separate her first finger from the other and use it for prodding.

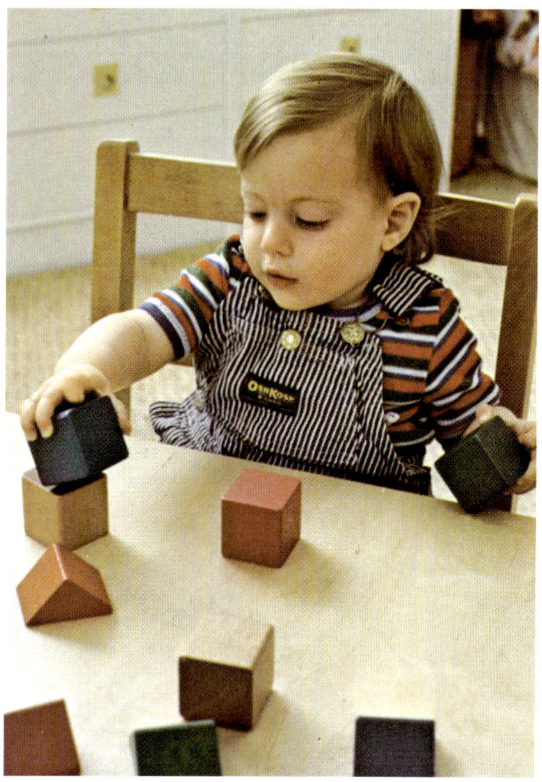

Building a tower of two bricks demonstrates all the manipulation skills which a baby has developed in his first year, including fine control of arm and finger movements and accurate judgment of distances.

Vision

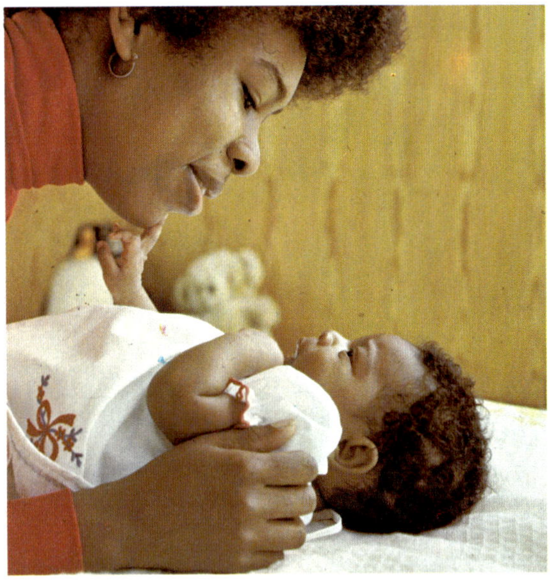

A newborn baby will respond to the mother's gaze by focusing on her face a short distance away.

Imagine being kept in a dark room for many months and then, suddenly, being released into the sunshine; a baby's experiences at birth must be very similar. It is known that the human eye is capable of discerning light and dark from about the seventh month of pregnancy. If you were to hold such a premature baby in your arms, he would turn away from the dark side of the room toward the well-lit window. The simplest way of testing whether a newborn baby responds to light is to shine a small flashlight into the child's eyes. He should blink, and you may be able to see his pupils becoming smaller. However, spontaneous scanning and following moving objects with the eyes is most likely in a dimly lit warm room.

It is not certain whether babies are able to see in color from birth. Adults have three color pigments – red, green and blue – in the cells at the back of their eyes. When light falls on these cells the pigments are stimulated, thus producing all the different colors seen. Color blindness occurs when one or more of the pigments are missing.

One of the first things a mother will do when she sees her newborn baby is to look into his eyes. Research has shown that newborn babies prefer to look at complex moving patterns, such as a face, with its curved features and constantly changing expressions. As a mother nurses a baby in her arms, the slight rocking movements make him open his eyes. The baby immediately focuses on his mother's face a short distance away, while she shows her great delight and encourages him to continue looking at her by smiling, moving her eyes and speaking. When a mother looks at her baby, she also tilts her head so that her face is in the same position as the child's. This position is called "*en face*". If you watch any mother as she feeds her baby you will see that she will automatically tilt her head forward and turn it slightly, so that she is looking into the baby's face, giving him the pleasure of seeing her.

The ability to see clearly depends on how well the eye can focus. At birth a baby finds it difficult to focus on objects at different distances. Instead he tends to maintain a fixed focus that only allows him to see things clearly if they are about 8 in (20 cm) or so away from his face. It is interesting that mothers naturally choose to hold their newborn babies at this distance from their face.

From birth a baby is bombarded with new sensations; everything the baby sees is new. Because he sees objects clearly only if they are within 8 in (20 cm), he is not overwhelmed by new visual information. This enables him to concentrate on learning about his immediate surroundings, particularly the person who feeds and cares for him. During the first few weeks of life, however, he quickly learns to

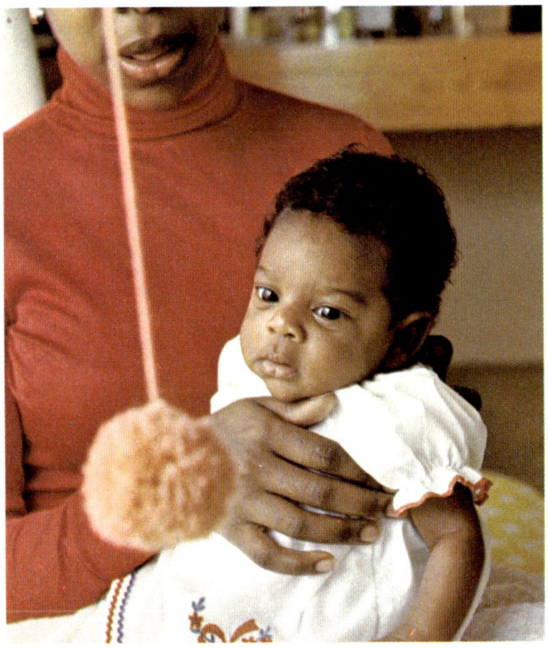

Here is a baby at six weeks, who is focusing on a brightly colored ball about 18 in (45 cm) away. If you move it from side to side, the baby's eyes will follow its movement.

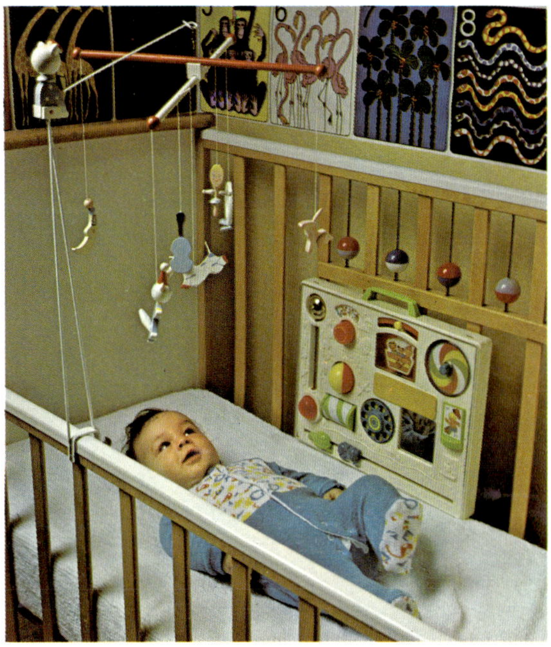

From three or four months, a baby will often stare for several minutes at a brightly colored toy a few feet away without trying to grab hold of it.

focus his eyes on more distant objects, and will look at them for a longer time and follow them if they move.

By six weeks, most babies will focus on an object held about 18 in (45 cm) or so away from their faces. If you dangle a brightly colored ball in front of a six-week-old baby at this distance, he will look fixedly at the ball for several seconds and will follow it with his eyes when it moves slowly from side to side. But the baby's attention can easily be distracted, for example by sounds. A noise will probably cause a reflex eye movement and make the baby look away. As the baby comes to see things more clearly, this in turn helps him to learn to control the movements of his head, and to keep it upright; once he can do this he can also look at objects for longer periods. A baby of three to four months will often stare for several minutes at an attractive toy a few feet away. He looks as though he would like to reach out and grasp it, but makes no attempt to do so. This prolonged staring is probably an important part of learning to recognize familiar objects. Recognition is an important part of learning to think and eventually to talk. The young baby gets excited when he learns to recognize what is going on around him – for instance the sight of his mother.

Once a baby is able to hold up his head steadily, he can learn to use both eyes together. If both eyes are focused on one point, visual pictures from each eye overlap and help him to judge the size and shape of objects, and their distance away from him. (An adult who loses the use of one eye, or who has one eye blindfolded, has difficulty in judging distances.) Good binocular vision is essential when a baby is learning to reach out and grasp his toys. He fixes his eyes on the toy, gauges how far it is away from him and can then guide his hand toward it.

By six months a baby should be able to move his eyes in any direction and follow the circular movements of a ball dangling from a piece of string. As he reaches out for a toy, you can see how well his eyes are helping to coordinate his hand movements. He should consistently move both eyes together and focus them on the same point, and should not squint. A simple way of testing whether a baby crosses his eyes is to hold a flashlight so that the baby stares at its light. The reflection of the light should be seen in the center of each pupil; if it is off-center in one eye, then that eye has a squint. Before six months many babies cross their eyes occasionally; after six months this squint is unusual. Although this is no cause for major concern, you should consult your doctor.

Between six and twelve months old, babies become particularly curious about new sights. When you take your baby into an unfamiliar room you will see how he or she looks around, and studies the new surroundings. Given a new toy he will immediately reach out for it and become absorbed in playing with it. This ability to concentrate on one thing at a time, shutting out all other stimuli, is important for learning. It may also account for a baby's apparent failure to respond during vision and hearing tests. Once the stimulus is well-known it fails to excite the baby's interest.

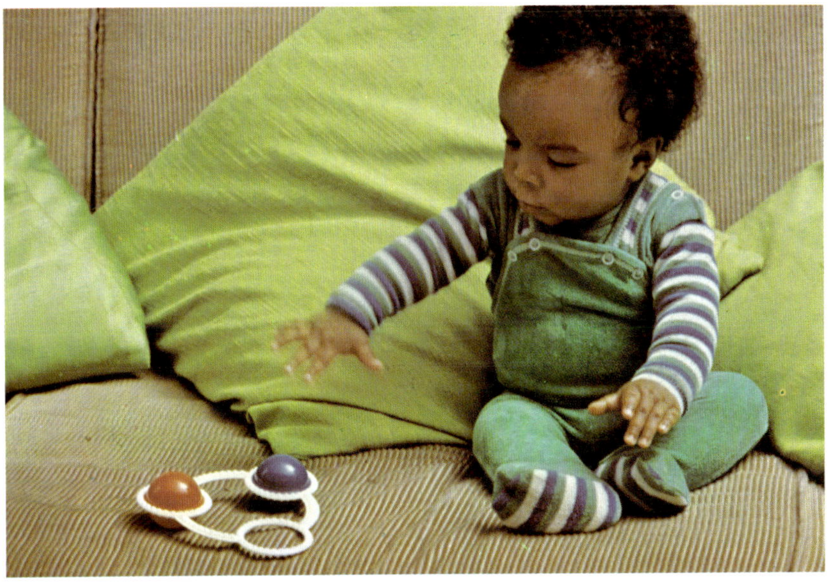

At six months, a baby learns to coordinate eyes and movements in order to reach out for a toy.

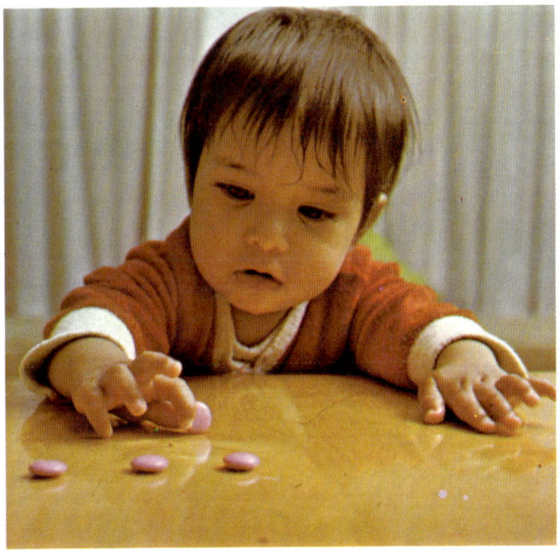

From eight months, a baby will be able to focus on something as small as a candy and will reach out to pick it up. This baby is about to pick up the candy between his first finger and thumb.

From eight months onward it is easier to measure how well a baby can see. For example, he should be able to see a small piece of food, like Cheerios, placed on a table in front of him, and try to pick it up and eat it.

Babies of one year can see the tiny round sprinkles used for decorating cakes and cookies. Put a few on a dark surface and see whether your baby points to them.

One method of testing distance vision is to roll white balls of varying sizes along a piece of dark carpet in front of the baby, and to watch the baby's eyes to see if he or she is following their movement. When this test is done in a doctor's office the baby usually sits on his mother's knee and the examiner rolls the ball at a distance of about 10 ft (3 m) away from them. Most babies of one year can see a ball $\frac{1}{8}$ in (3 mm) in diameter at this distance.

Hearing and speech

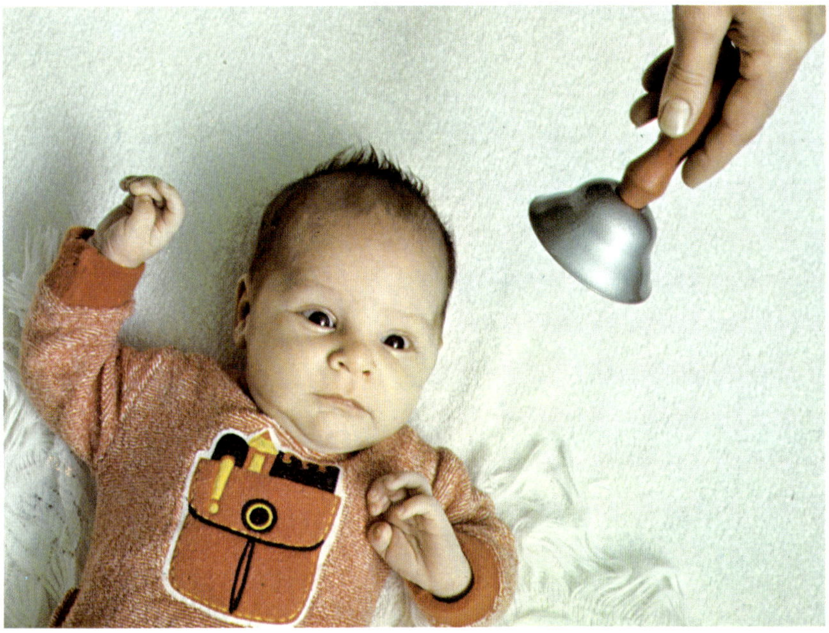

A newborn baby will respond to a sudden loud noise by appearing startled – that is, he will stop moving momentarily and widen his eyes.

Babies are able to hear long before birth. Research has shown that they move in response to sounds from as early as the twenty-sixth week of pregnancy. For the last three months before birth, a baby listens to the sound of his mother's voice, her heartbeat, the swishing of blood through the placenta and gurgling noises from the intestine. It is, therefore hardly surprising that recordings of these uterine noises, played to babies shortly after birth, have been shown experimentally to soothe them and stop their crying.

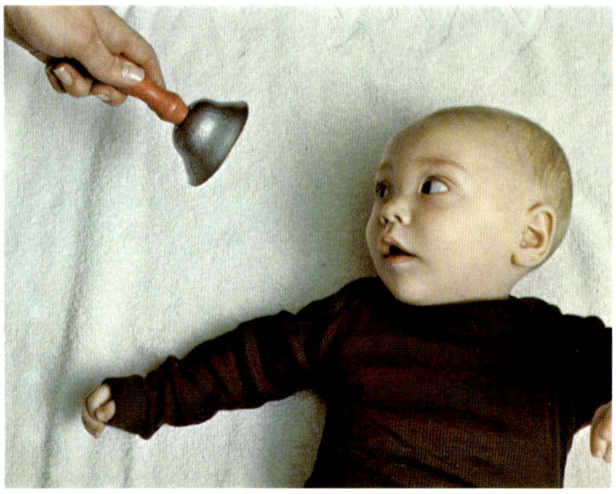

From four months onward, a baby will learn to locate the source of a sound and can turn toward it.

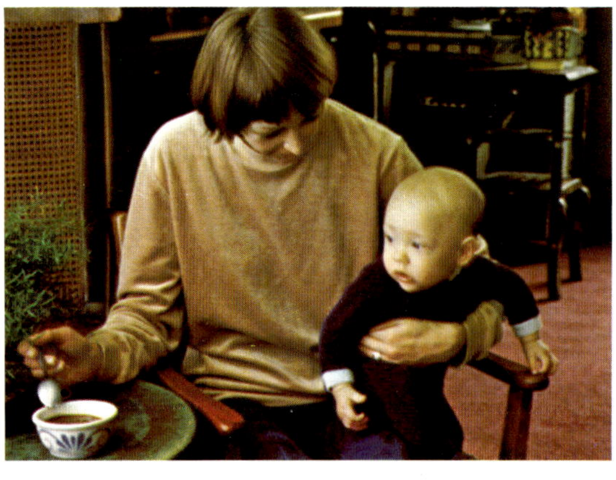

From four months onward a baby will learn to associate sounds with certain experiences; for example, he will become excited on hearing the sound of a spoon banging against a bowl.

Hearing in the first year

Newborn babies respond to sudden loud noises provided they are not deeply asleep or crying. They are often awake and alert shortly after a feeding, and this is a good time to test their response to sound. Make sure that the room is quiet and ask someone, who is out of sight, to make some sort of sharp noise – clap their hands or ring a small bell. The baby may momentarily stop moving and widen his eyes as if listening or, if the sound is very loud, he will probably appear startled and make tremulous movements with his limbs.

It is much more difficult to find out whether newborn babies hear quiet sounds but recent studies have shown that they respond to them with changes in heart rate and breathing pattern as well as by moving their limbs.

Babies seem to prefer high-pitched, musical sounds, and are more attentive to their mothers' voices than to the lower-pitched voices of their fathers. They move their limbs in time to these sounds and this rhythmic movement is thought to be rather similar to the nodding and affirmative noises adults make in conversation.

Over the first six months of life, you will notice that your baby becomes increasingly aware of the activities taking place around him and will try to see where sounds are coming from. Some babies are able to move their eyes toward the source of a sound by six weeks of age.

By four months most babies are able to control their head movements and have started turning their heads toward the source of a sound. At first a baby has to search for the sound but, gradually, he learns to turn his head directly to it. In addition, he learns to associate sounds with his experiences; he will become excited when he hears the sound of a spoon in a dish, because he knows he is going to be fed.

The seven-month-old baby should rapidly turn his head toward quiet sounds made at, and below, the level of his ear. By nine months he should be able to locate sounds made above the level of his ear. Your doctor will use this response to test your baby's hearing when he or she is seven months old. The doctor will try to use quiet sounds likely to interest the baby, such as a spoon being gently scraped around the inside of the cup, the rustle of tissue paper or a rattle. He will also, in a quiet voice, make "ps, ps, ps" and "cooee, cooee" noises. The sounds are made 1 to 2 ft (30 to 60 cm) away from the baby and on each side of his head, first at ear level, then below and then above. The noises should never be made directly behind the baby's head, because locating a sound depends on it being heard sooner and more loudly in one ear.

Hearing tests might seem easy to perform, but great care has to be taken or the results will be difficult to interpret. At seven months a

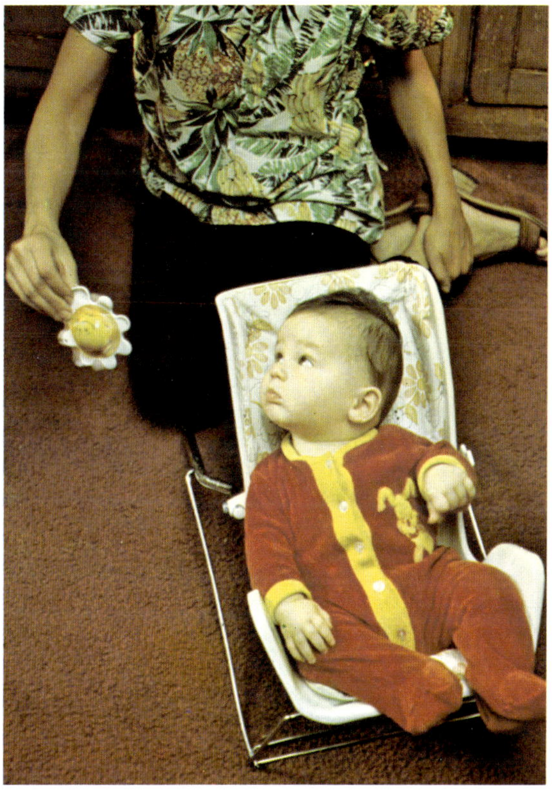

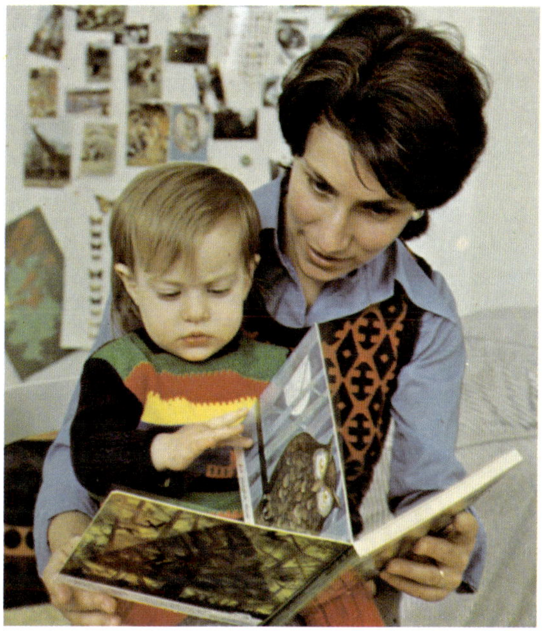

A seven-month-old baby turns his head quickly toward the source of quiet sounds, and can locate their position accurately.

Reading a story and looking at pictures give an ideal opportunity for the child to learn.

baby is very alert and may turn toward the examiner because he has seen the movement of the examiner's shadow or seen a reflection in a shiny surface, because he has caught sight of the rattle out of the corner of his eye, felt a draft or vibration, or is attracted by the doctor's cologne. A baby may fail to respond to the sound test because he is more involved in playing with a toy or watching other people in the room. If the environment is very noisy he may have difficulty in hearing the sound; or he may be bored with it, especially if he has heard it once or twice before.

The beginnings of speech

It is often thought that very young babies are unable to communicate their feelings until they have learned to speak, but this is not so. The newborn baby indicates his most urgent needs by crying, and his mother soon learns to distinguish between the different sounds which indicate hunger, pain, anger and pleasure. Babies also communicate with their eyes and imitative movements such as smiling, and by moving in rhythm with sounds.

A wonderful example of communication occurs when a mother or father picks up the newborn baby. The movement makes the baby open his eyes; he is attracted by the pattern of his mother's facial features and fixes his eyes on her face. She is delighted by his action and responds by smiling and speaking to him; he moves in rhythm with her speech and, after a few weeks, learns to smile back. This close contact of a baby and mother or father is important for learning. A baby's first sounds are attempts to imitate those which he hears. It is known that babies are more attentive to their mother's voice than to other sounds and, luckily, it is natural for a mother to talk to her baby as she feeds and changes him, and later when he is sitting playing on her knee. A quiet environment helps the learning process, because it is then easier for the baby to distinguish new sounds and to remain calm and attentive.

By the time he is six weeks old, the baby starts to make happy cooing noises. When feeding he practices coordinating his breathing, suckling and swallowing, and the movements of his lips and tongue. Soon the baby realizes he can modify his cooing sounds by moving his lips and tongue so that they interrupt the flow of air from the larynx, or voice box. These sounds, called "babble", are first heard at about three or four months, when they are rather repetitive. By six months they have a more tuneful quality.

With increasing practice a baby learns to mimic the sounds he hears most frequently. From eight months, strings of consonant sounds can be heard, such as "mamamamama" and "bababababa" made with the lips, and "dadadadada" and "nanananana" made with the tip of the tongue. When adults hear a baby making these sounds, they are pleased and their pleasure encourages the baby. They also say "mama" or "dada", and point to the appropriate person. Soon the baby learns to say just "mama", and not a string of consonants. By one year many babies are able to use one or two of these words knowing that they are talking about a particular person: sounds are becoming organized into language.

The child and the family

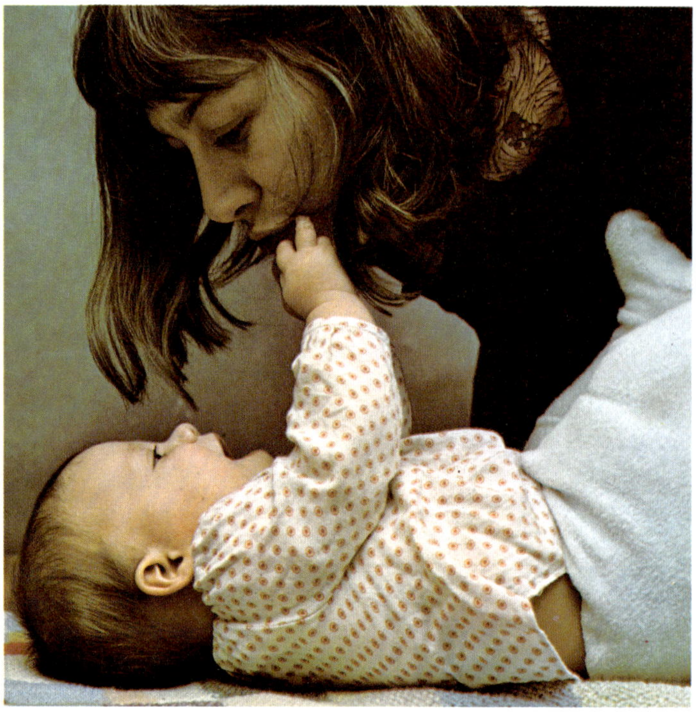

CHAPTER 15

Getting to know others

The new parents

Siblings and the new baby

Common problems with babies

A mothers' symposium

The newborn baby, like many animals, is entirely defenseless at birth. He cannot gather his food or even get it into his mouth. He cannot move or hide from predators, and he lacks any covering to protect himself from either cold or heat, rain or snow. It is therefore quite obvious that he must be protected by somebody. We naturally assume that his family will provide this protection, and it seems inconceivable that this should not happen. Every now and then, though, one hears of a baby being battered, abandoned or deserted, and one realizes that the feelings of warmth and attachment which seem so natural may not develop; they do not occur inevitably. If the early, and possibly the later, development of the child is to go well, it is important to understand the way in which this early attachment, which leads to the baby being protected, nursed and cared for, develops.

In a first pregnancy, even when planned and welcomed, the young mother has difficulty imagining the feelings that will develop for the baby when he is born. With an unplanned pregnancy, feelings of ambivalence may be even stronger. Once the baby is born, however, all such uncertainties are usually swept away. Even when the mother is planning to give the baby up for adoption, it is often astonishing to see how quickly doubts about this develop once she has the baby and rapidly "falls in love" with him. How does this happen? This intense bonding of mother and child happens spontaneously.

A young baby's cry is a peculiarly appealing signal, and very hard to ignore. Furthermore, the mother learns very rapidly, often within ten days, to distinguish her own baby's cry from that of other infants. Very early the baby likes to listen to human voices and begins to respond in preference to his

Cross references

See also	Chapter
Feeding in the first year	10
The new baby at home	11
Common problems in the newborn	12
Physical development	14

The baby uses his eyes, his hands and his voice to establish contact with the person who he now knows is his mother.

mother's voice above all other sounds. His mother responds to the baby's sounds and cries, by making baby noises herself. Automatically people tend to talk in rather high-pitched voices to babies, and it is possible that this artificial-sounding form of communication has some special significance and may be attractive to the infant to whom it is directed.

The newborn baby can see objects which are close to him clearly, and he seems to like the shape of the human face best (*see* chapter 14). He will spend longer periods of time looking at this than at any other shape, and the face he looks at is, almost inevitably, his mother's. The periods of time he will stare at her face may be quite short to start with, but they get longer, and at three or four weeks it is easy to observe a baby looking intensely at his mother. His mother instinctively puts her face in such a position that it is on the same level as the baby's face. Almost as soon as this intense gaze has been firmly established, the baby smiles at his mother. This may happen within the first ten days or not until six weeks or so. The baby's smile is enormously important, because of the feelings of reward it arouses in the mother.

How different are the personalities of babies from one another? Early signs of different temperament are, of course, to some extent limited to the way the child behaves in what are called the vegetative functions – eating and sleeping. Some babies are voracious eaters, suck strongly and demand a lot of food; others are slow and don't seem to want to take much. Patterns of sleep will normally vary greatly from one baby to another.

When an adult wakes up in the night he just turns over again and goes back to sleep but the baby who wakes every couple of hours immediately wonders where are those people he is getting to know – his parents – and cries out for them. You can see in this simple phenomenon how, right from the start, other people around him affect the baby's developing personality. In the United States, most parents expect the baby to sleep in his own crib, frequently in another room, and therefore the baby who wakes a lot at night can be very disturbing and difficult for them to manage. In other parts of the world where babies sleep in their mothers' beds from birth, when the infant wakes in the night he simply nurses at the breast for a minute or two, then goes back to sleep again immediately.

In other ways, too, the baby begins to express his personality very early. Some babies smile as soon as an adult approaches them, and burst into long streams of chuckling if anyone talks to them, whereas others may seem much more solemn and unresponsive. What is not really known is whether the smiling, laughing baby goes on to be the extrovert adult; and whether the solemn baby becomes the solemn and serious adult. The trouble is that the parents foster both reactions. As he gets older the child who laughs hears people say that "he's always laughing and smiling," and, probably to oblige the parents, he does. Likewise the non-laugher hears that "he's such a serious person," and this is the role he thinks he should take up. As the baby begins to express his personality in these ways early, however, his parents inevitably begin to have ideas about how the baby thinks and feels, and they create a picture of the child's personality or temperament. They should be aware that their expectations are directly communicated to the child who is in a critical state of personality development.

Getting to know others

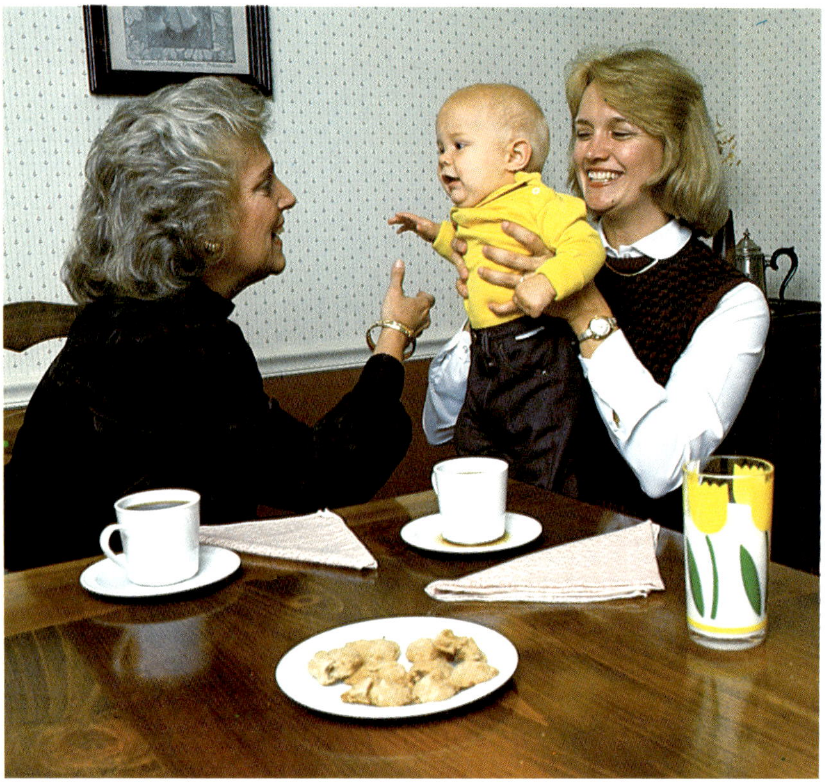

A baby is always ready to respond to the other members of the family, provided they make the first overtures.

The child can recognize his mother's smell, and probably her voice, quite early. But what exactly does this mean? Does the baby recognize her as a person? It is really very difficult to judge, since the child can't tell us what he is feeling – all we have to go on are our observations of his behavior.

In the first two or three months, it is quite easy for one sympathetic caretaker to take over from another in looking after the baby, and he shouldn't show any great signs of distress if this happens. At three months, a baby will smile as readily at a stranger's face as at his mother's and, indeed, will probably look at it for longer. This doesn't mean, of course, that he isn't interested in his mother, simply that the stranger's face presents a novel, and therefore particularly interesting, stimulus, whereas by this time he has begun to recognize his mother's face as familiar.

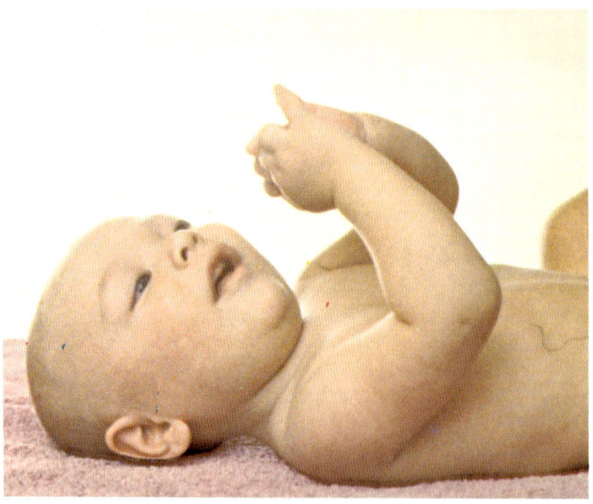

Learning where his own body begins and ends is an important step toward distinguishing between other people.

Obviously, before a baby can fully develop specific attachments and bonds with particular people, he has to make certain quite complex discoveries about the world. He must work out where his body starts and where it ends, and learn that objects, including people, continue to exist even when he can't see them. This understanding of the existence of objects when they are not there comes at about seven months. If you walk slowly around behind the baby, he will turn his head to follow you, and as soon as you have disappeared behind him he will turn his head around the other way to see if you are going to appear there. Before this age, he will lose interest once you get behind his easy line of vision.

Interestingly enough, it is at about seven months that we have the first real evidence that a strong bond has formed between mother and child. This has been demonstrated in various studies: for example, babies who had to go into the hospital for short periods, were observed to see at what age they became distressed. Quite a distinct break was found to occur at about seven months. Before that, separation from the mother did not elicit a major protest, and strangers were accepted as mother substitutes, whereas after that age they cried inconsolably when their mothers left them, and showed a vigorous response to the mothers when they reappeared. When a child went home from the hospital there was quite a long period of readjustment, during which there were clear indications that the baby was very anxious to have his mother stay near him.

Another way in which we can see that the baby is developing specific attachments and bonds, becomes apparent in his behavior to strangers. There is quite a change in the second half of the first year, when some infants may cry if a stranger approaches them, and will certainly not be disturbed if he leaves them. On the other hand, if the mother or father or other familiar adults go away, these babies will be visibly distressed: their protests and their affections are now directed toward specific people with whom they have formed strong attachments.

As the first year continues the range of sounds the baby makes expands enormously (*see* chapter 14). He likes to play games with people where he makes a string of sounds and expects them to respond. People who play these games with him are people he relates to, and indeed, toward the end of the first year, he may specifically begin to use some naming words, pointing to his mother, father and his brothers and sisters. Words are a means of developing the emotional bond which has been forming in so many ways, and they are further evidence that the baby is developing proper attachments.

It used to be thought that these attachments of the baby were primarily, inevitably, focused on the mother, and that the baby formed a bond with one person, and one person only, during this first year of life. Happily for fathers, this is not the case. The baby will form a bond with more than one person, and indeed, in an ordinary family, he may make demands on different members for different things. For example, he may want his mother to feed him, spooning the food in, but when it comes to bedtime he may want his father to carry him to his room and put him into his crib to sleep for the night.

Of course, the extent to which the baby's relationships will develop with the adults in his home depends as much on the adults as on the baby. He is ready to respond, but the adult must make the first overtures. For the father, this probably depends to a considerable extent on how closely he has been involved in the birth and subsequent day-to-day care of the child.

Grandma may be another important person in a baby's life; it may be her knee he likes to sit on in the morning after his bath and so on. By these simple observations we can tell that the baby has formed specific bonds and attachments during the first year of life and that these have been formed with specific people, usually members of his family. It is an advantage to the child, of course, that he can form attachments to more than one person, because if anything happens to his mother, usually his principal caretaker, it means that he will be able to get from someone else the emotional security and support that he needs.

A baby has to develop an idea about the permanence of objects, but of course it is more complicated than that. He has to understand that separate objects exist, and one of the first objects he studies with considerable fascination is himself.

At about three months one can watch the baby lying on his back, holding his hands in front of his face and looking at them (hand regard, or hand play). He moves his hands around, twisting them about, and generally seems fascinated by them. What is almost certainly happening is that he is relating the sensations that come in from his body to the visual information he has obtained by inspection. He learns that when he feels that wiggly movement of his fingers, the objects that he is looking at wiggle, and in time he realizes that his hands are part of himself. As his hand function develops, the baby uses his hands to explore things that are placed in front of them, and also, sometimes to his parent's embarrassment, to explore his own and other people's bodies. Things which stick out are natural objects of interest, and the little boy, when naked may hold, play with and explore his penis. A very common object of babies' interest, sometime after the six-month mark, is an ear, and parents are often worried about the way their children poke and play with their ears.

Perhaps this play simply represents the child's efforts to sort out in another way whether these sticking out objects are really part of him, or whether they are in fact like

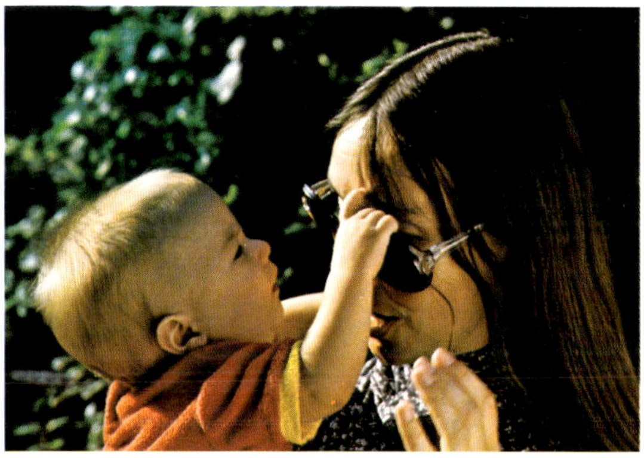

The baby will soon begin to explore other people, too. Glasses will probably fascinate him as he tries to determine whether they are part of a person, or separate objects.

those separate objects which people give him to play with. It is only when he has established this existence of his own body that he is ready to explore outside it. He can, in fact, make undirected swipes and hold onto objects very early and sometimes one sees a baby extending a hand toward an object at a very early age, but it is not until three or four months that he regularly reaches out for toys and rattles which are put in front of him and tries to get hold of them.

His own sense of himself allows him to make the necessary explorations of other people, when, for example the baby pulls at their clothes to see if they are attached; he is fascinated by glasses, which he wants to take off and handle. He may seem to be asking whether glasses are part of the body, or whether they are objects in their own right. He will continue this sort of exploration as he gets older.

We have seen that the baby in the newborn period has a strong primary walking response, that is, his body knows how to take systematic steps (*see* p. 130), but he can only do this if somebody holds him up and moves him along appropriately. He is quite strong enough to support his weight, he can see where he is going, and it is probable that his balancing organs are in full working order. Why then does he not walk? The reason is, of course, that all these different bits of equipment he has are not integrated with one another.

He does not realize that to walk he must

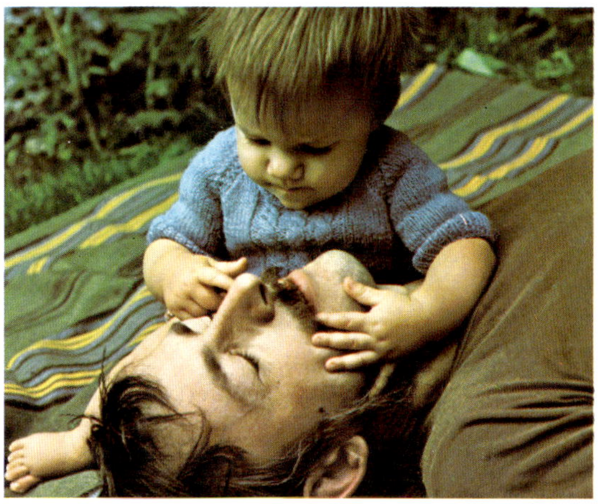

Hands can soon be used as tools to explore the baby's world. Other people's faces remain the most intriguing objects around a young baby.

support his weight first of all, and then that to move forward he must turn on that funny mechanism which moves his legs about, and that to guide himself he must use his vision to see where obstacles are and get around them. It is not very surprising that when he does start to walk, his first steps are sometimes hesitant and jerky, and he holds his hands up ready to catch himself, should he fall. Quickly, of course, all the different senses work together and he becomes a confident toddler.

This integration of the various parts of the central nervous system depends on growth and development within that system, that is to say, nerve fibers proliferating and joining up the different parts within the brain. It is for this reason that, although exercising and playing with a baby probably encourages the development of walking and may make him walk a month or so earlier than he would have done ordinarily, it won't make that much difference because a baby cannot walk until his brain is ready to do so. Indeed, if you don't exercise a baby and encourage him to walk, he will still walk by himself all the same.

This is not to imply that it is not a good thing to play with and handle babies: it certainly is. But it is doubtful whether it is worth spending a lot of time on any specific function, such as encouraging walking. It might be more important in order to develop walking, for example, to practice his visual activities. It is not really possible to tell what the baby is learning at any one time. What you can do is to provide a generally stimulating environment around him, rather than trying to affect specific items within his development.

The development of movement activities plays an important part in the development of the child's social competence, because apart from the physical aspects of his environment, it contains people, and once he can crawl or walk he is free to express his feelings about people as simply as possible, by coming toward them or going away. When he can make purposeful movements with his arms he can hold them out to be picked up, or he can take his hands away and turn his head to one side if he doesn't want to be touched.

If we have thought about the complexities of integrating various different parts of the body to get walking going, think how many more must be involved in achieving fluent speech. The child must be able to hear and decipher words that are said to him. He has then got to be able to decide what he wants to say himself and select the word to use meaningfully, and he then has to go through the complicated process of producing this word, which involves coordinating movements of his breathing, his vocal cords, his palate, his tongue, his lips, and getting all these going together at one and the same time. It is not surprising that, from an early age, babies like to make a lot of noise and practice sounds over and over again. Once they have got a word, in the second year, they may repeat it hundreds of times until they feel sure they can say it correctly.

The new parents

The arrival of a new baby, particularly the first, will have a profound effect on the relationship between the child's parents, who also have to form a relationship with their new baby. It is hard, during pregnancy, for a young couple to grasp just how changed their lives will be by the baby's arrival. Parenthood is probably the most important role a person will ever have to adopt, but it is also the one for which he or she is likely to have the least training. The job requires an enormous amount of energy, patience and flexibility but it can also provide tremendous rewards for both parents. The father's part is very important – parenthood is not solely a female responsibility. If he can involve himself with his wife in the care of their new child, both parents will find that, far from imposing a strain as they perhaps feared the baby will probably bring about a deepening and cementing of their relationship. It would be wrong, of course, to suggest that problems don't occur. They do. The crucial point is to be prepared for them and to see them for what they are – snags rather than insuperable difficulties.

The most mundane, but often the most common problem, is the change in family finances. Although many young married women work right up to the end of pregnancy, and some go back to work after a brief period, for many the arrival of the baby heralds the arrival of financial dependence on their partners. The family's income consequently drops at a time when expenses are increasing. If a couple can make financial plans in advance and discuss and agree on their priorities, it should be possible for them to deal with any financial tensions which arise in a spirit of cooperation rather than antagonism. Housing, too, needs careful forethought. A studio apartment is fine for two but if your nights are being disturbed, more space becomes a matter of urgency.

Some young mothers with small babies do become mildly to moderately depressed, a phenomenon which has been recognized with increasing frequency in recent years. There are, of course, biological changes too in the mother, as her body adapts to the non-pregnant state; there are hormonal changes going on, and many people believe that mothers are more emotional in the postpartum period (*see* chapter 8). The young mother will find that the arrival of the infant curtails her freedom of movement. It is not so easy to get out; simple household chores, easily done when alone, seem to take up all day. When her husband comes home in the evening, the young mother feels that she has achieved nothing, that their home is a mess and that she is not even able to do what she would like with her husband.

When his wife returned home with the baby, the husband may have imagined that, now she is "not working" and has only one small infant, to look after, who will sleep most of the time, his wife will be even better company than she has been before, that she won't be as tired

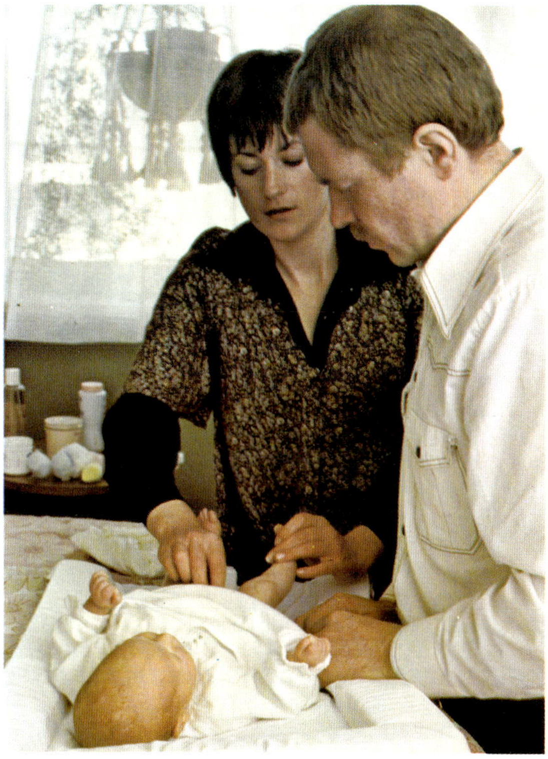

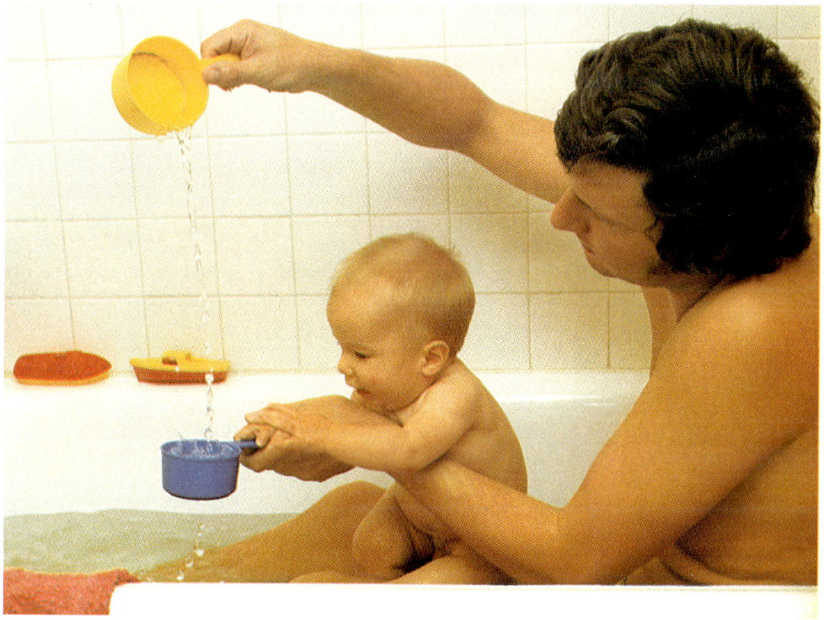

After the new baby has arrived, it takes time for both parents to get used to meeting the baby's needs.

The more involved the father is in the day-to-day care of the baby, the more rapidly the bond between them will develop.

and worn-out as she sometimes was when she had a full-time job.

To his amazement, he may find the reverse: his wife is now more exhausted than she ever was in the past, the confidence he recognized in her when she was at work seems to have disappeared, she doesn't seem to know how to cope with their new baby, which he has been fondly imagining will be largely her job. If his relationship with his wife is not to deteriorate, he must try to be tolerant and provide the support she needs until she has had time to become comfortable in her new role. Biological changes in the wife may have led to changes in sexual libido, and the stress and difficulties of the new relationship between the couple and the baby may also affect this important aspect of their marriage.

The parents, then, have to face great changes in their own relationship, which may not go well if they are taken by surprise by events. Clearly there is no reason for the relationship between the husband and wife to change, provided the baby has been planned and the parents have thought about the financial and housing problems. It is also helpful to find friends in a similar situation to provide mutual help and support, perhaps other young couples with children who may form groups to share some of the chores of looking after the baby to allow the mother independence. It is sad to see problems occurring, because they can interfere with what should be a period of real pleasure and satisfaction as the parents watch and interact with their infant as he or she develops.

As previously stressed the baby in fact has mechanisms which elicit "care-taking" behavior from adults around him. His cry, of course, is the most penetrating and distressing noise and it demands that he get attention. But equally his chuckles and smiles seem to elicit, from adults who want to be involved with him, behavior which would have surprised them a few months before. The father finds himself quite easily able to make curious high-pitched baby noises, which he previously found embarrassing when he watched others do the same thing with their children.

Where the couple is sharing the care of the child, the mother has the opportunity to get out and around and possibly continue some part of the active working life she enjoyed before the birth of the baby. When shared by both parents the period of early infancy is one of enormous satisfaction, because they feel that they alone are responsible, as indeed they are in a sense, for this miraculous unfolding and developing of a new human being.

A new mother can easily feel isolated with her baby, and become depressed. The company of other mothers can help to prevent this, and provides an opportunity to share any anxieties.

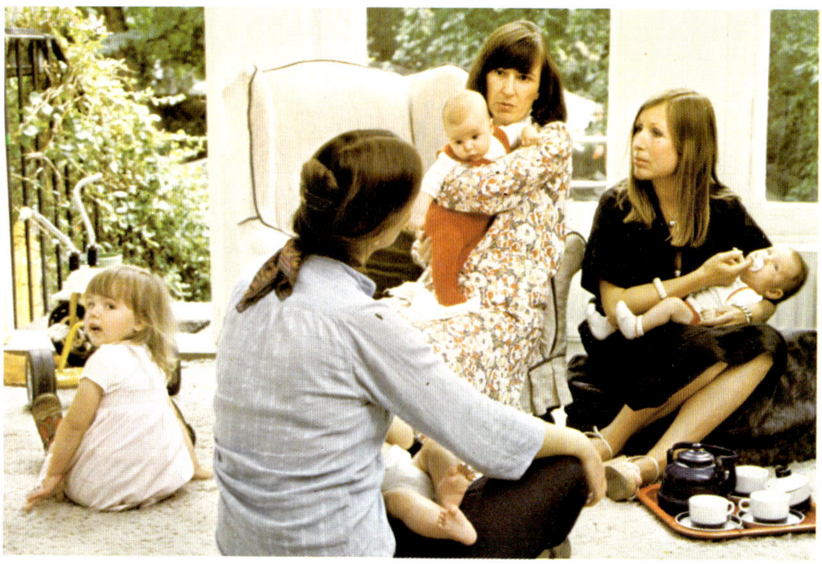

Siblings and the new baby

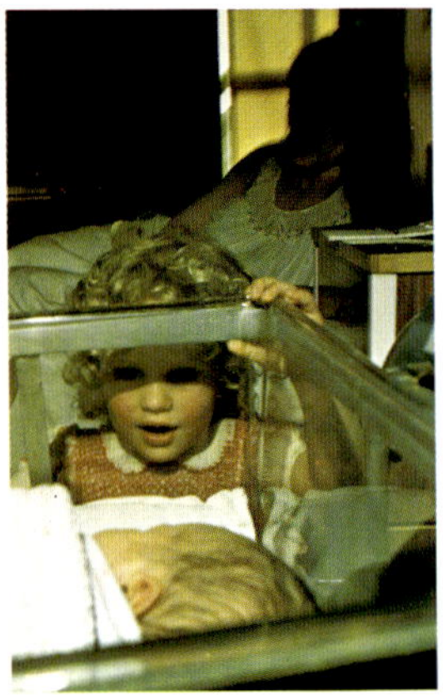

Despite knowing that a baby was "on the way" this toddler is clearly amazed at the sight of her new sister.

Second and subsequent children may often seem easier to manage than the first baby because the parents, now know what it's all about. But for the older children themselves, of course, the new baby is a surprise: however much the parents have prepared them, they often have little concept of what it's going to be like to have a brother or sister until the new child arrives. The behavior of the older children toward the new baby will vary according to their age, their sex, their own personality and the number of children there are already in the family.

When two children are born very close together, perhaps with a gap of barely a year between them, the parents have two babies on their hands and may have a one-year-old screaming for his food at the same time as the new baby is making demands. Such a combination is very exhausting for the parents, and the older child's "jealousy", if it can be called that, is very obvious. He doesn't want the mother to be feeding the baby when she ought to be feeding him.

This is a great strain, and the majority of studies suggest that, although most children born in a short interval do well, in general a longer gap between children is better. However, as these closely paired children grow up, they are very familiar with each other and often form closer ties than children who are more widely separated in age.

A more usual, and possibly wiser, gap between children is about two to three years. By this time, in terms of practical management, the two-year-old understands that he has to wait while mommy prepares his lunch, and so on, and can appreciate that sometimes the new baby has to be first and will, theoretically, wait patiently. Of course, in practice, the sight of the new baby receiving the attention that he has been used to, and apparently getting priority attention from his parents, may make him feel jealous and anxious. He fears this newcomer is going to displace him from his parents' affections. For example, although the older child may by this time be toilet trained, he may suddenly revert to wetting again. One two-year-old who had been "dry" for several months stood quietly wetting himself while watching his baby brother being breast-fed.

Older brothers and sisters may be surprised at how helpless the new baby is, but they will soon learn that he cannot be played with like a doll.

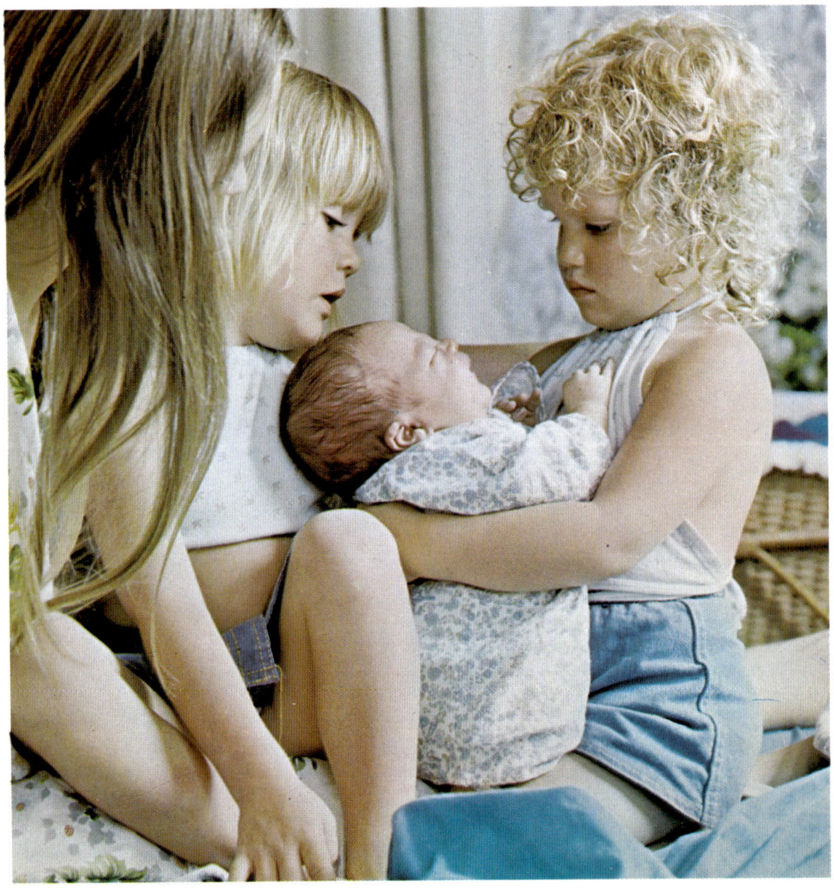

The feelings of jealousy of the toddler can often be overcome by the parents making sure that he is aware that he has certain privileges which the infant doesn't have. The father can play a very important role here by doing things like taking the toddler out for little expeditions of their own, while mother looks after the baby. But it is important, of course, to see that both parents give him special attention, so that he doesn't feel deserted for the new baby.

Plan how you are going to introduce the new baby to his older siblings. At the family's first hospital visit after the birth, try to have the baby in a crib beside you, so that you have your arms free for your older children. Small presents "from the new baby" are probably not a good idea, however, as any toddler will see through that piece of well meant deception: his new brother or sister is far too helpless to have been shopping! (It may also lead to his expecting a bribe in future delicate situations.) There is a lot of variation in the way the older child will react, and many toddlers enjoy participating in the caring routines for their younger siblings.

Even so, although the parents feel they are making every effort to help the toddler accept the new baby, there are great changes for a two-year-old when another baby arrives. Right up to the time when his mother disappears for a few days to acquire this "new" baby, whatever that is, the toddler has received the lion's share of his mother's attention. When he has called, she has come to him; when he has fallen and cried, she has given him immediate comfort. But now he discovers overnight that he is no longer able to command such immediate attention, and indeed comes second to somebody else. If this does not necessarily lead to feelings of jealousy toward the baby, it may lead to some feelings of resentment toward the mother. Of course there can be advantages for the older child in this changed situation. Inevitably he must learn to be more independent; he must play by himself or stand and watch while the mother feeds the baby, and therefore in terms of independence his character is bound to take a big leap.

Over a period of time, the child also recognizes his own superiority to the baby. He is bigger and more competent than the new infant, something which may surprise him if he expected the baby to have abilities right away, and so the very existence of the younger child does foster his own growing awareness of his capabilities.

Older children will again vary in their responses to a new baby. Little girls of four, five or six may long for babies, but be surprised that the baby cannot be played with like a doll, and put away when they themselves require attention. It is probably not a good idea to start a child at a day care center, nursery school or elementary school just at the time when the new baby arrives. Any child is almost bound to feel that this dismissal from the home is due to the new brother or sister. Behavior at home and beginning school may be difficult as a result. On the other hand, if the child has been settled in school or nursery school before the arrival of the new baby, with judicious management of the baby's day, it may be possible to see that the older child gets plenty of attention and does not really feel put upon by the new baby's routine.

So far, possible jealousies and difficulties which may arise with the birth of a new baby among older brothers and sisters have been emphasized but, in fact, for many children the arrival of a baby is a source of great pleasure.

In the first few months they may find the baby relatively uninteresting, but as he begins to sit up and take notice older brothers and sisters will enjoy playing with him enormously. They also seem to have far more patience than adults, and will endlessly retrieve a toy which a ten-month-old is joyously casting to the floor. As the baby gets bigger and by a year or fifteen months begins to move around, they will like to supervise his explorations and will become as attached and devoted to him as their parents are.

Indeed, we know that brothers and sisters do protect each other from stress within the family; that is to say, if one parent dies, or there is a divorce, the children provide emotional support for each other and prevent the development of disturbance. It is important in such emergencies to take every precaution that brothers and sisters are allowed to stay together for mutual support.

A very special example of a relationship between brothers and sisters is, of course, that which exists between twins. In this situation the infants need to realize from the start that everything has to be shared, but as they hopefully get equal amounts of attention from both mother and father, feelings of jealousy usually do not arise. Twins also have the stimulation of each other: each has a companion who is closely interested in him from the start of their lives, and it is not surprising to find that the relationship between the twins is often so important that it almost seems to interfere with the rest of their development. Thus twins often talk later than other children, although, as with all these observations, there is a wide degree of variation.

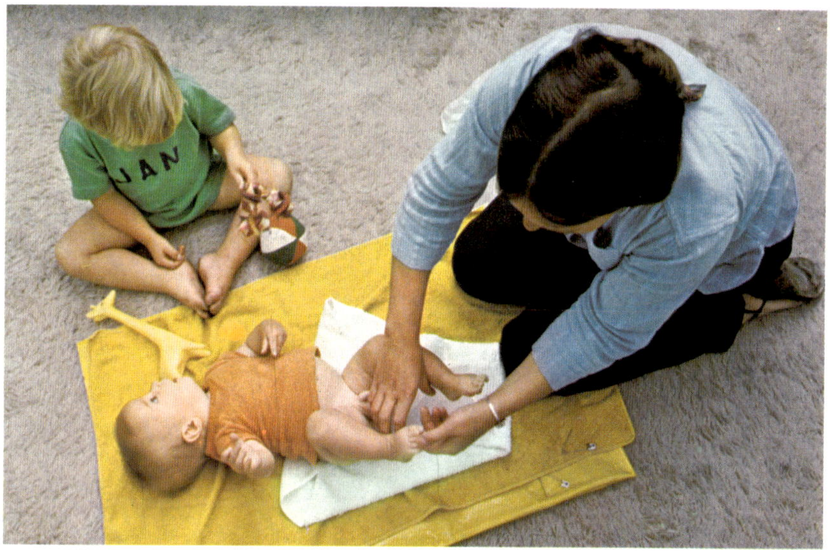

Letting a toddler "help" with caring for the new baby will prevent her feeling her place in the family has been usurped.

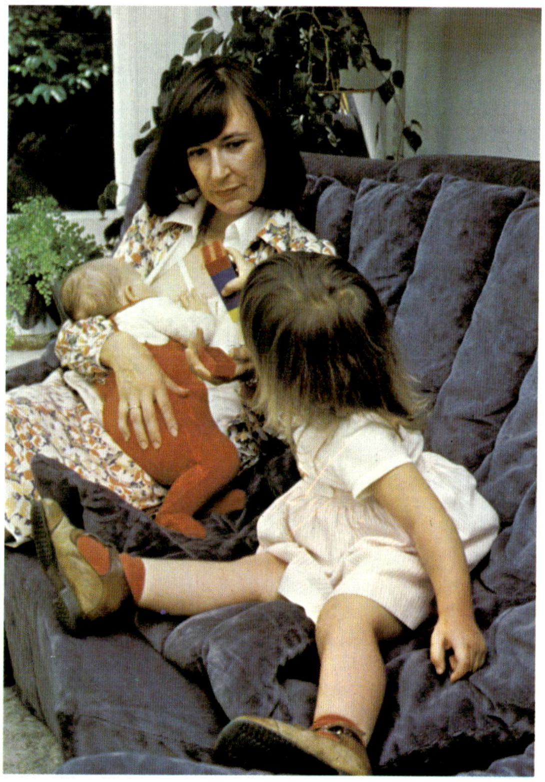

It may take time for a toddler to appreciate that her mother's attention now has to be shared. Occasional attempts at disruption are understandable.

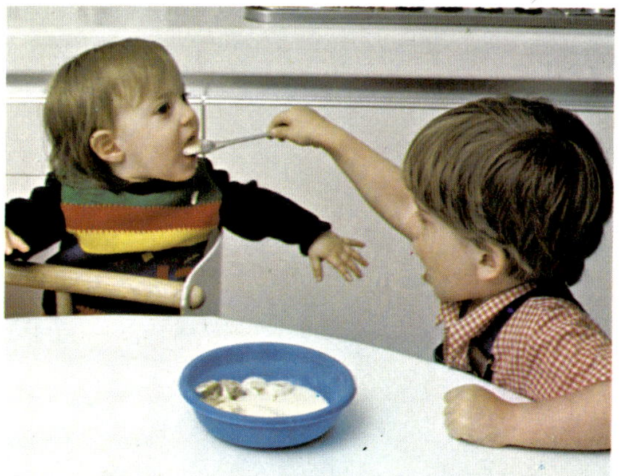

An older sibling will often show endless patience in playing with the baby and helping to teach him new skills.

Common problems with babies

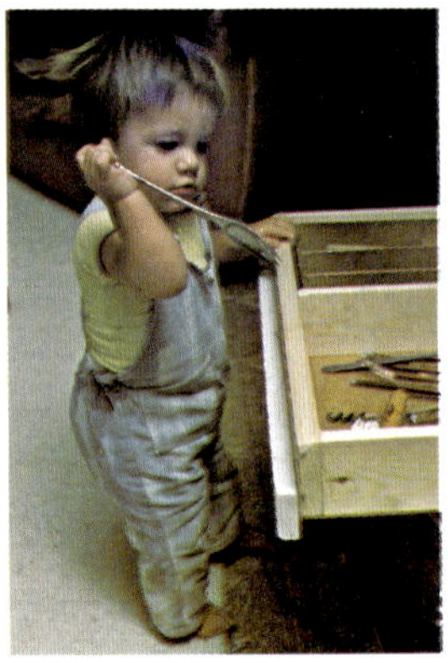

As the child gets older and more mobile, many fascinating and potentially dangerous corners of the home become accessible.

Most people think that babies sleep virtually 24 hours of the day when they are first born. In fact this is quite untrue. Even at birth the baby only spends an average of about 14 hours a day sleeping, with a good deal of time variation between babies. He can spend time lying in his crib doing nothing while his parents are under the impression that he is asleep. Although the child's demands for sleep will go on being more than the adult's, possibly up to as late as puberty, again there is tremendous variation between children. There is probably a general tendency for children to be made to spend much too long in bed, rather than the reverse.

The one-year-old will only sleep for about 12 hours out of the 24 and there is certainly no need for him to have a nap in the morning or afternoon if he doesn't want one. Many nursery schools still try to get children to sleep in the afternoon, and some children do like to take a little nap after lunch (like some adults). But if the child is active in the afternoon there is no point in getting him to lie down and pretend to sleep, a forced inactivity which may be very frustrating.

One of the most common causes of sleep problems is the parents' need to have the child out of the way for some hours. Many parents like their infants and young children to disappear fairly early in the evening so that they can have some time to themselves. This is fine, but expect your two-year-old, if you put him to bed at six o'clock, to wake at a similar hour in the morning, and don't expect him to do much sleeping, if any, during the day. It is much more practical to teach the child that you both need some privacy and that there are times when he should be doing something quietly on his own, rather than to try to force him into sleep, which, of course, will never succeed.

To add to the parents' problems, they may find they are becoming quite exhausted, if the baby is constantly awake at night and one who likes frequent feedings. Another change in the parents' lives may therefore have to be in their own patterns of sleep. The constant carrying, bending over, increased laundry and so on add up to physical exhaustion. When this is coupled with depression and the baby is difficult, the mother and father may find that they lack the energy and initiative to try to find out why their baby is being so difficult or to get any help. Domestic help, either by somebody in the family or from a professional source, for a week or two, may ease the parents through this difficult and exhausting initial period.

Greater motor control has its advantages, too. Once the baby can "sit up and take notice" he or she will enjoy a change of scene.

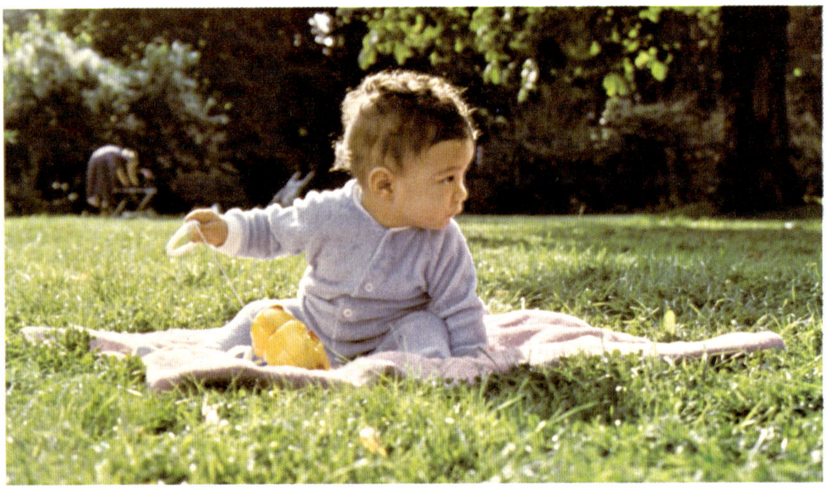

Colic is, of course, associated with sleep disturbance, but here the particular pattern is that the child usually cries and is restless and, indeed, seems to be in pain during the evening, perhaps from about eight until midnight, but then settles down and sleeps well through the night. The cause of colic remains somewhat obscure. It is more common in bottle-fed babies and is probably associated with swallowing too much air. The baby does really seem to be in pain: he draws up his legs, kicks and becomes red in the face, and he often passes a lot of gas. If you tap his tummy you can hear the gas inside him. Often, when the problem is quite a minor one, the child can be comforted by sitting him up or walking him up and down, but some children seem inconsolable and the family has to put up with two or three hours of frantic crying. Sometimes an adjustment in the way the child's day is organized will help with the problem, such as moving the bath time to the evening and giving him an opportunity to kick and move around more, which may help the passage of the gas. Sometimes a little mild medicine seems to ease the discomfort. In any case, the condition virtually always clears up by four to six months, although for the parents this short period of time can seem like a life sentence.

Babies go on having periods of being irritable and difficult throughout the first year. So too, of course, do adults: at different times of the day, week or month we are more or less easy to live with. The adult can explain his feelings, or at least those around him find it fairly easy to interpret his behavior; whereas the baby simply seems to cry or be difficult for no very good reason.

The parents want to know what is making their child unhappy, and a very common solution during the first year is to put any irritability which arises down to teething. Undoubtedly the child can have some minor disturbance when he is actually cutting his teeth, but on most occasions when "teething" is reported there is no evidence that the gums are inflamed or sore at all, and one must look elsewhere for the cause of the child's distress, although one does not always find an answer.

With the young baby, parents are often surprised how much social attention the child wants. He or she is not yet able to talk so why should one talk to him? Nor is he really able to play, so why should one give him toys? In fact, from the moment of birth, the baby is already involving himself in both these forms of social activity, although in a very simple way.

The sounds a baby makes in the first three months of life are all vowel sounds, but he builds up a big repertoire of them quite rapidly, and he likes to be involved in conversations with his family, occasionally at times in the day when other people have other things to do. This may be a moment when the child shows irritation.

By five or six months the baby is exploring objects, feeling them, putting them in his mouth to feel them with his tongue and taste them. This again is an activity which he cannot really do by himself. He wants attention, he wants someone to pick up the objects which he drops, he wants to vocalize about his explorations to someone who is paying some attention. He also likes straightforward social activities. He likes being carried around in someone's arms, being lifted up to look at things, being shown what's in the pots on the stove and seeing what his family is doing. He likes being cuddled and loved. When a six-month-old baby is lying on his back kicking his legs, it is not only for the pleasure of the movement but also for the pleasure of the social contact.

Some parents worry that they can spoil their children at this age, but in fact the evidence suggests that the more time you spend with a young baby, the more independent he will become later, so that one should not be at all worried about giving the young infant all the attention he demands – although it should be realized that it will not always be possible to meet his demands.

At some time he will of course learn to move. Most babies start crawling around about seven or eight months and this tremendously increases their range of exploring activities. It also increases their ability to control their social relationships; they can go and find their mother by now and, equally, they can go away from her.

Sometimes, when this first happens, the child may crawl into the next room and suddenly feel he has lost her. For the parents, the child's mobility begins to present problems with the precious objects around the house which the infant will get at, explore and pull down. Books come tumbling down from low shelves, ornaments can no longer be kept on low tables. For the child, it is very difficult to understand why his mother allows him to poke about in a cupboard full of pots and pans, but not in the cupboard next door which is full of fine china and glass. However, provided one can keep to relatively few restrictions, very early the baby will learn the meaning of the word "no". The sudden angry tone of voice will surprise him, but he will accept that this tone really does forbid him to touch the object in question.

The greater mobility, first of crawling, then of walking, allows the child to cut off a social relationship and eventually to go away, up to his own room or into another room and be separate from the adult with whom he has had such a close tie. He will explore this relationship endlessly in the second year of his life. But the increased motor skill will also mean that the child can pursue activities which were not such fun when he or she was less mobile. A small yard becomes an exciting place to explore, and happy hours can be spent in a sandbox which can easily be constructed in a corner of the back yard. From the sheltered world of the yard, the child begins to see beyond the fences, to meet neighboring children and explore relationships outside the family. Thus begins the process which will go on for another 10 or 15 years, of achieving an adult personality which allows him to be independent of his family, an independence which is best built on the secure base of the early years.

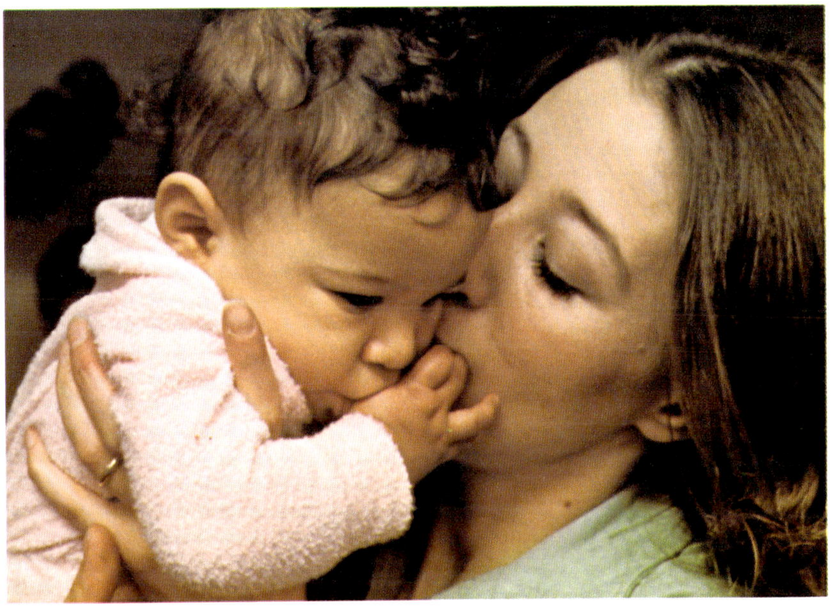

"Evening colic" is distressing both for the baby and for the parents. The baby can often be comforted by walking him up and down. The condition nearly always clears up by four to six months.

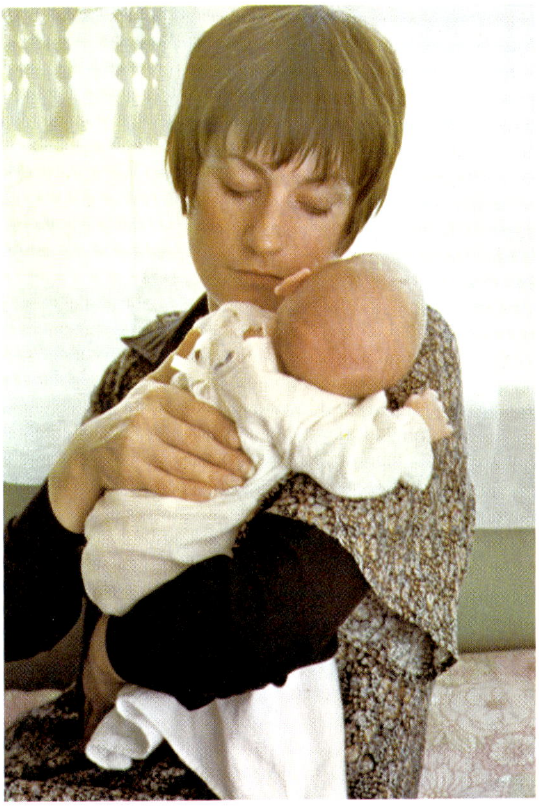

The parents' own lack of sleep can be one of the greatest problems to cope with in the early days. Help in the home can ease the situation until the baby's sleep pattern is established.

A mothers' symposium

In this changing world, new and exciting options for women are available. Strong family constellations and professional careers are not mutually exclusive. But certain trade-offs may be inevitable. Organization, cooperation and support systems are the mainstay of successful management for a couple balancing two careers and children. The ability to analyze your lifestyle periodically is vital to keeping life enjoyable. Here, four women discuss their life situations. Each is currently pregnant and has a young child at home. They are 26 to 34 years old. They share their experiences of coping with the complex task of combining a career and a family.

Joan: My major challenge with this pregnancy is my schedule. I'm a second year resident in internal medicine. Patient care rounds start at 7:00 am each morning and I'm on call at the hospital every third night. I get very tired. I also worry about how this pregnancy could affect my co-workers. For example, if I develop complications and have to be hospitalized, the other residents will have to take care of my patients and work my on-call nights. They already work too hard! It could really alienate me from the other residents. I'm the only one pregnant. My husband is a practicing pediatrician. We try to share home responsibilities equally, but, realistically the domestic responsibility is mostly mine, even though he is willing to help out.

Elizabeth: Well, I work at least 60 hours a week. I am trying to become a partner in my law firm. My husband can be a great help, but his career, to be honest, is his first priority. We haven't taken a vacation since our honeymoon. We are often in separate cities and see little of each other, let alone my child. The separations are necessary, but have put a strain on our time together with our child. On top of this, I often find conflicts between family obligations and my desire to advance my career. The decison to have a second child caused some tension. Because I was an only child I never wanted to have just one child. I know today there is a lot of information on raising an only child successfully, but I just didn't want this for myself. My husband felt we had enough to cope with already. He believes two or three children are impractical given our situation. He made me feel guilty, saying that another baby would diminish the time I now spend with our first child. Also, the demands at his office are increasing and he felt that he wouldn't be home enough to help out with the extra burdens of a second child.

Jennifer: I'm actually having an easier time with this pregnancy. Perhaps because I've been through it before and know what to expect. I like my job. It may not be quite so demanding as yours, Joan and Elizabeth, but perhaps I'm luckier in that respect. I'm a bank loan officer which entails lots of responsibility and some heavy decisions, but at least I can leave that all behind when my husband picks me up from work. He is an executive in maritime insurance. We both enjoy exercising. He jogs and I teach aerobics two nights a week at the Y. I absolutely love this class because it offers me personal time away from home and work. When I'm teaching, Jim, my husband, plays with our son which I think is very special for both of them.

Deborah: I am not quite sure where I fit in here. My life has a different emphasis. My husband Alan and I moved east after we graduated from college. He's a junior executive with a large company that sells computer systems to small businesses. It's a good job for him, but it requires lots of travel. I think when it's all added up Alan was on the road for almost 3 months last year. A career seems pretty much out of the question for me. I'm a homemaker, mother of a 2-year-old daughter, support person for my husband and now expecting a second child. There just isn't a free moment in the day it seems. I thought about a career as a senior in college, but Alan and I were married soon after graduation. I became pregnant right after we moved into our first apartment. One year later, Alan changed jobs and we moved again. Needless to say, I've been busy.

Joan: David and I realized a few years ago that our only solution was being organized every minute and investing in good help. We made a big mistake when our daughter Amy was born. We hired a cleaning lady and simply expected too much. She could not manage the many tasks that are part of making our type of household run. Now we have a live-in housekeeper – a must, because of our night-call schedules. It took time to find an agency and go through interviews but, boy, has it been worth the effort! She is very expensive, but she's extremely good with our child. We're really buying peace of mind.

Elizabeth: Well, you're the exception. I only have day help and I rely on babysitters when I have to work late. This is not ideal, I know. With so many different people looking after my son, I don't always have a secure feeling that the child is getting the best care. At least being cared for at home his surroundings stay constant. I tried a day care center, it was awful. What a wrenching experience each time Joe was dropped off. I just didn't have enough time to deal with this. I know out-of-home child care can work. I didn't give it a fair chance. Having someone come to our home seems best for now and certainly will be easier with a new baby.

Jennifer: I guess I'm lucky. My mother lives across the street. She loves a chance to care for our son. He is her first grandchild. When I started my job, I wasn't sure I was in favor of this. But now that I am working I realize how lucky we are. I never have to worry because I know it's a member of my family caring for my child. The only problem is that sometimes Billy gets confused as to who his real mother is. You know, it really does distress him. When I come home, I love to play with him. Sometimes he refuses to do things and says "Grammie doesn't make me do that." This really hurts. Occasionally, my mother and I disagree on how to discipline my son. He's only two and a half and already he knows he can stay up later when Grammie takes care of him.

Deborah: My situation is very different. I feel that the early years are the most important to a child. I don't think I could possibly leave my 2-year-old to someone else to raise while I was at work. Sometimes I envy women with family plus a stimulating career, but I wonder how they can truly have both – or if they're all really that fulfilled. I thoroughly enjoy my child and look forward to the next one. I don't think a career would be out of the question when the kids are off to school. Joan, how do you manage?

Joan: I make lists and more lists. I keep a running grocery list in the kitchen that we all add to and combine it with what supplies will be needed for the coming week. The final shopping list is in the same order as the items on our supermarket's shelves, aisle by aisle. It sure saves time and lessens temptation. We drop off the laundry and cleaning. It's fun, we chat and give any special instructions. I have the longest cord in existence on my kitchen phone. This way I can cook or clean up while tending to "those calls" that need to be made. It all comes together on Saturdays. Our child goes with us on the errands. It's hectic because if these chores don't get done on Saturdays they don't get done all week, but we make it a family day.

Elizabeth: We also use Saturday but we never finish our errands until late afternoon. Unless my husband is away on business, we always share these chores. Actually, I find Saturday quite frantic. But I try to devote Sunday to my child. Weekends are not a time of rest for us. Sometimes I begin work on Monday feeling exhausted.

Jennifer: My husband and I manage to do the shopping on a weekday evening, so we have the whole weekend to spend as a family. Sunday night supper is usually at one of our parents' homes.

Deborah: The weekend's a special time for us. We always try to work in a game of tennis. My husband's usually tired from the week's grind of traveling, but he really enjoys being with the family. If Alan has to do company entertaining, he can almost always do it during the week. We keep the weekends to ourselves. We both enjoy the outdoors and bring our daughter with us. This is almost always a good idea except this fall she caught a cold. Joan, what do you do if *your* child gets sick?

Joan: Illness really tests our system. Our housekeeper is very cool and astute. That takes some pressure off. There is much phoning as my husband and I decide who can get away from work. We try to do it 50 – 50, but it doesn't always work that way. I guess I'm fortunate he's a pediatrician and can handle illness. Not being on the scene – it's the hardest time for me. I have lots of guilt about not being home when illness or an accident happens. It's ironic, my job is caring for sick people and I can't always get away for my own child. I don't feel good about the way this is affecting our child. Sometimes I really wonder if we should have two full-time careers and young children.

Elizabeth: It does me in too. Our sitter always overreacts when my son gets sick. I am never quite certain of the severity of the problem. Consequently, I always feel I have to come home to make sure for myself. But, it's not considered acceptable for lawyers to run home to tend to household matters. Talk about guilt! This is an enormous source of anxiety for me.

Deborah: Gee, I'm not sure how I would cope if I weren't home when my child is ill.

Jennifer: I'm totally confident when my mother's there. She was a nurse before she retired, and she probably even does a better job than I would.

Joan: No matter how good the care, you still feel helpless if you're not on the scene.

Deborah: Elizabeth, how can you fit in all the prenatal visits?

Elizabeth: The firm lets you off for medical care. But I found a doctor who has evening office hours. I don't like being absent from work at this stage in my career. I must say, if I am kept waiting in the office I get furious – because I feel *my* time is so valuable.

Joan: Working in the hospital has its benefits. My doctor's office is there. His office pages me when it's time for my visit so I don't have to waste time in the waiting room. Bet you all think I don't need much time with my OB for questions. Honestly, I think I need this time more than many. Maybe I know too much and suspect that everything is happening to me and my baby. I'm less apprehensive with this pregnancy, but my imagination still runs wild on occasions. If you think having time for doctor's visits is tough, how about finding time to be alone with your husband!

Jennifer: My husband and I have private time together. Probably even more than all of you. Actually, this was more true before our first child. Now I feel he is concerned about my spending less time with him. He thinks I've become too involved with our child and the expected baby. I guess it will even get worse when the new baby comes home. It's kind of a competition for my attention. This has become a major source of tension in what is otherwise a very solid relationship, but I'm aware of it and we talk about it. That's what's most important, I feel, not to let little insecurities balloon into major divisions.

Deborah: We have a great deal of time together; but a lot of it involves entertaining business clients. Alan often talks of his career when I want to talk about us and the children. I miss private time with him alone.

Joan: As doctors, we realized early on how consuming a medical career could be. We plan carefully how we can manage time together. We get up very early to spend some private time together. When we are both home in the evening we put medicine aside, unless of course, the phone rings. We make the minutes with our child count, it's the quality of the time not the quantity that counts with us. After our child is tucked in bed, we talk, read, relax together. We try not to go off on separate projects. We know how important it is for us to share these moments.

Elizabeth: We try to do the same. But my husband travels so much I sometimes feel resentful. Fortunately, our spats are minor. My husband knows how tired I get right now with my pregnancy, job and family. I must say this pregnancy has been exhausting. I wish my firm recognized my need for a flexible work schedule at this time. I'm not asking for less work, just creative time management for talent who happens to be a young mother. Actually I'm ready to have this baby now!

Joan: With my luck, I'll probably be on duty when I go into labor. If so, it's easy to go just 3 floors down in the hospital. Having a live-in housekeeper will make my being in the hospital easier to manage. She knows the routines and, most important, our daughter knows and loves her. My husband will be with me in labor. He was a tremendous help last time. We've both done deliveries as medical students, so we know what to expect.

Elizabeth: My mother is coming to stay in our house when I go in the hospital. My husband has tried to plan his time so he will be home when the baby is due. Our lives absolutely have to connect for this event. I'll be very upset if the baby comes early and he's halfway across the country. I really need his support in labor. He is a tremendous help. He keeps me calm and encourages me. And our son is going to want his Daddy a lot when I'm away.

Jennifer: Mom will probably beat me to the hospital when I'm in labor. She is coming to see this delivery. We have arranged for a neighbor to take care of Billy.

Deborah: I guess I'm the only one with a definite schedule. I had a Cesarean last time after a long labor because my baby was too big for my pelvis. An ultrasound scan says this baby is even bigger so my doctor plans a repeat Cesarean a week before my due date. We are having my sister come to stay with our child. I'll probably be in the hospital six days and won't be up to much housework when I get home. My sister can stay for a week after I get home but my husband is going to pay for daily cleaning help for five or six weeks.

Joan: Do you plan to breast-feed?

Deborah: That's my plan. I know I'll be tired after the Cesarean, but, if I'm patient it will all work out. I breast-fed last time. It was one of the greatest experiences I have ever had – seeing my baby thrive and grow by feeding from my own body.

Jennifer: Oh, I agree. I had trouble with it, though, the last time. The nursery nurse gave me a lot of instructions and support. But, I still had trouble. I think I was just too anxious with the first baby. I'm determined to have it work this time. This may be our last baby, and I want to enjoy every minute of the experience.

Joan: Lots of career women are breast-feeding. Did you know you can pump your breasts and freeze the milk for feedings by someone else?

Elizabeth: Wrong! In my office it just can't happen. I'm not going to let anyone lay a guilt trip on me about this. Not at work, or in the hospital. I know what I can do and what I can't. It just simply wouldn't work. I can't leave conferences with clients to pump my breasts. Even if I could, there's no private place. It would only create additional frustration. There will be more of me left for the baby if I eliminate this hassle. I'm much better off using formula. Besides I really enjoy bottle feeding my baby.

Joan: I work with medical people so they are really in favor of breast feeding. There should be no problem. I am planning to return to work after 4 weeks. I will probably pump my breasts and have the housekeeper feed the baby during the day. She loves new babies. I'll breast-feed during the night because I really enjoy this relationship with my baby.

Jennifer: I breast-fed my baby for 3 days and never felt successful. This time I've been reading a lot about it and I feel more relaxed and confident. I'll try again, but if it doesn't go well, I'll switch to formula. After two good tries, I think I can make this change without feeling like I failed somehow.

Joan: My time, after the first week, seems almost like a vacation to me. It's cherished time with my family. Every minute will be special as I know I'm unlikely to have so much continuous and concentrated time with my children in the near future. Don't misunderstand, these weeks may not be all roses. Amy may not think a brother or sister is so swell, even though we have talked about the baby a lot. Her toilet training could take a tumble. Such things need time to be worked out. I'm hoping my month at home will give us all a good start. Elizabeth, does your firm give you maternity leave?

Elizabeth: I've checked with my law firm. I am entitled to 6 weeks off. But, I want to return in 3 weeks because there is a major corporate merger coming up that I have been working on for over a year. I want a family and I want to be a successful lawyer. I have been referred to as "the superwoman" by my friends. But I know that's just a myth. I found out the superwoman just doesn't exist when I had my first child. I knew there would be conflicts but I didn't realize how great they would be. Now just hearing the term "superwoman" makes me angry. I don't think people realize the enormous stress and the guilt involved in being a career woman, wife and mother. I really wanted a second child. Realistically, I may not be able to handle the responsibility of two small children and a very demanding career. Some things may have to change. Who knows – I may have to find a firm that offers a flexible work schedule.

Joan: I know that even with careful planning, organization and good help, there will still be stress. Just the fact that we have two children means twice the chance of having an illness. I only wish that our social system allowed more time off for new mothers. Just three months to six months would make a a world of difference.

Elizabeth: Well you know, our country is the only developed nation that sets such a low priority on having a newborn baby. Most other countries give substantial maternity leave with pay. Some even guarantee returning to work at an equivalent level of employment. That would be a joke in our law firm.

Jennifer: But it could work for many jobs. It would give the mother and the baby such a good start.

Joan: With the trend toward smaller families, you would think such a program should be possible in the United States. I mean, it should be economically feasible as long as the fathers didn't want three to six months also.

Jennifer: Well the father should have time with his newborn baby.

Joan: I couldn't agree more. Its just a question of what is affordable.

Deborah: Well, I think it is a marvelous idea. I knew career women had a lot of stresses when they started a family, but until now I didn't realize how great the pressures were. A substantial maternity leave could really change the whole picture – take the pressure off and improve the quality of life.

Elizabeth: Maybe there could be a program with substantial maternity leave for the mother and limited leave for the father. I doubt if it could be affordable for extended leave for both.

Joan: That would probably be excessive anyway. Throughout history one parent has raised the children. But the pressures today make it less possible for the other parent to spend a lot of time with the children. I only hope that we take time to realize how precious these moments with new babies are. The time passes so quickly. It's important to savor every minute.

Deborah: We really have different experiences and lifestyles. I am really happy with my role as a wife and mother. I now understand your roles better. I wouldn't trade places for anything, but I have developed a new respect for the complexity of your lives and all the different problems you have to deal with.

Joan: There is a fine line between an exciting, vigorous, full life and a horrible rat race. It seems to me that love, support and organization are the keys to keeping it sane. It would be very easy to allow the momentum of a vigorous life carry you over to a rat race or treadmill existence. I'll take advantage of my time at home with the new baby to reflect on our lives – get some perspective. Then when I return to the hospital I'll probably change some things so we can enjoy rather than survive.

Elizabeth: I think Joan has just said it all. You have to stop sometimes and analyze your way of life. There are things you can control and things you simply can't. Occasionally, I get cornered by the latter. You just have to concentrate on organizing the things you can control. Otherwise life is a treadmill. I'm sure my child knows when things are going well or poorly for me at the office. I mean, just the way I deal with him.

Jennifer: It's very interesting. We all have problems but they are different because our roles are different. There is no question, you can find yourself in a time crunch. I guess, how frequently that happens depends upon how you plan and manage the things you can control. I'm fortunate because Jim really pitches in and helps. Not just the doing but also the planning. I'm really glad we've had this opportunity to talk. I've learned a lot and look forward to this baby and continuing my career.

Chapter 16 Preventing accidents

Now that protection against and treatment of disease have so dramatically improved, accidents, both in the home and outside it, have become the most common cause of death in childhood. While all parents dread the possibility of their child having an accident, it is important to steer a middle course between adequate supervision and overprotectiveness. If you hover around anxiously every time your child attempts anything remotely adventurous, you run the risk of interfering with the natural development of his own sense of self-preservation. Unless you supervise him creatively, he may become too timid to enjoy himself with other children or defiant to the point of foolhardiness.

In the first year of life, a baby may put himself at risk by suddenly acquiring a new skill for which his parents are not prepared. Their easily contained infant suddenly starts crawling and poking around in potentially dangerous nooks and crannies previously safely out of reach. Look around your home with a view to his or her future safety: this alphabetical guide will help you to identify the danger areas. First aid instructions are given on pp. 208–211.

ANIMALS

A small baby is pretty defenseless against a dog or a cat. Even if you feel your pet is trustworthy, it is as well to avoid a situation where a pet and a baby are left alone together. Animals may be jealous of small babies.

It is wise to cover a baby carriage with a cat net if it is in the yard. This is not only a precaution against cats, but also against insects, if the mesh is fine enough.

The most docile pet can snap or scratch if provoked, so try to explain to a child that pets need gentle treatment.

ASPHYXIA

A child may die from suffocation when not enough oxygen can get into his lungs. A pillow is dangerous and unnecessary for a baby. It is possible for him to turn face down into it and therefore not get enough oxygen. This occurs rarely, but is sufficient reason for not using a pillow in a crib or carriage.

Never allow a child to play with a plastic bag. If he gets it over his head, it will stick close to the face so that he cannot breathe. Throw away plastic bags when you have finished with them, or keep them in a very safe place, preferably after making holes in them or tying a knot at the open end.

An old refrigerator can be very dangerous. Never keep one in the home or yard or leave one out to be collected, unless the door has been taken off. Never dump one in a vacant lot. A number of children have died after climbing inside old refrigerators to hide; they find themselves shut in and die from lack of air.

BURNS AND SCALDS

Unhappily, these cause many deaths in childhood and many admissions to the hospital. Even quite a small burn may mean several weeks in the hospital, with much misery and pain. Do your best to make your home as safe as you can.

Burns. A child's clothing can easily catch fire; buy only clothes that are made of fireproof material. If there isn't a special label, always ask if a material is safe when you buy something. Other items in a child's bedroom, such as the curtains, should also be made of safe material.

Any open fire should be carefully guarded from young children. It is important to have a screen which children cannot put their hands through and which is a reasonable distance from the fire. The best screens are secured to the wall and make sure that a child cannot crawl or climb into a fire. Fire tools are very dangerous and should be kept out of reach.

Electric heaters should be very carefully guarded indeed. Horrible burns can occur across the palm of the hand if a child puts a hand through a screen and grasps the electrical element. The electric current causes the hand to clench and he is unable to release it.

You will need to help your child to understand how dangerous fire is. Talk to him sternly if he plays with matches; it is a good idea to keep matches well out of his reach altogether.

Some space heaters are very unsafe if they are knocked over. If they must be used they should be placed in an area completely out of reach of any children. Better still, avoid the use of these heaters.

An iron is very dangerous if left unattended. A child may not realize that it is hot and can easily get burned badly by touching the bottom when the iron is switched on.

Fireworks. These are dangerous and should be kept well away from children – in fact, their sale is generally prohibited. Never allow a young child to play with fireworks. It is much safer to take them to a public display. The children can then watch and enjoy the excitement of fireworks without the risk of a burn or injury because of an explosion.

Scalds. These are even more common than burns and can easily occur, for example when a cup of coffee is spilled over a child. Be very careful when you are cooking. The handles of all pots should be turned inward. If they stick out over the front, a child can easily pull the handles and pour boiling water or fat over himself. There are pan guards on the market which prevent cooking pans from falling or being pulled off the top of the stove.

A tea or coffee pot is very unsafe if it is on a tablecloth. A common accident occurs when a child pulls the tablecloth and hot liquid from the pot or a cup tips over him or her. It is wiser not to use a tablecloth at all when there is a small child around. Make certain the pot and cups are near the center of the table, and that the table itself is steady.

When you fill the bathtub, always add cold water at the same time as hot. A child might climb into a bath of hot water before you add cold water.

CAR SAFETY

If you use a baby bed in the car, make sure that it is carefully strapped to the back seat. It must not fly off if you have to brake suddenly or bump into another car. A good restraint system should also prevent a child from falling out of the bed during impact or if the car turns upside down.

Never allow a small child to sit on your lap in the car; he may fly out of your hands and through the windshield if the car stops suddenly. Make it a firm rule that all children always travel in the back seat.

There are now very good children's car seats with a full harness. They can be anchored securely to the body of the car and fit on the back seat. Use a well-known, approved brand. Make certain that the car doors have a special "child-proof" lock system; they should shut firmly, so they cannot fly open while you are traveling.

CHOKING

You should never leave a baby with a propped up bottle, because this could be dangerous. Milk may get into the lungs and make him choke or cause an infection. Once your child starts solid food, do not leave him alone while he is eating. Small, hard pieces of food are particularly dangerous; so are nuts, especially peanuts. They are easily inhaled and can cause quite severe damage to the lungs. Babies can choke on things other than food. Try not to let a child play with objects small enough to go right into his mouth.

DROWNING

Small children can drown in a shallow pond. If you have an ornamental pond in your yard or nearby, make certain that it is fenced off or covered with wire mesh, or only allow them there with a responsible person. Don't leave a child alone in the bathtub.

Very small children or babies enjoy being taken to a swimming pool; you will need to be with them. If you enjoy swimming you may like to teach your child to swim at a very early age. Do not force your child to go in the pool if he or she is frightened. Use inflatable arm bands rather than a rubber ring for buoyancy. Always use life jackets on boat trips.

ELECTRICITY

Make certain that you have safe electric wiring throughout the house, so that your child cannot put his fingers into the sockets or plugs or pull loose wires and electrocute himself. If possible, plugs should be high up on the wall and out of a small child's reach; if not, special "dummy plugs" should be used to cover the sockets when not in use. Make certain that the electrical circuits are installed competently, that no wires are exposed, and that all cords are in a good condition.

An extension cord for a curling iron or a coffee pot is a particular danger. If it is not connected to the appliance, but left dangling with the electric current still on, a child may put it in his mouth and get severe electric burns on the tongue and lips.

FOREIGN BODIES

All babies and toddlers delight in inserting small objects in the various orifices of their bodies – ears, nose, mouth, vagina – none is exempt. For this reason it is best to keep small objects such as beads, stones and nuts out of their reach. Needles, pins, hairpins, buttons, etc., are particularly hazardous, and so are toys with small, detachable pieces such as glass eyes.

POISONING

Many children have to be admitted to the hospital because they have swallowed some drugs or a chemical. Usually, they are given some medicine to make them vomit or have their stomachs washed out. Some babies die as a result of poisoning. It is a serious problem and you should do all you can to keep chemicals out of the reach of children. This is becoming increasingly difficult, because of the number of household items that now contain chemicals. It is best to keep all potentially dangerous substances like cleaning preparations on a top shelf and locked up.

Drugs. Many drugs today look like candy; this is particularly true of iron pills. Drug manufacturers have done their best to make medicines and drugs palatable, but they are therefore more attractive to children. Drugs should always be kept out of the reach of children. You should have a medicine cabinet with a lock, placed high up on a wall. Try to remember that all medicines should be locked away in this cabinet and keep the key hidden.

Children are very inquisitive and may devise all sorts of schemes, like putting one chair on top of another, to get to out of reach cabinets. Consequently you should keep all pills in childproof bottles. Pills which are packed individually, in "blister packs", may be safer; each pill is in a bubble of plastic, which has to be broken before a pill is taken. It is then much more difficult for a child to take a large number of pills, because each one has to be taken out separately, rather than in handfuls from a bottle.

There are several common medicines which are extremely dangerous to children, and these include aspirin and iron. If you think your child has taken a large dose of drugs, do not hesitate to call the hospital or family doctor at once.

Other poisons. There are many chemicals in your house. Quite a dangerous one is bleach, which is often kept in an unlocked cabinet. This should be locked away like a medicine.

Never put any chemical into another bottle where it may be confused with a harmless liquid. Keep it in the original container or in a special bottle made for poisons. Some children have died because they took a drink from what they thought was a soda bottle, not realizing it was used for a chemical such as insect repellant or weed killer.

Be sure there are no bushes or trees in your yard (or houseplants) that bear poisonous berries or leaves. Be sure your child has no toys or furniture painted in toxic lead-based paint which he or she might suck. Avoid having chemicals in the house.

PREVENTING FALLS AND HEAD INJURIES

Heavy furniture like tables and cupboards should be secure, so that it cannot topple onto your child. Anything used by the child must be very stable; a high chair is a good example of something that could fall over. Most people now use a lower, more stable type of chair instead of the traditional high chair.

Remove loose or curled-up carpets, on which a child might slip or trip. Remember, newly waxed floors are also a potential hazard for toddlers.

Children are very adept at climbing up to windows. If there is any danger of a child falling out, you should fix safety locks or put up bars. It is not a good idea to fix bars on all your upstairs windows, however, because it might then be impossible to escape in a fire.

A young child can easily fall down a flight of stairs. Some people suggest putting a gate at the top of the stairs. It may still be possible for an enterprising and determined child to climb over the gate, and then fall down the stairs, in which case the fall would be even worse. A badly secured gate might also cause a fall. It is probably sensible to have a gate at the bottom of the stairs to prevent the child from crawling up them. Be sure the gate is constructed so that a small head cannot become trapped in it.

If you have a high crib put up the side of the crib before leaving it. A baby can easily roll off onto the floor. Be especially careful if you use a changing table for your baby; be sure never to leave the baby by himself on the table.

Whenever you take the baby out in a carriage or stroller, make sure he is strapped in firmly, especially if you happen to leave the carriage unattended. Once a baby can pull himself up it is only too easy for him to fall out of a carriage, which could lead to a nasty head injury. Do not overload a carriage or stroller with heavy shopping or another child, especially at the handle end. Make sure that the brake of a stroller is not within reach of a toddler.

Do not let a child run around with a potentially dangerous toy, such as a plastic whistle or a pencil in his mouth. If he were to fall, he might perforate his palate.

Do not allow a child to play near a glass door or partition. Falling heavily against the glass can cause serious injury, either by being cut or by impact.

RAILROADS

Railroad tracks are dangerous places for children. Unless there is adequate fencing, they can easily wander onto the track. A train may knock them down or they can be electrocuted on a third rail. If your house is next to a railroad, make certain that the fencing is secure and the children cannot get near the tracks.

ROAD SAFETY

Road accidents are only a minor cause of death under one year, although they cause many deaths and injuries to children over that age.

Many children get run over because they are allowed to play in an open street. Make sure that you have secure locks, out of a child's reach, on all doors leading outside so that your child does not wander out into the street. A young child should be accompanied when he goes out, particularly if he has to cross a street or road.

Even at a very early age, you should help your child to understand the rules that everyone must follow when crossing the street. Children should be taught to cross at a crosswalk or where there is a person on duty to control the traffic.

If you are driving, be very careful to watch out for children. They often run into the road from between parked cars; unless you are driving slowly, you will not have time to stop.

Be especially careful when you back a car out of a garage; you must make certain that there are no children playing in the driveway or road. Quite a number of children die each year because a car just backs over them.

SUNBURN

Small children are quite susceptible to sunburn. Take it easy in the first few days of a summer vacation in the sun. Half an hour at a time is quite enough. It is best to start with 10 to 18 minutes on the first day and increase slowly. Use suntan lotion to reduce risk of burning; keep a large hat and clothes handy, so you can dress the child as soon as he has had his quota of sun for the day. Keep small babies completely out of the direct sun. Reflected rays also burn. Remember that the redness caused by the sun often doesn't appear until long after the damge is done. Bad sunburn can result in vomiting and fever. If this happens, consult your doctor. Keep sunburned areas completely covered.

First aid

Minor accidents cannot be avoided entirely – especially falls and abrasions. But you must do your best to guard against major accidents by sensible safety precautions, especially in the house where most of them happen (*see previous pages*). This is an alphabetical checklist of basic first aid. Although children are particularly accident-prone, most of the advice is just as applicable to adults who have had an accident. With children, though, it is especially important to keep calm and be as reassuring as you can, no matter how alarmed you may be.

The first aid kit. Keep a first aid kit in a place where you can get at it easily, but your children can't. A high shelf in the kitchen is a good place if it is out of reach of mountaineering toddlers. Any clean tin box with a tightly fitting lid will do, but it should be clearly marked. The equipment should include:

1. Bandaids – assorted sizes
2. Gauze squares – large and small, for cleaning and dressing wounds
3. Gauze rolls for bandaging difficult areas
4. Non-stick sterile pads
5. Scissors for cutting tape and bandages
6. Adhesive tape
7. Antiseptic solution for cleaning wounds
8. Tweezers for removing splinters
9. Triangular bandage with two safety pins for a head dressing or a sling
10. Calamine lotion for soothing insect stings

Remember to replace immediately anything that is used. Many people add an antiseptic cream to their first aid kit, though this is not really necessary and can retard healing (*see* p. 210, **cuts and abrasions**).

ARTIFICIAL RESPIRATION

If a child has stopped breathing, you must give artificial respiration (mouth to mouth breathing) immediately and be prepared to continue as long as you can. You won't have time to look up instructions; learning the basic actions from a book is not as good as going to first aid classes, but could save a life.

Check breathing and pulse. Don't spend more than a few seconds on this. But make sure the child is not breathing – don't give artificial respiration if the child is still breathing, even faintly. If the heart has stopped beating **heart massage** is needed as well (*see* p. 209).

Start as soon as possible. Obviously, move him from a situation of danger, such as contact with a live electric appliance (*see* below, **electric shock**) or a gas-filled room. Otherwise, start right away. With a drowning child, don't waste time trying to get water out of his lungs. If you are getting out of the water, tip him head-down to drain out water, then give a few quick lung inflations when you reach waist-deep water.

Don't leave the child to get help. Until the child is breathing, don't leave him by himself. If necessary, carry the child with you to a telephone or a place where you can get help, stopping every few seconds to continue artificial respiration. Once breathing has started again, don't leave him for more than a minute in case it stops again.

When you have help, call for an emergency medical unit as soon as possible.

The best position. Lay the child on his back if possible. Clear out his mouth quickly with your finger. Tilt his head right back and pull his chin forward – this stops the tongue falling into the throat which would block the windpipe.

How to blow. First pinch the child's nostrils, so that when you breathe into his mouth the air won't escape through the nose. (With a baby you can put your mouth over both mouth and nose.) Take a deep breath, put your mouth over his open mouth, making sure the seal is airtight, and breathe out gently, looking sideways to see if the chest expands. Then take your mouth away. Wait till the chest has contracted and he has finished breathing out then blow again. Give the first five or six breaths quickly, then settle down to a rhythm – about one blow every six seconds.

If the abdomen rises, air is going into the stomach instead of the lungs. Check the position of his head – tilt it back further and pull the jaw further forward. If you can press his stomach with your hand this will help prevent air going there.

Be careful not to blow too hard for a small baby. Fill your cheeks with air and blow in the contents of your mouth. Watch the chest to make certain it moves.

How long to go on. Go on until medical help or the ambulance arrives. Do not give up if the child does not start breathing soon of his own accord. If you are with somebody else, take turns at giving artificial respiration.

When he does start to breathe for himself, keep him warm and still until medical help arrives, and stay by him in case his breathing stops again.

Heart massage. If the child turns blue and no heartbeat can be heard in the chest, external heart massage must be given as well as artificial respiration. It is very difficult for one person to do both; if you have to try, do them alternately – eight depressions of the chest and then two breaths of mouth to mouth breathing.

Lay the child flat on his back on the ground or floor. Place the heel of one hand on the lower part of his breastbone and place the other hand on top. One hand may be enough for a small child. Press down firmly, depressing the breastbone about 1 in (2.5 cm), then release it. Do this about once every three seconds. For babies, use only two fingers of one hand, and press the breastbone down about ½ in (1.5 cm), using about 30 or 40 presses a minute.

BITES

Animal bites should be carefully washed, dried and covered with a sterile dressing. The main danger is from tetanus. Unless you are quite certain the child's tetanus injections are up to date, take him or her to the doctor or to the Emergency Room of the nearest hospital immediately. (*See* chapter 17, **tetanus**.) If large or ragged, the wound will need stitching.

In the United States there is slight risk of rabies from an animal bite.

Scratches from cats do not usually need a dressing, but should be well washed and dried. If the scratch becomes yellow and drains, or will not heal, take the child to the doctor. There is danger from tetanus if the tetanus injections are not up to date.

BLEEDING

If blood is spurting rhythmically from a wound an artery has been cut and it is essential to stop the bleeding as soon as possible. This is done by pressure. Press hard with your fingers either on the wound, or just beside it, on the side between the wound and the heart. Take the child to the hospital immediately or call an ambulance. Keep up the pressure with your finger if the blood starts to flow again as soon as you remove them. If it slows, you can apply a dry dressing and a firmly tied bandage over the site. If the blood seeps through the bandage, don't take it off – apply another, tighter one, over the top and apply direct pressure.

The wounded child should not move around, and it helps if the injured part can be raised – held up in the air or rested on a cushion. Anyone losing a lot of blood is likely to suffer from **shock** (*see* p. 211).

A small cut can lose a lot of blood, but the blood often looks more than it really is. Apply a dressing – a bandage, a recently laundered handkerchief or a scarf or stocking will do – and if the blood does not stop press on the wound with your fingers. If this does not stop the bleeding, the wound may need stitching and the child should be taken to the doctor or Emergency Room.

BROKEN BONES

Sometimes it is obvious that a bone is broken. The limb bends in the wrong place, or there is a compound fracture with the bone penetrating through an open wound. The child must go straight to the hospital, but it is important first to prevent movement of the injured part, as this could do further damage to nerves and blood vessels. Simple ways to do this are bandaging a broken leg to the other leg, and tying a broken arm loosely to the body or putting it in a sling. A scarf or belt looped over the back of the neck makes an impromptu sling. In other words, use the body itself as a splint or support.

Do not give food or drink to the child – he may have to have an anesthetic.

Greenstick fracture. Children's bones often do not break right across, but bend, breaking on one side only like a young twig. This and some other types of broken bone may not be immediately obvious. The signs to look for are continuing pain and refusal to use the limb. Take the child to the Emergency Room of a hospital for an X ray, even if it is some days since the injury.

A head injury may fracture the skull. *See* **head injuries** below for signs indicating that you should take your child to the doctor.

ARTIFICIAL RESPIRATION

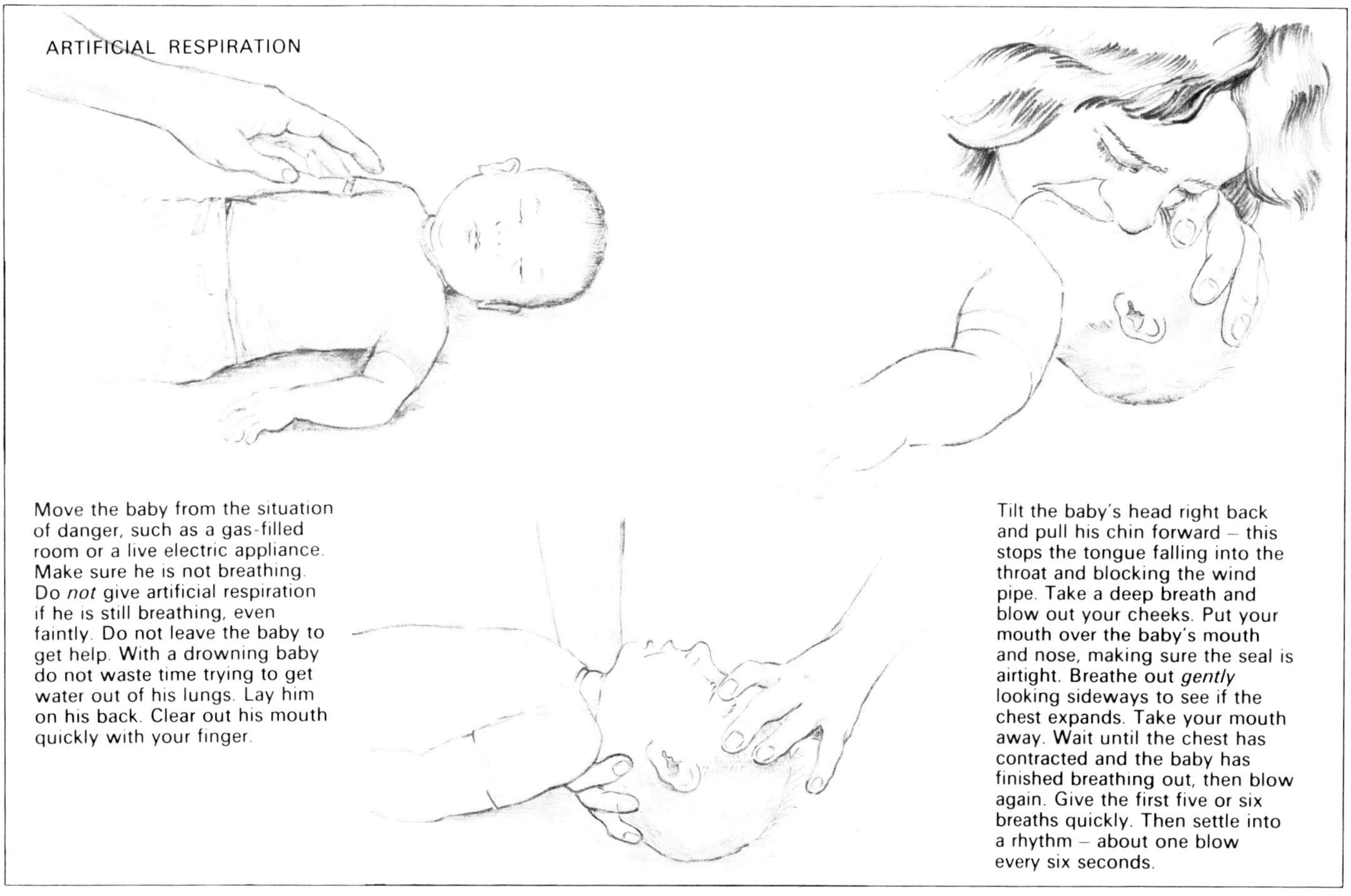

Move the baby from the situation of danger, such as a gas-filled room or a live electric appliance. Make sure he is not breathing. Do *not* give artificial respiration if he is still breathing, even faintly. Do not leave the baby to get help. With a drowning baby do not waste time trying to get water out of his lungs. Lay him on his back. Clear out his mouth quickly with your finger.

Tilt the baby's head right back and pull his chin forward – this stops the tongue falling into the throat and blocking the wind pipe. Take a deep breath and blow out your cheeks. Put your mouth over the baby's mouth and nose, making sure the seal is airtight. Breathe out *gently* looking sideways to see if the chest expands. Take your mouth away. Wait until the chest has contracted and the baby has finished breathing out, then blow again. Give the first five or six breaths quickly. Then settle into a rhythm – about one blow every six seconds.

BURNS AND SCALDS

If a child's clothes catch on fire, grab hold of him quickly and lay him on the ground. Cover him with any heavy cloth – a coat or rug – as quickly as possible, to put the flames out. If nothing is handy, roll on him yourself to extinguish the flames. If he runs around, his clothes will burn faster and his burns will be more severe.

Except for small burns – that is, under 1 in (2.5 cm) across – all burns and scalds should be seen by a doctor. Burns that do not look very serious can still cause **shock** (*see* p. 211).

People with severe burns should be taken to the Emergency Room of the nearest hospital as soon as possible. Do not remove clothing over a bad burn, unless it is smoldering – the heat will have sterilized it and it forms a temporary protection from germs in the air. Large uncovered burns should be covered loosely with a clean, dry, non-fluffy dressing as a first aid measure. A newly laundered pillowcase makes a good cover for burned arms and legs, a clean sheet for the body.

Do not give a badly burned child anything to eat or drink, unless the wait for medical attention is going to be longer than half an hour, when a few sips of water can be given.

With less serious burns, the burned part should be held under cold running water for five or ten minutes or until the pain ceases. If blisters form, a clean dry dressing should be applied. Do not burst the blisters. A recently washed and ironed handkerchief makes a simple sterile dressing. If no blisters form, no dressing is necessary. Do not apply jellies, ointments or creams.

Scalds. These can be serious, especially when the hot liquid soaks into the child's clothing and is held against the skin. If hot liquid is splashed on a child, take off his clothes as quickly as possible and then immerse the area in cold water. Be sure to take him to the doctor immediately unless the scald is very mild.

CHOKING

If your baby chokes on a piece of food or because his breathing becomes obstructed by any object in his throat or windpipe, immediately hold him upside down by the legs and pat him vigorously on the back. An older child can be bent over your knee with his head hanging down, or simply bent forward. This should dislodge the object and allow him to spit it out.

Do not attempt to hook out the obstruction with your finger, unless it is something like a large piece of meat or apple that can be easily grasped. You may push it further down and make things worse.

If the obstruction is not dislodged by this method and the baby is still choking, this is a medical emergency and you should call an ambulance or take him to the Emergency Room of the nearest hospital immediately. Don't stop trying to dislodge the obstruction. If he stops breathing, it is worth trying **artificial respiration** (*see* p. 208).

CONCUSSION *see* Head injuries

CONVULSIONS

Seizures or convulsions in children have two common causes. One is a high temperature, which can cause "febrile convulsions" in young children; the other is epilepsy – a tendency to fits – which can affect people of any age. In most convulsions a child loses consciousness, clenches his teeth and twitches and shakes all over. If standing he will fall to the ground. His eyes roll up and he may froth at the mouth. After a few minutes the fit ends and he falls asleep.

Never leave a child alone while he is having a convulsion. Stay with him and make sure he does not hurt himself against furniture or the fire. Don't try to restrain his limbs, and don't force anything between his teeth to stop him biting his tongue. Make sure he can breathe; turn him on his side and keep his chin forward to keep the airways clear.

When the fit is over, call the doctor. If the child has a high temperature, you can start to cool him by sponging with warm water once the convulsion is over, or use it to prevent a convulsion if his temperature rises to 103 °F (40 °C).

If the convulsion is immediately followed by another, or goes on for ten minutes or longer, this is an emergency and you should call a doctor or take him to a hospital as quickly as possible.

CUTS AND ABRASIONS

If a wound has bled and a scab has already started to form – as with many a scraped knee – leave the wound alone, except for cleaning any dirt or dried blood away from the surrounding skin. Dampening the scab with water or ointment encourages infection. Any dirt in the wound will usually come off with the scab.

If the wound is recent and still bleeding, and looks very dirty, wash it – tissues and hot water are clean and efficient, and an antiseptic can be added to the water. The best way to clean the skin around a wound is from the wound outward. Pat it dry and put on a sterile dressing. A large, deep or gaping wound should be covered with a dressing and taken to the hospital for cleaning and possibly stitching. (So should dirty cuts and scrapes on the face, which might leave scars.)

If a cut happened out of doors and the wound is dirty or deep and difficult to clean, there is a danger of tetanus infection, especially if it has animal droppings in it. If the child's tetanus immunization is not up to date, take him to the doctor or hospital immediately for an anti-tetanus injection (*see* chapter 17, **tetanus**).

Scalp wounds can bleed a lot, even if they are very small. As it is hard to keep a bandage or Band-aid on the head, even a small scalp wound may need stitching. If in doubt, ask your doctor or take the child to the hospital. If the cut is bleeding heavily, press on it with your fingers or thumb until it can be stitched.

Dressings and ointments. Bandages are only necessary to help stop bleeding, and to keep the wound clean while a scab is forming. Once a scab has formed a Band-aid is not necessary, and prevents the wound from drying. Do not put antiseptic ointments on a wound or scab as a matter of routine. They can be useful for cleaning a wound, but they cannot kill every germ. The ointments will only soften a scab and reduce its protective powers.

Infection. If the skin is reddened around the wound, and it remains painful, it may be infected and you should go to the doctor.

DISLOCATIONS AND SPRAINS

When the bones in a joint are displaced – as in dislocation – there is swelling and bruising, and possibly areas of numbness caused by damaged nerves. The joint may be deformed and painful to move. Prevent the child from moving the injured part and get him to a hospital as quickly as possible. Don't try to "put it back" – this may cause more damage. To keep him still, you can bandage the injured part in the most comfortable position.

As with a fracture, don't give anything to eat or drink – a general anesthetic may be needed.

In a sprain, the ligaments are torn or bruised but the bone ends are not actually displaced. The joint should be bandaged in the most comfortable position, and the child taken to a hospital. An X ray will usually be taken to make certain there is no fracture or dislocation.

DROWNING *see* Artificial respiration

ELECTRIC SHOCK

A mild shock will make the child pull his or her hand away and probably give him no more than a fright. Check the cause of the shock and make sure it does not happen again (*see* p. 207).

A bad electric shock may make the muscles clench so the child cannot pull his hand away, or he may lose consciousness. Don't touch his body or you will get a shock yourself. Quickly turn off at the wall switch, if you can, otherwise use any *dry, non-metal* object to push or pull him away, such as a broom, a rolled-up magazine or a yardstick. Dragging him by the clothes is another possibility, unless they are wet, but it is harder to avoid contact with his body.

If he is not breathing give **artificial respiration** (*see* p. 208). Shocks can cause **burns** (*see* above), which are often more serious than they look because although they can be small they are deep. Go to the doctor if in doubt about the seriousness of the burn.

EYE INJURIES

It is always safest to have an eye injury seen to by a doctor. However, if a harmful liquid gets into the eye, flush it immediately with clean water. Specks should be removed at once, either by drawing the upper lid down and away, allowing tears to wash out the eye, or with a sterile eye bath. If this is ineffective, go to your doctor or to a hospital Emergency Room.

FAINTING

If a child feels faint he should lie down or sit with his head between his knees. This encourages the blood supply to the brain. If he actually faints, he should recover in a few minutes after lying down. Loosen his collar and provide plenty of fresh air.

FALLS

If your child falls and injures a limb so that it is painful to move it, or if he sustains a deep cut that may need to be stitched, take him to your doctor or to the Emergency Room of the nearest hospital. See **cuts**, **broken bones**, and **dislocations and sprains** above for more details, and see **head injuries** below, especially if he has fallen from quite a height. It is more serious if he has hit his head on a hard surface.

FOREIGN BODIES

Don't try to retrieve an object stuck in a small child's ear unless you are quite sure you can remove it easily. It could be dangerous if it is pushed down into the ear. If you are in any doubt at all, take the child to the doctor or the nearest Emergency Room.

The same is true of objects stuck in the nostrils. If the child is old enough, it might be possible to remove the object with a pair of tweezers, but it is better to go to a doctor or Emergency Room. If you ask the child to blow his nose to dislodge the object, he may first breathe in hard, thus lodging the object more firmly.

Small children often swallow foreign bodies. Once swallowed, these objects are rarely a hazard – they simply traverse the intestine and reappear in the stool. If, however, it is medication that your baby has swallowed, or something sharp like a pin, then notify your doctor at once.

FRACTURES *see* Broken bones

HEAD INJURIES

If your child has a knock on the head you should watch his progress carefully. If he appears limp or drowsy immediately after the injury, or bleeds from the nose, ears or mouth, or if you think he has lost consciousness even for a moment, take him straight to the doctor or the Emergency Room of the nearest hospital. Keep him warm with a blanket.

If he has a head wound, you should take him to the Emergency Room to be examined and to have the wound sutured.

Even if he seems to be all right at first, you should still watch him carefully for 24 hours. If he becomes drowsy suddenly (apart from going to sleep in the ordinary way at bedtime), faints or begins to vomit, you should take him at once to your doctor or Emergency Room. If he goes to sleep after the fall, this may be no cause for alarm, especially in a baby, but check to make sure he is sleeping normally and not unconscious (*see* below, **unconsciousness**). Difficulty in breathing and persistent paleness are also indications for going to the doctor.

NOSEBLEEDS

Some children are more prone to nosebleeds than others, though any child can have one as a result of a fall or bump. The classic way to stop it is to have the child lie flat on his back. Do not extend his head backwards. Pinch the nose just above the nostrils by applying firm continuous pressure. The pressure must be applied for 10–15 minutes. The child may swallow some blood which might frighten him. So, remember to reassure him. If the bleeding doesn't stop with this measure call your doctor.

If the nosebleed is associated with a bad bump on the head, take the child to a doctor as soon as possible.

OBJECTS IN NOSE, EARS ETC. *see* Foreign bodies

POISONING

If you think your child has swallowed something poisonous, telephone your doctor, Poison Control Center or the Emergency Room of your nearest hospital at once, and ask their advice. Keep calm – do not give the child anything to drink or eat, and do not attempt to make him vomit.

If you take your child to the doctor or hospital, take with you some of the material you think he has swallowed – pills, berries, bleach or whatever it may be. Try to discover how much he has taken and when he took it, so that you can present an accurate account to the doctor. If the child vomits, take a sample of the vomitus with you also.

If the child is unconscious, lay him on his stomach, with his head turned to one side and tilted back, and the arm and leg of that side drawn up (the recovery position). This helps prevent choking if he should vomit.

If he is not breathing, give **artificial respiration** (*see* p. 208).

SCALDS *see* Burns and scalds

SHOCK

Severe shock is a state of circulatory collapse with low blood pressure, usually caused by a bad accident, or a serious illness. The symptoms are paleness, a cold sweat, quick shallow breathing and a rapid pulse (though it may sometimes be unusually slow). The child may vomit or faint.

Lay the child flat on his back, calm him and cover him with a blanket. Don't use hot water bottles – they divert the blood from the vital organs to the skin, and may make the shock worse. Don't give anything to eat or drink in severe shock, especially if the child has had an accident and is likely to need an anesthetic.

The word shock is also used for emotional shock. Most children are very upset after an accident and will need a great deal of comforting.

SPRAINS *see* Dislocations and sprains

STINGS

If your baby is stung, first see if the stinger has been left in and remove it with fine tweezers. Then, apply a cold sponge to give some pain relief, and calamine lotion will decrease any irritation. If the sting becomes very inflamed or swollen, consult your doctor about it. It is a good idea to see a doctor if a child is stung on or in the mouth, as the sting may affect his breathing.

Some people are very allergic to insect stings and go into a state of **shock** (*see* above). They should go to the hospital at once if stung.

SWALLOWED OBJECTS *see* Foreign Bodies

UNCONSCIOUSNESS

Unconsciousness, from any cause, is dangerous in itself because the child may choke on his tongue, or inhale vomitus and suffocate. The best position for an unconscious person – once you have made sure he or she is breathing – is lying on his front, with the head turned to one side and tilted back, and the leg and arm on the same side bent up to support that side. This is known as the recovery position. Then if he vomits, the vomit will flow out of his mouth without choking him.

Unconsciousness is not the same as being asleep, and the difference is usually obvious. An unconscious child will breathe differently, possibly snoring, and look different from a sleeping one. If you are not sure whether a child is asleep or unconscious – for instance, after a fall – try to wake him. If you cannot, he is unconscious. If you cannot wake him fully or he takes longer than usual to wake, these are also danger signs.

Obviously, if a person is unconscious, from whatever cause, the doctor should be called as soon as possible.

THE RECOVERY POSITION

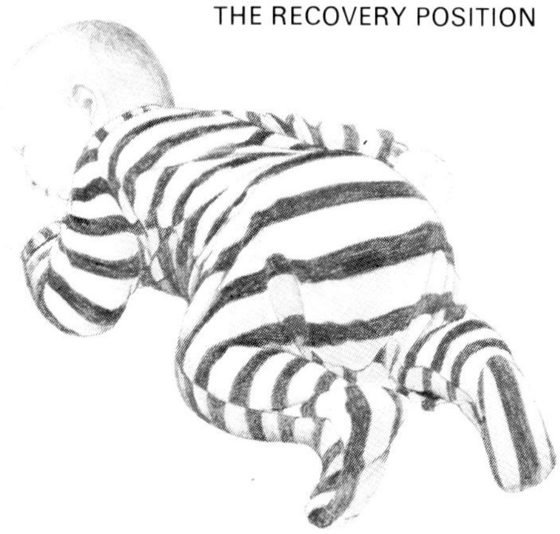

Chapter 17

A guide to your baby's health

It is sometimes difficult for you to know whether to call your doctor, take your baby to his office or request a housecall. This chapter gives an alphabetical checklist of the most common illnesses and problems in the first year or two of life, with advice on treatment (if necessary), and a brief note on whether or not to see a doctor. Often this depends on how severe the symptom is – as, for instance, with vomiting. This is obviously a matter where exact guidelines cannot be given. If you are worried about your baby, or unsure whether to contact the doctor, it's safest to call anyway. Discuss in advance with your doctor if he has a special time set aside to take telephone calls.

Both family practitioners and pediatricians realize that caring for small babies can be bewildering and frightening. They will be very happy to give advice about the social and emotional problems of family life as well as more practical help in child care. All of your own problems have a direct bearing on the happiness and well-being of your baby.

Seeing the doctor. Most sick children can be taken to the doctor's office and most doctors prefer to see their patients there. A child with a fever can be wrapped in a blanket in a car. Children with infectious diseases, such as chicken pox, measles or mumps, generally should not be brought to the office; however, many physicians do have an isolation area for such situations. Some children may be too ill to travel or may suffer from symptoms such as diarrhea that would make traveling very difficult. On these occasions you might ask the doctor for a housecall. It is important to realize that the most appropriate treatment for an ill child is more likely performed faster and better in a well-equipped physician's office or hospital.

Emergencies. When you feel that a medical emergency has arisen call the doctor at once. Should you be unable to reach your doctor's office, call the Emergency Room of your hospital for help. The following are some of the symptoms that may require immediate medical advice:

1. weakness, lassitude and unaccustomed apathy;
2. convulsions;
3. severe pain;
4. profuse and prolonged diarrhea and vomiting;
5. shortness of breath and difficulty in breathing;
6. bleeding which is difficult to stop;
7. serious accidents such as burns, scalds, head injuries, swallowing pills, poisons or solid objects.

If for some reason you are unable to contact your doctor then you should take your baby to the Emergency Room of the nearest hospital. If possible, have someone call to warn them that you are coming.

ANAL FISSURE

Such a tear in the lining of the anus is caused by passing hard stools. It is extremely painful and may make your baby scream when he has a bowel movement. Because it is so painful he may resist the urge to pass a stool, and this leads to further constipation. You may also notice spots of blood on the diaper.

Ask your doctor whether treatment is needed. Your baby will need more fluid to keep his stools soft, and a local anesthetic ointment can be applied to the fissure just before he has a bowel movement.

BALDNESS

Babies often rub off the hair from the back of their heads while lying in their cribs. This can result in a large bald area which is quite harmless. Normal hair will grow there again when the baby begins to sit up more.

BIRTHMARKS

These are not physically harmful, but they can cause much emotional upset and distress – more often to the parents than to the child who is affected. Most marks, but not all, disappear in time; these are discussed on pp. 128–9. Others, unfortunately, do not. These are the port wine stain, moles and freckles. It is fortunate that the port wine stain is the least common birthmark, since it does not fade away. It is dark red or purple and flat – occasionally its surface may be irregular. Usually these marks occur on the face or neck. Some are removed surgically, but greater success has been reported with the use of cosmetic camouflage creams.

Everyone has moles and freckles on their bodies – the average is about 30 per individual. They do not normally disappear and are small, brown or black, flat or raised

Some may sprout hair. They are harmless but if one is disfiguring it can usually be removed by a plastic surgeon.

BLADDER INFECTION *see* Cystitis

BLEEDING
Bleeding in the absence of injury is unusual. If it occurs you must consult your doctor. It is not normal for bleeding to occur from the nose, ear, gums, umbilicus, rectum or for blood to appear in the baby's urine.

BLOCKED TEAR DUCT
Most babies do not produce tears when they cry until they are about seven to ten days old, some may not produce tears until they are two or three months old.

The tear duct (or lachrymal duct) drains tears from the eye into the nose. If blocked, it can cause the eye to water persistently, or to discharge. Such blockage usually clears by the age of six months, and all that needs to be done is carefully to wipe away tears and debris with a clean tissue or absorbent cotton, dipped in cooled boiled water.

Occasionally blockage of the tear duct persists until after six months and has to be relieved by an ophthalmologist.

BLOOD IN STOOL
The most common cause of blood in stools is the passage of a hard stool that damages the lining of the bowel (*see* p. 212, **anal fissure**). If the bleeding is profuse, or your child is otherwise sick, consult your doctor.

BLUE BABIES
Congenital diseases of the heart that cause mixing of the blood from the two sides of the heart cause cyanotic or "blue babies". In these children the skin becomes bluish due to the dark, poorly oxygenated blood which is pumped around their bodies. A hole in a partition of the heart often underlies this disorder. Heart operations are sometimes necessary to correct the underlying malformation and can often produce dramatic improvement.

Not all babies with cardiac abnormalities are blue and most are diagnosed during one of the routine medical examinations your baby will undergo. Nor do all holes in the heart require an operation – some close by themselves in time.

BOTTOM, SORE *see* Diaper Rash

BOWLEGS
Most babies have slightly bowlegs for the first two years of life, and this condition disappears on its own.

BRAIN DAMAGE
A baby's brain can be damaged before, during or after birth. Before birth an infection, such as rubella (German measles), can injure the developing brain, or the placental function may deteriorate so that the brain receives insufficient nutrition to grow properly (*see* p. 47). A prolonged interruption of the oxygen supply to the brain during birth will also damage it. Physical injury may on rare occasions occur at that time. After birth, severe prolonged jaundice, persisting convulsions or severe dehydration may all damage brain tissue.

Brain damage can cause cerebral palsy which leads to the paralysis of certain muscles and may make the muscles flaccid and limp, or cause them to be spastic and rigid. Affected children may be mentally handicapped and may be deaf. Spastic children have rigid muscles which may make movement difficult and may make swallowing and feeding a problem.

Cerebral palsy should be suspected in the baby who is very difficult to feed and who moves his or her limbs very little or in a jerky fashion.

Much can be done to help the child with cerebral palsy and to help his parents to come to terms with his disorder. Teamwork is essential, with doctors, teachers and social workers cooperating with the parents and child.

BREAST ENLARGEMENT in the newborn
Maternal hormones cross the placenta and circulate in the baby's blood. One of their effects is to cause enlargement of the newborn baby's breasts. This occurs in both male and female babies. They may even secrete a milky substance. This is quite harmless – the breasts will revert to normal size on their own and must be left alone and not squeezed. These hormones may also cause vaginal bleeding for a few days in newborn baby girls.

BREATHING DIFFICULTIES
Difficulty in breathing is a medical emergency. You should contact your doctor at once if your child is fighting for his breath with rapid, heaving movements of the chest. Before the doctor arrives, be sure that your baby is not choking on an object that is blocking the upper end of his windpipe (*see* below, **choking**). Then make him comfortable by sitting him upright in your lap. If frightened, his breathing will become more difficult, so do your best to comfort him no matter how scared you are.

BRONCHIOLITIS
A viral lung infection seen in young babies up to 18 months of age. The small airways become narrowed due to swelling of the lining membrane. The child may wheeze and have difficulty breathing because of the obstructed airways. If severe, hospitalization for a few days may be required.

BRONCHITIS
Inflammation of the lining of the main tubes that pass into the lungs gives rise to the condition known as bronchitis. It can follow an infectious disease such as measles, whooping cough or a cold.

The main symptom is a cough and the baby's breathing may sound wheezy from mucus and inflammation in the bronchial tubes. You should take your baby to see the doctor if you think he has bronchitis. Sometimes, but not always, an antibiotic is necessary. The doctor will also be able to give you further advice as to how the mucus can be cleared from the bronchial tubes by simple physiotherapy.

BURNS AND SCALDS *see* p. 206

BURPING
Most babies swallow air as they eat, both with breast- and bottle feeding. At the end of the feeding they will burp if they are sat upright – to the satisfaction of all within hearing distance. Whether the baby is actually any better off is uncertain.

CEPHALHEMATOMA
This swelling may persist on the baby's head some two to three months after birth. It is caused by bruising during birth brought about by the stretching of the veins in the scalp as the baby's head passes through his mother's pelvis. The swelling is outside the skull and will not press on the brain. The edge of it may become bony and persist longer but it is quite harmless and disappears without treatment.

CEREBRAL PALSY *see* Brain Damage

CHICKEN POX *see* Infectious diseases

CHOKING
Coughing and sputtering may occur during feeding if your baby is receiving milk too quickly. Stop feeding the baby if he starts choking, as there is a danger that milk may pass down the windpipe (trachea) rather than the esophagus. Allow a few seconds to recover before feeding him again.

First aid for choking can be found in First aid p. 210.

CIRCUMCISION
Smegma, a cheeselike substance, is secreted by the skin of the head of the penis. This tends to collect in the space under the foreskin and may be a source of irritation or infection. By having your baby circumcised, the foreskin is removed and the smegma cannot accumulate. Thus, hygiene is simpler. Circumcision is not a medical necessity. It is a parental decision. However, if one male child is circumcised, it is advisable to treat all in the family the same.

Circumcision may be done in a number of ways. If done during the newborn period, it only causes a minimum of pain so anesthetics are not necessary. The operation takes approximately 10 minutes and the baby needs virtually no recovery period. Babies, given to their mothers minutes after a circumcision, look and act exactly the same as before the procedure.

When performing a circumcision some physicians use a Gomco clamp, which when carefully placed on the foreskin allows accurate removal of the redundant tissue. The clamp exerts pressure on the tissue so that there is rarely any bleeding. Other methods of circumcision are available.

Following a circumcision there may be slight bruising of the penis and the remaining foreskin is actually bruised and swollen. Other than keeping the area clean no special care is necessary. It is helpful to use a lubricant like Vaseline jelly so that the healing site does not stick to the diaper.

Some parents do not wish to have a circumcision done on their son. Careful cleaning of the area behind the foreskin during the bath is all that is necessary. Remember, the procedure is not done out of necessity unless there is a rare constriction of the foreskin such that retraction is difficult or impossible.

If a circumcision is to be done, it is easy in the newborn period. If your son requires a circumcision later in childhood, or as an adult, he can have much pain as well as difficult recovery period.

CLEFT LIP (Hare Lip)

The upper lip develops in two parts. These join together before birth. Occasionally this union does not occur and the baby is born with a cleft lip. The birth of a baby with a cleft lip is a great shock to his parents. They can be reassured however that it does not interfere with speech or feeding and that today plastic surgeons achieve wonderful results with almost unnoticeable scars. The operation is usually performed at about three months of age.

CLEFT PALATE

The palate, like the upper lip, also develops in two parts which unite before birth. If the union is incomplete the baby is born with a cleft palate – often he will have a cleft lip as well. Sometimes only the soft part of the palate is cleft and this is less a problem than if the bony part is affected. A baby with a cleft bony palate may have to wear a plate in the roof of his mouth for a few months. The palate is repaired by a plastic surgeon sometime in the first 18 months of life. There is no fixed time for this and the surgeon will decide the best time on an individual basis.

Cleft palate can interfere with feeding, but need not deter you from attempting to breast-feed your baby. Some babies with a cleft palate can bottle feed normally using an ordinary nipple, although others need a special nipple which fits over and blocks off the cleft palate. Special spoons are sometimes necessary for feeding.

Feeding a baby with a cleft palate can be time-consuming and makes great demands on the parents. If your baby is affected in this way discuss your difficulties freely and openly with your doctor or pediatrician. Most babies are treated successfully although some may require speech therapy later on to help them overcome any difficulties with voice production.

COLDS

Not all coughs and runny noses are caused by the common cold, but a great many are. This infection is caused by a highly contagious virus and there is little we can do to prevent it spreading from person to person; nor does catching one cold give protection against another. However, it seems prudent for non-family members with colds to avoid handling infants.

The symptoms include a watery discharge from the nose which may later become thicker and yellow, together with a blocked nose, a cough, and sometimes an elevated temperature.

If your baby catches a cold he will have difficulty breathing through the nose. This may make nursing and feeding difficult. Keep the nostrils clear by wiping away nasal secretions with soft tissues (never use cotton swabs). Nose drops will also give relief and make feeding easier if given about half an hour before a feeding. Never use these unless you have been advised to by your own doctor. If your baby has a fever you should consult your doctor, and also see him if your baby has a normal temperature but otherwise seems sick, for example, if he is listless, irritable, crying persistently or not eating well.

Tempra drops (acetaminophen) may make your baby feel more comfortable and help remove the feelings of wretchedness associated with a cold. Antibiotics are not necessary for the uncomplicated cold.

COLD SORES

These are caused by infection of the skin with a virus called **Herpes simplex**. They usually occur around the edges of the mouth as small blisters which become crusted. They may also affect the tongue and inside of the mouth where they can be very painful and may make your baby irritable and disinclined to eat.

No antibiotics are effective in getting rid of this condition, which usually lasts seven to ten days. A pain-relieving drug, such as Tempra (acetaminophen) may make your baby feel more comfortable. If the sore around the mouth becomes septic, then an antibiotic ointment may be necessary to eradicate this secondary infection. Your doctor will prescribe one.

Some children are prone to recurring episodes of cold sores around the mouth. The virus lies dormant in the skin and erupts whenever the child's resistance is lowered – for example, with a cold.

COLIC

This is a common cause of crying in the first few months of life. It does not affect all babies but some seem particularly prone to it. If your baby is subject to long bouts of crying and screaming, it is best if you take the child to your doctor rather than make this diagnosis for yourself.

Most attacks of colic tend to occur in the evening and are known as "evening colic". The baby screams continually for ten minutes or so, and may draw up his legs and kick in obvious discomfort. He is not consoled if he is picked up and cuddled. This episode passes only to be followed by another, five to ten minutes later. The baby may be on the point of falling asleep when another attack occurs and he begins screaming again. Others may follow for two to four hours. Parents are naturally very concerned to see their baby suffering such pain – especially as they seem so powerless to help. They may even feel like screaming themselves.

The causes of this colic are not known, though many fanciful ideas have been suggested. Fortunately, these episodes become less severe as the baby grows older, certainly by the age of six months.

If the colic is severe your doctor may be able to prescribe an antispasmodic drug. This is given about 20 minutes before evening and night feedings and often has a dramatically beneficial effect.

The important thing to realize is that this condition occurs in healthy babies and is not associated with any disease. It has no hazardous long-term effects on your child.

CONGENITAL DISORDERS

These are medical conditions which are present at birth. Some require treatment but many are not serious and will not harm your baby.

Some congenital abnormalities can be detected early in pregnancy by examining the amniotic fluid and by special blood tests. **Down's syndrome** and **spina bifida** can usually be predicted in this way.

There are three main groups of congenital disorder.

Inherited disorders. These result if the baby has acquired an abnormal gene from one or both of his parents (*see* pp. 21, 23). Cystic fibrosis and phenylketonuria are two conditions caused by such genes. If you have a baby with a genetic disorder, or if there is a history of such a condition in your family then you should get advice about the chances of your having affected children in future pregnancies. Your doctor is the first person to see. He may be able to give you all the information you need, or he may arrange for you to see a geneticist for further counseling (*see* p. 218, **genetic counseling**).

Environmental factors. Congenital abnormalities may be caused by environmental factors, which include some infections in pregnancy and the use of certain drugs by the mother during pregnancy (*see* p. 39). German measles (rubella) contracted in the first three months of pregnancy can cause deafness, blindness and abnormalities of the heart in the unborn child. Thalidomide was shown to affect the development of babies' limbs when taken in early pregnancy. The discovery of the terrible effects of this drug on the fetus highlighted the caution with which many drugs should be used in pregnancy. No drug should be taken by a pregnant woman without telling her doctor.

Unknown cause. The largest group of congenital disorders is the group for which no cause is known, and it includes birthmarks, hernias, undescended testicles, cleft plates, dislocated hips and **spina bifida** (*see* p. 223).

CONJUNCTIVITIS

This is the name given to inflammation of the conjunctiva – the layer of tissue which covers the eyeball and which lines the eyelids. This can result from an infection or can be due to an allergy. The affected eye is often red and discharges a sticky material. The eyelids are often stuck together after sleep.

If caused by an infection, conjunctivitis can be very contagious and spread throughout a household. This can be prevented by such precautions as not sharing towels and facecloths.

Conjunctivitis can easily be treated with eyedrops and eye ointment, but you should consult your doctor and he will advise you of the most suitable preparations. Eyesight is not damaged by an attack of conjunctivitis.

CONSTIPATION

There is no universal normal rate at which bowels should be emptied. Bowel function is individual – even at times idiosyncratic. Do not worry about your baby's bowel function. This is unproductive in every sense, and in later life your child, seeing how important his bowel movements are to you, may use this part of his repertoire to blackmail and manipulate you. However, alterations in an individual's normal habits may be significant and if, for example, a baby who normally has a bowel movement every day stops for two or three days, then you should consult your doctor. Remember, however, that it is quite usual for a breast-fed baby not to pass a stool for several days (*see* p. 165).

Sometimes a baby's stools become hard, dry and painful to pass. They may even tear the lining of the bowel and cause an **anal fissure** (*see* p. 212). To keep the stool soft give your baby more fluid, especially in hot weather. Drinks of water or fruit juice are best. A baby on solid food will benefit from puréed fruit. *Never* give your baby a cathartic.

A baby who has not had a bowel movement for two or three days and who begins to vomit may have developed an intestinal obstruction. He should be seen by your doctor as soon as possible.

CONVULSIONS (FITS)

These begin with loss of consciousness, draining of color from the face and twitching of the muscles of the face and limbs. Then the whole body may become rigid and may shake all over. Convulsions should never be ignored and must be reported to your doctor immediately – no matter what time of day or night.

Fits can be caused by a variety of conditions and it is best if your doctor sorts out what is happening. Until the doctor arrives, lay your baby on his side and make sure that he can breathe properly – do not lay him on his back, and make sure that his tongue does not flop back and stop his breathing. If the baby is feverish, sponge him down with warm water once the fit is over (*see* p. 225, **warm sponging**). Do not cover him with blankets and do not give him any medicine unless your doctor has advised this. Even if the convulsions stop of their own accord you should still report them to your doctor as soon as possible.

In some babies fits are caused simply by fever, which can be caused by infections such as the common cold, tonsillitis, earache or measles. These are called febrile convulsions. Other causes of convulsions are epilepsy and occasionally meningitis, for which urgent medical care is essential.

One important, but rare, type of convulsion at about six months of age produces very brief jerks of the whole body. They occur in bursts of jerks. If you see anything like this take your baby to the doctor.

Convulsions are quite common in the first week of life. They can be caused by brain damage at birth but most of them, especially at five to eight days, are caused by low blood calcium. They usually leave no after-effects.

See doctor immediately.

COUGH

A cough is a symptom, not a disease. The most common cause of a cough is a secretion that trickles down the back of the throat and irritates the pharynx and larynx. This explains why most coughs are worse when the child lies down.

Coughs do not always arise from irritation in the chest, though most parents describe their children's coughs as "chesty". Bronchitis, asthma and pneumonia will all cause a cough, but will also produce signs of illness, and a child who has a cough alone, and is otherwise well, is unlikely to be affected with any of these conditions.

If you are worried about your baby's cough, take him to see your doctor. You should always do this if your baby has a temperature, is wheezing, grunts when he breathes, or has difficulty in breathing. The doctor should see your baby if the cough has persisted for over a week.

See doctor.

CRADLE CAP

This can affect the heads of the best cared for babies and should not be considered a mark of neglect or mismanagement. It is common and, although unsightly, is not harmful. Yellow-brown flakes, or crusts, appear on the scalp and head and are also common over the fontanelle (soft spot). These are dried secretions from the sebaceous glands in the baby's skin.

Cradle cap can often be controlled if the baby's scalp is washed daily with gentle baby shampoos and lotions. Occasionally it is necessary to use special shampoos. Consult your physician.

CROUP

This is the name given to the crowing or croaking noise in your baby's throat as he breathes in. Some babies may make this noise from birth and it usually disappears some time during the first 18 months. However, it may follow a cold, when it is usually associated with laryngitis.

Croup following a cold is potentially serious and this is a condition for which you should seek the immediate advice of your doctor, even after office hours. This is especially necessary if your baby's breathing is difficult or labored.

The cause of the infection is a virus or bacteria which inflames the larynx and vocal cords and causes them to swell. This narrows the air passage to the lungs. First aid measures include propping the baby upright and increasing the humidity of the room by keeping a pan of water boiling and allowing the steam to circulate, or take him into the bathroom where a warm shower is running.

Croup is not usually treated with antibiotics. However, sometimes your baby may need to be admitted to the hospital to be treated more intensively for a day or two.

See doctor immediately.

CYSTIC FIBROSIS

This is an inherited disorder which results when a baby receives abnormal genes from both parents. It causes disorders in the mucus-producing glands in the lungs, in the pancreas and in the sweat glands in the skin. A baby with this disorder often suffers from repeated lung infections and from digestive upsets. He will pass bulky smelly stools, and will fail to thrive or gain weight.

A baby who is thought to have cystic fibrosis will need to be examined by a pediatrician. There is no cure for it, but treatment using pancreatic extracts, antibiotic medication and physiotherapy will help greatly.

CYSTITIS

Inflammation of the lining of the bladder is called cystitis; it is usually caused by an infection. In adults and older children the symptoms are pain and a burning sensation, and increased frequency in urination. Occasionally there may be blood present in the urine.

In babies these symptoms are difficult to detect, and cystitis in infants is often associated with a loss of appetite, vomiting, fever and failure to thrive. The diagnosis is made by examination of the urine and by attempting to culture the infecting bacteria in the laboratory. A clean specimen of urine is essential for this, and special sterile plastic cups are used. An alternative way is to obtain the specimen directly from the bladder by puncturing it through the abdominal wall with a thin needle and syringe. This procedure rarely causes the baby much discomfort.

Cystitis is treated by antibiotics. Further tests are sometimes advised to see if there is a reason for the bladder infection.

See doctor.

DEAFNESS

Hearing loss is a severe handicap to the developing child if it remains undetected. It is one of the functions that are carefully examined each time your baby has a developmental examination. If, at any time, you suspect your child is deaf, you should take him to see your family doctor. You might begin to suspect deafness if your baby does not respond to your voice unless he can see you.

Babies can be born with a hearing loss, and this is more likely if the mother suffered German measles (rubella) in the first few months of pregnancy. Recurring ear infections or fluid behind the eardrum may also lessen your baby's hearing ability. Most babies' hearing can be improved with treatment and occasionally special hearing aids are needed.

Failure to hear properly affects the development of speech and is a serious handicap to learning. For these reasons deafness must be detected early and treatment started promptly.

DEHYDRATION

This is a serious condition in small babies. It can result in brain damage, or even death, and is a particular hazard of severe diarrhea and/or vomiting. Excessive sweating can increase dehydration if your baby either has an elevated temperature or is in hot surroundings.

The combination of diarrhea and vomiting can soon lead to dehydration, so do not delay seeing your doctor if your baby develops these symptoms. This should be treated as a medical emergency.

The mouth of the dehydrated baby becomes dry and the eyes become sunken – notify your doctor immediately if your baby develops these features.

If your baby does become dehydrated he will need to be treated in the hospital and may be given fluids through a tube inserted into one of his veins.

Dehydration usually can be prevented by giving your baby adequate fluids. He will probably prefer cooled, boiled water or diluted fruit juice, but it doesn't matter what he drinks as long as he drinks some fluid. *See doctor immediately.*

DERMATITIS

Any inflammation of the skin, whatever the cause, is called dermatitis. *See* below, **eczema**, **diaper rash** and **skin care**.

DIAPER RASH

This can make your baby very unhappy and, if possible, you should do your best to prevent it. However, most babies develop it at some stage in their life, especially if their bowels are loose. Its presence is not a sign of maternal neglect nor mismanagement. It usually results when wet or soiled diapers are left on for long periods. Bacteria from the stools may act on the urine to produce ammonia – you may smell it when you change the baby's diaper. This irritates the baby's skin making it red and inflamed.

Diaper rash is prevented if diapers are removed as soon as they become soiled and if wet ones are not left on for too long. After soiling, the baby's bottom should be washed thoroughly with soap and warm water, or with special cleansing cream – pay particular attention to the folds in your baby's skin. Dry the bottom carefully before putting on a clean diaper.

If your baby has sensitive skin or seems to be developing diaper rash, then Desitin or baby ointment or Vaseline can be used to soothe the skin and to form a barrier between it and the urine. There are other excellent silicone barrier creams about which your doctor can advise you. Sometimes leaving the diaper off for a prolonged period helps diaper rash disappear, but make sure the room is warm if you decide to do this. Leaving off rubber pants is very helpful. Disposable diapers with liners which let the urine soak into the diaper but which remain dry next to the baby's skin, are also useful. And be sure that you thoroughly rinse soap and detergent from your diapers. A final rinse in a very weak solution of vinegar is a good way to neutralize any ammonia.

If your baby's diaper rash is slow to clear then you should take him to see your doctor. There may be another explanation for it, such as monilia. This requires treatment with antifungal creams, which your doctor will be able to prescribe. Seborrheic dermatitis is another cause of diaper rash, but this will be associated with a rash behind the ears and in the armpits, and often cradle cap. You should seek the advice of your doctor if you think your baby has this disorder. Treatment will probably require washing the scalp with a medicated shampoo and sometimes treating the diaper area with a steroid ointment.

DIARRHEA

This term means that the stools are more fluid than normal and often passed very frequently. If your baby is drinking normally, diarrhea is not usually anything to worry about, but nevertheless it is a good idea to take him to see your doctor. If your baby is not taking fluids, or if he is vomiting as well, then your doctor should see the baby as soon as possible as there is danger of **dehydration** (*see* above).

Uncomplicated diarrhea is best treated with clear fluids only – that is, water or fruit juice drinks. Milk and solid foods tend to make diarrhea last longer and should be avoided. Clear fluids should usually be given for two or three days. Your baby will come to no harm on this treatment and indeed may not even want milk or solid food if he has an upset tummy.

Antibiotics are rarely necessary for diarrhea. Antidiarrhea medicines such as Lomotil or Enterovioform should *never* be given to a small baby. Your doctor may regulate the baby's diet and if necessary prescribe medication.

DIPHTHERIA

Diphtheria is a lethal disease which your child should be routinely immunized against in the first year of life (*see* p. 226, **immunization**).

The infection begins with a sore throat and fever. Later hoarseness and weakness develop. A membrane may develop across the trachea (windpipe) and can obstruct breathing entirely. When this happens an opening through the neck into the windpipe has to be cut – a tracheotomy – otherwise the child may choke to death.

Fortunately this infectious disease is now very rarely seen in the United States, but it could return if many mothers neglect to have their children immunized.

DOWN'S SYNDROME

This is the proper name for the condition known as mongolism. It is an inherited disorder usually caused by an extra chromosome (*see* p. 22). The chances of having such a baby are increased in older mothers. Rarer types of the condition seem to run in families. If you have previously had a child with Down's syndrome or if any member of your spouse's family has been so affected, then you should discuss with your doctor the chances of having a mongol baby in a future pregnancy. He may advise you to see a geneticist for **genetic counseling** (*see* p. 218).

Down's syndrome can be diagnosed before birth and in early pregnancy by examining cells obtained from the amniotic fluid (*see* p. 59). The diagnosis is more commonly made at birth. These babies are rather floppy, with a tendency to sniffles and colds. The eyes are small and tend to be slanting and their faces rather flat.

Children with Down's syndrome are mentally handicapped, but many are able to achieve more now with the help of special schools and encouragement in early life.

The parents of a child with Down's syndrome can receive support from their local health organizations and education services and will not be alone in the difficult, though rewarding, task of looking after the baby. They will also gain much by meeting and helping other families with similarly affected children. Your own doctor or pediatrician will be able to put you in touch with organizations through which you can meet and learn from other families who have children with Down's syndrome.

DROWSINESS

All babies are drowsy when they are tired and before they go to sleep. If your baby is unusually drowsy then you should consult your doctor as soon as possible. This is especially so if your baby has other symptoms, such as a cough, diarrhea, vomiting, difficulty in breathing or an elevated temperature.

DRUGS

A small baby should not be given drugs or medicines, except on the advice of your doctor. Some preparations, such as aspirin, may be harmful in the first few months of life. If you feel that your baby has a condition that needs some sort of medication, then you should take him to see your doctor rather than prescribing something yourself.

DYSENTERY

Dysentery is an infection of the bowel that causes **diarrhea** (*see* above). It is contracted by eating food that has been contaminated by flies, or by hands that carry germs because they have not been washed after a bowel movement.

An adequate fluid intake is essential to prevent the development of **dehydration** (*see* above). Strict personal hygiene is also essential.

EARACHE

Many babies develop the habit of pulling their ears but this is not an indication of earache. A baby with earache is usually fretful and pale and may scream inconsolably from the pain.

Earache is usually due to **otitis media** (*see* p. 220) – an inflammation of that part of the ear behind the eardrum. This is caused by an infection and often follows a cold or measles. If you suspect your child has earache take him to your doctor as soon as possible. Treatment with a pain reliever and an antibiotic is usually effective. Ear infections can lead to perforated eardrums and partial deafness so all must be treated properly. The hearing of children who have had an ear infection must be checked to make sure that it has returned to normal.

Any discharge from the ear is abnormal and is an indication for you to consult your doctor. Never insert anything in the ear unless specifically directed to by the doctor. *See doctor immediately.*

ECZEMA

Infantile eczema usually begins as an irritating red area on the cheeks. It may become moist and drain, and may spread to other parts of the body. It is particularly common in the elbow creases and behind the knees.

Eczema itches and can make your baby very uncomfortable. He may scratch the rash so that it becomes infected. It is very difficult to prevent him from doing this. Eczema is in some way related to asthma and hay fever – all three may occur in one child or in other members of the family.

Consult your doctor if you think your child has eczema. He will be able to advise on how to wash your baby – soap can sometimes make eczema worse. Steroid creams are sometimes useful in controlling this skin condition.

Unfortunately there is no cure, but much can be done to relieve the symptoms of eczema and many babies outgrow it by three or four years of age. You can reduce the chances of eczema by breast-feeding for three months.

EPILEPSY

People who have epilepsy have episodes during which there is a temporary alteration in their level of consciousness. However not all such episodes are caused by epilepsy and some babies may develop them when they have a high temperature – these are called febrile convulsions (*see* **Convulsions** p. 215).

If your child has convulsions he should be seen by your own doctor who will probably arrange for him to be seen by a hospital specialist. An EEG (electroencephalogram) will help in reaching a diagnosis of epilepsy – this records the electrical activity of the brain and is usually done as an outpatient procedure. It is quite harmless and painless.

There are two main types of epilepsy – petit mal and grand mal. These differ in their effects on the child and are explained in detail below.

Petit mal. During these attacks the child loses consciousness for a second or two – he may look pale and vacant. He may stop talking in mid-sentence, and then continue after the fit as if nothing had happened. This may happen several times a day. The child does not fall down.

Grand mal. The child with grand mal has convulsions (*see* p. 215). These attacks can involve the whole body or just part of it. The affected person falls unconscious to the ground, clenches his teeth and often foams at the mouth. He then shakes violently often in a rhythmic way. In an attack the epileptic patient may pass urine and may bite his tongue.

During an attack the epileptic patient must be protected from harming himself; he is best laid on his side and it is particularly important to make sure he does not choke on his tongue and that he is able to breathe easily. If the convulsion goes on for ten minutes or more summon help from your doctor right away.

After the fit the epileptic person falls asleep and wakes up in an hour or two.

No cause for epilepsy can be found in most children though in some brain damage at birth may be responsible.

There is no cure for this disorder but the number of fits can be lessened by regularly giving affected children anti-convulsant medication such as phenobarbital and phenytoin.

If possible epileptic children should lead as normal a life as possible and should attend normal schools. Activities that would be hazardous should the child have a fit while engaging in them should be avoided, for example, cycling and rock climbing. But some, such as swimming, are safe if the child is in the water with a responsible adult.

Many parents feel guilty and ashamed if their child is found to have epilepsy. There is no cause or need to feel this way if your child is affected, as parents are in no way to blame and most epileptic children develop and behave normally.

EVENING COLIC *see* Colic

FALLS *see* First aid p. 211

FEEDING PROBLEMS *see* Chapter 10

FAT BABIES

No baby can become fat without eating more than he needs. There is a risk that fat babies will become obese adults and so will have an increased chance of developing a number of medical conditions. If you think your baby is too fat, discuss this with your doctor.

Fatness is easier to prevent than to treat. Do not give your baby milk feedings that are more concentrated than the manufacturer or your doctor advises. Give him a drink of water or fruit juice if he is thirsty rather than always milk. Cereal-containing foods are especially fattening, so limit this part of your baby's diet. Foods such as eggs, meat, fish, fruit, vegetables and cheese are less likely to make your baby fat and so should be offered as an alternative.

FEVERS

The normal body temperature is between 96 and 98.6°F (35.5–37°C). The temperature is slightly higher if taken rectally. This often rises when the body is infected with a virus or bacteria. Such an elevated temperature is called a fever. (For how to take your baby's temperature *see* below, **temperature**.)

The height to which the temperature rises is not an indication of the seriousness of the illness. A high temperature can be caused by something as commonplace as influenza or tonsillitis, where a slight rise in temperature may occur with a very serious illness. If your child seems generally sick yet has a normal temperature, you should still not hesitate to consult your doctor. Similarly do not panic if your baby's temperature is 100°F (38°C).

Fever is not a disease – it may, however, be the symptom of a disease, so it is best that you call your doctor for advice if the baby's temperature is elevated. Most babies with a fever may be safely wrapped in a blanket and taken by car to the doctor's office, where it will be easier for the doctor to examine the baby.

FISSURE *see* Anal fissure.

FITS *see* Convulsions; Epilepsy

FONTANELLE

The skull is formed by the fusion of separate bones. This is almost complete by birth except for small soft areas, called fontanelles. The fontanelle on top of the head is called the anterior fontanelle; it usually closes between 13 and 18 months. There is also a small gap at the back of the head – the posterior fontanelle. This closes at about two months.

The fontanelle does not need any special treatment. Do not worry – you cannot damage the brain underneath by washing the fontanelle.

The fontanelle is usually flat and sometimes pulsates – should it become very sunken or bulging, you should take your baby to see your doctor.

FOREIGN BODIES in the nose, ears etc. *see* First aid, p. 211.

GASTROENTERITIS

This infection of the stomach and bowels causes vomiting and diarrhea. The cause may be a virus or bacteria and is contagious. The spread is from feces to food, so that the baby's soiled diapers are a particular hazard. Anybody looking after a baby with gastroenteritis must be meticulous in washing his hands after nursing and cleaning his small patient or his diapers.

Babies with gastroenteritis quickly become dehydrated (*see* above, **dehydration**) as they lose much fluid from vomiting and diarrhea. A plentiful supply of clear fluids (water or fruit juice) is essential. Solid food and milk drinks tend to prolong the symptoms of gastroenteritis so they are best avoided.

Gastroenteritis is potentially dangerous, especially in the first few months of life. You should not hesitate to consult your doctor if your baby has such a bowel infection.
See doctor immediately.

GENETIC COUNSELING

Some diseases, such as hemophilia or cystic fibrosis, are inherited from one or both parents. If anyone in your family or your spouse's family has an inherited disorder or if you have previously had a child with a congenital illness (*see* above, **congenital disorders**), then you may want to know the risk that any of your future children will be so affected. Your doctor or pediatrician will be able to refer you to a medical center to discuss the matter with a specialist in genetic disorders. This is known as genetic counseling.

GERMAN MEASLES (RUBELLA) *see* Infectious diseases p. 228

GRINDING TEETH

Some children grind their teeth in their sleep. Nothing can be done to stop this and it does no harm.

GUMS

Patches of your baby's gums may be a little red and tender as teeth come through (*see* below, **teething**). This should only last a day or two and any discomfort will be relieved by a mild pain reliever, recommended by your doctor.

If your baby's gums are generally red and ulcerated so that he cannot eat or drink, then you should take him to see your doctor as he may have an infection of the mouth. Bleeding from the gums also merits your doctor's advice.

GUTHRIE TEST *see* Phenylketonuria

HAIR *see* Scalp care: Baldness

HARE LIP *see* Cleft lip

HEAD BANGING

Some babies bang their heads before going to sleep. This habit may begin at about nine months and may indicate feelings of insecurity in your child. Should it persist you should see your doctor and seek his opinion as to why your baby is behaving in this way and how he or she can be stopped.

Babies rarely do themselves physical injury by head banging but it is probably best to pad the inside of the crib.

HEART DISEASE *see* Blue babies

HEART MURMURS

The doctor may hear a heart murmur when he listens to your baby's heart with a stethoscope. A murmur is an extra sound generated by the heart. They are very common and most are harmless and insignificant and not an indication of a structural abnormality in the heart. However, it is sometimes necessary to investigate heart murmurs further by doing chest X rays. Doppler flow studies and an electrocardiogram to be certain that the murmur is an innocent one. Occasionally it is necessary to see a child over a period of years to make sure of this.

HEAT RASH *see* Prickly heat

HERNIA

A hernia, or rupture, is a protrusion beneath the skin caused when the contents of the abdomen bulge through a weak point in the abdominal muscles. Hernias can occur in a number of places.

An **umbilical hernia** results when the contents of the abdomen protrude through the gap in the muscles through which the umbilical cord passed. These are very common and can be quite large: they may bulge even more when the baby cries. They are quite harmless and usually disappear without any treatment at all in the first year or two.

An **inguinal hernia** may be felt or seen as a lump in the groin or scrotum. It is more common in boys than girls and may be associated with an undescended testis (*see* below, **testes**). There is a high risk that an inguinal hernia will become blocked and strangulated – that is, cut off from its own blood supply. This can damage the intestine and is a very dangerous condition.

If you notice a lump in your baby's groin or scrotum you should take him to see your doctor as soon as possible. The lump will not cure itself. The doctor will arrange for your baby to see a surgeon for an operation. The small hernia is easily repaired and your baby will recover soon afterward.

HIVES

Urticaria, or hives, are names for this itchy skin rash, which appears as white weals surrounded by an area of redness. These may be of any size or shape and can occur at any site on the body. The condition is very itchy but usually disappears in a few hours. However, the weals may continue to appear intermittently over a period of some days. Some children seem particularly susceptible to these attacks.

Hives may follow stings or insect bites. It is sometimes caused by an allergy to foods, such as shellfish or strawberries. Allergies to a drug, such as pencillin or aspirin, can also trigger off such an attack. Emotional factors may be involved, but in most patients the cause is never known.

Calamine lotion soothes the irritation of hives. If the itching is particularly severe, your doctor may prescribe an antihistamine.

Hives are a very inconvenient complaint but fortunately usually of no serious consequence.

HOARSENESS

Hoarseness and **croup** (*see* above) are both caused by laryngitis and inflammation of the vocal cords. Both usually follow a cold. If the baby has difficulty in breathing associated with hoarseness you should contact your doctor at once.

HOLE IN THE HEART

An operation may be necessary to correct this malformation, although some holes in the heart close by themselves in time. A baby with a hole in the heart may become cyanosed (*see* p. 213 **blue babies**) due to poorly oxygenated blood being pumped around the body.

HYDROCEPHALUS

The condition is caused by an abnormal accumulation of cerebrospinal fluid (CSF) within the skull. The fluid presses on the brain and interferes with its function, and at the same time pushes the skull bones outward. The baby has a greatly enlarged head. Hydrocephalus can develop before birth and is often associated with **spina bifida** (*see* below). If it is untreated,mental handicap can develop.

The treatment of hydrocephalus is by operation. A valve is inserted that drains the excess CSF from the brain into a vein in the neck or into the peritineal cavity.

IMMUNIZATION *see* p. 226.

IMPETIGO

Impetigo is caused by a bacterial infection of the skin. It starts as red spots, which weep and then become covered in dirty yellow "honeycomb" crusts. It spreads quickly and is very contagious. If you think your baby has impetigo take him to your doctor, who will recommend special treatment. Do not allow any member of the family to share a towel or facecloth with anybody who has impetigo.

INSECT STINGS *see* First aid, p. 211

INTUSSUSCEPTION

Fortunately this is a very rare condition. It causes severe abdominal pain and occasionally blood in the stools. Intussusception occurs in babies between the ages of three months and two years and is a form of intestinal obstruction. It is brought about when a portion of the intestinal wall passes down through the middle of its adjacent part. This is forced forward giving rise to severe bouts of pain as it moves on. The baby screams and becomes very pale during these attacks but can seem quite well and even fall asleep in between. Vomiting and blood in the stool may develop.

Babies with intussusception are usually older than those with **colic** (*see* above). If you think that your baby has developed this condition notify your doctor at once. An operation is sometimes necessary to pull back the piece of intestine causing the trouble.
See doctor immediately.

IRON
An adequate intake of iron is needed so that the body can make hemoglobin and to prevent anemia. The normal baby gets iron from its mother in the last months of pregnancy and stores enough for the first six months of life. At about this time he then starts mixed feeding and is given iron in his food. Meat, liver, egg yolk and green vegetables are all rich in iron. If weaning is postponed until after six months then there is a chance that iron deficiency anemia may develop, and iron supplements may be necessary.

Premature babies have poor stores of iron and have to be given supplements of iron from about one month onward.

Your doctor or pediatrician will advise you if he thinks that your baby needs iron supplements.

ISOLATION *see* Infectious diseases, p. 228

JAUNDICE
Jaundice is not a disease in itself, but a symptom of a number of different conditions. The jaundiced baby has almost yellow skin and the whites of the eyes are also affected. These appearances are due to the collection of a compound called bilirubin.

Bilirubin is formed when the red blood cells are broken down at the end of their life: it is then excreted in the bile by the liver into the intestine. Many babies become jaundiced in the first few days of life (*see* chapter 12), as their livers are immature and cannot excrete all the bilirubin that has formed at that time. Within a few days liver function improves so that the jaundice disappears without any treatment.

Jaundice should always be reported to your doctor. He may arrange blood tests to be sure that the level of bilirubin in your baby's blood does not rise too high, as this can cause damage to the brain. Jaundice may make your baby rather sleepy and slow to feed but it rarely causes any problems. If it becomes severe then your baby may need to have a blood transfusion in which some of the bilirubin-rich blood is drawn off and replaced with normal blood. This is called an exchange transfusion and it is repeated until his bilirubin is below the dangerous range. Less severe elevation may be treated by physiotherapy, placing your baby under ultraviolet light.

KOPLIK'S SPOTS
These spots, which are white and look like grains of salt, are an early sign of measles. They develop in the lining of the mouth inside the cheeks and are usually present before the skin rash is seen. The doctor will look for these spots if he suspects your child is developing measles.

LARYNGITIS
Inflammation of the larynx is usually caused by a viral or bacterial infection and occasionally occurs following a cold. The symptoms are **hoarseness** and **croup** (*see* above). Laryngitis can cause narrowing of the air passage into the lungs and difficulty in breathing. This can be dangerous and if it occurs you should contact your doctor at once. The baby may need to be taken to the doctor's office or hospital emergency room. Increasing the humidity of the air will help breathing. Do this by running a warm shower and sitting in the bathroom holding the baby.
See doctor immediately.

LAZY EYE *see* Squint

LEAD POISONING
Lead, if eaten, can cause anemia, convulsions, kidney damage and brain damage. The most common source in infancy is paint. Be sure, therefore, that there is no lead-containing paint on your child's furniture, especially the crib or bed, or on his toys.

LUMBAR PUNCTURE *see* Meningitis

MALARIA
The frequency of overseas travel has meant that this tropical disease is occasionally seen in the United States and other western countries. It is caused by a parasitic organism carried by a mosquito and transmitted to man by mosquito bites. The symptoms of malaria usually develop about two weeks after infection but they can take many months before they show themselves. A fever occurring every two or three days is the most common first symptom of malaria, together with headache and drowsiness. Convulsions and coma may eventually develop.

If your child develops a fever after you return from a malarial region you should consult your doctor at once and tell him where you have been. Malaria can be simply and effectively treated, yet without treatment can be fatal. If you plan to take your child to a foreign country, be sure to consult with your physician early. Special immunizations or prophylactic drugs may be advisable.

MALNUTRITION
Malnutrition in babies is still common in developing countries and is caused mainly by a deficiency of protein. Other deficiency diseases include anemia, due to lack of iron, and rickets, which is caused by lack of vitamin D.

Babies of normal birth weight have an adequate store of iron and do not require iron supplements (*see* above, **iron**). Premature babies do not have such an iron store and need supplements of iron after birth. From six months onward a diet containing meat, egg yolk and green vegetables supplies all the iron the developing baby needs.

Vitamin C is given in the form of fruit juices from about one month onward. Never boil these drinks as this destroys vitamin C.

Vitamins A and D are found in fish oils, such as cod liver oil, and this is usually given to babies from the first month onward. However, it should not be given to babies who are bottle-fed with milk already fortified with vitamin D, as it is possible to give too much of this vitamin and to make the baby ill.

In industrialized countries the most common form of malnutrition is too much food rather than too little, resulting in overweight babies (*see* p. 217, **fat babies**).

MEASLES *see* Infectious diseases, p. 228

MEATAL ULCER
A small ulcer may form at the tip of the penis in circumcised baby boys and is due to rubbing by wet diapers. In the uncircumcised, the foreskin prevents such irritation. The ulcer may extend into the urethra and is very painful when urine passes over it. This causes the baby to scream as he empties his bladder.

If you think your baby has a meatal ulcer then take him to see your doctor. He will prescribe an ointment which forms a barrier between the urine and the tender ulcer until the ulcer has healed. A local anesthetic ointment can also be applied to give relief.
See doctor immediately.

MEDICINES, ADMINISTRATION OF
Giving medicines to small babies can sometimes be very difficult. If your baby will take the medicine in a little syrup off a teaspoon this is the best way. Otherwise, make it into a drink with a small amount of cooled, boiled water and give it to the baby from a bottle or cup.

Never force medicine into your baby, especially if he is crying, for he may then inhale it. This is particularly dangerous with oily preparations such as cod liver oil, as these can cause pneumonia if they reach the lungs.

MENINGITIS
The meninges are the thin membranes that cover the brain and spinal cord. When they are inflamed the child is said to have meningitis. Such inflammation can be caused by bacterial or viral infections.

The symptoms of meningitis include fever, vomiting, irritability, drowsiness, apathy and convulsions. Blood spots may appear in the skin. The diagnosis of meningitis in babies can be very difficult – the baby will be very sick and the doctor on examination may find little explanation. A lumbar puncture and analysis of the cerebrospinal fluid will give the diagnosis.

Provided there is no delay in beginning treatment with antibiotics, a baby with meningitis usually recovers. It is nevertheless a very serious infection. It can result in partial deafness and so the baby's hearing must be carefully tested on recovery, and for some time afterward.
See doctor immediately.

MONGOLISM *see* Down's syndrome

MUMPS
This virus infection is rare in small babies. The child with mumps has a fever and the salivary glands situated over the angle of the jaw (the parotids) become swollen and tender and cause discomfort (*see* p. 230, **infectious diseases**).

NASAL DISCHARGE
Your baby's nose may discharge a clear fluid if he has been crying or if he has a cold. Some babies seem to have this most of the time and are said to be "sniffly". They grow out of this and it does no harm. Wipe away any discharge from the baby's nose with a soft tissue and this will ease his breathing.

If the nasal discharge becomes green or yellow take your baby to see the doctor and discuss with him whether further treatment might be necessary.

NASAL OBSTRUCTION
Small babies have difficulty sucking and feeding if their noses become blocked. *Never* attempt to unblock your baby's nose with cotton swabs, as you may do damage. If the obstruction persists and distresses your baby, take the child to your doctor. He will advise on how this symptom is best relieved. He may prescribe nose drops, but never use these on your baby unless the doctor has instructed you to do so.

NAVEL *see* Umbilicus

NOSEBLEEDS
Bleeding from the nose is unusual in small babies and deserves advice from your doctor. Occasionally it results if a toddler has pushed something like a bean or bead into his nostril. Sometimes a small blood vessel inside the nostril becomes damaged and bleeds. Your doctor will advise on the best treatment for this.

As a first measure, get the child to lean over a bowl and breathe through his mouth until the bleeding stops. Pinching the lower part of the nose for several minutes between your thumb and forefinger can also help.

OBESITY *see* Fat babies

OTITIS MEDIA
This is the name given to inflammation of the middle ear – that is, that part of the ear immediately behind the eardrum. It is the most common cause of earache in children and can make a small baby scream inconsolably with pain. The small baby with otitis media may have more general symptoms, and there may be no reason to suspect the ears as the source of infection. For example, he or she may have diarrhea or vomiting, or simply be unwilling to eat.

Otitis media often develops after the common cold, mumps, scarlet fever or measles. The diagnosis is made when the doctor views the eardrum with an otoscope and sees that it is red and inflamed, bulging outward, and that the bones of the middle ear are no longer visualized. To facilitate diagnosis a tympanogram may be performed. At a later stage the eardrum may rupture and cause a discharge to appear.

If you think your child has earache, take him to see your doctor as soon as possible. If your child is in severe pain you may need to call your doctor night or day for his advice on the further management of the condition. A pain-relieving drug, such as Tempra drops or, for older children, aspirin, will be needed, and an antibiotic is nearly always prescribed to eradicate the underlying infection. Ear drops should only be used on medical advice. A child with otitis media should show a degree of improvement within 24–48 hours of starting prescribed medication.

Otitis media can cause a temporary damage to hearing, which may persist for some weeks. Take your child to see the doctor until he is satisfied that the hearing has returned to normal.
See doctor immediately.

PALLOR
A pale color may be an indication that your baby is anemic, although this is not always so; it can be that he simply has a light-colored complexion. The diagnosis of anemia depends on a blood test, so if you think your baby is anemic you should discuss this with your doctor.

Babies sometimes turn pale during bouts of severe pain as with **intussusception** (*see* above) or during a **convulsion** (*see* above). Both these conditions need further immediate medical advice.

PENICILLIN
Penicillin was the first antibiotic to be discovered and developed for routine medical use. It is able to destroy certain bacteria in the body and is used in the treatment of infections such as tonsillitis. Like all antibiotics, it is not effective against viral infections such as the common cold.

Some people suffer allergic reactions to penicillin, such as asthma or **hives**. They should use an alternative antibiotic, and must warn doctors not to prescribe penicillin for them.

PENIS
The penis of small baby boys rarely requires much attention. **Circumcision** (*see* chapter 12 and p. 213) is best done shortly after birth.

The foreskin protects the tip of the penis from irritation of urine-soaked diapers. Its removal can sometimes lead to a small sore at the opening of the penis – a **meatal ulcer** (*see* p. 219).

If the baby has not been circumcised, gentle retraction of the foreskin will permit cleaning away the smegma that collects there. If the baby has been circumcised, less smegma collects and proper hygiene is a simple matter. In some countries these hygienic measures are not employed.

Erection of the penis occurs in baby boys, and you may notice this sometimes, for instance when changing diapers. This is quite normal.

PERITONITIS
This is an inflammation of the thin tissue, the peritoneum, that lines the inside of the abdominal wall and covers the abdominal organs.

Peritonitis is usually a complication of certain diseases of the abdominal organs, for example appendicitis or a perforated peptic ulcer, or an obstructed inguinal hernia (*see* p. 218, **hernia**).

The baby with peritonitis is seriously ill and may be listless and semicomatose. He or she requires urgent treatment in the hospital.

PERTUSSIS *see* Whooping cough; Infectious diseases, p. 228

PETS
Some animals, such as dogs and cats, may resent the arrival of a new baby as much as older brothers and sisters, so do not decrease the attention you give your pet when the baby is born.

There are a few conditions that dogs and cats can pass to small babies. These include fleas, **ringworm** (*see* below) and **worms** (*see* below). There is also the risk of bites and scratches from these animals. You should therefore never let your pets into the baby's crib or carriage and should cover the carriage with a cat net when it is in the garden. Never leave your baby and pets unattended together.

PHENYLKETONURIA
This is a rare inherited disease in which the baby lacks the specific enzyme needed to deal with the chemical compound known as phenylalanine. It can lead to mental deficiency. The condition can be detected by such a test as the Guthrie test, which is routinely performed on a sample of the baby's blood.

Babies with phenylketonuria are then fed a special diet until their brains have finished developing and in this way are able to develop normally. Without such a diet irreversible mental handicap would be the inevitable result.

Couples who produce a baby with phenylketonuria must both possess a recessive gene for this disorder, and there is a one in four chance that subsequent children will also be affected. These parents would benefit from **genetic counseling** (*see* p. 218).

PNEUMONIA

Infection of the tissues of the lung itself is called pneumonia. This condition may be confined to one area or lobe of the lung (lobar pneumonia) or it may be generalized throughout one or both lungs (bronchiopneumonia).

The child with pneumonia may have a cough and an elevated temperature. Breathing may be rapid and shallow and the child may grunt with each breath. There are many medical conditions that can be the cause of these symptoms, so it is best if you consult your doctor if your child develops any of them.

Pneumonia may be a complication of the common cold, or measles, or whooping cough. It may develop after gastroenteritis, or if your child has inhaled food or some other foreign body, or if his resistance has been already lowered following a previous illness.

Fortunately, pneumonia will usually respond to treatment with antibiotics. Indeed, the response is so good that most children can be cared for at home and do not need to go into the hospital. Adequate intake of fluids must be maintained and the doctor may ask you to perform some simple physiotherapy on your child to help the infected mucus in the lungs to drain out. He will show you how to do this.

POISONING *see* First aid, p. 211

POLIOMYELITIS

As a result of the immunization of babies against polio, this infectious disease has almost disappeared from western countries. It is nevertheless a serious infection which can kill and cripple.

The disease is usually contracted by eating food contaminated with the virus. It used to be more common in the summer months and was thought to be associated with the increased number of flies at that time of the year, as these insects carry the virus from the feces of those with the disease to other people's food. Polio can also be contracted by inhalation of the virus.

The incubation period for polio is about three weeks, and anyone in contact with a case should be kept in quarantine for 21 days.

Polio may be a mild illness resembling influenza, but it can be very serious and muscle paralysis can develop. If the muscles of the chest wall are affected, breathing may become impossible, and artificial respiration may be necessary. After acute infection the polio victim may be badly crippled, because the damaged nerves cannot be repaired and the muscles they serve become weak and wasted.

Immunization against polio is strongly recommended in infancy (*see* p. 226, **immunization**) and for anybody, adult or child, traveling in the tropics. If you or your husband have never been immunized against polio, you should consult your physician before your baby is immunized.

PRICKLY HEAT

Some babies develop itchy red spots and small blisters in hot weather – this is particularly common in hot, moist, tropical climates. The face, neck and upper trunk are mainly affected. Excessive sweating is the main cause of prickly heat and frequent cool baths will prevent and give relief from this condition. Talcum powder or calamine lotion are also soothing.

Prevent your baby from becoming overheated and sweating excessively by not overdressing him, and also by not using too many blankets in hot weather. A cotton shirt next to his skin will be better for him than a woolen one.

PYLORIC STENOSIS

The pylorus is the outlet of the stomach and leads to the duodenum. In some babies, for reasons no one understands, the muscle lining the pylorus becomes thickened and the channel through it becomes narrower. This may interfere with the passage of food from the stomach and lead to vomiting.

The vomiting associated with pyloric stenosis is said to be "projectile", and the contents of the stomach are often brought up with such force that they are propelled several feet. Such vomiting after feedings usually begins at the age of two or three weeks. Pyloric stenosis rarely develops in a baby over the age of six weeks. It is more common in little boys and seems to run in families.

If your small baby vomits most of his feedings regularly, consult your doctor, even if the baby is otherwise quite well. Your doctor may want to see the baby at a time when you are feeding him so that he can examine the baby's abdomen. In this way the doctor may be able to feel the thickened pyloric muscle and the diagnosis will be clear.

Babies who have pyloric stenosis become very hungry, and if the vomiting is prolonged they can become seriously ill. Usually a small and relatively simple operation is needed to relieve the obstruction. The baby is in the hospital for a very short period of time and thereafter his progress is normal.

QUARANTINE

Most infectious diseases are most contagious shortly before the characteristic signs of the disease appear, and in the early stages of the disease. The incubation period is the time between the initial contact with the disease and the first signs of the disease appearing in the patient. It is therefore possible to catch an infectious disease from somebody near the end of their incubation period before they themselves know they have it. For this reason, the strict period of isolation for the benefit of others should be from the time of initial contact with the disease, or as soon as you discover you have been in contact with it, until the end of your incubation period. If, after that time, there are no signs of infection, then the period of quarantine is over; if signs of infection do appear, isolation is necessary for a further period depending on the disease (*see* p. 228, **infectious diseases**).

Strict quarantine precautions for the infectious diseases of childhood are now rarely applied throughout a possible incubation period, although the isolation of known cases of an infectious disease is still recommended. However, for serious infections, such as polio for instance, strict quarantine from the time of initial contact with a case is recommended. Quarantine precautions should also be stricter if there is a risk to women in early pregnancy. Thus a person susceptible to German measles (rubella) who has been in contact with this disease should avoid contact with a susceptible woman who is in the first three months of her pregnancy. Similarly, susceptible contacts should keep away from all small babies.

REGURGITATION *see* Vomiting

RH-DISEASE

A woman with Rh-negative blood who has a partner with Rh-positive blood may conceive a child who is Rh-positive. Some of this child's blood may pass across the placenta into the mother's circulation toward the end of pregnancy or in labor, and she may produce antibodies to Rh-positive blood cells. Usually by then her baby will have been born so that problems will only arise in subsequent pregnancies of Rh-positive babies. The first pregnancy is complicated in 1–2 per cent.

Fortunately there has now been devised a special injection that is given to all Rh-negative mothers who have Rh-positive babies at 28 weeks' gestation and right after delivery. This is known as the anti-Rh injection. It destroys any of the baby's Rh-positive blood cells that may have entered the mother's circulation before they have stimulated her antibody producing system to produce anti-Rh antibodies. In this way complications can be prevented in the current and subsequent pregnancies.

There are still some Rh-negative women whose blood contains anti-Rh antibodies and who will conceive Rh-positive babies. These antibodies can cross the placenta into the unborn baby's blood and may destroy his blood cells. This may cause severe anemia and jaundice – heart failure and brain damage may result and many babies die, often before they are born. The diagnosis is usually made before birth – the obstetrician checks the blood group of the pregnant mother and also looks for Rh antibodies. If the obstetrician suspects your baby is affected he may do an amniocentesis and if indicated arrange transfusion for your baby while it is still in the uterus. He will almost certainly deliver your baby early and your baby will thereafter be carefully cared for by the hospital pediatrician.

If your baby is jaundiced (*see* p. 219) the pediatrician will arrange blood tests to ensure that the bilirubin in the baby's blood does not reach a level that could cause brain damage. If the bilirubin level rises too high then an exchange blood transfusion will be necessary – small volumes of the baby's blood are drawn off and replaced by Rh-negative blood. In this way maternal antibodies and bilirubin are diluted out of the baby's blood and the chances of brain damage are eliminated.

Rh-disease is now rarely seen because of the effectiveness of the anti-D injection given to Rh-negative mothers at 28 weeks and immediately after the delivery of an Rh-positive baby. All Rh-negative mothers should be sure that they receive this when necessary and thereby prevent Rh complications in the current and future pregnancies.

RICKETS

A deficiency in vitamin D causes rickets. Rickets leads to a softening of the bones, and the baby develops bowlegs and swelling at the wrist, ankles and over the ribs. It is now extremely rare in the United States, as most babies are given vitamin D supplements, either in fortified milk preparations or vitamin drops. Your doctor will advise you when to give vitamin D to your baby and how much to give. Do not give more than the recommended dose as an excess of vitamin D can be harmful.

RINGWORM

Ringworm, a fungal infection of the skin, is not, as the name suggests, a worm infestation. It begins as a small red sore which grows bigger. Healing then begins at the center as the infection spreads out in a circular fashion, and this gives rise to the characteristic rash. These patches can occur anywhere on the body.

The fungi that cause ringworm can also affect the hair and may cause bald patches on the scalp.

Ringworm is very contagious and spreads easily throughout a family, so do not share combs, brushes or towels if you suspect your child has this condition. Ringworm also occurs in animals – cats or dogs may be the source of the infection – so have pets examined by your veterinarian if anyone in your family develops ringworm.

If you suspect your baby has ringworm, take him or her to your doctor. He will prescribe something, perhaps an ointment, to be applied directly to the circular patches, and he may also give you an antifungal antibiotic should the scalp also be affected by the disease.

ROSEOLA INFANTUM

This is a mild, common condition that occurs in babies and toddlers. It begins with a very high temperature and sometimes a cough, and may make your baby very miserable. By the third or fourth day, the temperature suddenly returns to normal and the baby looks much better. At that time a bright red rash with spots the size of a pin head, appears all over the body. By then the baby will be quite well.

There are no complications with this condition and no specific treatment is needed although your doctor may prescribe medication to lower the temperature and make your baby feel more comfortable.

RUBELLA *see* Infectious diseases, p. 228

RUPTURE *see* Hernia

SCABIES

This very itchy skin condition is caused by a small mite that burrows into the skin. It is contracted by close contact with someone who has scabies or from infected clothes and bedding. The rash of scabies consists of red spots that may blister and crust over the backs of the hands, between the fingers, around the wrists and ankles, and on the trunk. Scratching may cause these spots to become infected.

If you think your baby has scabies, then take him to your doctor. He will prescribe a special paint, such as benzylbenzoate, for you to paint on the baby's skin and on the skin of the other members of the household.

SCALDS *see* First aid, p. 210

SCALP CARE

Wash your baby's scalp with soap or baby shampoo twice a week; wash the **fontanelle** (*see* above) in the usual way. You cannot damage it by doing this. Rinse away all traces of shampoo with clean water. Dry the scalp gently with a towel. Some babies have a tendency to collect thick flaky crusts on the scalp – this is called **cradle cap** (*see* above). These babies may need to have their scalp washed more often than twice a week with a medicated shampoo. Bathing a baby is described in chapter 11.

SCARLET FEVER

Scarlet fever begins with a raised temperature and a sore throat. Nausea and vomiting may then develop. The tongue is usually covered with a white coating and on the second day the rash appears. This begins as pinpoint red spots on the chest and neck, and gradually spreads all over the body. The area around the mouth may remain pale. After three days the rash gradually fades and a week later fine scales of skin may be shed from the hands and feet.

Scarlet fever is commonly caused by the same bacteria that causes tonsillitis – the **streptococcus**. It is therefore treated with penicillin or erythromycin. Scarlet fever is a variant of tonsillitis and no more serious than that. **Otitis media** (*see* above) may be a complication and acute nephritis or rheumatic fever may develop if this complication is not treated.

SCREAMING

Small babies may scream for the same reasons as they cry (*see* chapter 12). If you are unable to console your baby it may be because he is in pain. Conditions such as **colic** (*see* above), **otitis media** (*see* above) and acute **intussusception** (*see* above) may make a baby scream in this way. You should therefore consult your doctor if you are at a loss to explain your baby's behavior.

SCROTUM

The scrotum should contain two testes (testicles). If your baby boy's does not, then take him to your doctor – he may have undescended testis (*see* below, **testes**).

If you think your son's scrotum is enlarged, consult your doctor about this also. It may be due to a small **hydrocele** (*see* chapter 12) which is a harmless collection of fluid around the testis, or to an inguinal **hernia** (*see* above) which will require a small operation to prevent complications.

SEBORRHEIC DERMATITIS

This condition may develop from **cradle cap** (*see* above) though it can develop without this. Both have a common cause, namely excessive secretions from the sebaceous glands in the skin. In adults this causes dandruff. In babies seborrheic dermatitis can give rise to a moist scaly red rash on the forehead and above the ears, and in the creases of the groin, under the arms and around the neck. If your baby has such a rash then take him to your doctor and he will advise on further care.

SEPTIC SPOTS *see* Chapter 12

SKIN CARE

Most babies' skin can be washed in soap and warm water and no special oils or lotions are normally needed. If your baby has a skin disorder such as **eczema** (*see* above) then you may be advised not to use soap, and to wash your baby only in clear water or with a special emulsifying ointment.

The skin of some babies may react to the detergent in which you wash their clothes – enzyme washing powders may cause particularly severe reactions. It is best to wash diapers and clothes in pure soap flakes or powders as these are less likely to cause sensitivity reactions.

SLEEP

It is impossible to say definitely how much sleep a baby needs. Some need more than others, as with adults. Most babies ensure for themselves that they have as much sleep as they need. The newborn baby sleeps most of the time and only wakes up for feedings. As he or she grows older, less sleep is required.

Your baby should be protected from drafts and extremes of temperature when asleep. Some days he can sleep out of doors if it is not too damp, cold or foggy. For the first three months or so he can sleep in a crib or carriage in his parents' room; thereafter, if possible, he is best on his own. You can always look in on him from time to time or listen via a simple baby alarm system.

If your baby cries in the night, he may be hungry, or too cold or too hot, or uncomfortable with a wet or soiled diaper, or he may simply be lonely. Once these needs have been dealt with he should be put back to bed after a short cuddle – and it is hoped that he will then go back to sleep, although he may cry for 15 minutes or so.

How long he should be left to cry is difficult to say. Your own doctor should be consulted about the baby who persistently cries for long periods in the night. He may be able to prescribe some medicine to make the baby sleepy and help break the habit. Such medicine should only be given for a few days and the baby must not be treated with it indefinitely. While a baby who is awake during the day should be given things to do – toys and rattles to hold or mobiles and balloons to look at – and should be able to watch all that is going on in the family around him, games and prolonged social sessions should be avoided in the small hours, unless that is what the parents want!

If your baby cries loudly and for a long time and is not comforted when picked up and nursed, then he may be in pain. If you think that this is so, notify your doctor at once.

SMALLPOX VACCINATION
Vaccination against smallpox is no longer performed as part of the routine immunization program of infancy. Smallpox has been officially eradicated in the world and vaccination is no longer necessary. This represents a major public health triumph.

SNEEZING
The lining of a baby's nose is very sensitive and, once irritated, it can trigger off sneezing very easily. All babies sneeze frequently. If yours does, it does not mean the child has a cold unless there are other signs (*see* above **colds**).

SNIFFLES
The noses of some babies seem to produce an excess of mucus and run all the time. Keep the nose of such a baby clear, using soft tissue. This is all that is needed, as this is not a serious symptom and does not mean the baby has a perpetual cold. Nose drops are not recommended.

SPASTIC CHILDREN
The spastic child has sustained brain damage before, during or after birth. The effects will depend on the areas of the brain that have been damaged.

Usually there are defects in movement and posture known as cerebral palsy. There may be muscle rigidity or the muscles may be flaccid and limp. This may lead to difficulty in walking and moving the arms. Involuntary movements may also develop.

The spastic child is sometimes mentally handicapped and some may have difficulty hearing. Blindness is uncommon but some spastic children may have epileptic fits.

The child with such brain damage, and his parents, can benefit greatly from the skills of teachers, social workers, doctors and nurses trained specially to look after these children, and to make sure that they reach their maximum potential.

SPINA BIFIDA
This is a congenital disorder of the lower spine in which the spinal cord is exposed on the surface of the back or is covered by a sac of fluid. Neurologic involvement can range from minimal to severe. The legs may become paralyzed and the baby may lose control of his bowels and bladder, so that urine and feces leak. Although the defect on the back can be repaired by surgery the consequences remain irreversible.

Some children with this condition develop **hydrocephalus** (*see* above) which may affect the function of the brain, so mental handicap may be added to their already serious problems (*see* above, **brain damage**).

If a mother has a baby with spina bifida, she has a chance of recurrence of 3–5 per cent in future pregnancies. Antenatal detection of this condition is possible by testing the mother's blood at 16–18 weeks for an elevation in alpha fetoprotein which suggests the presence of spina bifida. Additionally, ultrasound scanning is helpful to detect spina bifida or anencephaly, another neural tube defect.

SQUINT (STRABISMUS)
Most babies seem to have a squint, or strabismus, in the first three months of life before they have acquired a proper control of their eye muscles. If you think your baby is squinting, even if only for a moment, after the age of three months, then you should take the child to see your doctor. He may want your child to see an eye specialist; babies are usually referred to a specialist after six months of age.

If a squint persists, the squinting eye may become blind. For this reason squints must be detected early so that prompt treatment can be started. Fortunately, the sooner treatment is begun, the more simple and more effective it is.

If your baby has a squint he may have to wear a patch over his good eye. In this way he is forced to use the weaker squinting eye, which then becomes more efficient. The older child may wear glasses in which one lens has been made opaque, and he may be given exercises for the eye muscles. Sometimes an operation to lengthen or shorten the eye muscles is needed, but this is unlikely if the squint is detected and treated as soon as possible.

An appearance of squinting in some babies may be due to folds of skin that lie over the inner part of the eye. But don't diagnose this yourself; take your baby to see the doctor if you suspect he has a squint.

Babies are usually tested for squint at the doctor's office, but nevertheless do not assume that this has been done, and take your child to see your doctor if at any time you suspect a squint. The diagnosis and treatment are so simple if started early, and the consequence of leaving it untreated – one blind eye – is all the more sad, because it could have been prevented.

STICKY EYES
Conjunctivitis (*see* above) is a common cause of a baby's eyelids sticking together. If it does not respond to simple treatment, such as wiping away any discharge with a piece of absorbent cotton soaked in cooled boiled water, then your baby should see a doctor. Antibiotic eye drops or ointment may be needed to clear up a mild infection. Sticky eyes do not affect a baby's eyesight in any way.

STOMACH UPSETS
Do not be alarmed if your baby vomits once or twice or has one bout of diarrhea, especially if the child seems otherwise well. However, if he vomits repeatedly, or has many profuse liquid stools, you should consult your doctor (*see* above, **diarrhea**, and below **vomiting**). Small babies can lose a lot of fluid through vomiting and diarrhea and can soon become dehydrated (*see* p. 216, **dehydration**).

STOOLS
Unless you think your baby has **diarrhea** (*see* above), do not become too preoccupied with the color, smell or consistency of your baby's stools. However, if you are in any doubt whether the baby's bowels are behaving normally (*see* p. 164), do not hesitate to consult your doctor. This is especially necessary if he or she shows any other signs of being sick.

STRABISMUS *see* Squint

STYES
The hair follicle of an eyelash may become infected and a tender swelling, called a stye, results, which looks like a small boil. Pain is relieved by holding a hot compress or clean washcloth against the stye, and it sometimes helps if the eyelash of the infected follicle can be removed. Some children suffer repeatedly.

An antibiotic eye ointment or penicillin tablets may be needed to treat a severe stye, so consult your doctor if your child has a stye that is not responding to treatment.

SUDDEN INFANT DEATH SYNDROME (SIDS)
An unexplained and sudden crib death of a baby between 3 weeks and 7 months. The child may have a slight cold, with no fever or unusual symptoms, thus no apparent need to consult a doctor. Postmortem examination often reveals no adequate explanation of the cause of death. Shock to parents can be shattering, guilt and depression overwhelming. Counseling for the deceased child's family is often needed.

TEARS *see* Blocked tear duct

TEETH CARE
Your baby's first teeth will emerge during his first year of life (*see* below, **teething**).

They should be cleaned each day using a clean piece of gauze. As your baby grows older a soft toothbrush can be used.

TEETHING

The first tooth can come through at any time during the first year; the age at which this occurs varies tremendously. Rarely, a baby may be born with a tooth. Occasionally the child is over one year old before the first tooth emerges. Neither variation need cause concern.

The average age at which the first tooth appears is six months, and the first tooth to erupt is one of the lower central incisors. The upper central incisors follow about a month later, and adjacent teeth two to three months after that. Most children have six teeth by the time they are one year old. Variations occur, however, and are nothing to worry about (*see* also p. 183).

The eruption of teeth through the bone of the jaw and the gum can be uncomfortable and seems to be more so for some babies than others. Many babies are not upset at all when cutting teeth, but some are irritable and cry a great deal as a result of the pain thay have in their mouths. They may also salivate excessively and may soak their clothes in this way. Painful gums may also cause sleep disturbance, make feeding uncomfortable, and lead to a preference for softer foods. Such a baby may get some relief from a mild painkiller, such as Tempra drops. If this fails to relieve his symptoms, take him to see your doctor and discuss further care with him. Teething powders and other remedies are not recommended.

Teething is associated with many myths and dangerous old wives' tales. It is tempting to suggest that any symptom which develops at about the age of six months must be due to teething. This is unwise. Teething does not cause serious illness; it is not responsible for convulsions, fever, listlessness, rashes, diarrhea, vomiting or loss of appetite. Doctors still see babies whose symptoms of serious illness have been wrongly thought to be due to teething, and which, because of this, have been brought for medical care rather late. If you have any doubt about your baby's symptoms, do not hesitate to take him to see your doctor.

TEMPRA DROPS

Tempra (acetaminophen) is an effective, mild pain reliever. It will also lower an elevated temperature and may be given to prevent febrile convulsions (*see* **convulsions**). It can be given to small babies in the appropriate dose, usually 0.6 cc (60 mg) every six hours. Drops are given to the baby with a calibrated dropper. It should not be continued more than two days. It is preferred to aspirin for babies under one year and can be purchased without a prescription.

TEMPERATURE

Baby's room temperature. Your baby's room should be neither too hot nor too cold; the ideal temperature is about 65°F (18°C), to about 70°F (21°C) in the first two weeks. Try to make sure that there are no rapid nor extreme variations in temperature throughout the 24 hours.

Feedings. Foods must never be too hot or they may damage the lining of your baby's mouth. Always test the temperature of each feeding. Most mothers feed babies milk at blood heat – that is, a temperature which feels neither hot nor cold when a few drops are sprinkled on the back of the hand or inside of the wrist. There is, however, no harm in giving babies cold food, even straight from the refrigerator.

Body temperature. The average body temperature is 98.6°F (37°C) when taken by mouth, though it is quite normal for it to be a little above or below this. If your baby has a temperature markedly above this then he has a **fever** (*see* above). This does not mean he or she is seriously ill – indeed, it is quite common. Simple conditions can cause a fever – but if your baby shows other signs of illness then consult your doctor. If your baby's temperature is normal but he is otherwise ill, still consult your doctor. Do not be reassured by a normal temperature – many diseases do not cause fever.

Taking a baby's temperature. To take your baby's temperature you will need a clinical thermometer. Before use, shake down the mercury into the bulb at the lower end. Then enclose the bulb between the folds of skin either in the baby's groin or under his armpit. Some authorities recommend taking the temperature rectally. Hold it in place for about three minutes and then read off the temperature. After each use, rinse the thermometer in cold (never hot) water.

TESTES (TESTICLES)

Both testes have usually descended into the scrotum before birth, although this may be delayed in those babies born before term. Both testes should be in the scrotum by three years of age; if they are not, your son should see a doctor. An operation may be necessary by the age of five or six to bring the testes into the scrotum and thereby ensure normal development and function.

TETANUS

Tetanus is a serious infection that causes muscle spasms and occasionally death. The organisms live in animal manure, but can survive elsewhere out of doors. The disease is acquired through dirty, contaminated cuts, especially deep puncture wounds that cannot be cleaned easily, for instance from a rusty nail. Anyone who has these injuries and has not had up-to-date tetanus immunization will need to have an anti-tetanus injection when the wound is being dressed as a precaution.

Tetanus vaccine is also incorporated into the triple vaccine which is given routinely to all babies in the first year of life (*see* p. 226, **immunization**). A booster is usually given before starting school, and should be given every ten years from then on.

THALIDOMIDE

This sedative drug is no longer prescribed, as its use during pregnancy has been associated with congenital abnormalities in the limbs of babies.

THIRST

Small babies get thirsty and should be offered a drink of boiled water or fruit juice at least once a day. Your baby will enjoy drinks more often than this in hot weather or if he has a fever.

THREE-MONTH-COLIC *see* Colic

THRUSH (MONILIA)

If your baby seems to be in pain during feeding and you notice that his tongue or gums are covered with a thick white fur, then he has most probably developed thrush. Take your baby to your doctor and he will be able to prescribe Nystatin suspension for you to apply to your baby's mouth. Thrush is caused by a fungus and is very easily cured.

Babies can acquire thrush from incompletely sterilized feeding utensils, or from the mother if she has a vaginal discharge caused by thrush. Your doctor will be able to prescribe for this also if necessary.

Thrush can cause **diaper rash** (*see* above), which also responds to treatment with Nystatin ointment.

THUMB SUCKING

All babies enjoy sucking their thumb or fingers – many indulge in this even before they are born. Some do it more than others and it is not necessarily an indication of hunger. It is harmless and no attempts need be made to stop it.

TONGUE-TIE

The tongues of some babies seem to be closely fixed to the floor of the mouth and parents worry that eating and speaking will be affected. These fears are groundless; the tongue grows in the first year of life so that it can protrude quite normally.

TRIPLE VACCINE *see* Immunization

TUBERCULOSIS *see* Immunization

TYPHOID *see* Immunization

URINARY INFECTIONS

These occur rarely in small babies and usually there are no symptoms that would suggest that the infection is in the urinary system. General symptoms such as fever, irritability and loss of appetite are common, and the doctor may find little to explain these symptoms when he examines your baby. However, an examination of a sample of urine under a microscope or attempts to culture the infecting germ may give the diagnosis.

Urinary tract infections usually respond promptly to treatment with antibiotics such as ampicillin. Should your baby have repeated urinary infections, your doctor will order further investigations, including special X rays, to see whether or not there is some underlying cause for the infection. He will then advise you and arrange for these investigations.

URINE

The frequency with which a baby passes urine varies and is usually less in hot weather when more fluid has been lost in sweating. Be sure that your baby is given adequate volumes of fluid in hot weather to maintain a steady moderate production of urine. If you think your baby has stopped passing urine altogether, it is important that you consult your pediatrician or doctor as soon as possible.

A baby's urine is usually clear, though it may be a more concentrated golden color from time to time. You may notice that your baby's urine is more concentrated first thing in the morning – this is quite normal. The urine may seem more concentrated in hot weather, and this is an indication that your baby is not taking enough fluids. If your baby's urine forms a white deposit after standing for a period of time, do not be alarmed. The white deposit is phosphates and urates, and their presence is quite normal. Similarly a pink spot on the diaper is sometimes caused by uric acid – a normal constituent of urine and should not be a cause for concern.

You may also notice a smell to your baby's urine. A smell of ammonia is normal and is due to the breakdown of the urea in the urine to ammonia. A fishy smell may indicate a urinary tract infection – you should consult your doctor about this at the first opportunity.

It is not normal for a baby to scream or to be in pain when he or she passes urine. If your child has this symptom take him to see your doctor. The baby may have a sore on the tip of the penis (a **meatal ulcer**, *see* above) or soreness around the vulva. A **diaper rash** (*see* above) may also occasionally give rise to this symptom, as may **cystitis** (*see* above).

URTICARIA *see* Hives

VISION

Newborn babies are thought only to be able to focus at about 10 in. They will look at your face and will turn toward light. Gradually they see more detail and learn to focus more accurately; vision is not fully developed until the baby reaches about six months of age.

VITAMINS

The most important vitamins a baby needs are vitamins A, B, C and D. He will obtain sufficient vitamin A and B from the milk he takes, be it breast or cow's milk. Supplements of vitaimin C and D, however, are usually given and many doctors and pediatricians give vitamins A and B in addition, just to be on the safe side.

A deficiency of vitamin C causes scurvy. There is enough vitamin C in breast milk for most babies' requirements, but cow's milk is deficient in this vitamin. Vitamin C may be given as orange juice, but many physicians prefer multivitamin preparations because orange juice can cause an allergy in some infants. If you do give vitamin C as orange juice, start this when your baby is about one month old. Never boil the juice because vitamin C will be destroyed by boiling.

A deficiency of vitamin D can lead to rickets (*see* above). Most babies need about 400 units of added vitamin D a day if breast fed, or if fed unmodified cow's milk. Most modern formulas are fortified with vitamin D, so check with your doctor whether or not your baby needs supplements, as to give too much vitamin D can be harmful.

Low birth weight babies always need supplements of vitamin D, and are usually also given A and C.

Vitamin D is given as vitamin drops (sometimes in preparations which also contain vitamin A) or as cod liver oil. If needed these supplements should be started when your baby is between two and four weeks old.

Vitamin supplements can usually be stopped when the baby is on a mixed diet – in which case he will be receiving an adequate intake of all required vitamins in his regular meals.

VOMITING

Most babies regurgitate small volumes of milk at some time – some do this quite regularly. This is usually of no serious significance, especially if the baby is otherwise well and growing normally. If a baby has an acute illness in which he suddenly begins vomiting most of his food, then you should take him to your doctor as soon as possible. This is especially necessary if he has other symptoms such as a fever or diarrhea, or is listless. Prolonged vomiting can cause **dehydration** (*see* above) so consult your doctor at once, even if it is after office hours.

Dehydration is especially likely to occur if the vomiting is also associated with diarrhea. If your baby is vomiting *and* has not had a bowel movement for at least 24 hours then this condition may also be serious, as it is possible that there is some intestinal obstruction. You should therefore consult your doctor as soon as possible.

Vomiting in such babies does not always indicate a stomach upset; it can be caused by many conditions, including tonsillitis, **otitis media, pneumonia** or a urinary tract infection. So if your baby is vomiting and seems generally sick you should seek your doctor's advice as soon as possible to determine the underlying cause.

Pyloric stenosis (*see* above) is another cause of vomiting in the first few weeks of life. The baby with this condition is generally well, but is very hungry because he is unable to keep down his feedings, in his stomach. Seek the advice of your doctor as soon as possible if you think your baby has this disorder.

WARM SPONGING

This procedure is used to reduce an elevated temperature. It is particularly useful to make the baby more comfortable during a debrile illness. Warm sponging also helps to make the child with a fever much less restless and uncomfortable.

Undress your baby and sit or lay him on a towel or waterproof sheet. Use lukewarm water (not cold water) and apply this all over his body using a cloth or a sponge. Allow the body to dry by itself. The procedure takes about ten minutes and can be repeated every hour if necessary.

WAX IN THE EARS

Wax is normally produced by the outer part of the ears, where it may collect. It is quite harmless and only becomes a problem when well-meaning parents attempt to remove it with hairpins or cotton swabs. Do not try to remove wax from your baby's ears in this way or you may cause damage. Do not use ear drops either, except on the instruction of your doctor.

If you feel you have cause to be worried, discuss it with your doctor.

WEIGHT GAIN

A baby's health and progress are best judged by the way he behaves – is he happy, alert and full of energy? His weight is only one guide to his progress. Don't be alarmed if your baby seems to be gaining weight slowly but is otherwise well. Similarly, don't be falsely reassured if his weight gain is satisfactory but there is something about him that worries you. Discuss your worry with your doctor or pediatrician.

Most doctors do not attach much importance to a baby's pattern of weight gain unless it is too rapid, when the need to prevent obesity (*see* above, **fat babies**) will determine the future management of the baby. Loss of weight, however, is not normal in small babies – consult your doctor if your baby is losing weight.

WHOOPING COUGH *see* Infectious diseases

WORMS

If your baby has worms you can see them in his stools. Don't be alarmed or ashamed if this occurs, as any child can catch worms and they are not to be seen in any way as a sign of neglect by a child's parents.

The most common worm in the United States is the pinworm. These look like small white threads between $\frac{1}{4}$ and $\frac{1}{2}$ in (0.5 and 1 cm) in length. In tropical countries roundworms, hookworms and tapeworms are more common. Once recognized, all worm infestations can be easily and effectively treated.

X RAYS

Don't be alarmed if your baby requires a series of X rays. The dose of radiation used when an X ray is taken is extremely small and not likely to cause complications in later life.

Immunization

The number of diseases against which immunization has been developed is fairly small. The principal ones in the United States are diphtheria, polio, whooping cough, tetanus and rubella (German measles), measles and mumps. Immunization programs will, of course, vary from country to country and a typical U.S. program is given on page 227. Your doctor may wish to modify this schedule slightly. The underlying aims of the program remain the same, however: to give as much protection as possible against the diseases in question by using the minimum number of injections necessary, and causing as little reaction as possible. Although the number of vaccinations given is kept as low as possible, it may still seem as if your baby is constantly having to undergo injections. You may question whether such an elaborate program of protection is really necessary, particularly since many diseases have almost completely disappeared, or been eradicated, in this country. However, it is only by a continuing careful immunization program of all children that these potential killers are, and will be, kept at bay. Unless there are clear medical indications that your child should definitely not have a particular vaccine – and only your doctor can decide this – you have a responsibility to the community as a whole to make sure that your baby is immunized and that the immunization program is complete. Once this basic step has been taken, it is most important that you maintain a check and update any immunizations, where necessary. Instill the concept into your children so they make a point on carrying on with this protection throughout their lives.

Very simply, immunization works by persuading the body to produce antibodies needed to fight a specific infection. By giving a weakened form of the germ causing the infection, the body is stimulated to produce sufficient antibodies without having to suffer the disease itself. If the germs then attack the body a second time, in a stronger form, the body is already protected. It is very important that you keep a careful, up-to-date record of your baby's vaccinations and that you tell your doctor of any symptoms, however minor, which might mean postponing an injection for at least a short time.

Basic immunization program

A comprehensive timetable for immunization is presented on p. 227. But it seems wise to give a brief summary of the recommendations of the American Academy of Pediatrics for the routine immunization of infants in the United States. This schedule may be used both for premature and small-for-gestational-age infants. There are no seasonal restrictions.

Routine immunization is begun at two months of age with DTP (diphtheria and tetanus toxoids and pertussis vaccine) and TOPV (trivalent oral poliovirus vaccine). They may be given at the same time. It makes no difference whether the mother is breast- or bottle feeding.

Both the DTP and TOPV are repeated at four months of age.

The DTP is repeated at six months. If the area has a high endemic level of poliomyelitis, the TOPV may be repeated at this time as well.

At 15 months the child may be immunized against measles, mumps and rubella with a single injection. Immunizing against rubella is especially important in girls because developing this infection during early pregnancy may cause birth defects. Immunizing against mumps is especially important in boys because mumps can cause serious orchitis (inflammation of the testicles) or pain and swelling of the testicles in later life.

At 18 months the DTP injection and the oral TOPV are repeated. Both these immunization procedures should be repeated once more between the ages of four and six years.

This recommended immunization schedule is published in the 1982 Report of the Committee on Infectious Disease of the American Academy of Pediatrics. The recommendations are based on the experience and knowledge of experts in pediatric infectious disease. Your doctor or pediatric clinic may follow an immunization schedule that varies slightly from this. Additionally, when other factors are taken into consideration, such as the health of your child or changing patterns of infectious disease, changes in the recommended immunization schedule may be necessary.

It is important to note that an interruption in the schedule does not cause failure to achieve final immunity provided the recommended number of immunizations is given. Furthermore, any interruption that occurs in the immunization schedule does not require starting the whole process all over again.

Immunization should not normally have any adverse effect on your baby. But, if after an injection the child becomes exceptionally irritable or sick, or develops a fever, then you should let your doctor know as soon as possible. Don't be concerned if a small lump develops at the site of the injection. This lump will always disappear in time.

Unimmunized children

Children who did not receive any immunizations against infectious disease as infants will usually be immunized on an accelerated schedule. Your doctor will discuss this possibility with you and will work out a schedule for your child.

Optional vaccinations

There is a number of other diseases against which a child can be vaccinated, although this is not always recommended. Your own doctor or pediatrician will advise what is best for your child.

Tuberculosis. B.C.G. vaccine is recommended by some authorities for all children who live in or plan extensive travel to areas where tuberculosis is prevalent. This vaccine is sometimes given to newborn babies if a member of the household in which they live has recently developed this infection. The infant given B.C.G. vaccine is separated from the potentially contagious individuals until it becomes tuberculin positive.

Rubella. Immunization against rubella (German measles) is recommended for all girls and it is usually given between the ages of 15 months and puberty. Immunization is also given to women who have no natural immunity to this infection, but these women must be careful to avoid pregnancy for at least three months after the injection.

Influenza. Immunization against influenza is not normally recommended for children unless they suffer from serious heart or lung disease.

Tuberculin Testing – The initial test is normally done at the age of 12 months or at the time the measles-mumps-rubella immunization is given at 15 months.The frequency of any repeated tuberculin tests depends entirely upon the possible risk of the individual patient to exposure from the infection.

Immunization for travel overseas

Requirements for travel overseas vary from time to time, so that only a general guide can be given. Your doctor will be able to give you more up-to-date advice if you think that you and your family are going to need immunization prior to going on a trip. It is worth noting that you should consult your doctor in good time as a program of injections can take up to six weeks. Your local Department of Health should have access to the most up-to-date information on which specific immunizations are necessary for travel to any area in the world.

The following summarizes a few of the infectious diseases that you will require immunization against, and the areas of the world for which such immunization is necessary.

Smallpox. Vaccination of babies (and adults) is no longer done in the United States, since this very serious disease has now been completely eradicated throughout the world, after an intensive immunization program by the World Health Organization that ended in 1979.

Yellow fever. A certificate of vaccination will be required for those traveling to and from Central Africa and certain tropical regions of South America. Immunization is best avoided for babies under nine months old and for those allergic to egg protein. Your own doctor will be unable to administer yellow fever vaccine, and you will have to attend a yellow fever vaccine center – your doctor should be able to give you the address of the vaccine center closest to you.

Cholera. Immunization against cholera is advised for travelers to areas where this infectious disease has been identified by the World Health Organization – this includes some countries in Asia, the Middle East and Africa, for example. Immunization against cholera is most definitely not recommended for babies who are under one year of age.

Typhoid This disease is common in the developing world, so immunization against it is advised for travelers to most countries outside North America and Europe. Immunization is not recommended for babies under one year old. Cholera and typhoid are usually spread from person to person via food and water. If you are in an area where these infections occur, you should boil all water before drinking, cooking or cleaning your teeth. Remember that ice (if it is available at all) will have been made from water that may have been contaminated and should be avoided for safety's sake. Raw vegetables, salads and ice cream can easily be contaminated and should be avoided.

Similarly, eating raw shellfish and underdone meat or fish is not recommended. The maintaining of a high standard of personal hygiene is of the greatest importance when in those areas.

Polio. A booster dose of polio vaccine is recommended to all travelers outside Europe and North America.

Malaria. There is no injection which will protect anyone against malaria. This is a widespread disease in some parts of Asia, Africa and South America. If traveling to any of these areas, your doctor will be able to discuss with you the details of preventive treatment against this disease such as anti-malarial pills.

*RECOMMENDED SCHEDULE FOR ACTIVE IMMUNIZATION OF NORMAL INFANTS AND CHILDREN

Age	Diphtheria, Tetanus and Whooping Cough	Poliomyelitis	Measles, Rubella, Mumps
2 months	DTP	TOPV	
4 months	DTP	TOPV	
6 months	DTP	third dose optional for areas of polio endemicity	
15 months			Will be given as: measles-rubella or measles-mumps-rubella combined vaccines
18 months	DTP	TOPV	
4–6 years	DTP	TOPV	
14–16 years	Td		

DTP – diphtheria and tetanus toxoids combined with pertussis (whooping cough) Vaccine. It is administered as an injection and may cause a red swelling at the injection site. If the baby is sick it is best to postpone the injection until the baby is better. This should never be given to a baby who has previously had fits or convulsions, screaming episodes or collapse following administration of pertussis-containing vaccine. In such instances your doctor may consider an immunization not containing the pertussis portion.

TOPV – trivalent oral poliovirus vaccine. It is recommended to administer it on this schedule to breast-fed as well as bottle-fed infants. Over 400 million doses have been administered in the United States.

Td – combined diptheria and tetanus toxoids. Should be repeated every ten years.

Measles – measles – mumps – rubella vaccine may be administered as an injection at 15 months of age.

***Source:** "Red Book", 1982.
American Academy of Pediatrics.

Infectious diseases

Up to several months of age babies have some protection against the common infectious diseases of childhood that their mothers have had, such as measles, mumps, chicken pox, scarlet fever and German measles. The antibodies in the mother's blood cross the placenta into the baby's circulation during pregnancy and provide what is termed "passive" immunization. The exception to this is whooping cough against which "active" immunization will be provided under the immunization program (see page 227). Such protection cannot be provided against all the common infectious diseases, however, so young babies ought not to be exposed to infection from older children for whom these diseases are of little consequence.

The infectious diseases commonly associated with childhood are contagious – that is, they spread directly from one child to the next. Susceptible children who come into contact with any of those infected are almost certain to catch it. A child who has had one infectious disease is unlikely to contract it again. He is naturally immune to it. Artificial immunity can be acquired by **immunization** (see above) using inactive viruses or bacteria.

Maiming and life-threatening diseases such as diptheria, polio, whooping cough and tetanus are now very rare, and immunization in infancy has contributed greatly to their decline. The lesser infectious diseases are very common and can make your child miserable for a week or two. They rarely have any serious consequences. Since they are highly infectious they are usually acquired in childhood when mixing with other children begins. They also tend to occur in minor epidemics.

The *incubation period* of an infectious disease is the time between catching the infection and showing signs of the disease. The isolation period is the length of time that a child with a disease has to be kept away from other people so that they do not become infected. It is best to protect babies and children who are already ill by keeping them away from anyone with the disease. Otherwise there is little point in strict quarantine precautions.

In the incubation period you may not realize that your child has one of these diseases. He may be generally sick and off-color, listless and apathetic. Even your doctor may not be able to make the diagnosis until the characteristic signs of, say, chicken pox have developed. However, if you suspect your child has an infectious fever, then it is not advisable to take him to the doctor's office because of the risk of spreading the infection in the waiting room to other children who are already ill. Telephone the doctor and let him decide what to do; he should always be notified if you suspect your child has an infectious disease. He will advise you on further care needed.

The table below indicates the characteristics of the most common infectious diseases of childhood.

CHARACTERISTICS OF THE COMMON INFECTIOUS DISEASES OF CHILDHOOD

Disease	Incubation period	Rash and other features	Treatment	Isolation period
Chicken pox	10–21 days	Small, itchy red spots, first on the face and limbs and then predominantly on the trunk. Later these develop into watery blisters and then form crusts.	Calamine lotion soothes the rash. An antihistamine may help the child to sleep.	1 week from the onset of the rash.
*German Measles	14–21 days	Small pink pinhead spots spread rapidly over face and trunk and disappear by the third day. The child may have symptoms of a cold and enlarged glands in the neck.	Aspirin (or Tempra drops for a small baby) may make the child feel more comfortable.	Until rash has disappeared avoid contact with any pregnant woman who is not protected against this infectious disease; particularly those in the first three months of their pregnancy.
*Measles (Rubeola)	10–12 days	Begins with symptoms of a cold with cough, runny nose, watery inflamed eyes and an elevated temperature. Dark red spots first appear behind the ears and spread to the face, limbs and trunk. These spots begin as pinhead size, but later join together and become blotchy.	Aspirin (or Tempra drops for a small baby). Antibiotics will be needed if a chest or ear infection develops.	From the fifth day of incubation period to the third day of the rash.
*Mumps	14–21 days	At first the child is off-color with general aches and an elevated temperature. A painful swelling may then develop at one or both sides of the face or under the jaw. Opening the mouth may be uncomfortable.	A pain relieving drug such as aspirin (Tempra drops for a small baby). A hot compress held over the swelling is soothing.	Until one week after the swelling has subsided. Avoid contact with adult males who have not had the mumps.
Scarlet Fever	2–5 days	Begins with a sore throat, elevated temperature, headache and often vomiting. Stomachache may also be a feature. The skin is flushed and dry with a pale area around the mouth. The rash consists of small bright red dots packed closely together. The skin flakes off toward the end of the infection; this is quite harmless.	Aspirin (Tempra drops for a small baby) together with an antibiotic such as penicillin.	One day after beginning antibiotics.
*Whooping cough (Pertussis)	5–21 days	Begins with a cold and cough for a few days. Spasms of continuing coughing then develop – often on the same breath. As the child breathes in, a characteristic whoop may be heard. It does not arise in all patients with whooping cough, however. These bouts of severe coughing can cause vomiting and may make feeding difficult.	Antibiotics are occasionally effective in cutting short an attack of whooping cough. Cough syrup is rarely effective in easing the cough. Ensure an adequate intake of fluids – for example with fruit juices.	Four weeks from the beginning of the cough. Shorter period if treated with antibiotics. Avoid contact with small babies and toddlers.

*Effective vaccines are now available against these infectious diseases. Discuss with your doctor a program of immunization for your baby.

a look to the future

Have you ever wondered where our national priorities are? Our newborn babies are our most important resource. The very future of our nation depends upon the favorable outcome to the pregnancies in the United States. And yet, what is the state of this concern? Few insurance policies offer comprehensive benefits to pregnant women. Pregnancy is usually treated by the insurance company as something that should not have happened to a responsible couple. Outpatient care and antepartum testing are not always covered. And the pregnancy may be covered by a flat amount instead of realistic coverage of the expenses. When insurance executives are asked why there is a low priority on pregnancy, they answer, "The couple has nine months to plan for it, don't they?" That reflects their mentality and gives a strong picture of their priorities!

We could always turn to the government for help. But the money that is spent on pregnancy management is pitifully small compared to that spent upon the newborn and the infant. Why are we not looking realistically at the prospects of prevention? Perhaps one reason is that the fetus doesn't vote. The average legislator is a male and often far beyond the age of starting a family. His concern for prostatism and baldness could easily overshadow his concern for a couple having a baby. Every responsible couple should know the views of their local politicians concerning health-care delivery for those having babies. But do they? Worrying about gun control, oil spills or even the national debt is minor compared to having concern for the potential outcome of pregnancies. Couples should question politicians carefully on their position on preventative measures for pregnant patients. It is crucial that there be recognition and support for the availability of such items as antenatal evaluation of physical, psychological, nutritional and genetic factors, nutritional guidance in pregnancy, multiphasic screening tests to evaluate maternal and fetal risks and access for prospective parents to the appropriate levels of care. If there is little understanding or concern by the politicians in this area, it is unlikely that they will manage other societal issues humanistically. With the greater number of women actively involved in politics and the expanding awareness of women's issues, we should see increasing concern for the preventive aspects of childbearing which start before pregnancy.

Perinatal associations of health-care professionals and consumers have become an important force in effecting health-care legislation. As a direct result of their involvement, now almost all of the states require that if a couple has a premature baby it be covered by medical insurance from the moment of birth. Were you aware of the small print in most insurance policies? It commonly stated the newborn was not covered until the baby was six weeks old. What good did that do for the couple with a premature baby or a term baby with serious problems? The first time that the couple knows they are not covered is after the baby with the problem is born. Good sense tells us that, ethically, small print should rightfully have been written in large print. In the future the insurance companies should cover a pregnancy completely. Actually, a visit to the doctor and counseling before getting pregnant should be covered. If the policy does not cover such commonsense items, it should be compelled to state so in bold print. The consumer has rights that must be recognized and respected.

Not all of the responsibility should be on the government or the insurance company. The couple has a responsibility to enter pregnancy in an optimum condition: the fetus must be given every chance to reach its full potential. To do this the couple must be willing to enter pregnancy with the mother in her best physical and mental condition. She should have a well-planned program of exercise, diet and rest. She should be prepared to curtail or, better yet, omit potentially harmful agents like alcohol and tobacco. She should be committed to the concept that she will not take over-the-counter medications or prescription medications unless advised to do so by her doctor. In short, she should be ready to devote nine months to providing an optimal environment for the development of the baby.

Ideally, the patient should see her doctor within six weeks from her last normal menstrual period. In this way, baseline laboratory testing can be performed. In the future, hopefully, this will include comprehensive screening for any problems that could arise during the pregnancy. Obviously, not all problems lend themselves to screening so early in pregnancy. The physician must still be vigilant in order to detect any new problems arising during a pregnancy.

During the initial visit to the doctor, the patient will be classified as high risk or, hopefully, low risk. If she is classified in the latter category she will receive routine antenatal care and delivery in a community hospital. If she has a pregnancy that is classified as high risk, she will be referred to the appropriate specialists for sophisticated care.

Approximately three decades ago, neonatal intensive care units were organized in the United States. They have proven to be extremely valuable in the care of the premature, the small-for-dates baby, the infant of the diabetic mother and other newborns with complications. About two decades ago high risk pregnancy units were organized to care for those specialized problems that required sophisticated testing and intensive care. As the neonatal and the obstetrical units were developed, the concept of regionalization was also developed. This concept espoused the use of a tertiary perinatal center by numerous secondary and primary care hospitals. If the patient's problems required diagnostic testing or sophisticated management the patient would be referred to such a center for care. If, following evaluation, the problem was such that it could easily be managed at the local level the patient would be referred back to her doctor.

For a number of reasons this concept was accepted better in some areas than others. Sometimes it required consumer pressure to effect a necessary referral. Other times a frankly bad outcome and malpractice suit prompted the use of the referral system. Ideally, this system should be available to all couples in the United States. If there is a major problem with transportation to such a facility, what better use of government funds could there be than to provide whatever is needed to effect comprehensive, excellent antenatal care?

Once a serious or life-threatening problem is identified the mother should automatically be delivered in the tertiary care center where, around the clock, sophisticated perinatal care is available. The delivery would be attended by a highly trained neonatologist and his team.

When the baby is born the neonatal team can transfer a sick newborn to a neonatal intensive care unit where sophisticated management can be rendered. Such intensive care units are not merely a collection of complicated life-sustaining and monitoring instruments. The intensive care unit is a highly specialized organization of health professionals. It is this round-the-clock availability of trained personnel that makes the tertiary care center unique. This type of care cannot be provided at the community level because of the extraordinary personnel requirements.

In the setting of all this technology, there should be a strong effort to maintain a humanistic approach to medicine. The staff must be trained to have a high level of sensitivity, so that they can recognize and tend to the stress couples may be experiencing. The hospital administration must be quick to recognize the level of stress that accompanies this sort of professional involvement. The nursing personnel must periodically be rotated out of the intensive care units so that they do not experience the devastating phenomenon of psychological burnout. This has terminated many a brilliant intensive care nursing career.

Women abound in the workplace. Employers need to meet women halfway on the childbearing issue. Part-time options and flexible scheduling need to be available to young mothers. It is only civilized to provide maternity leave that includes job security. Consideration must be given to paternity leave requests. We perform no service to society by continuing the myth that two-career families carry no risk to the child. Out-of-home child care is a critical issue. Quality daycare centers must become more available, accessible, and affordable to all. The public is going to have to be willing to stand up and be counted. These changes are coming, but they are coming too slowly. They cost money. But what better way could we spend our money than on the most precious resource of the future – our children?

resources

This list includes a wide selection of community and health-oriented resources. Some relate specifically to pregnancy and childbirth; others are general, but may be useful to the pregnant woman or new mother. Remember that in many cases we have listed national headquarters – do look in your local telephone directory for addresses in your area.

ALCOHOL ABUSE

Alcoholics Anonymous
P.O. Box 459
Grand Central Station
New York, NY 10163

Alcohol abuse in relative or friend

Al-Anon Family Group Headquarters, Inc.
P.O. Box 182
Madison Square Station
New York, NY 10159

Use and abuse during pregnancy

National Clearinghouse for Alcohol Information
P.O. Box 2345
Rockville, MD 20852

ALTERNATIVE BIRTH SETTINGS

National Association of Parents and Professionals for Safe Alternatives in Childbirth
(NAPSAC)
P.O. Box 267
Marble Hill, MO 63764

Family-centered maternity care

The Cybele Society
Suite 414, Peyton Building
Spokane, WA 99201

BIRTH CONTROL

Planned Parenthood Federation of America, Inc.
810 Seventh Avenue
New York, NY 10019
(212) 541-7800 (800) 223-3303

Zero Population Growth, Inc.
1346 Connecticut Ave, NW
Washington, DC 20036
(202) 785-0100

BIRTH DEFECTS

March of Dimes Birth Defects Foundation
Box 2000
White Plains, NY 10602

National Center for Education in Maternal and Child Health
Georgetown University
3520 Prospect Street, NW
Washington, DC 20007
(202) 625-8400

BREAST CANCER REHABILITATION

Reach to Recovery
American Cancer Society
19 W. 56th Street
New York, NY 10019
(212) 586-8700

BREAST FEEDING

La Leche League International
9616 Minneapolis Avenue
Franklin Park, IL 60134

CHILDBIRTH EDUCATION

Dick-Read

Read Natural Childbirth Foundation, Inc.
1300 S Eliseo Drive
Greenbrae, CA 94904

Husband-coached childbirth

The American Academy of Husband-Coached Childbirth
P.O. Box 5224
Sherman Oaks, CA 91413

Lamaze

American Society for Psychoprophylaxis in Obstetrics, Inc. (ASPO)
1411 K Street, NW
Washington, DC 20005

General

International Childbirth Education Association
P.O. Box 20048
Minneapolis, MN 55420

DRUG ABUSE

Information

Food and Drug Administration
5600 Fishers Lane, Room 15B-32
Rockville, MD 20857

Prevention

National Institute of Drug Abuse
Prevention Branch
5600 Fishers Lane, Room 10A-30
Rockville, MD 20857

Treatment

Second Genesis, Inc.
4720 Montgomery Lane
Bethesda, MD 20814
(301) 656-1545

EXERCISE

Young Men's Christian Association of U.S.A. (YMCA)
101 North Wacker Drive
Chicago, IL 60601
(312) 977-0031

Young Women's Christian Association Headquarters (YWCA)
726 Broadway
New York, NY 10003
(212) 614-2700

HEALTH PROBLEMS

American Academy of Child Psychiatry
3615 Wisconsin Ave, NW
Washington, DC 20016
(202) 966-7300

Arthritis Foundation
1901 Fort Myer Drive (Room 507)
Arlington, VA 32209
(703) 276-7555

American Dental Association
Bureau of Health Education
211 East Chicago Avenue
Chicago, IL 60611

American Heart Association
2233 Wisconsin Avenue NW (Suite 200)
Washington, DC 20007
(202) 337-6400

American Public Health Association
1015 15th Street, NW
Washington, DC 20005
(202) 789-5600

Cystic Fibrosis Foundation
8401 Corporate Drive, Suite 110
Landover, MD 20785
(301) 459-8444

Epilepsy Foundation of America
815 15th Street, NW Suite 528
Washington, DC 20005
(202) 638-5229

High Blood Pressure Information Center
120/80 National Institutes of Health
Bethesda, MD 20205

Leukemia Society of America, Inc.
733 3rd Avenue
New York, NY 20017
(212) 573-8484

Muscular Dystrophy Association
1800 Massachusetts Avenue, NW
(Suite 100)
Washington, DC 20036
(202) 466-7450

National Kidney Foundation
2233 Wisconsin Avenue, NW (Suite 320)
Washington, DC 20007
(202) 337-6600

National Multiple Sclerosis Society
1200 15th Street, NW (Suite 601)
Washington, DC 20005
(202) 296-5363

National Society for Autistic Children
1234 Massachusetts Avenue, NW
(Suite 1017)
Washington, DC 20005
(202) 783-0125

Howard University for Sickle Cell Disease
2121 Georgia Avenue, NW
Washington, DC 20059
(202) 636-7930

National Spinal Cord Injury Association
2550 M Street, NW
Washington, DC 20007
(202) 296-2934

Reye's Syndrome Foundation
425 13th Street, NW
Washington, DC 20004
(800) 233-7393

Retinitis Pigmentosa Foundation
6021 Neilwood Drive
Rockville, MD 20852
(301) 881-3776

Tay-Sachs Foundation
11728 Becket Street
Rockville, MD
(301) 279-5878

United Cerebral Palsy Association, Inc.
425 I Street, NW Suite 141
Washington, DC 20001
(202) 842-1266

INFERTILITY
American Fertility Society
2131 Magnolia Avenue (Suite 201)
Birmingham, AL 35256
(205) 251-9764

INFORMATION GENERAL
American Academy of Child Psychiatry
3615 Wisconsin Avenue, NW
Washington, DC 20016
(202) 966-7300

American Academy of Family Physicians
600 Maryland Avenue, SW
(Suite 770)
Washington, DC 20024
(202) 488-7448

American College of Obstetricians and Gynecologists
600 Maryland Avenue, SW
(Suite 300 East)
Washington, DC 20024
(202) 638-5577

NUTRITION
The American Dietetic Association
430 North Michigan Avenue
Chicago, IL 60611

Department of Foods and Nutrition
American Medical Association
1101 Vermont Avenue, NW
Washington, DC 20005
(202) 789-7400

PARENTING
American Red Cross
431 18th Street NW
Washington, DC 20005
(202) 737-8300

Consult your physician or OB Clinic

PREGNANCY
Resource Center
American College of Obstetricians and Gynecologists
600 Maryland Avenue, SW
Washington, DC 20024

Office of Maternal and Child Health
US Dept. of Health and Human Services
5600 Fishers Lane, Room 7-39
Rockville, MD 20857

RAPE
National Center for the Prevention and Control of Rape
5600 Fishers Lane, Room 15-99
Rockville, MD 20857

Consult local phone directory for listing of "Rape/Crisis Center"

RUNAWAYS
National Network of Runaway and Youth Services, Inc.
905 6th Street, SW (Suite 612)
Washington, DC 20024
(202) 488-0739

SEXUALITY AND SEX COUNSELING
American Association of Sex Educators, Counselors, and Therapists
600 Maryland Avenue, SW
Washington, DC 20024

Sex Information and Education Council of the U.S.
80 Fifth Avenue (Suite 801)
New York, NW 10011

SEXUALLY TRANSMITTED DISEASES
Technical Information Services
Center for Prevention Services
Centers for Disease Control
Atlanta, GA 30333

SMOKING
American Lung Association
1740 Broadway
New York, NY 10019
(212) 245-8000

American Cancer Society, Inc.
777 Third Avenue
New York, NY 10017
(212) 371-2900

American Heart Association
7320 Greenville Avenue
Dallas, Texas 72531
(214) 750-5334

Smokenders
3708 Mt. Diablo Blvd (Suite 100)
Lafayette, CA 94549

STERILIZATION
Planned Parenthood Federation of America, Inc.
810 Seventh Avenue
New York, NY 10019
(212) 541-7800

SOCIAL SERVICE ORGANIZATIONS
American Red Cross
431 18th Street, NW
Washington, DC 20005
(202) 737-8300

Association for Retarded Citizens of the United States
1522 K Street, NW (Suite 516)
Washington, DC 20005
(202) 785-3388

Child Welfare League of America
1346 Connecticut Avenue, NW
(Suite 320)
Washington, DC 20036
(202) 833-2850

Family Service Association of America
1346 Connecticut Avenue, NW
(Suite 712)
Washington, DC 20036
(202) 822-8390

The Salvation Army
503 E Street, NW
Washington, DC 20001
(202) 783-4050
(202) 783-4058 (emergency service)

United Way of America
701 North Fairfax Street
Alexandria, VA 22314-2045
(202) 836-7100

WEIGHT LOSS
Weight Watchers International
800 Community Drive
Manhasset, NY 10030

Consult your physician

WOMEN'S ISSUES
National Organization for Women
425 13th Street, NW (Suite 723)
Washington, DC 20004
(202) 347-2279

National Women's Health Report
P.O. Box 25307
Georgetown Station
Washington, DC 20007

Parents Without Partners, Inc.
Washington, DC
(202) 638-1320

Women's Legal Defense Fund, Inc.
2000 P Street, NW (Suite 400)
Washington, DC 20036
(202) 887-0364

acknowledgments

We should like to extend our thanks and appreciation to the following institutions for the help and advice they have given us in the preparation of this book: Queen Charlotte's Hospital, Royal Free Hospital, St. Mary's Hospital, Paddington Green Hospital, Family Planning Association, Georgetown University Hospital, Washington D.C.

ARTISTS

14/15 Jon Wells
16/17 Eric Jewell Associates (tl); Jon Wells (c); Terry Allen Design (b)
18/19 Jon Wells
20/21 Terry Allen Design (tl, bl, tr); Pippa Clarke/Linda Wagner (br)
22 Pippa Clarke/Linda Wagner
23 Valerie Wright
26 John Hind and Venner Artists (1); Venner Artists (bc)
27 Roy Flooks
30 Terry Cheverton and Venner Artists
31 Jon Wells
32 Venner Artists
33 Terry Cheverton
34 Venner Artists
35 Candida Amsden
37 Terry Cheverton
40 Venner Artists
46/47 Venner Artists
48 Candida Amsden
49 Terry Cheverton
50/51 Candida Amsden
53 Eric Jewell Associates (tr); Terry Cheverton (cr, bl)
72/73 Venner Artists (tl, tr, cr); Eric Jewell Associates (bl)
74/75 Venner Artists
76 Terry Cheverton
78 Venner Artists
83 Venner Artists
89 Venner Artists
90 Venner Artists
92 Eric Jewell Associates
104/105 Terry Cheverton
106/107 Terry Cheverton (bl, tr); Venner Artists (bl, tr); Venner Artists (br)
108 Terry Cheverton
109 Venner Artists
112 Venner Artists
115 Eric Jewell Associates
127 Terry Cheverton (tl); Eric Jewell Associates (tr)
142 Candida Amsden
146 Sue Rose
148 Candida Amsden
159 Candida Amsden
172/173 Sue Rose (bl); Candida Amsden (br)
181/182 Eric Jewell Associates
183 Terry Cheverton
209 Sue Rose

PHOTOGRAPHERS

1/5 Sandra Lousada
6/7 Bill Carter
8/11 Sandra Lousada
12 B.B.C. Television
15 Manfred Kage/Bruce Coleman Ltd (tr); Gene Cox/Micro Colour International (c, b)
17 John Pryce-Davies
19 Manfred Kage/Bruce Coleman Ltd (tr); Gene Cox/Micro Colour International (c)
22 Gene Cox/Micro Colour International
24 Claude Rives/Transworld Feature Syndicate
28/29 John Troha/Black Star
30 Bill Carter
32 Gene Cox/Micro Colour International
33 Bill Carter
36/37 Robert Golden
38 Medcom Inc.
40/41 Sandra Lousada
42/43 Robert Vente (tl); John Troha/Black Star (bl, br)
44 Carlo Bevilacqua/Euro Colour Library
47 Michael Bennett
48/49 Carlo Bevilacqua/Euro Colour Library (tl); Carnegie Institution of Washington, Department of Embryology, Davis Division (bl, br); Michael Bennett (tr)
50/51 Ronald Benzie
52 John T. Queenan
54/55 John T. Queenan (tfl, tl); Shaun Skelly/Daily Telegraph Colour Library (tcl); John Troha/Black Star (bl, br)
56/57 John Troha/Black Star (tl); Shaun Skelly/Daily Telegraph Colour Library (br); Michael Bennett (tcr)
70 John Troha/Black Star
76 Sandra Lousada
77 Bay Hippisley
78/81 Sandra Lousada
84 John Troha/Black Star
86/87 Mike St. Maur Shiel (tl, tr); John Troha/Black Star (bl)
88-92 Robert Golden
94/95 John Troha/Black Star
100 Howard Sochurek/John Hillelson Agency
102/103 John Troha/Black Star
104 Shaun Skelly
105 Royal Free Hospital
106 Shaun Skelly
107 Royal Free Hospital
108 Brian Seed/Aspect Picture Library
110 Richard Greenhill
114 John Troha/Black Star
116/117 John Troha/Black Star
118/119 Bay Hippisley
124 John Troha/Black Star
126 Suzanne Arms/1976 Jeroboam Inc.
127 Shaun Skelly (tl)
128/129 Shaun Skelly
130/131 Bay Hippisley
132/133 John Troha/Black Star (tl, tr); Bay Hippisley (bl); Shaun Skelly (br)
135 London Express News and Features
136 Claire Leimbach
138 Clay Perry
139 Bay Hippisley
140 Richard Greenhill
141 Sally Greenhill
143 John Troha/Black Star
145/147 Bay Hippisley
148/149 Richard Greenhill
150/154 Richard Greenhill
155 John Troha/Black Star
157 John Troha/Black Star
158/159 Sandra Lousada
160 Bay Hippisley
161 Courtesy of Peaudouce
168 Richard Greenhill
170 Richard Greenhill (tl); John Troha/Black Star (br)
171/175 Richard Greenhill
176/177 Bay Hippisley
178 Richard Greenhill
180 Michael Joseph
183 Richard Greenhill
184/185 Richard Greenhill
186 Richard Greenhill (tl, bl, br); Roger Perry (tr)
187 Richard Greenhill
188 Richard Greenhill
189/192 Richard Greenhill
194/195 John Troha/Black Star (tl); Richard Greenhill (tr, bl, br)
197 Richard Greenhill
198 Michael Joseph (tl, bl)
199/201 Richard Greenhill

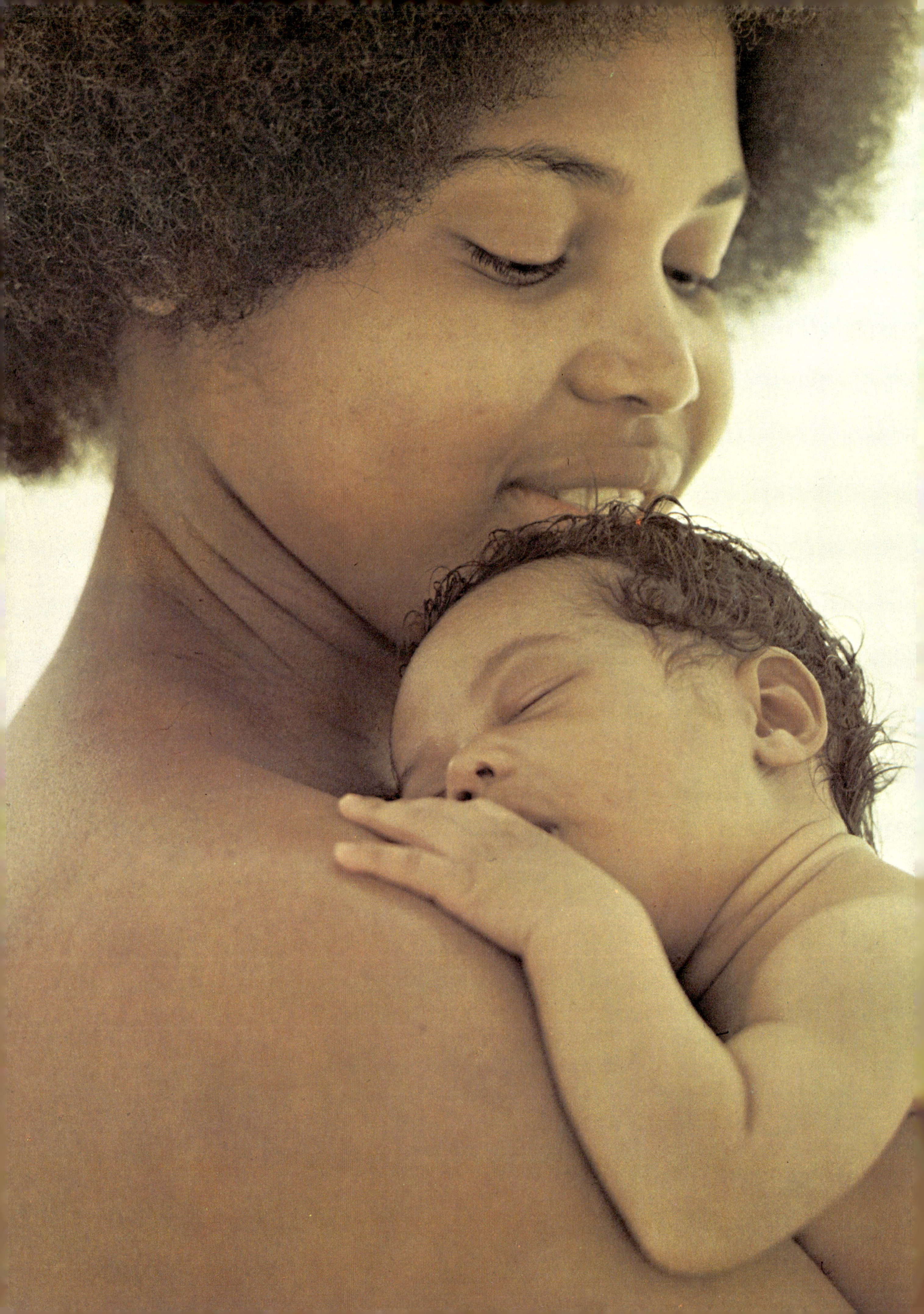

index

Page numbers in *italics* refer to the illustrations and captions

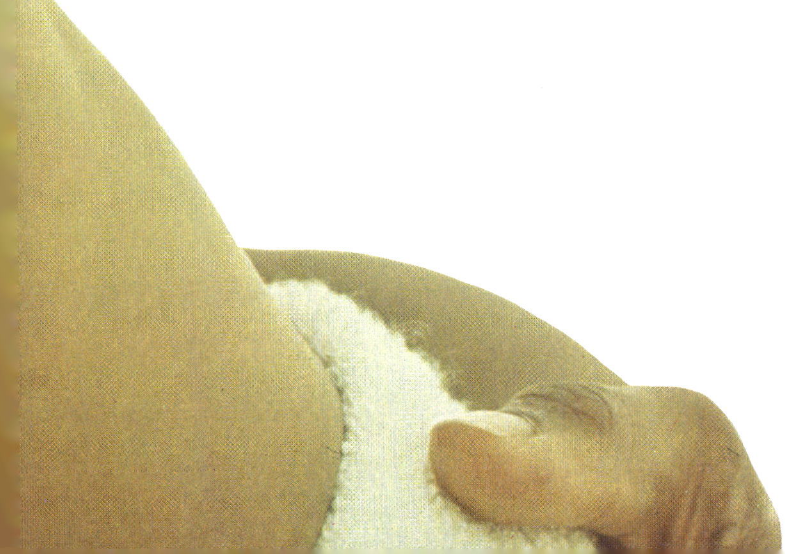